PARKLAND TRAUMA HANDBOOK

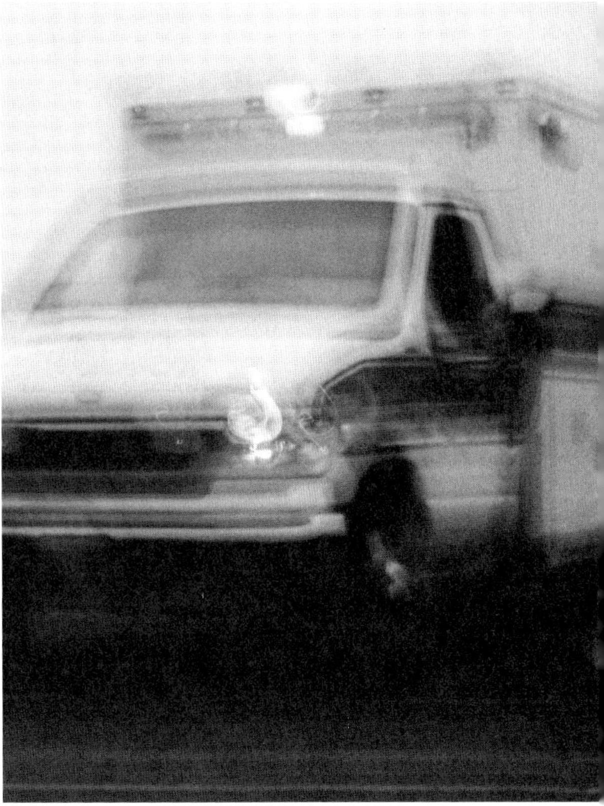

third
EDITION

PARKLAND TRAUMA HANDBOOK

EDITED BY

Alexander L. Eastman, MD
*Chief Resident in General Surgery
Parkland Memorial Hospital
Department of Surgery
University of Texas Southwestern Medical Center
Dallas, Texas*

David H. Rosenbaum, MD
*Chief Resident in General Surgery
Parkland Memorial Hospital
Department of Surgery
University of Texas Southwestern Medical Center
Dallas, Texas*

Erwin R. Thal, MD, FACS
*Professor of Surgery
Division of Burns, Trauma, and Critical Care
University of Texas Southwestern Medical Center
Senior Attending Surgeon
Parkland Memorial Hospital
Dallas, Texas*

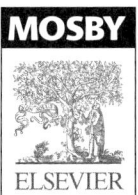

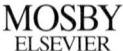

1600 John F. Kennedy Boulevard
Suite 1800
Philadelphia, Pennsylvania 19103-2899

PARKLAND TRAUMA HANDBOOK ISBN: 978-0-323-05226-9

Copyright © 2009 by Mosby, Inc., an affiliate of Elsevier Inc.
Copyright © 1999 by Mosby International Ltd.

All rights reserved. No part of this publication may be reproduced or transmitted in any form or by any means, electronic or mechanical, including photocopying, recording, or any information storage and retrieval system, without permission in writing from the publisher. Permissions may be sought directly from Elsevier's Rights Department: phone: (+1) 215 239 3804 (US) or (+44) 1865 843830 (UK); fax: (+44) 1865 853333; e-mail: healthpermissions@elsevier.com. You may also complete your request on-line via the Elsevier website at http://www.elsevier.com/permissions.

Notice

Knowledge and best practice in this field are constantly changing. As new research and experience broaden our knowledge, changes in practice, treatment, and drug therapy may become necessary or appropriate. Readers are advised to check the most current information provided (i) on procedures featured or (ii) by the manufacturer of each product to be administered, to verify the recommended dose or formula, the method and duration of administration, and contraindications. It is the responsibility of the practitioner, relying on his or her own experience and knowledge of the patient, to make diagnoses, to determine dosages and the best treatment for each individual patient, and to take all appropriate safety precautions. To the fullest extent of the law, neither the publisher nor the authors assume any liability for any injury and/or damage to persons or property arising out of or related to any use of the material contained in this book.

Library of Congress Cataloging-in-Publication Data
Parkland trauma handbook/edited by Alexander L. Eastman, David H. Rosenbaum, Erwin R. Thal. -- 3rd ed.
  p. ; cm.
 Includes bibliographical references and index.
 ISBN 978-0-323-05226-9
 1. Traumatology--Handbooks, manuals, etc. 2. Blunt trauma--Handbooks, manuals, etc. 3. Wounds and injuries--Handbooks, manuals, etc. I. Eastman, Alexander L. II. Rosenbaum, David H. III. Thal, Erwin R. IV. Parkland Memorial Hospital (Dallas, Tex.) V. Title: Trauma handbook.
  [DNLM: 1. Wounds and Injuries--diagnosis--Handbooks. 2. Wounds and Injuries--therapy--Handbooks. WO 39 P2485 2009]
  RD93.P3 2009
  617.1--dc22 2008041754

Acquisitions Editor: James Merritt
Publishing Services Manager: Tina Rebane
Design Direction: Gene Harris

Printed in the United States of America
Last digit is the print number: 9 8 7 6 5 4 3 2 1

Working together to grow
libraries in developing countries
www.elsevier.com | www.bookaid.org | www.sabre.org

ELSEVIER BOOK AID International Sabre Foundation

Contributors

Adam C. Alder, MD
Resident in General Surgery

Severn Barloco, MD
Resident in General Surgery

Adam W. Beck, MD
Resident in General Surgery

Christopher Bell, MD
Resident in General Surgery

Jennifer Blumetti, MD
Resident in General Surgery

Amy Brazda, MD
Resident in General Surgery

Scott Brakenridge, MD
Resident in General Surgery

Harshal Broker, MD
Resident in General Surgery

James A. Chambers, MD, MPH & TM
Resident in General Surgery

Kevin Crawford, MD
Resident in General Surgery

David Curtis, MD
Resident in General Surgery

Nabil N. Dagher, MD
Resident in General Surgery

Sean Dineen, MD
Resident in General Surgery

Alexander Eastman, MD
Resident in General Surgery

Henry Ellis, MD
Resident in Orthopaedic Surgery

Kousta I. Foteh, MD
Resident in General Surgery

Joshua L. Gary, MD
Resident in General Surgery

Robert Garza, MD
Resident in General Surgery

Makram Gedeon, MD
Resident in General Surgery

Richard M. Gillespie, MD
Resident in General Surgery

Julie Grimes, MD
Resident in Obstetrics and gynecology

Jason Hall, MD
Resident in General Surgery

Alan E. Harzman, MD
Resident in General Surgery

Richard Hershberger, MD
Resident in General Surgery

Arsalla Islam, MD
Resident in General Surgery

Radha Iyengar, MD
Resident in General Surgery

Samuel Jacks, MD
Resident in General Surgery

Kshama Jaiswal, MD
Resident in General Surgery

Lauren Kane, MD
Resident in General Surgery

Jarrod King, MD
Resident in Orthopaedic Surgery

Contributors

Jorie Klein, RN
Director, Trauma and Disaster Services

Rohit K. Khosla, MD
Resident in Plastic Surgery

Marc Labat, MD
Resident in Emergency Medicine

Lee Ann Lau, MD
Resident in General Surgery

Avron Lipschitz, MD
Resident in General Surgery

Clifann McCarley, RN, BNS
Trauma Nurse-Clinician

Jennifer L. McDougal, MD
Resident in General Surgery

Barbra S. Miller, MD
Resident in General Surgery

Meredith Miller, MD
Resident in General Surgery

Ian Mitchell, MD
Resident in General Surgery

Brian Oleksy, DDS, MD
Resident in Oral and Maxillofacial Surgery

Craig Olson, MD
Resident in General Surgery

Matthias Peltz, MD
Resident in Thoracic Surgery

Damon S. Pierce, MD
Resident in General Surgery

Christina Roland, MD
Resident in General Surgery

Josh Roller, MD
Resident in General Surgery

David H. Rosenbaum, MD
Resident in General Surgery

Frances Rosenbaum, MD
Resident in Obstetrics and Gynecology

Kelly Schmidt, MD
Resident in Neurological Surgery

Paul Schumacher, MD
Resident in General Surgery

Tif Siragusa, MD
Resident in General Surgery

Stephen Smith, MD
Resident in Vascular Surgery

Taylor Smith, MD
Resident in General Surgery

Lance E. Stuke, MD
Resident in General Surgery

Patrick T. Sweeney, MD
Resident in General Surgery

Hemangini Thakar, MD
Resident in Plastic Surgery

Steven A. Vela, MD
Resident in General Surgery

Krishna Venkatesh, MD
Resident in General Surgery

Lance Walsh, MD, PhD
Resident in Urologic Surgery

Stacey Woodruff, MD
Resident in General Surgery

Foreword

We are pleased to present the third edition of the *Parkland Trauma Handbook*. Again, the manual presents the basic tenets of trauma management and updates protocols to meet current standards. The treatment of multiply injured patients remains a team effort and is best provided by adhering to trauma systems that cover the spectrum from prevention to rehabilitation. This team includes physicians from all specialties and support personnel from several disciplines. Essential ingredients for success include the reflective assessment of outcomes based on registry-generated data, pristine performance improvement and patient safety activity, well-designed research projects, and administrative and professional commitment, all led by the general (trauma) surgeon who serves as the "captain of the ship."

This new handbook reflects the considerable changes that have occurred since the last edition. Improvements in imaging, proliferation of nonoperative management, the introduction of minimally invasive procedures, as well as improvements in the general overall care of the patient, have accelerated in recent years. Efforts in trauma prevention have been reflected in changing patterns of injury. Along with the advances in technology comes a responsibility to be cost effective as one travels down the diagnostic highway.

The *Parkland Trauma Handbook* is designed to assist young surgeons in training, general and specialty surgeons who do not treat a large number of injured patients, support personnel, and other colleagues in the management of these difficult cases. The principles and guidelines are based on the experience of a large Level 1 trauma center and the text has been written in its entirety by our excellent surgical housestaff. The handbook is a practical guide to be used in the management of trauma patients.

This edition has been edited by two of our excellent chief residents, Alex Eastman and David Rosenbaum, and facilitated by the ever-present, senior mentorship of Dr. Erwin Thal. The *Parkland Trauma Handbook* continues to emerge from the forefront of trauma care, written by those who deliver that care every day and every night at one of the country's busiest trauma centers. We are proud to present this fine piece of work.

Robert V. Rege, MD
Chair, Department of Surgery
The University of Texas Southwestern Medical Center
Dallas, Texas

Preface

The chief surgical resident is the most senior house officer at Parkland Memorial Hospital. His or her expertise is a sought-after commodity in the treatment of the severely injured, sick, or dying. As a result of their experiences at Parkland, the Parkland "trauma chief" tends to walk a little taller as he or she roams the wards and intensive care units at night. Since its inception, the *Parkland Trauma Handbook* has served as a guiding light, helping us transition from wide-eyed Interns to seasoned surgical professionals.

Revision of a work of this nature is daunting, and as is the case with many other of our traditions, the work of those who have come before us is unparalleled. The original manual, from Mike Lopez, was genius. It was only improved by that of Fiemu Nwariaku, who set the standard high, making it challenging for us to revise and update his work. His guidance at the beginning of this process was invaluable. In terms of mentorship, the leadership of Dr. Thal is unparalleled. He is a true giant in the field and a fantastic mentor, advisor, and friend (not to mention a merciless editor).

As we worked through the revisions, the contributions of several people made this book possible. First, the surgical residents of Parkland Memorial Hospital are an extraordinary group of men and women. We thank each of them for their contributions and persistence.

Dianne Wynne, Dr. Thal's right hand and more, deserves more thanks than we can offer. For pushing us to stay on track, and more importantly, for keeping Dr. Thal in line, we are indebted. We also owe Jim Merritt and Tina Rebane at Elsevier our sincere thanks, for without their guidance and tremendous patience this project would have never made it to completion.

We talk so often of the days when surgical giants walked the halls of Parkland Memorial Hospital and other leading medical centers. Our giants include Dr. Jules Cahan, Dr. Stephen R.T. Evans, Dr. Joseph Minei, Dr. Erwin Thal, Dr. Mike Cornell, Dr. John Cargile, Dr. Kelvin Johnigan, Dr. William Cheadle, Dr. Hiram Polk and Dr. J. David Richardson. To each of you, who have invested your time, energy, and vast resources into shaping us as surgeons, we hope in some small way our efforts with this manual will show you the beginnings of the fruits of your labors.

Lastly, to the people of Dallas, Texas, who continue to place their trust in us and further our education by their continued patronage of our services 24 hours a day, 365 days a year at Parkland Memorial Hospital, thank you. We hope this book in its newest rendition will continue to prepare men and women who when you need us, will don their boots and head to the Trauma Hall walking tall.

Alexander L. Eastman, MD
David H. Rosenbaum, MD

Foreword from the First Edition

Parkland Memorial Hospital is nationally recognized as a leader in the care of injured patients. Underpinning this recognition is a well established approach to the care of trauma patients. This approach is based on (1) an understanding of the pathophysiology of injury; (2) consistent application of established surgical principles; (3) ongoing evaluation of careful clinical studies; (4) knowledge of the surgical literature; and (5) decades of direct experience with the care of injured patients. This approach is carried out by a multidisciplinary team of surgeons led by general surgeons. The general surgery chief resident and the surgery specialty chief residents, under the careful supervision of experienced attending surgeons, play key roles in this system.

The Parkland surgical residents have developed formal and informal methods for transmitting this approach to each other. This handbook is the result of a suggestion by Miguel (Mike) Lopez-Viego that this information be codified into a handbook which could provide this information to surgical residents and students at Parkland and nationally. The result is a handbook written by residents for residents. Erwin Thal has played the role of an attending in a masterful fashion. He has made suggestions regarding organization, encouraged and occasionally cajoled the residents to meet deadlines. He has reviewed the manuscripts, made suggestions and provided a consistency in style and approach.

The result is this handbook which emphasizes a practical and consistent approach to the management of injured patients. It can be read from cover to cover or used as a pocket reference for immediate information on individual problems.

The handbook promises to be a major benefit to students, residents and to injured patients.

Drs Thal, Lopez and all the residents from the surgical specialties at Parkland are to be congratulated on this effort and the outstanding result.

James Carrico MD
Professor and Chairman
Department of Surgery
UT Southwestern Medical Center
Dallas, Texas

Preface from the First Edition

This handbook is the result of the collaborative efforts of senior surgical residents and fellows from Parkland Memorial Hospital. The goal of this project was to construct a practical, portable, trauma reference source that would be of use to medical students, residents, and practicing physicians on a daily basis.

The material in this handbook is based solely on sound and established principles of trauma care. Where possible, we have included brief reviews of the historical, anatomic, and physiologic basis for the diagnostic and management regimens we recommend. The information in our book is tempered by the experiences and policies of the trauma services at Parkland Memorial Hospital. These, to a large extent, are based on decades of experience with the care of injured patients.

The authors of this text collectively dedicate this project to our teachers, past and present, senior residents and professors alike. For they provided us with the independence to manage complicated trauma patients and thus learn the art of trauma care through high volume personal experiences. These were always supported by an academic environment that was strict and demanding, but always constructive and supportive.

The support and guidance of Dr. C. James Carrico and Dr Erwin Thal during this project were critical to its completion and exemplify the dedication of the faculty at Southwestern Medical School to the field of trauma. We are also grateful for the support of Susie Baxter, Anne Gunter and Nancy at Mosby-Year Book.

The contributing authors also consider this handbook a salute to our professor and friend and our constant source of surgical wisdom, Robert N. McClelland, a man whose greatest interest has always been the education of surgeons and the advancement of surgical knowledge.

Miguel A. Lopez-Viego

Contents

1 Epidemiology of Trauma   1
James A. Chambers, MD, MPH & TM

2 Trauma Systems   5
Alexander L. Eastman, MD

3 Trauma Performance Improvement and Patient Safety   11
*Christina Roland, MD, Jorie Klein, RN,
and Clifann McCarley, RN, BNS*

4 Advanced Trauma Life Support   16
Adam C. Alder, MD

5 Trauma Scoring Systems   18
Jennifer L. McDougal, MD

6 Mechanisms of Injury   24
James A. Chambers, MD, MPH & TM

7 All-Hazards Disaster Preparedness and Mitigation   29
Alexander Eastman, MD

8 Initial Assessment of the Trauma Patient   31
Severn Barloco, MD, and Hemangini Thakar, MD

9 Shock   43
Hema Thakar, MD, and Jennifer Blumetti, MD

10 Transfusion Therapy   50
Harshal Broker, MD, and Samuel Jacks, MD

11 Emergency Department Diagnostic Modalities   60
Makram Gedeon, MD

12 Ultrasound in Trauma   71
Radha Iyengar, MD

13 Catheters and Tubes   75
Lauren Kane, MD

14 Damage Control Surgery   93
Craig Olson, MD, and Alexander L. Eastman, MD

Contents

15 Neurologic Trauma 97
Kelly Schmidt, MD

16 Soft Tissue Injuries of the Face 109
Hema Thakar, MD, and Jennifer Blumetti, MD

17 Facial Fractures I—Upper Facial Skeleton 123
Avron Lipschitz, MD, and Brian Oleksy, DDS, MD

18 Facial Fractures II: Maxillary, Midfacial, and Mandibular Fractures 137
Avron Lipschitz, MD, and Brian Oleksy, DDS, MD

19 Ophthalmic Injuries 148
Fiemu E. Nwariaku, MD

20 Neck Injuries 157
Jennifer L. McDougal, MD

21 Thoracic Trauma 165
Adam W. Beck, MD

22 Diaphragmatic Injury 180
David H. Rosenbaum, MD

23 Esophageal Trauma 183
Richard Hershberger, MD, and Stacey Woodruff, MD

24 Gastric Trauma 188
Lance E. Stuke, MD, and Kousta I. Foteh, MD

25 Pancreatic and Duodenal Trauma 193
Adam W. Beck, MD

26 Small Bowel Trauma 204
Barbra S. Miller, MD

27 Liver and Biliary Tract Trauma 210
David Curtis, MD

28 Splenic Trauma 225
Scott Brakenridge, MD, and Christopher Bell, MD

29 Colon and Rectal Trauma 235
Josh Roller, MD

30 Renal Trauma 243
Lance Walsh, MD, PhD

31 Radiologic Evaluation of the Genitourinary Tract in Trauma 250
Lance Walsh, MD, PhD

32 Genital and Perineal Trauma 254
Meredith Miller, MD

33 Extremity Vascular Trauma 259
Damon S. Pierce, MD

34 Abdominal Vascular Injury 264
Stephen Smith, MD

35 Thermal, Chemical, and Cold Injuries 273
Robert Garza, MD

36 Principles of Fractures and Dislocations 287
Richard M. Gillespie, MD, and Joshua L. Gary, MD

37 Complications of Musculoskeletal Trauma 290
Lee Ann Lau, MD

38 Fractures of the Pelvis and Acetabulum 303
Arsalla Islam, MD, and Jarrod King, MD

39 Fractures and Dislocations of the Lower Extremity 312
Krishna Venkatesh, MD

40 Knee Ligament Injuries 334
Krishna Venkatesh, MD

41 Foot and Ankle Injuries 342
Taylor Smith, MD, and Henry Ellis, MD

42 Upper Extremity Fractures and Dislocations 347
Taylor Smith, MD, and Henry Ellis, MD

43 Hand Injuries and Infections 360
Rohit K. Khosla, MD, and Tif Siragusa, MD

44 Fractures in Children 379
Amy Brazda, MD, and Kevin Crawford, MD

45 Bites 396
Marc Labat, MD

46 Trauma in the Pregnant Patient 403
Julie Grimes, MD, and Frances Rosenbaum, MD

47 Pediatric Trauma 410
Ian Mitchell, MD, and Kshama Jaiswal, MD

48 Geriatric Trauma 416
Severn Barloco, MD

49 Anesthesia in Trauma 419
Nabil N. Dagher, MD

50 Cardiovascular Support and Management in the Intensive Care Unit 425
Sean Dineen, MD, and Paul Schumacher, MD

51 Bedside Procedures in the Surgical Intensive Care Unit 434
Steven A. Vela, MD, and Kousta I. Foteh, MD

52 Pulmonary Disorders 438
Makram Gedeon, MD

53 Disorders of Thermoregulation in the Intensive Care Unit 453
Jason Hall, MD

54 Disorders of Acid-Base, Fluids, and Electrolytes 461
Sean Dineen, MD, and Paul Schumacher, MD

55 Infection in the Surgical Intensive Care unit 474
Alan E. Harzman, MD

56 Metabolism and Nutrition 495
Radha Iyengar, MD

57 Organ Donation and Management of the Organ Donor 501
Matthias Peltz, MD

Index 509

Epidemiology of Trauma

James A. Chambers, MD, MPH & TM

I. INCIDENCE

A. Since the early 20th century, blunt and penetrating trauma have increased in incidence and impact in the United States, resulting in a tremendous public health challenge.
1. Trauma is the fourth leading cause of death overall (~150,000 deaths/year) and the leading cause of death in persons ages 1 to 44 years. More deaths result from trauma than from all other causes combined in persons ages 1 to 34 years.
2. Additionally, 28 million persons (~10% of the US population) are evaluated for trauma in emergency departments annually, with 1.5 million being admitted to the hospital.

B. Trauma constitutes a significant and rising problem in the remainder of the world as well, predominantly from intentional injuries (violence). The number of unintentional injuries is rising as well as more countries industrialize.

1. **Violence**
    a. Each year, 1.6 million deaths are caused by violence worldwide. Intentional injury is the leading cause of death among persons ages 15 to 44 worldwide. Fourteen percent of all males and 7% of all females die as a result of violent injury.
    b. Approximately 50% of violent deaths are suicides, 33% are homicides, and 20% result from armed conflict.
    c. Young males (ages 15 to 29 years) are at highest risk of homicide (19.4/100,000) with males older than 60 years at highest risk for suicide (44.9/100,000).
    d. Significant geographic/cultural variation exists:
        i. In Africa and the Americas, homicide is three times more common than suicide.
        ii. In Southeast Asia and Europe, suicide is twice as common as homicide.
        iii. In Western Pacific countries, suicide is almost six times more common than homicide.

2. **Unintentional injury**
    a. Mechanisms of injury traditionally seen in the developing world include burns and simple nonindustrial work-related injury, but with increasing technology, motor vehicle crashes are rapidly becoming a major source of morbidity and mortality.

II. ETIOLOGY AND PATTERNS OF INJURY (CURRENT FOR YEAR 2002 IN THE UNITED STATES UNLESS OTHERWISE STATED)

A. Age/gender
1. More than three-fourths of emergency department trauma visits, half of trauma hospitalizations, and half of trauma fatalities are in persons under 45 years of age.
2. Patients 65 years and older are at highest risk of having injuries requiring hospitalization or resulting in death. Those older than 75 years are at particular risk of dying as a result of sustained injuries.
3. Male gender is a risk factor for trauma up to age 65 years at which time females surpass the male risk. Overall, males are 40% more likely than females to sustain significant injuries.

B. Mechanisms (consistent with Parkland Memorial Hospital admissions)
1. Fatalities
   a. Motor vehicles: 31%
   b. Firearms: 19%
   c. Poisonings: 13%
   d. Falls: 9%
   e. Pediatric-specific
      i. In preadolescent patients, drowning and burns are second only to motor vehicle collisions as causes of death.
   f. Chronology of fatal injury
      i. 50% die at the scene or en route to a hospital.
      ii. 30% die as a result of neurologic injury within 2 to 48 hours after injury.
      iii. 20% die of infection or multiorgan system failure within days to weeks after injury.
2. Nonfatal injury (93.6% unintentional; ratio of nonfatal:fatal injuries 200:1)
   a. Falls
   b. Motor vehicle crashes
   c. Firearms

C. Causes
1. Motor vehicle collisions: 42,500 deaths, 350,000 hospitalizations, and 4 million emergency department visits stem from motor vehicle crashes each year. All age groups except increasingly mobile over age 85 seniors are experiencing slowly decreasing death rates. Males are twice as likely as females to sustain a fatal injury, except for those ages 15 to 44 years, when they are three times as likely to die as a result of a motor vehicle collision.
   a. Factors include speed, vehicle instability, braking, road design, and intoxication.
      i. Shoulder and lap belts decrease front seat fatalities by 45%, and fatalities are further decreased by airbags.
      ii. Alcohol is a factor in 50% of fatal collisions involving persons ages 15 to 34 years, and alcohol is especially associated with motorcycle deaths.

2. Firearms
    a. In many US index cities, firearm-related fatalities outnumber motor vehicle deaths. In 1999, more than half of the deaths from firearms were suicides, 38% were homicides, and 3% were unintentional. The majority (88%) of firearm homicides in 1999 involved handguns.
    b. Males and young persons are most affected.
    c. Suicides increased between 1980 and 1999, and most were gun-related.
3. Falls
    a. Although falls caused only 9% of injury deaths in 1999, they account for over a third of all injury hospitalizations and for one fourth of all injury-related visits to emergency departments.
    b. Falls are the leading cause of nonfatal injuries in children under the age of 5 years.
    c. Men up to the age of 45 years account for the majority of injuries resulting from falls, but after the age of 45 years females more commonly sustain significant injuries from falls. Falls are the most common causes of nonfatal injuries in the elderly and account for almost 80% of elderly trauma admissions.

D. Factors
1. Violence
    a. Two million reported violent (intentional) injuries occur per year in the United States, and 31% of trauma deaths stem from violence. Violence in the urban setting independently correlates with socioeconomic depression.
        i. 63% are from suicide, of which 57% involve firearms.
        ii. 37% are from homicide, of which 64% involve firearms.
2. Occupation
    a. Approximately 6,000 occupation-related deaths occur annually. The transportation industry accounts for the majority of these deaths.
    b. 13 million occupation-related injuries are reported each year, with almost half resulting in long-term disability. The highest rates occur in nursing and personal care sectors.

III. IMPACT

A. More total life is lost from trauma in the United States before the age of 75 years than from any other cause.
B. Total lifetime costs incurred by trauma account for an estimated $260 billion (1995 US dollars) annually.
C. Lost quality of life/lost productivity is difficult to quantify.

IV. PREVENTION

A. Prevention must consider:
1. All three parts of the epidemiologic triad (host, agent, environment)

2. Opportunities for intervention in terms of phases are pre-event, event, and post-event. (Half of deaths occur at the scene of the event or en route to a hospital.) Severe, irreversible neurologic damage accounts for the majority of the remainder.
3. Mechanisms of intervention include engineering, education, and legislation.

B. Trends:
1. Public health success: Since the early 20th century, the death rate (deaths/miles traveled) has been reduced nine-fold, and occupation-related, unintentional deaths have decreased 87%.
2. In the past several decades, homicide rates have fluctuated but suicide rates have remained stable; the number of deaths resulting from firearms has decreased overall, except in adolescents and young adults, in whom firearm-related deaths have increased.

V. SUGGESTED READINGS

Blum RW, Nelson-Mmari K: The health of young people in a global context. J Adolesc Health 35(5):402-418, 2004.

Centers for Disease Control and Prevention: Web-Based Injury Statistics Query and Reporting System (WISQARS). www.cdc.gov/ncipc/wisqars (most recent data from 2002).

Centers for Disease Control and Prevention: National Injury Surveillance System – All Injury Program (NEISS-AIP). MMWR 50(17):340-346, 2001.

Cinat ME, Wilson SE, Lush S, Atkins C: Significant correlation of trauma epidemiology with the economic conditions of community. Arch Surg 139:1350-1355, 2004.

Hansen KS, Morild I, Engesaeter LB, Viste A: Epidemiology of severely and fatally injured patients in western part of Norway. Scand J Surg 93:198-203, 2004.

Kobusingye O, Guwatudde D, Lett R: Injury patterns in rural and urban Uganda. Injury Prevent 7:46-50, 2001.

Moore EE, Feliciano DV, Mattox KL: Trauma, 5th ed. New York, McGraw-Hill, 2003.

Otieno T, Woodfield JC, Bird P, Hill AG: Trauma in rural Kenya. Injury 35:1228-1233, 2004.

Sieling BA, Beem K, Hoffman MT, et al: Trauma in nonagenarians and centenarians: Review of 137 consecutive patients. Am Surg 70:793-796, 2004.

World Health Organization: World Report on Violence and Health. Geneva, WHO, 2002.

World Health Organization: The World Health Report 2003 – Shaping the Future. Geneva, WHO, 2003.

World Health Organization: Global Strengthening of Care for the Wounded. Bull World Health Organ 82(4), 2004.

Trauma Systems

Alexander L. Eastman, MD

I. HISTORICAL DEVELOPMENTS

A. The beginnings of a trauma system in the United States can be found during the American Civil War when emphasis on the rapid treatment of injured soldiers dictated the organization of medical staff, transport crew, and field hospitals.
B. Major innovations in the development of organized trauma care stem from military conflicts.
1. Rapid transport and treatment were further refined in subsequent wars.
2. Notable improvements occurred during the following conflicts:
    a. Korean War—the introduction of helicopters delivering wounded soldiers directly to mobile army surgical hospitals located near the front lines.
    b. Vietnam War—further refinement of field transport system.
    c. Operation Desert Shield/Storm—widespread use of Forward Surgical Teams (FSTs), specialized units that provide surgical stabilization immediately behind front lines.

C. Several notable publications:
1. Accidental Death and Disability: The Neglected Disease of Modern Society (1966)—first widespread civilian acceptance of the notion of organized trauma systems.
2. Injury in America – A Continuing Public Health Problem (1985)—promoted awareness of the staggering societal costs of trauma and of the widespread lack of organized care for trauma victims.

D. Important legislation:
1. The Emergency Medical Services System Act (1973)—provided financial incentives to states to coordinate regionalized emergency medical services (EMS) activities.
2. The Trauma Care Systems Planning and Development Act (1990)—The first federal funding for the development of statewide trauma systems.

II. RATIONALE FOR REGIONALIZED CARE

A. Numerous studies have confirmed improved patient outcome and decreased mortality following trauma if medical care is provided by a specialized trauma center.
1. Most notably, the comparison of the preventable death rates in Orange County, California, where patients were delivered to the nearest hospital, and in San Francisco, California, where patients were delivered to the designated trauma center. This legendary study by West and associates illustrates the benefits of regionalized trauma care.
    a. The preventable death rate in Orange County was approximately 73%, in contrast to 1 preventable death in San Francisco.

TABLE 2-1
COMPARISION OF NON-CNS TRUMATIC DEATHS[a]

	San Francisco 1974		Orange County, California						
			1974[b]		1978–1979		1980–1981		
							Trauma Center[b]		Nontrauma Center
Category	n	%	n	%	n	%	n	%	n	%
Preventable deaths	0/16	0	22/30	73	15/21	71	2/23	9	4/6	67
Appropriate operation performed	15/16	94	6/30	20	3/21	14	16/18	89	1/5	20
Hemorrhagic deaths (no surgery performed)	1/16	6	17/30	57	14/21	67	1/14	7	1/2	50

[a] From West JT., Cables R., Gazziniga A. Impact of regionalization: The Orange County Experience. *Arch Surg* 1983; 118:740–744.
[b] Region with an organized system of trauma care.

b. Following the implementation of trauma centers in Orange County, the preventable death rate declined to 9% (Table 2-1).

III. STRUCTURE OF TRAUMA SYSTEMS

A. The trauma system should provide well-organized plans and protocols to meet the following goals of regionalized care:
1. Access
2. Prehospital care and triage
3. Acute care at specialized centers
4. Rehabilitation

B. Eight essential characteristics of an inclusive, regional trauma system have been identified based on recommendations of the American College of Surgeons:
1. Authority to designate trauma centers granted to a lead agency
2. A formal process used for trauma center designation
3. American College of Surgeons guidelines applied to trauma centers
4. Trauma center survey performed by an out-of-area survey team
5. Designated trauma centers limited in number based on community need
6. Written criteria established to determine hospital triage
7. Trauma centers undergo ongoing evaluation and monitoring
8. Trauma centers availability structured on statewide or regional basis

C. Hospitals included within a trauma system must provide care and resources commensurate with their designated level.

IV. AMERICA COLLEGE OF SURGEONS VERIFICATION REVIEW CRITERIA FOR TRAUMA CENTERS

The American College of Surgeons has revised the verification review criteria (VRC) for trauma centers. Type I and Type II VRC are considered essential for a hospital to be verified as a Level I trauma center, but Type II requirements are considered less urgent. A full explanation of the verification review process and verification site visit can be found in American College of Surgeons Committee on Trauma: Resources for the Optimal Care of the Injured Patient. Chicago: American College of Surgeons, 2006, or online at http://www.facs.org/trauma/vrc1.html.

Level I facilities must have surgical specialists available, including orthopaedic surgery, plastic surgery, obstetric and gynecologic surgery, ophthalmology, otolaryngology, and urology.

The following are some of the Type I criteria for Level I trauma centers:
1. The hospital must have the commitment of the institutional governing body and medical staff to become a trauma center. There must be sufficient infrastructure and support to the trauma service to ensure adequate provision of care.

2. A Level I trauma center must meet admission volume performance requirements.
3. A trauma director must have responsibility and authority for determining each general surgeon's ability to participate on the trauma panel based on an annual review.
4. The trauma medical director must be either board-certified or an American College of Surgeons fellow.
5. The trauma medical director participates in trauma calls and has the authority to correct deficiencies in trauma care and to exclude from the trauma team those trauma team members who do not meet specified criteria.
6. There is a multidisciplinary peer review committee chaired by the trauma medical director or designee, with participation from general surgery, orthopaedic surgery, neurosurgery, emergency medicine, and anesthesia.
7. Surgical commitment is essential for a properly functioning trauma center.
8. A general surgeon must be in-house 24 hours a day and is expected to be in the emergency department on patient arrival, with adequate notification from the field.
9. The trauma surgeon on call must be dedicated to the trauma center while on duty.
10. Seriously injured patients are admitted or evaluated by an identifiable surgical service staffed by credentialed providers.
11. The emergency department has a designated emergency physician director supported by an appropriate number of physicians to ensure immediate care for injured patients.
12. A neurosurgical liaison is designated.
13. Neurotrauma care is promptly and continuously available for severe traumatic brain injury and spinal cord injury and for less severe head and spine injuries when necessary. An attending neurosurgeon is promptly available to the hospital's trauma service when neurosurgical consultation is requested, and there is a formally arranged contingency plan in case the capability of the neurosurgeon, hospital, or system to care for neurotrauma patients is overwhelmed.
14. Sufficient equipment and operative capabilities for orthopaedic trauma care must be available.
15. Plastic surgery, hand surgery, and spinal injury care are available at Level I trauma centers.
16. Anesthesiology services are promptly available for emergency operations or airway problems.

17. There is an anesthesiologist liaison to the trauma department, and anesthesia services are available in-house 24 hours a day.
18. The post anesthesia care unit has qualified nurses available 24 hours a day as needed.
19. Radiologists are promptly available, when requested, for the interpretation of radiographs, performance of complex imaging studies, or interventional procedures. Conventional radiography and CT are available in trauma centers 24 hours per day.
20. Physicians must be available to care for critically ill trauma patients 24 hours a day.
21. The ICU has the necessary equipment to monitor and resuscitate patients.
22. Laboratory services are available 24 hours a day for standard analyses such as of blood, urine, and other body fluids. The capablility for coagulation studies, blood gases, and microbiology must also be available 24 hours a day.
23. The blood bank must be capable of blood typing and cross matching and must have a supply of red blood cells, fresh frozen plasma, platelets, cryoprecipitate, and appropriate coagulation factors as needed for injured patients.
24. The trauma service retains responsibility for patients and coordinates all therapeutic decisions appropriate for its level. The trauma surgeon is kept informed of all management decisions.
25. Patients in Level I facilites have in-house physician coverage for intensive care at all times.
26. The intensive care unit has the necessary equipment to monitor and resuscitate patients, and qualified nurses are available 24 hours per day to provide care in the intensive care unit.
27. The trauma center collects and analyzes trauma registry data and uses corrective strategies to define the results of analysis.
28. The results of analysis and corrective strategies are documented.

V. SUGGESTED READINGS

American College of Surgeons Committee on Trauma: Resources for Optimal Care of the Injured Patient. Chicago, American College of Surgeons, 2006.

Arroyo J, Crosby L: Basic rescue and resuscitation – Trauma system concept in the United States. Clin Orthop Rel Res 318, 1995.

Bazzoli G, Madura K, Cooper G, et al: Progress in the development of trauma systems in the United States JAMA 273:395-401, 1995.

Eastman AB, Bishop G, Walsh J, et al: The economic status of trauma centers on the eve of health care reform. J Trauma 36(6), 1994.

Moore E: Trauma systems, trauma centers, and trauma surgeons: Opportunity in managed competition. J Trauma 39(1), 1995.

West J, Cales R, Gazziniga A: Impact of regionalization: The Orange County experience. Arch Surg 118:740-744, 1983.

West J, Williams M, Trunkey D, Wolferth C: Trauma systems: Current status – future challenges. JAMA 259:3597-3600, 1988.

Trauma Performance Improvement and Patient Safety

Christina Roland, MD, Jorie Klein, RN, and Clifann McCarley, RN, BNS

I. PURPOSE

- **A.** To ensure that all essential criteria required for level I trauma center verification by the American College of Surgeons Committee on Trauma, the state and regional health services, JCAHO, and the institutional program are met.
- **B.** To ensure that quality, efficient, effective, and cost-appropriate care is delivered to the trauma patient.
- **C.** To ensure that those individuals who receive services provided by the trauma program are satisfied with the services rendered.
- **D.** To strive for optimal patient outcomes.

II. DEFINITIONS

- **A.** Trauma medical director—faculty trauma surgeon providing direction and leadership to trauma program.
- **B.** Director of trauma services (nursing)—nursing director of all inpatient trauma programs at Parkland Memorial Hospital.
- **C.** Trauma services staff—dedicated, specially trained trauma nurses who provide continuous care and case management from initial trauma center resuscitation through hospital discharge.
- **D.** Trauma service structure—see the institution's organizational chart.

III. PROTOCOL

- **A.** The Trauma Performance Improvement and Patient Safety (TPIPS) Protocol includes the review of all patients who meet criteria for:
1. Level I, II, or III trauma activation
2. All admitted trauma patients
3. Trauma patients who are transferred in or out of Parkland Memorial Hospital
4. All trauma patients who die as a result of their injuries
- **B.** Trauma services staff perform rounds on all trauma patients daily.
- **C.** Care managers review each trauma patient's care for the following:
1. Coordination of care
2. Timeliness of care
3. Appropriateness of care
4. Compliance with established standard of care
5. Quality of care
6. Outcomes, including complications
7. Service to patient and family

8. Cost of care and system performance
D. All deviations from the standard of care, unusual occurrences, issues of cost of care, and patient safety or satisfaction issues are identified and documented on the performance improvement tracking forms.
1. Each complication is graded using the following grading system:
   a. Grade I complication: non-life-threatening alteration in care, no residual disability, and necessitating only a minor, bedside procedure.
   b. Grade II complication: potentially life-threatening, but no residual disability. May require an invasive procedure.
   c. Grade III complication: residual disability, may require organ resection, and may produce persistence of life-threatening condition.
   d. Grade IV complication: death or a nonsurvivable outcome.
2. All deaths undergo a multidisciplinary trauma attending peer review.
   a. Each death is defined as:
      i. Nonpreventable: injuries are nonsurvivable with optimal care.
      ii. Potentially preventable: injuries are severe but survivable with optimal care.
      iii. Preventable: injuries are physiologically survivable with optimal care.
3. All deaths and variances/complications have a standard of practice score assessed. Each case is reviewed to define if the standard of practice was followed. The scores utilized are as follows;
   a. 1–practice guidelines were followed, time delays are appropriate.
   b. 2–practice guidelines were not followed, minor deviation occurred.
   c. 3–practice guidelines were not followed, significant deviation in care occurred.
   d. 4–significant deviations in standards of practice occurred, which are defined as error in judgment, delay in diagnosis or interpretation, or error in technique.
   e. 5–practice guidelines are not formally defined.
4. Each complication/variance is reviewed to define the contributing factors. The contributing factors are categorized as:
   a. System inadequacy due to volume, capacity, or capabilities
   b. Patient disease process related to injury or comorbid disease
   c. Patient cooperation
   d. Language barrier
   e. Provider outcome
   f. Unable to define contributing factors
5. Trauma team activation reports are generated from the trauma services staff and reviewed by the trauma medical director and director of trauma nursing during the weekly TPIPS meeting. Delays in faculty/team response are specifically reviewed to define system issues versus provider issues.
E. Weekly Trauma Performance Improvement review meeting
1. All deaths, complications, and variances and all system delays are presented and reviewed by the housestaff, trauma medical director, and trauma nursing director.
2. Consulting trauma, orthopaedic, and neurosurgery teams review the findings prior to the weekly meeting.

3. All TPIPS meetings are closed to visitors and students to maintain patient privacy and confidentiality.

F. Weekly trauma multidisciplinary peer review conference

1. This meeting is utilized to close all open issues from the weekly TPIPS meeting.
2. Trauma residents are responsible for the presentation of each case.
3. Case presentations provide a brief overview of:
   a. Mechanism or injury
   b. Prehospital interventions and response
   c. Vital signs, revised trauma score (RTS), Glasgow Coma score
   d. Level of trauma activation and response time
   e. ABC (airway, breathing, and circulation) assessment and interventions, priorities of care, diagnostic priorities, and progression of care to include the specific issues identified by the trauma medical director.
   f. The resident is expected to have relevant published data regarding the specific issues of the case.
   g. Each case's discussion and documentation are entered into the trauma registry for inclusion in the performance review process.

G. All trauma patients meeting level I, II, or III trauma activation criteria are expected to have an emergency department disposition (out of the emergency department, into hospital bed) within 6 hours of trauma team activation. Variations in the disposition time are documented.

1. The trauma service managers document all admission/observation patients who are not discharged or converted in the established time frame.
2. The service managers also identify all patients in the system with a hospital stay greater than 5 days.

H. Trauma transfers

1. All patients transferred to Parkland Memorial Hospital trauma unit are reviewed for appropriateness of the transfer.
2. All transferring facilities receive a follow-up form regarding the patient's injuries, management, compliance to EMTALA guidelines, and if the transfer required a higher level of care. The form also includes some outcome information and whether or not the transfer was valid.
3. Each facility receives a form called Trauma Facility Transfer Review Tool. Returned forms are reviewed and trended for issues.

I. On a scheduled basis, paramedics who arrive with a trauma patient are asked to complete an EMS Trauma Satisfaction Survey.

J. The trauma midlevel providers who discharge trauma patients provide the trauma patient/family members with a form called Parkland Trauma Service Department Patient Satisfaction Survey.

IV. TRAUMA PERFORMANCE IMPROVEMENT REPORTS

A. The trauma medical director, director of trauma nursing services, and trauma service managers generate monthly and quarterly reports that are reviewed at the trauma executive committee meeting.

B. The senior vice president for surgical services presents an overview and summary of the trauma performance improvement activities to the Clinical Improvement Committee, Clinical Operations Committee, and the Board as needed.
C. The trauma registry coordinator provides monthly reports to assist in the compilation of performance improvement reports and provides a report reflecting the registry's monthly medical record completion.
D. Each trauma service manager completes a monthly trauma service performance summary. The summary is completed by the 20th day of each month. The trauma service manager reviews the summary with the trauma faculty and director.
E. Services provided through the Injury Prevention Programs and Trauma Outreach Education are reviewed through the trauma performance improvement process for the quality of the course, relevance of the course, and link to trends in trauma care. Monthly reports are included on the Trauma Executive Committee's agenda for review.

V. TRAUMA REGISTRY REVIEW

A. The trauma registry coordinator completes monthly audits to review record completeness and accuracy of the registrars for interrater reliability.
B. Reports are included in the trauma performance improvement process and reporting structure.
C. Individuals seeking data from the trauma registry must follow the trauma registry procedures. Individuals must complete a data registry form, define the use of the data, and gain required signatures before data will be processed. Data that are to be included in a trauma report that is to be distributed outside the Parkland Memorial Hospital trauma program or has the potential for publication require institutional review board approval.
D. The trauma registry coordinator is responsible for tracking and filing all data requests and the actual report that is released.

VI. RECORD KEEPING

A. All performance improvement documentation is coordinated in a dedicated notebook.
B. All case reviews, documentation, and follow-up documentation are organized, maintained, and secured in the director's office.
C. All documents produced for reports will be numbered for tracking purposes and returned. All copies other than the original are shredded.

VII. MONITORING

A. The trauma services staff monitor the defined North Central Texas Regional Trauma Advisory Council's (RAC) system performance standards.
B. Items defined as variance to the established RAC guidelines are referred to the RAC's system performance improvement committee using the defined referral guidelines and tools.
C. Trauma service managers complete the system review tool and forward it to the director of trauma nursing to prepare for RAC review.
D. Items referred are tracked for closure.
E. All items are processed through the trauma performance improvement meeting for review and defined action plan.

VIII. DIVERSION REVIEW

A. Trauma services staff monitor the request for trauma diversion.
B. The trauma nurse-clinician on call completes the diversion tracking/status tool.
C. The diversion tool and outcome are reviewed, tracked, and trended through the trauma performance improvement plan.

IX. SUGGESTED READINGS

American College of Surgeons, Committee on Trauma: Resources for Optimal Care of the Injured Patient. Chicago, American College of Surgeons, 1999.

American College of Surgeons, Committee on Trauma: Trauma Performance Improvement, A How-to Handbook. Chicago, American College of Surgeons, 1999.

Fitzpatrick MK, McMaster J: Performance Improvement in Trauma Care, Trauma Nursing: From Resuscitation Through Rehabilitation, 3rd ed. Philadelphia, WB Saunders, pp 34-47.

Joint Commission on Accreditation of Healthcare Organizations: Joint Commission Accreditation Manual. Oakbrook Terrance, IL, JCAHO, 1998.

Society of Trauma Nurses: Trauma Outcomes Performance Improvement Course. Chicago, Society of Trauma Nurses, 2004.

Advanced Trauma Life Support

Adam C. Alder, MD

I. HISTORY/INTRODUCTION

A. Advanced Trauma Life Support (ATLS) course is a continuing medical education program that was adopted by the American College of Surgeons Committee on Trauma in 1979.
B. Care during the "golden hour" is the primary focus of ATLS, when rapid assessment, resuscitation, and often operative intervention improve survival and decrease associated morbidity dramatically. ATLS protocols, when initiated at a trauma center, can improve the performance of the previously described procedures and may improve short-term mortality as well.
C. ATLS is updated periodically, most recently in 2004, to include more interactive sessions.
D. The course goals are as follows:
1. To educate the physician first responder in initial assessment and resuscitation of the multiply injured trauma patient.
    a. Studies have shown these changes have improved education and performance of participants.[1,2]
2. To standardize the acute care of the multiply injured patient across multiple specialties and disciplines.
3. To improve the process of care and mortality at hospitals that have adopted the ATLS course as mandatory training.[3]
4. To improve/facilitate the rapid transfer of injured patients to the appropriate level of trauma care.

II. COURSE STRUCTURE

A. The ATLS course is supervised by the Committee on Trauma of the American College of Surgeons.
B. The student course is intended for physicians only. Non-physicians may participate by auditing the course with written approval of the state/provincial Committee on Trauma chairperson. (Note: At Parkland Memorial Hospital, all trauma nurse-clinicians participate in the didactic portions of the course as a part of the Advance Trauma Nursing Certification (ATCN) program.)
C. At Parkland Memorial Hospital, we currently enroll all of our surgical interns in the ATLS course during the week before they begin their internship.
D. All slides, manuals, skill station radiographs, and testing materials are distributed by the American College of Surgeons.

E. Course participants must attend the entire course, demonstrate knowledge in core contents and skill stations, and have a written test score over 80% for successful completion.
F. Reverification is required every 4 years by successful completion of a refresher course.

III. REQUIRED SKILLS

A. ATLS focuses on prompt, accurate initial diagnostic assessment and immediate, appropriate therapeutic maneuvers. The skills felt to be critical are as follows:
1. Rapid initial assessment
2. Resuscitation and stabilization in an organized fashion
3. Determination of need for transfer to a trauma center
4. Arrangement of interhospital transfer
5. Delivery of optimal care to the trauma patient

IV. REFERENCES

1. Ali J, Adam R, Pierre I:. Comparison of performance two years after the old and new (interactive) ATLS courses. J Surg Res 97:71-75, 2001.
   This prospective cohort study compares the cognitive and clinical performance of providers who have completed the current and former ATLS courses. There was no significant difference between the cognitive performance scores, but in both the OSCE and approach portions of the clinical performance scores, the new interactive course helped providers perform at a higher level.
2. Kennedy DWG, Gentlemen D: The ATLS course: A survey of 228 ATLS providers. Emerg Med J 18:55-58, 2001
   This survey of 228 ATLS providers reveals that 97% of respondents felt their clinical practice had been improved by attending the new interactive ATLS course, 25% reporting this to be a large improvement.
3. Olson CJ, Arthur M, Mullins RJ: Influence of trauma system implementation on process of care delivered to seriously injured patients in rural trauma centers. Surgery 130:273-279, 2001.
   Process of care (an alternative to mortality analysis) was significantly improved in Oregon trauma centers after passing a mandate that all providers in a trauma center be ATLS certified.

V. SUGGESTED READINGS

Van Olden GD, Meeuwis D, Bolhuis HW, et al: Advanced trauma life support study: Quality of diagnostic and therapeutic procedures. J Trauma 57:381-384, 2004.
Prospective cohort study from the Netherlands comparing adequacy of procedures related to resuscitation of trauma patients before and after initiation of ATLS training among providers. These authors report that procedures were more adequate except for use of oxygen and full exposure, which were equivalent, after initiation of ATLS.

Trauma Scoring Systems

Jennifer L. McDougal, MD

I. OVERVIEW

Trauma scoring systems attempt to quantify diverse injuries in order to predict patient outcomes. Injury scoring systems are either physiologic, anatomic, or a combination of these measures. There is a general consensus that such scoring systems provide a standardized tool for epidemiologic studies and for comparison of treatment modalities across a broad trauma population.

II. COMMON TRAUMA SCORING SYSTEMS

- **A. The Glasgow Coma Score (GCS)** is a commonly used index for evaluating the level of consciousness and overall status of the central nervous system (Table 5-1). Three physiologic categories (eye-opening, verbal response, and motor response) are assessed and the total score (3 to 15) is determined by the sum of the highest value the patient achieves in each category. The GCS is helpful because it can be rapidly calculated in the field, and it correlates with mortality.
- **B. The Revised Trauma Score (RTS),** derived from the original Trauma Score described by Champion and associates in 1981, combines the GCS with systolic blood pressure (SBP) and respiratory rate (RR), each

TABLE 5-1
GLASGOW COMA SCALE

Eye opening	
Spontaneous	4
To voice	3
To pain	2
None	1
Verbal response	
Oriented	5
Confused	4
Inappropriate words	3
Incomprehensible sounds	2
None	1
Motor response	
Obeys commands	6
Localizes pain	5
Withdraws from pain	4
Flexion to pain	3
Extension to pain	2
None	1

TABLE 5-2
REVISED TRAUMA SCORE

Assessment	Method	Coding
Respiratory rate	Count total breaths in 15 seconds and multiply by 4	10–29 = 4 >29 = 3 6–9 = 2 1–5 = 1 0 = 0
Systolic blood pressure	Measure systolic cuff pressure on either arm by auscultation or palpation	>89 = 4 76–89 = 3 50–75 = 2 1–49 = 1 0 = 0

Glasgow Coma Scale
 (see Table 5-1)
GCS conversion scale:
13–15 = 4
9–12 = 3
6–8 = 2
4–5 = 1
<4 = 0

on a scale from 0 to 4 (Table 5-2). In the prehospital setting, any category with a score of less than 11 necessitates transfer to a trauma center. As an in-hospital tool, the RTS has been shown to correlate well with patient outcomes (Figure 5-1).

$$RTS = 0.9368 \, (GCS) + 0.7326 \, (SBP) + 0.2908 \, (RR)$$

C. **The Acute Physiology and Chronic Health Evaluation (APACHE)** classification is a physiologic score employed extensively to assess both medical and surgical intensive care patients. The APACHE system considers preadmission health status, age, and physiologic state during the first 24 hours of intensive care unit stay. This system does not seem to correlate well with evaluation of trauma patients but is used widely in the research arena to compare varied patient populations.

D. **The Systemic Inflammatory Response Syndrome Score (SIRS**, Table 5-3) is calculated using patient temperature, heart rate, respiratory rate, and white blood cell count. Hypothermia appears to be the most significant predictor of mortality.

E. **The Abbreviated Injury Score (AIS)** divides the body into six separate regions (head and neck, face, thorax, abdomen, bony pelvis and extremities, external structures) and assigns each a severity value (1 to 6, 1 being minor and 6 almost always fatal). The Injury Severity Score (ISS) is calculated as the sum of the squares of the three highest AIS scores (Table 5-4), and ranges from 1 to 75. Any victim with an AIS of 6 is automatically given an ISS of 75. The ISS correlates well with mortality but is limited in that it cannot account for multiple severe

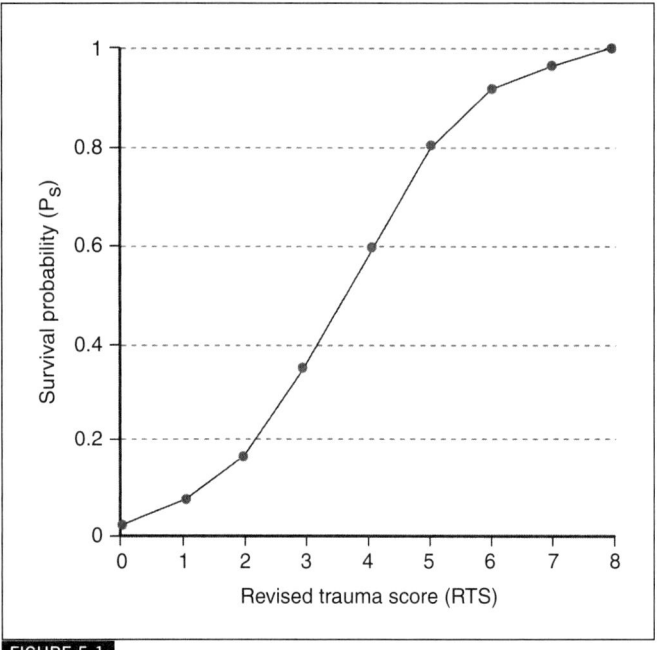

FIGURE 5-1
Survival probability (P_s) vs Revised Trauma Score. (From Champion H, Sacco W, Copes W: Trauma scoring. In Moore EE, Mattox KL, Feliciano DV [eds]: Trauma, 3rd ed. Stamford, CT, Appleton & Lange, 1996, pp 53-67.)

TABLE 5-3
SYSTEMIC INFLAMMATORY RESPONSE SYNDROME SCORE

Score Variable	Points
Fever or hypothermia	1
(temperature >38°C or <36°C)	
Tachycardia	1
(heart rate >90)	
Tachypnea	1
(respiratory rate >20, $Paco_2$ <32 mm Hg)	
Abnormal white blood cell count	1
(>12,000 mm^3 or <4,000 mm^3, or 10% bands)	
Maximum total SIRS score	4
** (SIRS is defined as ≥2)	

TABLE 5-4
EXAMPLE CALCULATION OF INJURY SEVERITY SCORE

Body Region	Injury	AIS Score	ISS
Abdomen	Ruptured spleen	2	
Chest	Fractured ribs	2	$2^2 + 2^2 + 3^2 = 17$
Extremity	Fractured femur	3	

injuries in a single region. Figures 5-2 and 5-3 demonstrate the use of ISS in comparing patients with both blunt and penetrating injuries.

F. The Pediatric Trauma Score (PTS) is a system for children and is similar to the RTS. It has six components: weight, airway, systolic blood pressure, central nervous system, open wound, and skeletal injury. Each component is given a score ranging from -1 to +2. Generally, patients with a PTS of less than 8 will benefit from transfer to a pediatric trauma center.

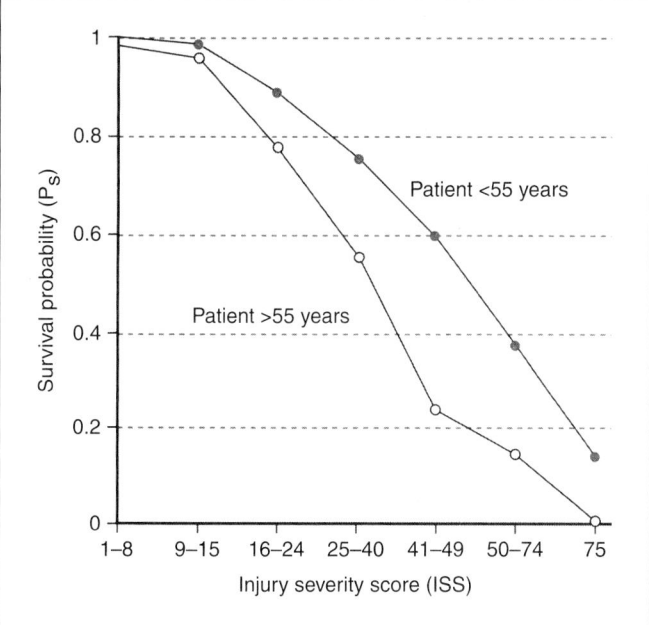

FIGURE 5-2

Survival probability vs Injury Severity Score in patients with blunt injuries. (From Champion H, Sacco W, Copes W: Trauma scoring. In Moore EE, Mattox KL, Feliciano DV [eds]: Trauma, 3rd ed. Stamford, CT, Appleton & Lange, 1996, pp 53-67.)

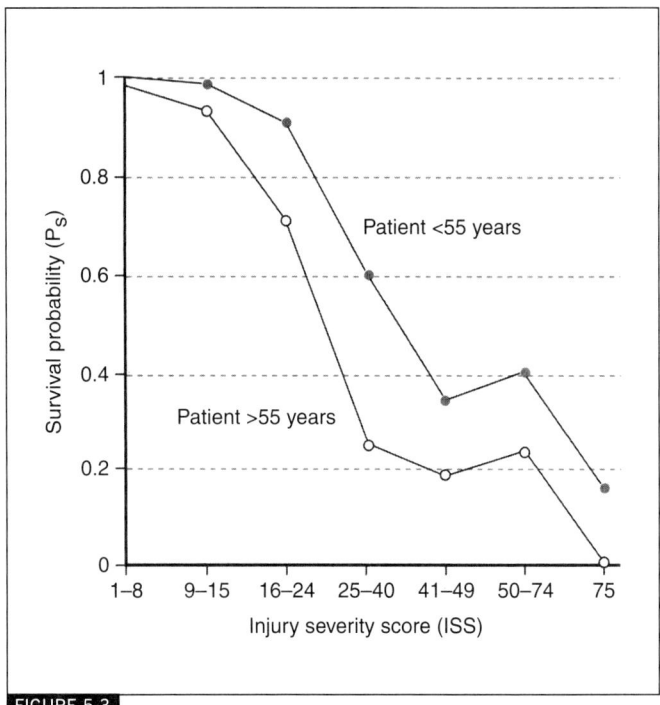

FIGURE 5-3

Survival probability vs Injury Severity Score in pateints with penetrating injuries. (From Champion H, Sacco W, Copes W: Trauma scoring. In Moore EE, Mattox KL, Feliciano DV [eds]: Trauma, 3rd ed. Stamford, CT, Appleton & Lange, 1996, pp 53-67.)

III. PERFORMANCE IMPROVEMENT AND TRAUMA REGISTRY

Data collection and frequent audit of prehospital and in-hospital care will ensure that trauma patient outcomes are comparable to national standards. Trauma registries provide an extremely useful tool in the hospital quality improvement program. Availability of this information will also allow evaluation of the impact of instituting injury prevention programs.

In keeping with the recommendations of the American College of Surgeons Committee on Trauma, the trauma services at Parkland Memorial Hospital are part of a national trauma registry. Certain audit filters identify those patients that require in-depth review. These include length of stay in the emergency department, time elapsing to obtain a head CT scan in patients with altered mental status, time to operation in hemodynamically unstable patients, time elapsed for consultant services to assess and treat patients, and so forth.

Audit filters will identify patients with a delay or error in diagnosis, error in judgment, error in technique, or inappropriate care. System problems and protocol procedures can also be monitored.

All deaths are classified as nonpreventable, possibly preventable, or preventable. This information can be used for trending of care and addressing special problems, and is essential for the survey committees when reviewing trauma systems and hospitals for initial or repeat credentialing. This registry activity is coordinated between the trauma medical director and the trauma nurse coordinator.

IV. SUGGESTED READINGS

Flint L, Richardson J: Organization for trauma care. In: Richardson J, Polk H, Flint L (eds): Trauma: Clinical Care and Pathophysiology. Chicago, Year Book, pp 8-9.

Maurer A, Morris A: Injury severity scoring. In: Moore E, Feliciano D, Mattox K (eds): Trauma, 5th ed. New York, McGraw-Hill, 2003, pp 87-90.

Mechanisms of Injury

James A. Chambers, MD, MPH & TM

I. GENERAL ASPECTS

A. *Trauma* is derived from the Greek word *tpauma* (wound), while *ballistics* comes from the Greek word βάλλο (to throw). Both terms thus imply a transfer of energy via particles (electromagnetic, gas, solid, etc.) from the environment to the patient (thermal, chemical, mechanical, etc.). This energy transfer results in anatomic and/or physiologic derangement.

B. The severity of the injury is influenced by a number of factors:
1. Type, intensity, and duration of exposure to the external energy source
   a. The results of trauma from multiple energy sources may be synergistic (e.g., blunt trauma and burn).
2. Physical properties of the involved tissue(s)
3. Age and comorbidities of the patient
4. Individual (phenotypic) variations in inflammatory response to physiologic insults
5. Length of time between injury and intervention

C. Mechanisms of injury are broadly categorized as blunt or penetrating.
1. Correct differentiation between the two catagories is significant in that the sequelae of each fall into different patterns of presentation and treatment. Frequently, however, components of both are simultaneously encountered in an injury.

II. PHYSICS OF BLUNT TRAUMA

A. Crushing (compressive strain): force applied to a fixed structure (or opposing forces pinning a structure between them). Such stress can deform tissue and disrupt viscera.

B. Shearing: opposite forces applied across different points of a structure.

C. Tensile: opposing forces pulling on (apart) the same structure

D. Commonly encountered mechanisms and pattern of injury
1. Motor vehicle collisions
   a. Fatality risk, from greatest to least, is as follows: front impact > side impact > rollover > rear impact (related to dispersion of energy).
      i. Fatality most strongly correlates with brain injury. This is most effectively prevented with car restraints (additive benefits of seat belts and airbags).
   b. Specific injuries and injury pattern:
      i. Front impact: head/neck injury from impact to window or shoulder restraint, chest injury from impact to steering column, feet/leg impact to floorboard/dash, posterior dislocation of hip
      ii. Side impact: Injuries to thorax and abdomen are most common with lateral impact collisions.

iii. Rollover: varied, random injury pattern
  iv. Rear impact: hyperextension of neck
  v. Ejection: mortality increases because the vehicle is not available to absorb energy. It is associated with higher ISS, central nervous system injury, and intensive care unit admission.
2. Motor-pedestrian collisions
   a. The injury pattern is related to the relative heights of the pedestrian and the vehicle bumper. Most frequently, the majority of force impacts around the knee, and usually there are lesser injuries to the head and the trunk and ribs unless the person is thrown on the vehicle's hood or windshield.
3. Falls:
   a. The severity of injury increases with the height of the fall and varies according to the position of the person at the time of impact as well as according to the landing surface. Orthopaedic injury, particularly spinal trauma, as well as shearing and compressive thoracoabdominal injuries should also be suspected in falls.
4. Pediatric trauma
   a. Children have proportionately larger heads and sustain brain and cervical spine injuries more oten than adults.
   b. Pediatric orthopaedic trauma differs due to the presence of physes and more compliant bones. Relatively more energy is required to induce fractures in children.
   c. Child abuse/neglect must always be suspected in cases with discordance between histories and with burns, multiple or spiral fractures, retinal hemorrhage, and internal organ damage without a significant mechanism by history.
5. Geriatric trauma
   a. Not only do the elderly frequently experience different types of trauma than younger patients (e.g., falls), but they also have a significantly higher mortality when corrected for trauma severity.

III. PENETRATING TRAUMA

A. Compared with blunt trauma, organ involvement by penetrating trauma is more a function of surface area or volume than inherent tissue characteristics or anatomic fixation. Hence, penetrating injuries to the abdomen most frequently involve the intestines rather than the spleen or liver.

B. Ballistics
1. There are four determining factors of missile damage:
   a. Mass
   b. Velocity of projectile
      i. As kinetic energy = mv^2, energy increases exponentially with velocity, but only linearly with mass.
   c. Construction of bullet
      i. Bullet construction: jacketed (required for civilian use), deformable (increases impact surface area), or hollow point (fragments upon impact)

d. Flight characteristics
      i. Yaw: deviation from longitudinal axis in flight path increases damage.
      ii. Tumbling: end-over-end rotation of projectile around its center of mass (effectively, undamped yaw) increases damage.
2. Composition of target
   a. Elasticity: ability of tissue to restore itself to initial shape/size after stress
      i. More elastic tissues (e.g., muscle, lung) tend to absorb less injury and thus sustain less damage than less elastic tissues (e.g., bone, solid organ parenchyma – kidney, spleen, liver). Additionally, denser tissues tend to absorb more energy and thus receive greater injury than less dense tissues.

B. Two characteristics of damage from penetrating missiles
1. **Permanent cavity**: direct compressive damage (determined by mass, deforming, yaw/tumbling, fragmenting). Impacted dense objects such as bone may shatter and become secondary projectiles, thus multiplying damage.
2. **Temporary cavity** (region of "stretch" induced by the shock wave of the passing projectile)
   a. Significant compression and shear can injure blood vessels, nerves, and even viscera without directly contacting the projectile. Intestinal perforation from non-intraperitoneal high-velocity gunshot wounds have been reported. High-velocity weapons (e.g., hunting or military rifles) produce significantly more cavitation effect than lower-velocity weapons (e.g., handguns, Uzis).
   b. It should be noted that some academic authorities have begun to incorporate aspects of the Red Cross classification of war wounds in approaching extremity civilian gunshot injuries in the United States. This places more emphasis on the appearance and features of the wound (skin wounds, the presence of a cavity or metallic foreign bodies, fracture, neurovascular injury, metallic) than on characteristics of the weapon used.

V. MISCELLANEOUS

A. Blast
1. Primary: stress along tissue planes of varying physical characteristics results in compressive and shearing strain. Strain leads to vascular injury, avulsion of organs, and perforation of membranes. Specific examples of pneumothorax, bowel rupture, and tympanic membrane perforation are commonly cited.
2. Secondary: injuries may result from objects in the environment that are accelerated by the blast and impact tissue.
3. Tertiary: refers to movement of the body by a blast force that results in crushing, laceration, and other such injuries.
4. Quarternary: covers injury from associated mechanisms at the time of injury (thermal damage, inhalation, etc.)

B. Nonlethal weapons

1. Multiple types of "nonlethal" or "less-than-lethal" weapons are being (and have been) developed for civilian law enforcement and military use in the United States and abroad. Authorized government users are trained to deploy these weapons under very specific circumstances with tactical limitations such as firing distance or no blows to head. Usage outside these parameters increases the potential for lethal injuries (depending on the weapon system).
2. Rubber bullets (and buckshot) have been developed for long rifle and handgun (and shotgun/grenade) fire.
3. Bean-bag projectiles may be fired from a shotgun and at approximately 20 feet impart momentum of 4 to 5 Newtons, comparable to a hand-thrown baseball at 30 feet. (Typical baton blows are 7 to 11 Newtons.)
4. TASER (conducted energy device); newer, advanced TASERs have evolved significantly from early "stun guns" of the 1970s, applying very high frequency (with high voltage, low current) electricity to stop combative behavior. Injury in healthy volunteers is rare, and published reviews of TASER-associated deaths almost uniformly report individuals who were using illicit drugs (particularly cocaine or PCP) and had generally been subjected to other physical trauma before arrest; several have had prior histories of cardiac disease. Causality has thus not been definitively linked to any patient death. However, patients may be brought to the emergency department for barb removal. Further, TASER use in pregnancy has been anecdotally linked to miscarriage.
5. In the United States, use of pepper (Capsaicin) spray is legal and the spray has also been packaged for "paintball gun" firing.

C. Burns

1. Thermal burns are frequently complicated by blunt trauma in industrial, home, or vehicle fires. Standard ATLS management of all burn victims is mandatory.
2. Electrical burns often create deceptively innocuous-appearing wounds with extensive deep damage. High-voltage electric injury can induce muscle spasms of sufficient magnitude to cause fractures (e.g., of spinal column).

D. Nuclear radiation

1. Alpha radiation is composed of two protons and two neutrons. Alpha energy cannot penetrate the stratum corneum and is injurious only to open wounds or to respiratory or intestinal epithelia when inhaled or ingested.
2. Beta radiation is composed of charged particles lighter than those for alpha. They can cause "beta burns" to the skin, but penetration is superficial. Again, ingestion or inhalation could lead to more significant injury.
3. Gamma radiation is able to penetrate deep tissues to involve the bone marrow and central nervous system, resulting in severe, potentially lethal syndromes from whole-body irradiation.

4. Neutron radiation, like gamma radiation, easily penetrates human tissue. Although uncharged (unlike gamma), neutron irradiation is more destructive, resulting from direct collision with nuclei.
5. Combined radiation energy: a nuclear detonation could result in injury from thermal pulse, direct blast overpressure, and damage from secondary projectiles in addition to radiation exposure (primary, secondary, tertiary, and quarternary blast injuries, as described above).

VI. SUGGESTED READINGS

Bleetman A, Steyn R, Lee C: Introduction of the TASER into British policing: Implications for UK emergency departments: An overview of electronic weaponry. Emerg Med J. 21(2):136-40, 2004.

Coupland RM: The Red Cross classification of war wounds: The E.X.C.F.V.M. scoring system. World J Surg. 16(5):910-917, 1992.

Galbraith KA: Combat casualties in the first decade of the 21st century – new and emerging weapon systems. JR Army Med Corps 147(1):7-14, 2001.

Gugala Z, Lindsey RW: Classification of gunshot injuries in civilians. Clin Orthop 408:65-81, 2003.

Helling TS, Watkins M, Evans LL, Nelson PW, et al: Low falls: An underappreciated mechanism of injury. J Trauma 46(3):453-456, 1999.

Kenny JM, Heal S, Grossman M (Pennsylvania State University Applied Research Laboratory): The Attribute-Based Evaluation (ABE) of less-than-lethal, extended-range, impact munitions. State College, PA, Pennsylvania State University, 2001.

Lewer N, Davison N: Non-lethal technologies – an overview. Disarmament Forum 1:37-51, 2005.

Mahajna A, Aboud N, Harbaji I, et al: Blunt and penetrating injuries caused by rubber bullets during the Israeli-Arab conflict in October, 2000: A retrospective study. Lancet 359(9320):1795-1800, 2002.

Moore EE, Feliciano DV, Mattox KL: Trauma, 5th ed.. New York, McGraw-Hill, 2003.

Orange County Sherriff's Office: Taser Task Force Medical Findings. Orange County, FL, Orange County Sherriff's Office, 2004.

Ricks RC, Berger ME, O'Hara FM: The Medical Basis for Radiation Accident Preparedness: The Clinical Care of Victims. Philadelphia, Taylor & Francis, 2002.

Santaniello JM, Luchette FA, Esposito TJ, et al: Ten year experience of burn, trauma, and combined burn/trauma injuries comparing outcomes. J Trauma 57(4):696-701, 2004.

Sharma OP, Oswanski MF, White PW: Injuries to the colon from blast effect of penetrating extra-peritoneal thoracoabdominal trauma. Injury 35(3):320-324, 2004.

Tuggle DW: Blast injury. J Okla State Med Assoc 96(9):419-421, 2003.

US Department of Defense Air Sea Land Application Center: Multiservice Procedures for the Tactical Employment of Nonlethal Weapons. (FM 90-40, MCRP 3-15.8, NWP 3-07.31, USCG PUB 3-07.31), Oct 1998.

US Department of Defense, Military Medical Operations Office, Armed Forces Radiobiologic Institute: Medical Management of Radiological Casualties Handbook. Bethesda, US Department of Defense, 1999.

All-Hazards Disaster Preparedness and Mitigation

Alexander L. Eastman, MD

I. DISASTER MANAGEMENT

A. Contending with disasters maximally stresses the resources and capabilities of a trauma system. Guidelines in Resources for Optimal Care of the Injured Patient, developed by the American College of Surgeons Committee on Trauma, provide basic recommendations for disaster management planning.
B. Incident Command Systems (ICS): Hospital Emergency Incident Command Systems (HEICS) must be exercised and used.
C. Allowing personnel to perform their regular duties, albeit under different and potentially austere conditions, provides for best outcomes.

II. HOSPITAL DISASTER COMMITTEE

Hospitals should designate a disaster committee composed of representatives of all hospital departments. This disaster committee serves the following functions:
1. Planning and innovation regarding disaster preparedness
2. Coordination during disaster conditions
3. Advocacy for hospital-based disaster programs
4. Providing education to hospital staff regarding planning and preparedness efforts

III. DISASTER PLANS

The disaster plans should reflect the potential disasters for the region and differentiate between multiple and mass casualties with graded responses. These plans should also integrate local or regional disaster agencies to ensure a coordinated response. Lastly, the plan should reflect realistic response and care capabilities of the institution.

IV. INVENTORY OF AVAILABLE AND DESIRED SUPPLIES

The inventory of available and desired supplies, including blood bank products, should be determined and arrangements with the Red Cross or other blood banks should be well established.

V. HOSPITAL SPACE CONSIDERATIONS

Space for response activities should be designated within the hospital and should include areas for triage, critical stabilization, hazardous chemical or radioactive material decontamination, nonsalvageable patients, operations and minor procedures, and a morgue. Specified space should also be reserved for an administrative control center, a communications headquarters, and a counseling area.

VI. THE DISASTER PROTOCOL

The disaster protocol should assign all personnel, preferably working in teams of physicians, nurses, and administrators, with specific duties and work areas. The personnel also should include a hospital disaster commander and a triage physician who is an experienced trauma surgeon. A specified disaster site team should be available if field triage and treatment are requested. Finally, personnel requirements include security staff and a public relations person.

VII. DISASTER PLAN ENACTMENT

Disaster plan enactment should ideally be practiced twice annually at a minimum, followed by critical evaluation of system performance.

VIII. REVIEW OF THE DISASTER PLAN

The disaster plan and accompanying supporting information (telephone and contact numbers) should be reviewed on a quarterly basis to ensure that all information is current and accurate.

IX. SUGGESTED READING

Eastman AL, Rinnert KJ, Nameth IR, Fowler RL, Minei JP: Alternate site surge capacity in times of public health disaster maintains trauma center and emergency department integrity: Hurricane Katrina. J Trauma 63: 253–257, 2007.

Initial Assessment of the Trauma Patient

Severn Barloco, MD, and Hemangini Thakar, MD

The goal of the initial assessment of the trauma patient is to avoid preventable deaths by rapidly identifying and treating potentially life-threatening injuries. The primary and secondary surveys proceed according to Advanced Trauma Life Support protocol. Strict adherence to these algorithms minimizes the incidence of missed life-threatening injuries.

I. PRIMARY SURVEY–ABCs OF TRAUMA CARE

The primary survey takes place simultaneously with any emergent resuscitation of the patient. Reevaluation of the patient is continuous, and the primary survey may be repeated several times during the initial assessment. The primary survey includes the following components:

A. Airway/cervical spine
1. Airway compromise is rapidly fatal, and thus assessment of the airway is given the highest priority.
2. Management objectives are to maintain the intact airway or to establish an airway if it is not patent or is questionable.
   a. NOTE: Asking the patient questions on arrival to the emergency department is an easy way to ensure airway patency.
3. Look for chest wall expansion, and listen/feel for air movement at the patient's nose and mouth.
4. The patient's mouth should be opened and examined to make sure that a foreign body or a flaccid tongue has not acutely occluded the airway. The chin lift or jaw thrust maneuvers may help facilitate ventilation in an obtunded patient; an oral or nasal airway may also be useful.
5. In all trauma patients, the cervical spine demands careful attention. The cervical spine should be stabilized until it is proven to be normal, either by radiologic studies or by examination of an awake and oriented patient with a normal physical examination (e.g., nontender to palpation). Stabilization of the spine is usually best accomplished with a cervical collar.
6. **Basic airway maneuvers:**
   a. Supplemental oxygen (Fio_2 >0.85) via non-rebreather mask or nasal cannula
   b. Chin lift and jaw thrust
   c. Suction to remove secretions
   d. Nasopharyngeal or orophayngeal airway
7. Advanced airway maneuvers:
   a. Rapid-sequence intubation (RSI). This is the preferred method for intubation of trauma patients who are not comatose. RSI seeks

to prevent aspiration during emergency intubation. There are four steps:
  i. Preoxygenation—100% oxygen is administered to an adult for a minimum of 8 vital capacity breaths. This is usually performed while equipment is being prepared. The Sellick maneuver (cricothyroid pressure) is started during this phase and continued until successful endotracheal intubation has been confirmed.
  ii. Pretreatment—during this phase, medications are administered to the patient to attenuate the effects of intubation. Fentanyl (3-5 μg/kg) can reduce sympathetic response especially in patients with concomitant head injury. Lidocaine (1.5 mg/kg) is used to counteract bronchospasm and increased intracranial pressures. Atropine is always used in children (0.02 mg/kg) to prevent bradycardia and asystole in children under the age of 10 years. Indications for using pretreatment medications are relative, and this stage can be skipped in urgent cases. Three minutes should be allowed to elapse before induction.
  iii. Sedation/paralysis—during this stage, a powerful sedative is administered followed immediatedly by a paralytic. At Parkland Memorial Hospital, the preferred agent is etomidate (0.2-0.4 mg/kg IV). This is followed by succinylcholine (1.5 mg/kg IV) unless contraindicated secondary to a potentially hyperkalemic state. In the case of the latter, vecuronium (0.1 mg/kg IV) can be used.
  iv. Endotracheal intubation—the largest tube possible is used (this facilitates later care and weaning in the intensive care unit).
 b. Supraglottic intubation
 c. Surgical airway (cricothyroidotomy, tracheostomy)
8. Four groups of patients generally require advanced maneuvers:
 a. Apnea
 b. Upper airway obstruction unable to be corrected with simple airway maneuvers (see above, 6a-d).
 c. Altered mental status—Glasgow Coma Score (GCS) <9
 d. Respiratory distress—e.g., stridor or respiratory rate >40
9. Orotracheal intubation. When performed with in-line cervical spine stabilization it is our preferred method of obtaining a definitive airway. Preoxygenation to maintain oxygen saturation close to 100% is required prior to intubation by any method.
 a. Nasotracheal intubation is an alternative that requires that the patient be spontaneously breathing and is only attempted if there are no suspected basilar skull or cervical spine fractures. (It is used infrequently at Parkland Memorial Hospital.)
  i. A small tube is introduced at a right angle to the face into a naris after local anesthetic is applied to the nasopharynx. It is then advanced until maximal breath sounds are appreciated, approximately 14 to 16 cm in an adult. At this point, the tip is just above the glottis and the tube is further advanced during inspiration.

I. Primary Survey–ABCs of Trauma Care

   ii. Placement is then confirmed with capnography and auscultation. If the trachea has not been entered and the tube is anterior in position, the tube is then retracted and advanced with the head in a flexed position. If it is lateral, the tube is retracted and rotated, then advanced.
   iii. It is our practice to change the nasotracheal tube to a larger oropharyngeal tube when the patient has been stabilized.
10. Supraglottic intubation. The combitube (Sheridan catheter, Argyle, NY) is becoming more common as an adjunct to difficult airways performed in the prehospital environment. It is a supraglottic airway device designed to be placed blindly. The tube has two lumens and two balloons that are used to protect the airway (see Figure 8-1). It is contraindicated in individuals shorter than 5 feet and those with an intact gag reflex, esophageal disease or a known caustic ingestion. At Parkland Memorial Hospital, we change these tubes to an oral endotracheal tube once the patient is stable upon presentation to the emergency department.
11. Cricothyroidotomy. The most difficult aspect of a cricothyroidotomy is identifying and maintaining the surgical landmarks. The following technique reduces that difficulty.
    a. The surgeon first identifies the cricothyroid membrane (Fig. 8-2) and immobilizes it between the thumb and middle finger of his or her non-dominant hand with the index finger placed on the thyroid notch (Fig. 8-3).
    b. Throughout the procedure the surgeon never moves this hand; thus the cricothyroid membrane is always localized.
    c. An incision is made down to the cricothyroid membrane using a scalpel with the dominant hand (Fig. 8-4). The blade is swept in an upward motion away from the practitioner as it is removed, making a transverse incision through the cricothyroid membrane. The blade can then be introduced back into the wound and the incision extended a short distance towards the practitioner. The focus of the procedure is to rapidly secure an airway for the patient; thus, hemostasis is a secondary concern.
    d. The cricothyroid membrane can then be opened further by placing the scalpel handle through the membrane and turning the scalpel 90 degrees. A 6-0 endotracheal tube or a No. 4 or No. 6 tracheostomy tube is then inserted (Fig. 8-5).
    e. Alternatively, a vertical incision in the neck can be made and carried down to the cricothyroid membrane. Either method (transverse neck incision or vertical neck incision) is acceptable.
12. Needle cricothyroidotomy
    a. Needle cricothyroidotomy is performed by placing a large IV cannula in the trachea and connecting it to oxygen.
    b. A Y connector makes the exhalation step easier.
    c. The patient is then ventilated for 1 second and allowed to exhale for 4 seconds.
    d. Hypercarbia limits this technique to 30 to 45 minutes of ventilation.

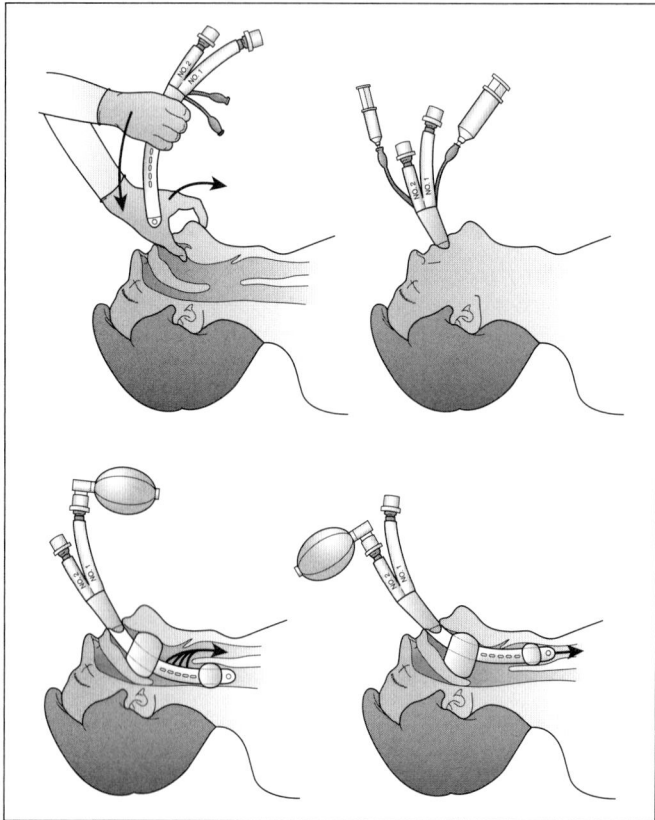

FIGURE 8-1

Combitube insertion. *(Adapted from Miller RD (ed): Anesthesia, 6th ed. Philadelphia, Saunders, 2005).*

    e. Surgical cricothyroidotomy is contraindicated in children younger than 13 years. Needle cricothyroidotomy may be the only option available until a formal tracheostomy can be performed.

    f. A needle cricothyroidotomy can be performed in the emergency department until a definitive airway can be obtained.

B. Breathing

1. Look for chest movement and listen to breath sounds.
2. If breath sounds are unequal, assessment of the tracheal position will determine if there is mediastinal shift, which may indicate the presence of tension pneumothorax or massive hemothorax.
3. These should be treated immediately by chest tube placement prior to proceeding with the remainder of the evaluation. In the case of tension

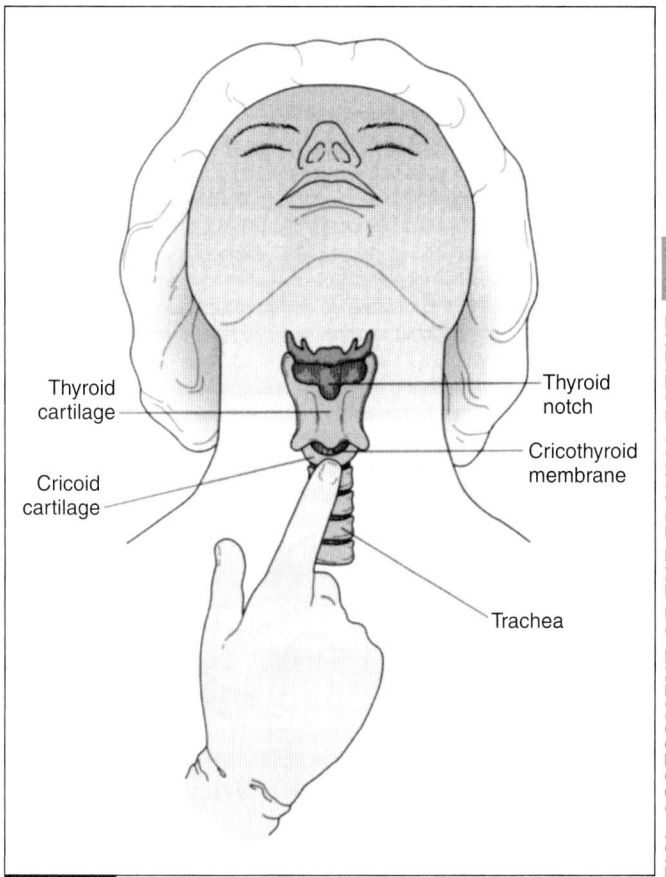

FIGURE 8-2

Surgical cricothyroidotomy.

pneumothorax, needle decompression prior to chest tube placement can be a temporizing, life-saving measure.

C. Circulation

1. Assessment of circulation begins by observing the patient's skin color and feeling the temperature of the skin.
2. Cool, clammy skin, pallor, and weak pulses are indicative of hypovolemic shock. In contrast, warm and dry extremities are characteristic of spinal shock.
3. Evaluation should also include listening for heart sounds, palpation of peripheral pulses, and blood pressure measurement.

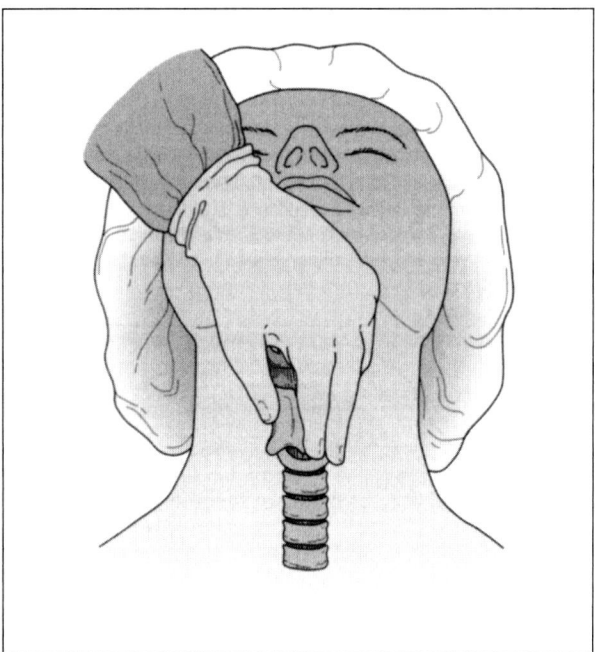

FIGURE 8-3

See text.

4. Management of circulatory deficits is begun by immediate vascular access with large-bore (14- or 16-gauge, if possible) intravenous catheters and administration of 2 liters of crystalloid solution (see Chapter 9).
5. At Parkland Memorial Hospital, we do not routinely obtain central venous access as initial first choice except in patients in whom upper extremity access is not possible or in patients with massive intra-abdominal hemorrhage.

D. Disability

1. A brief, focused neurologic examination will rapidly evaluate for the presence of significant intracranial injuries that may require operation.
2. The Glasgow Coma Score (GCS) is obtained; patients with a GCS of 8 or less are intubated to protect the airway.
3. In addition we perform a rapid examination of the pupils and document gross motor function in all extremities.

E. Exposure

1. The incidence of late diagnosis of significant injuries in the trauma patient can be minimized by exposure and by a careful examination of the patient's body.

I. Primary Survey—ABCs of Trauma Care

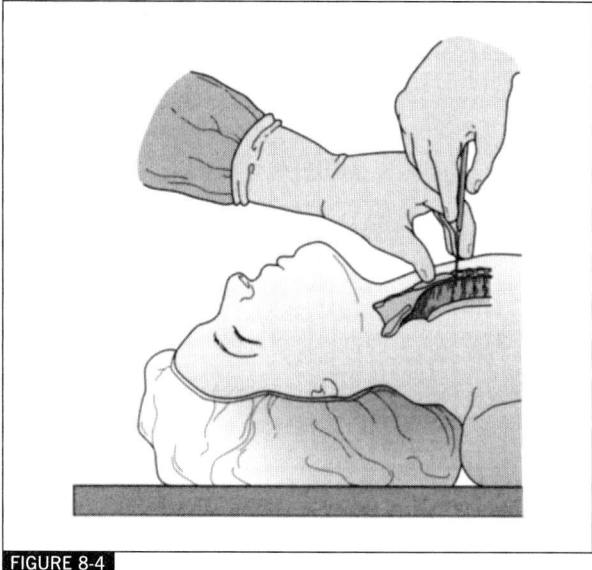

FIGURE 8-4
See text.

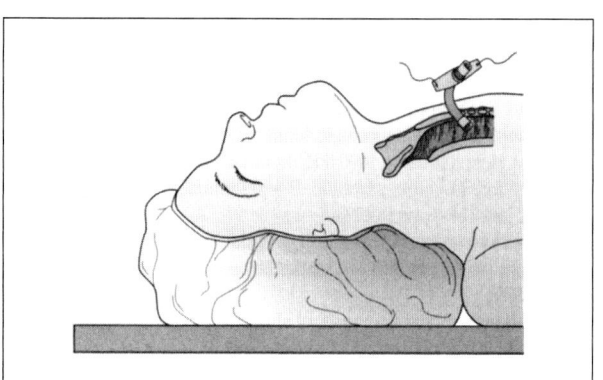

FIGURE 8-5
See text.

2. All of the patient's clothes are removed, the patient is log-rolled, the back is assessed, a rectal examination is performed, and the backboard is removed during this step.
3. We have identified hair-bearing areas such as the axillae, perineum, and head as high risk for missed penetrating injuries.
4. Avoiding hypothermia is a concurrent goal, especially in burn patients, since they do not possess normal skin homeostasis.
5. Warming is initially achieved using warm blankets or warm air devices.
6. All trauma resuscitation rooms at Parkland Memorial Hospital are kept at 75°F or warmer.

F. Other aspects of initial assessment
1. Intravenous fluid resuscitation followed by blood transfusion if indicated
2. Insertion of a nasogastric tube
3. Foley catheter–urine dipstick analysis
4. HemoCue – obtained for each patient on arrival; in patients without urgent indication for surgery (e.g., hemodynamically normal patients), HemoCue readings are obtained at 10 and 20 minutes after arrival while intravenous fluid resuscitation is ongoing.

II. SECONDARY SURVEY

A. The secondary survey, or complete history and physical examination of the injured patient, does not begin until the primary survey has been completed and the resuscitation phase has begun.
1. A minority of patients will continue to remain unstable after resuscitation and will require emergent operative intervention to control hemorrhage or to evacuate lesions that are creating a mass effect within the cranial vault.
2. The majority of patients, however, are hemodynamically normal.
3. These patients undergo a complete history and thorough head-to-toe physical examination.
4. The secondary survey includes special procedures such as x-rays, laboratory tests, ultrasound studies, CT scans, and peritoneal lavage. Chest, pelvic, and cervical spine radiographs take precedence over other studies.
5. A nasogastric tube should be inserted, if not contraindicated, prior to obtaining a chest x-ray.
6. During the secondary survey, the "ABCs" should be constantly reassessed and interventions made as indicated.

B. History and mechanism of injury
1. Obtain pertinent past medical history.
2. AMPLE: A = allergies, M = medications, P = past illnesses, L = last meal, E = events of injury.
3. Ask the emergency medical technicians for historical events.

C. Vital signs
1. Narrow pulse pressure and tachycardia are the earliest signs of hypovolemia.

2. Pulse: orthostatic changes, tachycardia, and arrhythmias are monitored.
3. Hypotension is a late sign of hypovolemia.
4. Respiration: look for apnea or tachypnea.
5. Temperature: look for hypothermia or hyperthermia.

D. Head
1. Skull: Inspect and palpate for skull fractures and perform repeated neurologic examination.
2. Eyes: Check pupillary size and for conjunctival or fundal hemorrhages, lens dislocation, hyphema, contact lenses, raccoon sign, globe entrapment, and nystagmus. A quick visual check can be done by asking the patient to read the print on the side of an intravenous bag with each eye.
3. Ears: Check for hemotympanum, perforation, cerebrospinal fluid (CSF) leak, and Battle's sign.
4. Nose: Check for cerebrospinal fluid leak, septal deviation, septal hematoma, fracture.
5. Mouth: Check for aspiration, hemorrhage, laceration, dental injuries, and foreign bodies.

E. Maxillofacial
1. Maxillofacial trauma is associated with two life-threatening conditions: airway obstruction and hemorrhage.
2. Patients with midface fractures may also have fractures of the cribriform plate, and should have gastric intubation performed by the oral route only (e.g., orogastric tube).

F. Cervical spine and neck
1. Principles
   a. All patients with maxillofacial trauma caused by blunt force should be presumed to have a cervical spine injury.
   b. The neck must be protected until a fracture can be excluded, either by non-tender examination of an alert, oriented, nonintoxicated patient or by radiographic evaluation (plain films, computed tomography [CT], magnetic resonance imaging [MRI]) of the obtunded patient.
   c. Following manual stabilization of the neck, however, the cervical collar should be unfastened temporarily to allow adequate examination of the neck. The absence of a neurologic deficit or pain does not rule out injury to the cervical spine.
2. Assessment
   a. Inspection for jugular venous distention, tracheal deviation, hemorrhage, penetrating wounds, and hematoma
   b. Palpation for deformity, fracture, crepitance, masses, and thrill
   c. Auscultation for stridor and bruit
3. Diagnostic radiography
   a. Adequate cervical spine radiograph (on which you must see the C7-T1 junction) or CT scan. CT scan is preferred at Parkland Memorial Hospital.
4. Management
   a. Adequate immobilization of the cervical spine must be maintained until the definitive treatment of any injuries.

G. Chest
1. Assessment
   a. Look for symmetrical excursions, deformity, flail chest, retraction, penetrating wound, sucking chest wound, contusions, and hematomas.
   b. Listen high on the anterior chest for pneumothorax; listen low on the posterior chest for hemothorax, decreased breath sounds, and distant heart tones. Breath sounds are often best heard in the axillae.
   c. Feel each rib and both clavicles individually for crepitus or fracture.
2. Therapeutic and diagnostic techniques
   a. Chest radiograph
   b. Pleural decompression (chest tube thoracostomy)
   c. Needle thoracentesis
   d. Pericardiocentesis (rarely used)
   e. Focused abdominal sonography for trauma (FAST) evaluation of tamponade

H. Breast
1. Breast examination is performed on all patients as part of the secondary survey.
2. The axillary tail of Spence is avoided during tube thoracostomy.

I. Abdomen
1. Principles
   a. The abdomen can present a diagnostic challenge for even the most experienced clinician.
   b. Distention is a late sign. A 1-cm change in abdominal girth may account for as much as 3 L of blood loss.
   c. Initial examination and frequent reevaluation are paramount to the management of abdominal trauma.
2. Assessment
   a. Look for penetrating wound, hemorrhage, hematoma, contusion, and distention.
   b. Listen for bowel sounds and bruits.
   c. Feel for tenderness, rebound, crepitus, masses, and thrill.
3. Diagnostic Studies
   a. FAST
      i. Its utility lies in its ability to detect fluid (e.g., blood) in the pericardium or abdomen with high sensitivity.
      ii. FAST is most sensitive in patients with precordial/transthoracic wounds and in hypotensive patients with blunt abdominal trauma.
      iii. Its ability to diagnose solid organ injury or to assess retroperitoneal structures is limited.
      iv. Lower rib fractures, subcutaneous air, and patient body habitus may interfere with examination.
   b. Peritoneal lavage:
      i. Must be considered in patients with altered sensorium from trauma, alcohol, or drugs

ii. Should be considered for patients undergoing anesthesia for other procedures (orthopaedic or neurosurgical), because the abdominal examination is unreliable
iii. Indicated in hemodynamically abnormal patients with a negative FAST
   c. Local wound exploration for stab wounds to anterior abdominal wall
   d. CT scan with IV but no oral contrast
   e. Exploratory laparotomy, if indicated

J. Rectum and perineum
1. Principles
   a. Examination performed in all patients
   b. Is usually performed during primary survey while patient is log-rolled to minimize patient movement
2. Assessment
   a. Anal sphincter tone
   b. Rectal blood
   c. Bowel wall integrity
   d. Prostate position
   e. Blood at the urinary meatus
   f. Scrotal or perineal hematoma
   g. Vaginal wall integrity
3. Management
   a. Foley catheter, if there is no blood at meatus, no high-riding prostate gland, and no scrotal or perineal hematoma.
   b. If any of these are present, a retrograde urethrogram is obtained prior to inserting the catheter.

K. Back (generally performed at end of primary survey)
1. Palpate each spinous process for bony deformity.
2. Look for evidence of blunt or penetrating trauma.

L. Extremities and fractures
1. Assessment
   a. Inspection for deformities, expanding hematoma, and open wound
   b. Palpation for tenderness, crepitus, abnormal movement, fracture, and pulses
2. Management
   a. Use of splints (traction splints if indicated)
   b. Tetanus prophylaxis as indicated
   c. Pain relief, as appropriate (usually IV morphine in 2-mg increments)

M. Neurologic
1. Assessment
   a. Reassess Glasgow Coma Score.
   b. Sensory and motor evaluation
   c. Paralysis or paresis
2. Management
   a. Adequate immobilization of the entire patient
   b. Neurosurgical consultation, if indicated

N. Vascular
1. Assessment
   a. Palpate or evaluate by Doppler ultrasound all extremity pulses; however, the presence of a pulse does not rule out an arterial injury.
   b. Record details of vascular examination.
   c. Capillary refill
   d. Signs of a vascular injury
      i. Bleeding
      ii. Expanding hematoma
      iii. Bruit or thrill
      iv. Abnormal pulse examination
      v. Impaired distal circulation
   e. Evaluate for compartment syndrome.
      i. Decreased sensation
      ii. Increasing pain
   f. Continued reevaluation
2. Management
   a. Measurement of extremity pressure indices
   b. Angiogram if arterial injury is suspected in hemodynamically normal patient
   c. Fasciotomies, if indicated
   d. Amputation, if indicated
   e. Photographic evidence and a documented second opinion are usually helpful.

O. Summary
1. Primary survey
   a. Airway
   b. Breathing
   c. Circulation
   d. Disability
   e. Environmental/exposure
   f. Simultaneous resuscitation and stabilization
2. Secondary survey
   a. Complete history and physical examination
3. Adjunctive studies
4. Prioritize management.
5. Reassess and reprioritize.

III. SUGGESTED READINGS

American College of Surgeons Committee on Trauma: Advanced Trauma Life Support for Doctors. Chicago, IL, American College of Surgeons, 1997.

American College of Surgeons: Ultrasound in the Acute Setting. Chicago, IL, American College of Surgeons, 2004.

Dutton RP, McCunn M: Anesthesia for trauma. In Miller RD (ed): Anesthesia, 6th ed. Philadelphia, Saunders, 2005, pp 2451-2496.

Parks SN: Initial assessment. In Moore EE, Feliciano DV, Mattox KL (eds): Trauma, 5th ed. New York, McGraw-Hill, 2003, pp 445-458.

Shock

Hema Thakar, MD, and Jennifer Blumetti, MD

I. DEFINITION

Shock is defined as the clinical state characterized by inadequate tissue perfusion. Untreated, hypoperfusion leads to organ failure and patient death. The ability to recognize and treat shock and its underlying causes is essential in trauma care (Table 9-1).

II. INITIAL ASSESMENT

Following the establishment of an adequate airway and ventilation, the circulatory system is evaluated. Vital signs and physical examination, combined with a simultaneously obtained pertinent history, are essential in the diagnosis and treatment of shock.

III. INITIAL TREATMENT

A. Vascular access
1. Peripheral intravenous access should be obtained with two large-bore IV catheters (16-gauge or larger). Our first choice of access site is in the antecubital fossae bilaterally.
2. In the hypotensive intensive care unit patient, our practice includes the placement of central venous access catheters in the subclavian vein. Previously, saphenous vein cutdowns were more commonly used if upper extremity peripheral access was unobtainable, and this is still a useful technique. For procedure protocols, refer to Chapter 13, Catheters and Tubes.
3. Large-bore, short catheters provide the means for the most rapid instillation of intravenous fluids. For this reason, standard double- or triple-lumen central venous catheters are not used in resuscitation. Vein size has no clinical effect on the rate of fluid administration.
4. Rapid infusers such as a "Level One" allow the administration of up to 1 L of warmed fluid per minute.

B. Fluid challenge
1. Initial fluid resuscitation begins with a bolus infusion of 2 L of lactated Ringer's solution. Lactated Ringer's solution is typically used because it is a balanced salt solution. Patients who have ceased bleeding tend to respond to the fluid challenge, but patients who respond transiently may have ongoing blood loss.

C. Transfusion
1. Blood is obtained for type and crossmatching during insertion of the catheters. However, the patient in shock may require the immediate transfusion of unmatched blood products.

TABLE 9-1
CHARACTERISTICS OF SHOCK STATES

Physiologic sign	Hypovolemic	Cardiogenic Myocardial	Cardiogenic Mechanical	Neurogenic	Septic
Pulse	+	+	+	nl or −	+
Blood pressure	−	− to nl	−	−	−
Respiratory rate	+	+	++	nl/+	++
Urine output	−	−	−	−	−
Neck veins	Flat	Distended	Distended	Flat	Flat
Skin temperature	Cold	Cold	Cold	Warm	Warm
Skin sensation	Clammy	Clammy	Clammy	Dry	Moist/dry
Cardiac index	+/−	−	−	+/−	++
Central venous pressure	−	+	++	−	nl/+
Pulmonary capillary wedge pressure	−	++	+	−	−/nl
Systemic vascular resistance	++	++	++	−	−
Response to volume	+++	−	+	+	+

− = decreased; + = Increased; nl = normal

2. In hemorrhagic shock, blood is administered after the 2-L fluid challenge. Care is taken not to overload the patients with crystalloid.

IV. TYPES OF SHOCK

Classification of the types of shock allows better understanding of the pathophysiology and treatment of inadequate tissue perfusion.

A. Hypovolemic (hemorrhagic) shock
1. **Definition**. Hypovolemic (hemorrhagic) shock is the result of acute blood loss or the loss of plasma and extracellular fluid with a reduction in the circulating intravascular volume. This is the most common form of shock in the trauma patient.
2. **Pathophysiology**
   a. Compensatory mechanisms for acute intravascular volume loss include sympathetic and adrenal responses. Sympathetic response results in increased heart rate and peripheral vascular resistance to maintain cardiac output.
   b. Vasoconstriction results in a redistribution of blood flow to the heart and brain. Simultaneous venoconstriction prevents blood from pooling in the venous capacitance vessels.
   c. As the volume deficit grows, the pulse pressure narrows with a rise in diastolic pressure secondary to sympathetic discharge. Continued hemorrhage leads to a fall in systolic pressure and progressive hypotension as compensatory mechanisms are overwhelmed.

d. As perfusion decreases, cells shift from aerobic to anaerobic metabolism. This results in an increase in lactic acid production and a fall in pH.
e. Altered cell membrane permeability and the inability to maintain electrolyte gradients lead to sodium and water shifts into the cell, with further depletion of the extracellular fluid volume. Without correction of shock, these water shifts lead to cellular swelling and subsequently cell death.

3. **Classification of hemorrhagic shock**. Advanced Trauma Life Support (ATLS) guidelines describe four classes of hemorrhage based on percentage of acute blood volume loss (Table 9-2). Hemorrhagic shock is classified as follows:
   a. Class I hemorrhage: loss of up to 15% of blood volume
   b. Class II hemorrhage: 15% to 30% blood loss, approximately 800 to 1500 mL of blood in a 70-kg patient
   c. Class III hemorrhage: 30% to 40% blood loss, approximately 2,000 mL
   d. Class IV hemorrhage: greater than 40% blood loss

4. **Treatment of hemorrhagic shock**
   a. Primary treatment is aimed at correcting and stopping the underlying cause of hemorrhage. Control of external hemorrhage is accomplished by direct digital pressure.
   b. Resuscitation is begun with 1 to 2 L of lactated Ringer's solution.
      i. Crystalloid fluid resuscitation reduces the necessity for blood transfusion in many patients with mild to moderate shock.
      ii. Patients with ongoing hemorrhage may initially respond to a fluid bolus but will subsequently deteriorate unless the source of hemorrhage is controlled.

TABLE 9-2
HEMORRHAGIC SHOCK[a]

Physiologic sign	Class 1	Class II	Class III	Class IV
Blood loss (% blood volume)	>15	15–30	30–40	≥40
Pulse rate (b.p.m.)	<100	>100	>120	>140
Blood pressure	Normal	Normal	Decreased	Decreased
Pulse pressure (diastolic)	Normal	Narrowed	Narrowed	Very narrow or absent
Capillary refill	Normal	Delayed	Delayed	Delayed
Skin	Normal	Cool, pale	Cool, pale	Cold, ashen with mottling
Respiratory rate	14–20	20–30	30–40	>35
Urine output (mL/h)	>30	20–30	5–15	Negligible
Mental status	Slightly anxious	Mildly anxious, thirsty	Anxious and confused, or apathetic	Lethargy progressing to coma

[a] Modified from American College of Surgeons. *Advanced Trauma Life Support Program*, Chicago; 1988:72.

iii. Trauma patients with hemorrhagic shock and continued signs of hypoperfusion require packed red blood cell replacement. When crossmatched or type-specific blood is not available, universal donor type O, Rh-negative blood is administered.
iv. Hypertonic saline solutions and colloid volume expanders (albumin, dextran, hydroxyethyl starch) are not used at Parkland Memorial Hospital in the initial resuscitation of trauma patients.
v. Failure to respond to adequate crystalloid and blood administration indicates the need for immediate surgical intervention to control exsanguination. Alternative causes of shock (cardiogenic, obstructive, or distributive) must be considered.
vi. Thoracic aortic cross-clamping is not advocated. If a patient decompensates in the operating room, rapid celiotomy and intra-abdominal control of the aorta at the diaphragm are accomplished.
vii. Vasopressors are not used in initial resuscitation.

5. **End-points of resuscitation**
   a. Frequent reevaluation of the patient during the resuscitation period is necessary to determine the adequacy of treatment.
   b. Adequate volume resuscitation is measured by the following parameters:
      i. Heart rate
      ii. Pulse pressure
      iii. Blood pressure
      iv. Level of mentation
      v. Skin perfusion
      vi. Urine output
   c. Base deficit and serum lactate are sensitive indicators of the degree of anaerobic metabolism during shock and volume deficit. A persistent or worsening base deficit signals ongoing hemorrhage and should prompt continuous resuscitation. Lactate can be used similarly.
   d. In difficult resuscitations, hemodynamic monitoring with a central venous pressure or pulmonary artery catheter may assist in following volume status and managing superimposed cardiac dysfunction or septic shock.

B. Cardiogenic shock
1. **Definition**. Cardiogenic shock is a manifestation of failure of the heart as a pump secondary to myocardial dysfunction, arrhythmias, or structural factors. History, physical examination, selective hemodynamic monitoring, diagnostic tests, and a high index of clinical suspicion all play a vital role in determining the cause of cardiogenic shock.
2. **Pathophysiology**
   a. Myocardial damage may occur following rapid deceleration injury to the thorax.
   b. Myocardial infarction may occur, especially in the elderly population with atherosclerosis.

c. Depressed myocardial function results in increased heart rate and cardiac contractility from catecholamine release in an effort to maintain cardiac output. Increased peripheral vasoconstriction helps to maintain blood pressure as well.
   d. Without intervention, the resultant increase in oxygen demand and decrease in diastolic filling will lead to worsening myocardial ischemia.
3. **Treatment**
   a. Patients must be adequately volume resuscitated prior to initiation of inotropic support.
   b. A central venous pressure or pulmonary artery catheter is used to monitor and guide resuscitation in these patients.
   c. Constant electrocardiographic monitoring is necessary to detect dysrhythmias accompanying myocardial contusion or infarction, which must be treated promptly.

C. Obstructive shock

1. **Definition**. Obstructive shock occurs when blood flow to the heart is obstructed. Mechanical obstruction of cardiac output following trauma most frequently results from cardiac tamponade or tension pneumothorax.
2. **Pathophysiology**
   a. Obstruction leads to inadequate diastolic filling or systolic dysfunction due to increased afterload.
   b. Cardiac tamponade causes impaired diastolic filling secondary to increased pericardial pressure.
      i. It is characterized by hypotension, muffled heart tones, narrow pulse pressure, and distended neck veins, accompanied by tachycardia, a paradoxical pulse, and central cyanosis.
      ii. It occurs most commonly following penetrating thoracic trauma, although it is occasionally encountered in a patient with blunt chest injuries.
      iii. Diagnostic tools include focused abdominal sonography for trauma (FAST) examination and chest radiography.
   c. Tension pneumothorax causes increased intrathoracic pressure with a resultant decrease in venous return.
      i. It may mimic cardiac tamponade in presentation, with hypotension, tachycardia, evidence of elevated central venous pressure, and jugular venous distention.
      ii. This is a clinical diagnosis and not a radiographic diagnosis. It should be strongly suspected in the trauma patient with markedly decreased or absent breath sounds with hyperresonance to percussion on the affected side and tracheal deviation to the opposite side.
3. **Treatment**
   a. In the unstable patient, therapeutic pericardiocentesis is a temporizing maneuver. Emergent thoracotomy or sternotomy is required for definitive treatment and repair of cardiac injuries.

Emergency department thoracotomy is indicated in the patient with suspected tamponade following penetrating thoracic trauma who presents following a witnessed cardiac arrest.
  b. For tension pneumothorax, the practice at Parkland Memorial Hospital is to rapidly place a thoracostomy tube in the fourth intercostal space of the affected side. If a thoracostomy tube is not *immediately* available, needle thoracostomy in the second intercostal space should be performed. This must, however, be followed with proper thoracostomy tube placement.

D. Distributive shock

1. **Definition**. This type of shock is marked by decreased peripheral vascular resistance either from sepsis or loss of sympathetic tone from spinal cord injury.
2. **Pathophysiology**
   a. Venodilation leads to a decrease in preload with a normal or elevated cardiac output.
   b. Neurogenic shock is caused by a loss of sympathetic tone causing a relative hypovolemia and hypotension with a wide pulse pressure and dry, warm skin. It is almost always associated with spinal cord injury in the trauma patient, although high spinal anesthesia with loss of vasomotor tone can also occur. It is not caused by an isolated head injury, and another source of shock in these patients must be sought (usually hemorrhagic).
   c. Septic shock is uncommon immediately after trauma, but it is the most common cause of death in intensive care unit patients. Sepsis occurs secondary to bacteremia and the consequent development of cardiovascular insufficiency and vasodilatation. Initially, the septic patient is in a hyperdynamic state with decreased systemic vascular resistance, increased cardiac output, and increased oxygen consumption. However, over time, cardiac output will decrease. Progression to multiorgan failure and death is not uncommon.
3. **Treatment**
   a. Initial treatment is the same as for hypovolemia with fluid administration.
   b. Vasopressors may be used to support arterial pressure only after intravascular volume is restored.
   c. Hemodynamic monitoring is often helpful.
   d. In septic shock, identification and elimination of the infectious source are vital. Surgical debridement or drainage must be performed when indicated.
   e. Aggressive treatment of hyperglycemia to maintain blood glucose between 80 to 110 mg/dL has been shown to decrease morbidity and mortality in sepsis, regardless of whether the patient has a history of diabetes. Treatment should include an insulin drip to maintain blood glucose in this range.

f. Steroids are indicated only in the patient with documented adrenal insufficiency and should not be given to all patients with septic shock.
   i. Patients with adrenal insufficiency benefit from physiologic doses of steroids. Adrenal insufficiency should be suspected when a patient has hypotension refractory to pressors.
   ii. Baseline serum cortisol is obtained. Adrenal insufficiency is defined as a value less than 25 μg/dL. If the results are normal, then other causes of hypotension should be investigated.
   iii. Cosyntropin stimulation test can assist in diagnosing the patient with relative adrenal insufficiency. A dose of 250 μg of cosyntropin is given intravenously and the cortisol levels are measured at 0, 30, and 60 minutes. An increase in cortisol *less* than 9 μg/dL is indicative of adrenal insufficiency.
   iv. If adrenal insufficiency is confirmed, treatment should be started immediately. Treatment consists of hydrocortisone 100 mg IV 3 times a day for 7 days. Patients can be given dexamethasone while undergoing cosyntropin stimulation because it does not interfere with the test. Once the results return, the patient should then be switched to hydrocortisone.
   v. At Parkland Memorial Hospital steroids are only given for documented adrenal insufficiency.

E. Spinal shock
1. This is not treated unless the patient is symptomatic.
2. The patient's legs can be elevated to provide some autotransfusion.
3. Vasopressors are given only if the above fail.

V. SUGGESTED READINGS

Dellinger RP, et al: Surviving sepsis campaign: Guidelines for management of severe sepsis and septic shock. Crit Care Med 32(3), 2004.

Hotchkiss RS, et al: Medical progress: The pathophysiology and treatment of sepsis. N Engl J Med 348(2), 2003.

Marik P, et al: Adrenal insuffiency during septic shock. Crit Care Med 31(1), 2003.

Transfusion Therapy

Harshal Broker, MD, and Samuel Jacks, MD

I. INTRODUCTION

Over ten million units of blood are transfused each year in the United States. Transfusion therapy remains one of the most common and important treatment modalities in the acute management of trauma. The trauma surgeon's approach to and understanding of transfusion therapy remain critical and evolving components of trauma care.

II. INDICATIONS

A. Restoration of intravascular volume
1. This is the most common indication for red blood cell transfusion. Empiric transfusion with packed red blood cells (PRBC) is indicated in the emergency department when the patient remains hypotensive (systolic blood pressure < 90) after sufficient crystalloid administration (usually 2000 mL) and no other source of hypotension is identified.
2. Type-specific and, if necessary, type O Rh-negative blood is administered in this situation en route to the operating room or intensive care unit. Patients with class II hemorrhage (15% to 30% blood volume loss) usually do not require transfusion if their source of hemorrhage is controlled.
3. Blood transfusion is always necessary in patients with obvious evidence of hypoperfusion (class III and IV shock).
4. Most patients who are hypotensive from a hemorrhagic source have lost at least 2000 mL of blood.

B. Restoration of oxygen-carrying capacity
1. A **hemoglobin of 7 g/dL** (Hct 20 to 21) is well tolerated in most trauma patients and is an acceptable end-point once surgical lesions are corrected and hemostasis is achieved.
2. A **hemoglobin of 10 g/dL** (Hct 30) may be optimal in the elderly or in patients with evidence of cardiovascular compromise.
3. This **"transfusion trigger"** should be individualized based on multiple factors including:
   - Mental status changes
   - Tachycardia
   - Respiratory rate
   - Blood pressure
   - Cardiac output/index
   - Arterial pH
   - Base deficit
   - Urine output

C. Correction of coagulopathy. Coagulopathy is an expected finding in patients with massive transfusions (>10 units), hypothermia, crystalloid over-resuscitation, and prolonged shock. The etiology is multifactorial, and implicating factors include hypothermia-induced platelet dysfunction, dilutional thrombocytopenia, and dilution of clotting factors. Studies have documented diminished platelet metabolism, including thromboxane production, at temperatures < 34°C. Initial therapy involves rapid rewarming of the patient to maintain core temperatures >35°C, followed by correction of abnormal coagulation studies (Fig. 10-1).

1. **Transfusion triggers:**
   - Platelets. In the resuscitation phase, platelets should be kept above 100,000/μL. When the patient is fully resuscitated, platelet counts of 20,000 to 40,000/μL are acceptable, as long as there is no bleeding.
   - Fresh frozen plasma (FFP). Prothrombin time (PT)/International Normalized Ratio (INR), or partial thromboplastin time (PTT) values greater than 1.5 × normal indicate a need for fresh frozen plasma. Vitamin K may also be used as an adjunct. Of note, normal values for

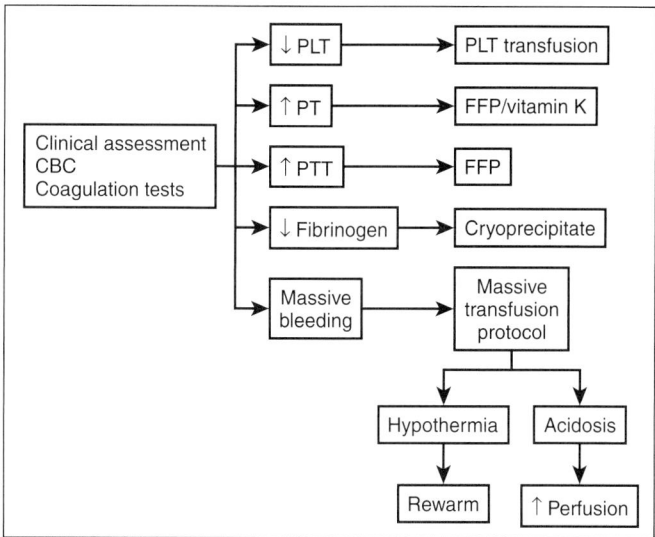

FIGURE 10-1

Correction of abnormal coagulation studies.

PT/INR and PTT are not accurate in the hypothermic patient, and normothermia must be corrected in order to assess the degree of coagulopathy adequately.
- Cryoprecipitate. This is indicated when fibrinogen levels are low.
- Recombinant factor VIIa (rfVIIa). This is given if there is persistent bleeding in spite of standard therapy.

III. BLOOD PRODUCTS

A. Packed red blood cells. This component is obtained after centrifugation of whole blood.
- PRBCs are used to replenish volume and oxygen-carrying capacity.
- Each unit is 200 to 300 mL in volume.
- PRBCs are usually stored in sodium citrate anticoagulant solution, which functions by binding calcium, thus depleting calcium levels. Citrate is converted to lactate and then bicarbonate in the patient, which provides an alkaline load.
- Although PRBCs are prepared by centrifugation, up to 40% of a unit may consist of leukocytes, plasma, and platelets. Washed red blood cells are available, which are further depleted of leukocytes, platelets, and plasma. Washed red blood cells may be useful in preventing nonhemolytic febrile reaction that is caused by host antibodies to foreign leukocytes.

B. Whole blood. Theoretically, this is the ideal transfusion product because it contains a full complement of red blood cells, platelets, and coagulation proteins. This product has limited utility in the trauma patient; when whole blood is stored for longer than 24 to 48 hours, there is significant platelet dysfunction and decrease in clotting factor activity. Whole blood is generally not available because of the valuable utilization of its components.

C. Platelets. Platelets are obtained from the buffy coat layer after centrifugation of whole blood.
- Platelets can be stored frozen for up to 5 days.
- Platelet transfusions are usually administered in 6-unit increments.

D. Fresh frozen plasma. FFP is obtained immediately after freezing of the supernatant, left after removal of red blood cells and the buffy coat layer.
- FFP contains high levels of coagulation factors including II, V, VII, IX, and XI but may require up to 45 minutes to thaw and should be used promptly.
- FFP is used liberally at Parkland Memorial Hospital in coagulopathic patients with solid organ injuries (liver or spleen) or intracranial hemorrhage.

E. Cryoprecipitate. In the past, cryoprecipitate has been used infrequently in acute trauma. However, there has been a trend in recent years to include cryoprecipitate when massive transfusion is needed and in patients with hypofibrinogenemia.

- Cryoprecipitate contains concentrated factor VIII, von Willebrand factor, and fibrinogen. It is most useful in specific conditions such as:
  a. Hypofibrinogenemia
  b. von Willebrand disease
  c. Hemophilia A
  d. Factor XIII deficiency

F. Activated factor VII. Although a recombinant form of activated factor VII (rVIIa) has traditionally been used only in the treatment of hemophilia disorders, there is growing evidence and experience in using rVIIa in the acutely bleeding trauma patient. **Note:** rVIIa is very expensive.
- Activated factor VII has been demonstrated to inhibit fibrinolysis, to promote a more stable fibrin plug, and to enhance platelet adhesion and activation. It enhances thrombin generation on activated platelets and therefore may be of benefit in providing hemostasis in patients with profuse bleeding or impaired thrombin generation.
- At Parkland Memorial Hospital, factor VIIa is included in the massive transfusion protocol.

IV. COMPLICATIONS OF BLOOD TRANSFUSION

A. Iatrogenic. Administration of incompatible blood or use of an incompatible carrier can lead to transfusion complications.

TABLE 10-1
BLOOD PRODUCTS

Blood Product	Characteristics
Whole blood	(500 mL); 35%-40% hematocrit (Hct); no platelets or coagulation factors active; frequently unavailable
Packed red blood cells	(300 mL); 65%-80% Hct; no platelets, white blood cells, or plasma. Children are frequently transfused in 10-mL/kg volumes.
Leukocyte-poor red blood cells	(300 mL); 65%-80% Hct; 70% leukocytes removed; for patients with frequent febrile reactions
Washed red blood cells	(300 mL); 65%-80% Hct; 85% leukocytes and 99% plasma removed; for patients with allergic reaction to plasma protein in donor blood
Frozen red blood cells	(250 mL); 65-80% Hct; 3-year shelf-life storage of rare blood or autologous donor cells.
Platelets	(40-70 mL); 5.5×10^3 platelets per unit. Each unit should raise platelet count 5000-10,000; 6-10 units are usually given at a time.
Fresh frozen plasma	(180-300 mL); 200 units of factor VIII and 200-400 mg of fibrinogen per unit; must be used within 6 hours of thawing; requires ABO typing; adequate source of all coagulation proteins
Cryoprecipitate	>80 units of factor VIII (VIII:C); good source of factor VIII:vWF and fibrinogen in <15 mL plasma

- Improper patient infusion and clerical errors are important causes of inappropriate transfusion.
- When hypotonic or calcium-containing solutions are used (e.g., 5% dextrose or lactated Ringer's solution), red blood cell clumping, hemolysis, and clot formation may occur.
- Blood should be infused through lines carrying isotonic fluid, such as normal saline or Plasmalyte.

B. Immunologic. The incidence of hemolytic reactions is 0.03% to 2% per unit. It is fatal in 1/100,000.

1. **Acute hemolytic reaction** is the result of transfusion of ABO-incompatible blood.
   - Hypotension, fever, chills, hemoglobinuria, confusion, chest pain, back pain, dyspnea, and bleeding diathesis mark this reaction.
   - The transfusion should be stopped and the patient's blood sent for free hemoglobin and haptoglobin levels and a Coomb's test.
   - Treatment is supportive, with maintenance of good urine output.
2. **Delayed hemolytic reaction** is due to prior sensitization in a patient who has a nondetectable level of antibody at the time of typing.
   - These patients present with indirect hyperbilirubinemia and hemoglobinuria several days after transfusion.
   - This reaction is generally well tolerated and milder than the former.
3. **Febrile reactions** are probably due to antileukocyte antibodies and are seen in patients who have had prior transfusions. Although this is a mild reaction, an acute hemolytic reaction must be ruled out before transfusion is continued.
4. **Nonhemolytic allergic reactions** are seen in 1% to 4% per unit transfusion. These reactions generally occur in patients who have not had previous transfusions and may be caused by reaction to leukocytes or plasma proteins.
   - The reaction is usually mild, with urticaria, fever, hives, and bronchospasm, but may be severe and may even present with anaphylaxis.
   - Treatment is supportive: antihistamine (diphenhydramine, 25 mg IV), epinephrine (1:1000; 0.1 to 0.5 mg IM or SC every 10 to 15 minutes), and IV steroids (hydrocortisone, 40 to 100 mg) may be indicated.
5. **Immunosuppression** is becoming a more recognized complication of blood transfusion.
   - Data from cardiac surgery, colon cancer, and renal transplant studies show decreased T-lymphocyte proliferation, reversed CD4/CD8 ratio, depression of natural killer cells, decreased B-lymphocyte reactivity against antigens, and decreased macrophage phagocytosis.
   - Given these findings, the risks of immunosuppression should be taken into consideration when deciding to transfuse. However, fear of immunosuppression should not override the need for appropriate blood replacement in the acute setting.

IV. Complications of Blood Transfusion

C. **Infections**. The advancement of technologies dedicated to the screening of infectious diseases has greatly increased the safety of the blood supply. Nucleic amplification testing (NAT) is now performed on virtually all blood collected in the United States for detection of HIV and hepatitis C. Future advances in screening techniques will likely lead to a lower incidence of hepatitis B.
1. **Viral contamination** per unit transfusion is reported as:
   a. **HIV**: 1/1 to 2 million
   b. **Hepatitis B:** 1/200,000
   c. **Hepatitis C**: 1/1 to 2 million
   d. **Human T-cell lymphocytotrophic virus (HTLV) types I and II:** 1/1 to 2 million
   e. **West Nile virus:** 1/1 million in endemic areas
   f. **Cytomegalovirus** (CMV) is the most common virus transmitted with transfusions in the United States. Because it is endemic, routine screening for CMV is not performed. However, CMV transmission by transfusion requires transfer of infected leukocytes, and with the transition to an all-leukocyte-reduced blood supply, CMV transmission is becoming less frequent.
      - Immunocompromised patients (e.g., transplant patients) should receive leukocyte-reduced or CMV-screened blood products.
2. **Bacterial contamination** per unit transfusion is reported as:
   a. Transfusions of products with bacterial contaminants (e.g., syphilis, malaria, *Yersinia enterocolitica, Babesia microti, Trypanosoma cruzi*): 1/5 million
   b. The onset of fever, chills, and hypotension shortly after transfusion make the distinction from acute allergic or hemolytic reaction difficult. These patients may become very ill and may need to be treated with broad-spectrum antimicrobial agents and supportive care.

D. **Metabolic complications**
1. **Potassium**
   a. Packed red blood cells contain 30 to 40 mEq per unit after 3 weeks of storage secondary to cell lysis. Hyperkalemia can be induced in the setting of massive transfusion.
2. **Calcium**
   a. Citrate, the preservative used in blood products, binds to calcium to prevent clotting during storage.
   b. At infusion rates >1 unit per 5 minutes, hypocalcemia may occur. This may cause hypotension, myocardial depression, arrhythmias, and coagulopathy.
   c. Treatment is slow IV calcium gluconate (0.45 mEq elemental calcium) per 100 mL of citrated blood transfused.
3. **Acid-base**
   a. Stored PRBCs contain citrate, which is converted by the liver to bicarbonate, thus perpetuating an alkalotic effect.

4. **Hypothermia**
   a. Defined as temperature <34°C (PRBCs are stored at 1° to 6°C and have a shelf-life of 35 days.)
   b. Infusion of cold blood products augments heat loss caused by exposure and has several detrimental effects including:
      i. Acidosis
      ii. Leftward shift of the oxygen dissociation curve
      iii. Increased oxygen affinity
      iv. Impaired platelet function
      v. Myocardial depression
      vi. Arrhythmias
      vii. Respiratory depression
   c. Thus, when transfusing large amounts of blood products, heated IV tubing should be used.
E. **Disseminated intravascular coagulation (DIC)**
1. Red blood cell adenosine diphosphate (ADP) and membrane phospholipoprotein activate the procoagulant system via factor XII and complement. Diffuse microvascular thrombosis, consuming platelets and coagulation factors, occurs. Simultaneous fibrinolysis releases fibrin split products into the circulation.
   a. The etiology of DIC includes:
      i. Massive transfusion
      ii. Sepsis
      iii. Crush injury
      iv. Multiple injuries
   b. Clinical features include:
      i. Fever
      ii. Hypotension
      iii. Acidosis
      iv. Proteinuria
      v. Hypoxia
   c. Laboratory features include:
      i. Thrombocytopenia (<80,000/mm^3)
      ii. Decreased fibrinogen (0.8 g/L)
      iii. Prolonged PT and PTT
      iv. Elevated fibrin-degradation products or D-dimers
      v. Fragmented red blood cells on smear
   d. Treatment involves aggressive hemodynamic support and removal of underlying cause (transfusion of compatible washed PRBCs). If these measures fail we have used IV heparin infusion (titrated to maintain international normalized ratio (INR) between 1.1 and 1.5), antithrombin III, or epsilon-aminocaproic acid (Amicar) with variable success. The onset of DIC portends a poor prognosis. Mortality is high mainly due to end-organ damage and failure.
F. **Transfusion related acute lung injury (TRALI).** TRALI is defined as noncardiogenic pulmonary edema temporally related to transfusion therapy.

1. Diagnosis requires exclusion of other diagnoses (such as sepsis, volume overload, cardiogenic pulmonary edema).
2. Pathogenesis may be explained by a two-hit hypothesis, with the first hit being a predisposing inflammatory condition and the second hit involving the passive transfer of neutrophil or HLA antibodies from the donor or the transfusion of biologically active lipids from older cellular blood products.
3. The first hit involves priming the adherence of neutrophils to the pulmonary endothelium. Examples of the first hit can include surgery, sepsis, trauma, massive transfusions, cardiac disease, and possibly multiparity.
4. The second hit activates these primed neutrophils, resulting in the release of the reactive oxygen species that cause capillary leak and pulmonary edema.
5. Treatment is supportive with outcomes better than for most other causes of acute lung injury. Management should be guided by the use of a pulmonary artery catheter (PAC) to show that fluids are not needed within a normal wedge. Volume overload must be excluded to differentiate TRALI from phenomena such as shock lung or adult respiratrory distress syndrome after massive transfusion.
6. Mortality rate can be as high as 5% to 8%.

E. Acute respiratory distress syndrome (ARDS)
1. This syndrome occurs in patients with an average incidence of 0.02% per unit blood transfused.
2. It can occur with any blood product containing plasma, and signs usually appear during transfusion or within 3 to 4 hours.
3. The clinical features include fever, chills, hypotension, and progressive respiratory insufficiency.
4. Hypoxemia is refractory to supplemental oxygen, and ARDS can be avoided by transfusing washed PRBCs in symptomatic patients.
5. Treatment consists of aggressive pulmonary support and possibly mechanical ventilation.
6. The syndrome follows a milder course when caused by transfusion, usually resolving within 48 to 96 hours.
7. The mortality rate is significantly lower than mortality of ARDS associated with other etiologies (10% vs 60%).

V. MASSIVE TRANSFUSION PROTOCOL

The development of massive transfusion protocols has standardized the approach to correcting blood loss in acute situations. These protocols are of the utmost use and importance in effective trauma care. The massive transfusion protocol is intended to be initiated in an operating room setting and is activated when blood loss is anticipated to exceed 5 units/hour or 10 units/procedure. Data to determine the effectiveness of these protocols are actively being analyzed.

TABLE 10-2
MASSIVE TRANSFUSION PROTOCOL

Shipment	RBC	TP	PLT	CR	rVIIa
1a	5 (O-Neg)	2 (AB)			
1b	5	2			
2	5	2	1		2.4 mg
3	5	2		10	
4	5	2	1		2.4 mg
5	5	2			
6	5	2	1	10	2.4 mg
7	5	2			
8	5	2	1		
9	5	2		10	
10	5	2	1		

The replacement of blood loss in the acute trauma setting begins with un-crossmatched type O-negative blood and should be switched to type-specific crossmatched blood as soon as it becomes available.

Table 10-2 is an example of the Massive Transfusion Protocol in use at Parkland Memorial Hospital.

VI. BLOOD SUBSTITUTES

As of now, red blood cell transfusion is the only available method for restoring blood's oxygen-carrying capacity. Several blood substitutes are currently in clinical trials and fall into two categories: (1) molecules that incorporate hemoglobin in their structure (hemoglobin-based oxygen carriers) and (2) synthetic molecules (perfluorocarbon and porphyrins), which carry oxygen and carbon dioxide. These products are likely to change the dynamics of hemorrhagic shock in the future.

VII. PEARLS AND PITFALLS

A. **Hypothermia.** Prevention and treatment of hypothermia are essential to achieving hemostasis and avoiding physiologic impairments.
B. **Infectious risk.** Prophylactic platelet and fresh-frozen plasma transfusions carry infectious risk and are not warranted unless there is thrombocytopenia and acidosis is corrected.
C. **Factor depletion.** PT, PTT, and fibrinogen are reliable predictors of factor depletion and should be used to assess the need for replacement of clotting factors.

VIII. SUGGESTED READINGS

Goodnough LT, Brecher ME, Kanter MH, AuBuchon JP: Transfusion medicine. First of two parts–Blood transfusion. N Engl J Med 340(6):438-447, 1999.

Peterson S, Weinberg J: In Moore E, Mattox K, Feliciano D (eds): Trauma, 5th ed. New York, McGraw-Hill, 2003, pp 227-237.

Rutherford E, Skeete D, Schooler W, Fakhry S: In Townsend C, Beauchamp R, Evers B. Mattox K (eds): Sabiston Textbook of Surgery, 17th ed. Philadelphia, Saunders; 2004, pp 113-136.

Spence R, Mintz P: In Mintz P (ed): Transfusion Therapy: Clinical Principles and Practice, 2nd ed. Bethesda, MD, AABB Press 2005, pp 203-241.

Emergency Department Diagnostic Modalities

Makram Gedeon, MD

At Parkland Memorial Hospital, the initial evaluation of the trauma victim is a highly organized team approach that incorporates the trauma surgeon, emergency physician, and trauma nurses, among others.

Diagnostic studies in the emergency department are adjuncts to the primary and secondary surveys. The clinical state of the patient should be the main drive behind obtaining diagnostic studies, the purpose of which shifts from one of cavitary triage looking for hemorrhage in the unstable patient to one of injury detection and definition in the more stable one.

This chapter provides a brief overview of the diagnostic tools used in the emergency department to evaluate the acutely injured trauma patient.

I. PLAIN FILMS

Screening chest and pelvis radiographs are obtained in the trauma bay following the primary survey. Additional plain films are ordered as indicated by the history and the physical examination.

A. Chest
1. The chest film is an effective screening modality for the detection of pneumothorax, hemothorax, fractures, and mediastinal abnormalities.
2. It is obtained with the patient in the supine position after a nasogastric tube has been inserted.
3. Certain clues on the chest film point to a possible thoracic great vessel injury and should be sought (Table 11-1)
4. A coned-down view is sometimes obtained to better assess the mediastinum.
5. Pneumothorax is best appreciated on inspiration-expiration films.

B. Cervical spine
1. A cervical collar is placed in all blunt trauma victims.
2. A screening lateral view showing the base of the skull, all seven cervical vertebrae, and the first thoracic vertebra will demonstrate most cervical spine injuries.
3. In stable patients, the cervical spine is evaluated by CT scan.

C. Pelvis
1. Screening anteroposterior (AP) films are obtained in all multitrauma victims.
2. If a fracture is present, inlet, outlet, and Judet views are obtained.
3. At Parkland Memorial Hospital, we use the Young-Burgess classification for pelvic fractures as this pertains to severity (Table 11-2).
4. A pelvic binder is used in patients with unstable pelvic fractures (specifically with LCII, LCIII, APCII, APCIII, and vertical shear fractures), as well as in patients over the age of 55 years.

TABLE 11-1
RADIOGRAPHIC ABNORMALITIES AND CLUES ASSOCIATED WITH THORACIC GREAT VESSEL INJURY

Fractures
Sternum
Scapula
Multiple left ribs
Clavicle in multisystem-injured patients
First rib

Mediastinal clues
Obliteration of the aortic contour
Widening of the mediastinum (>8 cm)
Depression of the mainstem bronchus >140 degrees from trachea
Loss of prevertebral pleural stripe
Calcium layering at the aortic knob
"Funny looking" mediastinum
Deviation of the nasogastric tube in the esophagus
Lateral displacement of the trachea

Other findings
Apical pleural hematoma
Massive left hemothorax
Obvious blunt injury to the diaphragm

Lateral chest x-ray
Anterior displacement of the trachea
Loss of the aortic and pulmonary window

From Moore EE, Feliciano DV, Mattox KL: Trauma, 5th ed. New York, McGraw-Hill, 2003, p 575.

D. Extremity radiographs
1. Ordered as indicated by the physical examination

E. Clearing the cervical spine
1. Life-threatening hemodynamic and pulmonary issues should be addressed before a lengthy cervical spine evaluation is undertaken.
2. The patient who is awake, alert, oriented, and not intoxicated, without distracting pain or neurologic deficit, and who has no neck pain is considered to have a stable cervical spine and does not need routine imaging. An attempt is made to clear the neck clinically:
   a. The neck is examined for midline tenderness.
   b. The patient is asked to gently flex/extend and rotate the neck.
   c. If there is no neck pain with the above maneuvers, the cervical spine is cleared.
3. All other patients require a thin-cut axial CT scan with sagittal reconstruction in the areas with questionable findings on plain films.

TABLE 11-2
YOUNG-BURGESS CLASSIFICATION OF PELVIC FRACTURES

Category	Characteristics/Stability	
LC (LATERAL COMPRESSION)	*Transverse fracture of pubic rami, ipsilateral or contralateral to posterior injury*	
	I-Sacral compression on side of impact	Stable
	II-Crescent (iliac wing) fracture on side of impact	Rotationally unstable, vertically stable
	III-LCI or LCII on side of impact; contralateral open-book (APC) injury	Unstable
APC (ANTEROPOSTERIOR COMPRESSION)	*Symphyseal diastasis of longitudinal rami fractures*	
	I-Slight widening of pubic symphysis or anterior SI joint; stretched but intact anterior SI, sacrotuberous and sacrospinous ligaments; intact posterior SI ligaments	Stable
	II-Widened anterior SI joint; disrupted anterior SI, sacrotuberous and sacrospinous ligaments; intact posterior SI ligaments	Rotationally unstable, vertically stable
	III-Complete SI joint disruption with lateral displacement; disrupted anterior SI, sacrotuberous and sacrospinous ligaments; disrupted posterior SI ligaments	Rotationally unstable, vertically unstable
VS (VERTICAL SHEAR)	Symphyseal diastasis or vertical displacement anteriorly and posteriorly, usually through the SI joint, occasionally through the iliac wing or sacrum	Rotationally unstable, vertically unstable
CM (COMBINED MECHANISM)	Combination of other injury patterns, LC/VS being the most common	Variable stability

Adapted from Cameron JL: Current Surgical Therapy, 8th ed. Philadelphia, Mosby, 2004, p 996.

4. If obtained, plain films are considered adequate technically if:
   a. The lateral view shows the base of the skull to the upper border of T1.
   b. The open mouth view reveals the lateral masses of C1 and the odontoid process.
   c. The AP view shows the spinous processes of C2 to T1.
5. The radiographs should be read by a physician with expertise in interpreting the studies.
6. If the radiographs are normal but the patient complains of significant neck pain, flexion/extension films are obtained to rule out ligamentous injuries.
7. An MRI of the cervical spine should be ordered in patients with neurologic deficits referable to the cervical spine.
8. Patients who are obtunded (or sedated) are considered to have a stable cervical spine if both an adequate three-view cervical spine series and a thin-cut axial CT with sagittal reconstruction through C1 and C2 are normal.
9. The cervical collar is maintained in the intoxicated patient and in the patient with distracting pain, and an attempt to clear the neck clinically is made later when the patient is alert and oriented and the cause for the distracting pain is addressed.

II. ULTRASOUND

Ultrasound is a noninvasive, operator-dependent modality that has gained widespread use in trauma since the 1990s. The examination is performed at the bedside within minutes and during the secondary survey while the patient is being simultaneously resuscitated.

A. The range of frequencies used in medical diagnostic ultrasound is 2.5 to 10 Hz.
1. Lower frequencies have better tissue penetration than higher frequencies: A 3.5-Hz probe is used to image intra-abdominal organs and free intra-abdominal fluid.
2. Higher frequencies give better image resolution: A 5- to 8-Hz probe is used to examine the sternum for fractures and pleural spaces for hemothorax or pneumothorax.

B. The **F**ocused **A**ssessment for the **S**onographic Examination of the **T**rauma Patient (FAST) is performed by sequentially surveying the pericardial sac and abdominal cavity for free fluid (blood).

C. The first view is the **subxiphoid view** (alternatively, left parasternal).
1. Examines the heart and pericardium
2. Gain is set so that blood in the heart appears anechoic.
3. Used to look for hemopericardium (Fig. 11-1)
   a. A negative examination does not rule out a cardiac injury because blood could be decompressing into the chest if the pericardium is torn.
   b. A positive examination is an indication for exploration (thoracotomy perfromed in the emergency department if the patient is in extremis).

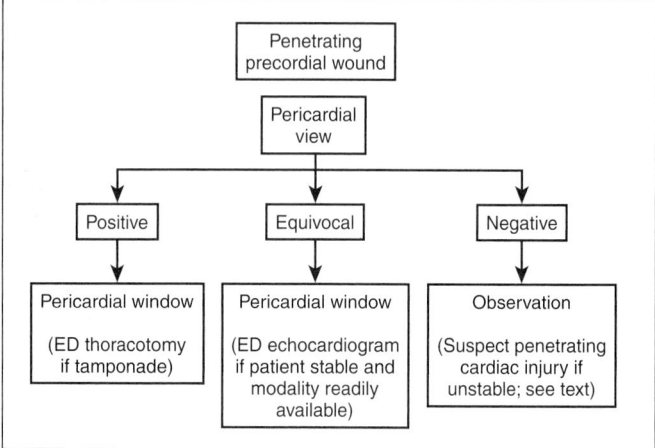

FIGURE 11-1

FAST in penetrating torso wounds. *(Adapted from Moore EE, Feliciano DV, Mattox ICL: Trauma, 5th ed.* New York, McGraw-Hill, 2003, *p 318).*

4. In blunt trauma arrest, the pericardial ultrasound determines the presence of a reversible cause of the hemodynamic compromise.
D. An **examination of the dependent portions of the abdominal cavity** is performed next.
1. The right upper quadrant view looks at the hepatorenal recess, or Morrison's pouch. Regardless of the intra-abdominal organ injured, this is the view most likely to show free intra-abdominal fluid if present.
2. The left upper quadrant view examines the splenorenal recess. The cooperative patient is asked to take a deep breath because this moves the kidney and spleen below the ribs.
3. The pelvis (bladder) view looks at the rectovesical/rectouterine space (pouch of Douglas). A full bladder provides a better acoustic window.
4. A positive FAST examination in an unstable patient with blunt trauma to the abdomen mandates laparotomy (Fig. 11-2).
E. An **examination of both lower thoracic cavities and sternum** can also be performed, looking for hemothorax, pneumothorax, and sternal fractures.
F. FAST is not useful for the evaluation of penetrating abdominal injuries, retroperitoneal injuries, or suspected hollow viscus injuries.

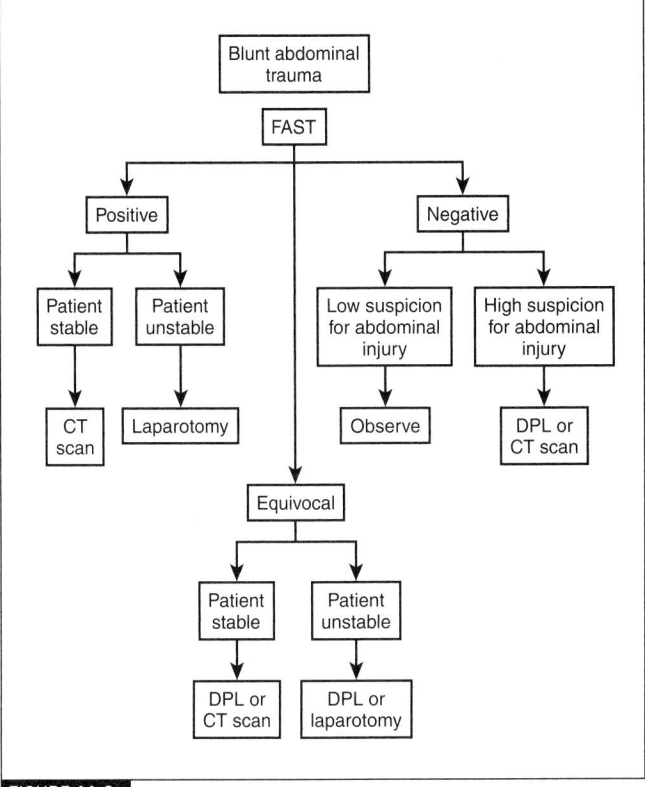

FIGURE 11-2

FAST in blunt abdominal trauma. DPL = diagnostic peritoneal lavage. *(Adapted from Moore EE, Feliciano DV, Mattox KL:Trauma, 5th ed. New York, McGraw-Hill, 2003, p 318).*

G. FAST can be difficult to interpret in obese patients and those with extensive subcutaneous emphysema.

III. DIAGNOSTIC PERITONEAL LAVAGE

Diagnostic peritoneal lavage (DPL) was introduced in 1965 as an expeditious and accurate method of identifying intra-abdominal hemorrhage. It is highly sensitive in that regard. However, it is invasive and fails to identify the exact source of bleeding. Because of this and the widespread use of ultrasound and CT, DPL has been relied on with decreasing frequency over the years.

A. Used in unstable patients with an equivocal or negative FAST. It can also be used when FAST or CT is unavailable in a stable patient.
B. Useful for the evaluation of hemoperitoneum and hollow viscus/mesenteric injuries
C. Not sensitive for retroperitoneal or diaphragm injuries
D. Helps in the evaluation of anterior abdominal stab wounds
E. Other characteristics:
1. DPL can be performed with either the open or percutaneous technique.
2. The percutaneous technique is easier and faster to perform but has a higher rate of complications.
3. At Parkland Memorial Hospital, the percutaneous technique is used with conversion to open in case of difficulty.
4. Infraumbilical DPL is preferred.
5. Supraumbilical access is preferred in pregnant patients to avoid injuring a gravid uterus and in patients with pelvic fractures to avoid sampling a pelvic hematoma (causing a false-positive result).
6. **Open technique:**
   a. The abdomen is surgically prepped and draped. A Foley catheter and a nasogastric tube are inserted. Local anesthesia is used.
   b. A vertical incision is made one third of the way between the umbilicus and the symphysis pubis, and the midline fascia is incised. The peritoneum is opened and a dialysis catheter is placed and aspirated using a 10-mL syringe. If 10 mL of gross blood is aspirated, the test is considered positive.
   c. Otherwise the catheter is directed toward the pelvis and 1 L (or 10 mL/kg in children) of normal saline or lactated Ringer's solution is infused.
   d. The fluid is then siphoned back into the empty infusion bag placed below the level of the body (the bag has to be vented to allow fluid to flow).
   e. Part of the fluid recovered is sent for laboratory analysis.
7. **Percutaneous technique:**
   a. The Seldinger technique is used to gain access to the peritoneal cavity. An 18-gauge needle is inserted, through which a guidewire is advanced and directed toward the pelvis.
   b. The needle is withdrawn, a small skin incision is performed, and the dialysis catheter is advanced over the guidewire, which is then removed.
   c. The same steps as those for open DPL are then performed.
F. The test is considered positive if:
1. 10 mL of gross blood is aspirated.
2. The fluid examination is positive for bile or particulate matter.
3. The cell count is more than 100,000 red blood cells/mm^3 or 500 white blood cells/mm^3.
4. The fluid amylase is greater than the serum amylase.

IV. COMPUTED TOMOGRAPHY

CT scanning has become integral to the evaluation of the trauma victim. It should be emphasized that CT scans should be obtained only in hemodynamically stable patients after the primary and secondary surveys are completed. Sending a patient to the CT scanner should be regarded as a departmental transfer during which the patient is continuously monitored.

A. Head and cervical spine CT
1. Indications for head CT include:
   a. A history of significant head trauma.
   b. Loss of consciousness
   c. Decreased Glasgow Coma Score (GCS)
   d. Inability to reliably examine the patient (e.g., the patient is intoxicated, sedated, or intubated)
2. The head CT is obtained without contrast.
3. Without a reliable physical examination, the neck is cleared by obtaining a CT scan rather than relying on plain films.

B. A **face CT** is obtained whenever the mechanism of injury or the physical examination suggests facial fractures. This is sometimes postponed until after the cervical spine has been cleared because some scanners require coronal scanning for image reconstruction.

C. Neck CTA
1. This is an IV contrast-enhanced, thin-cut CT used for screening blunt cerebro-vascular injuries (carotid/vertebral). Certain criteria should alert the surgeon to a possible blunt cerebrovascular (BCV) injury (Table 11-3).

D. Chest CT/CTA
1. Obtained in patients with questionable plain films or whenever thoracic great vessel injury is suspected

E. Abdomen CT/CT cystogram
1. Sensitive for solid organ and retroperitoneal injuries. Not sensitive for hollow viscus and mesenteric injuries
2. Most useful in stable patients who have a positive or equivocal FAST examination or equivocal physical findings

TABLE 11-3
CRITERIA FOR BLUNT CEREBROVASCULAR INJURY

Cervical spine fracture
Neurologic examination not explained by brain imaging
Horner's syndrome
LeFort II or III facial fractures
Skull base fracture involving the foramen lacerum
Neck soft tissue injury (e.g., seat belt injury or hanging)

Adapted from Miller PR, Fabian T, et al: Prospective screening for blunt cerebrovascular injuries: Analysis of diagnostic modalities and outcomes. Ann Surg 236:387, 2002.

3. IV contrast is used. Oral contrast is added when a duodenal injury is suggested by the initial scan.
4. CT with triple contrast (PO, IV, and rectal) helps in evaluating back and flank stab wounds.
5. CT with delayed excretory phase images the kidneys and ureters. Contrast can be injected retrograde through the Foley catheter to image the bladder (CT cystogram).

F. Bony pelvis/extremity CT scan
1. Noncontrasted and ordered when plain films demonstrate fractures (consult with the orthopaedic service)
2. If pelvic fractures are suspected, oral contrast is not used as it may obscure the fracture and delay operative repair.

V. ANGIOGRAPHY

A. Can be both diagnostic and therapeutic
B. Indications include:
1. An abnormal extremity vascular examination or decreased ankle-brachial index (ABI)
2. Evaluation of penetrating neck injuries (zones I and III)
3. Management of pelvic fractures with significant blood loss
4. Suspected vascular injury in the neck or chest
5. Splenic or hepatic blush and/or bleeding seen on CT (in the hemodynamically stable patient).

VI. MAGNETIC RESONANCE IMAGING

1. Has a limited role in the emergency department
2. Obtained to define the level and extent of a spinal cord injury
3. Helps in determining cervical spine ligamentous injuries

VII. UROLOGIC IMAGING

A. Kidney
1. CT with IV contrast is more sensitive than intravenous pyelogram (IVP) in the detection of renal injuries. This is obtained when gross hematuria is present.
2. IVP has a role in operative procedures to demonstrate contralateral kidney function when nephrectomy is contemplated.

B. Ureters
1. Spiral CT images, delayed 5 to 8 minutes after the injection of IV contrast, are obtained.
2. Failure of the ureters to opacify or extravasation of contrast should raise suspicion of injury.

C. Bladder
1. Bladder injury is suspected when gross hematuria, pelvic fractures, or pelvic fluid is present.
2. Conventional stress cystography and CT cystography have equivalent sensitivities.
3. Stress cystogram is performed by filling the bladder retrograde through the Foley catheter with iodinated contrast to a standard volume of 300 to 400 mL and obtaining a plain radiograph.
4. Alternatively a CT scan is done (CT cystogram).

D. Urethra
1. Injury in males is suspected when blood is present at the meatus, when the prostate is abnormal (high riding) on the digital rectal examination, when a perineal or scrotal hematoma is present, or when the Foley catheter is difficult to insert.
2. The presence of vaginal bleeding in females should heighten suspicion for urethral injury.
3. A retrograde urethrogram is obtained.
4. A bulb syringe is partially inserted in the distal urethra.
5. 30 mL of iodinated contrast is injected.
6. A plain radiograph is simultaneously obtained.

VIII. MISCELLANEOUS

A. Local wound exploration
1. Used in the evaluation of stab wounds to the anterior abdomen
2. Thoracoabdominal stab wounds are excluded from exploration to avoid causing pneumothorax.
3. Exploration is performed at the bedside under local anesthesia and using sterile technique.
4. The wound edges are extended with a scalpel and the tract is followed until its end is identified.
5. If the wound penetrates the posterior abdominal wall fascia (posterior rectus fascia above and transversalis fascia below the arcuate line), there is a possibility of peritoneal violation and intraabdominal injury.

B. Echocardiogram and electrocardiogram
1. An echocardiogram is indicated when the FAST examination is equivocal in the stable patient with a penetrating precordial wound.
2. A 12-lead electrocardiogram is obtained when blunt myocardial injury is suspected.

C. Esophagram
1. Obtained when esophageal injury is suspected.
2. First, water-soluble contrast is used, followed by thin barium.
3. In the noncooperative patient, contrast can be instilled in the nasogastric tube.

D. Rigid proctoscopy/sigmoidoscopy
1. Done whenever a rectal injury is suggested by the history or abnormal digital rectal examination (rectal defect or positive guaiac)
2. Difficult to perform in the trauma bay due to patient discomfort
3. Best done after induction of anesthesia in the patient going to the operating room

E. Joint injection
1. Methylene blue or saline injected to assess joint integrity
2. Usually done by the orthopaedic service

IX. SUGGESTED READINGS

Advanced Trauma Life Support for Doctors, Student Course Manual, 6th ed. Chicago, American College of Surgeons, 1997.

Cameron JL: Current Surgical Therapy, 8th ed. Philadelphia, Mosby, 2004, pp 904-909, 925-931.

EAST Trauma guidelines, Identifying Cervical Spine Injuries Following Trauma, www.east.org, Year 2000 Update.

Eastman AL, et al: CTA screening for blunt cervical vascular injury: It's ready for primetime. J Trauma, 60(5): 925-929, 2006.

Hoff WS, et al: Practice management guidelines for the evaluation of blunt abdominal trauma: The EAST Practice Management Guidelines Work Group. J Trauma 53:602-615, 2002.

Moore EE, Feliciano DV, Mattox KL: Trauma, 5th ed. New York, McGraw-Hill, 2003, Chapters 15, 16, 25, 28, 29, 37.

Schneidereit NP, et al: Utility of screening for blunt vascular neck injuries with computed tomographic angiography. J Trauma 60:209-216, 2006.

Stassen NA, et al: Reevaluation of diagnostic procedures for transmediastinal gunshot wounds. J Trauma 53:635-638, 2002.

Ultrasound in Trauma

Radha Iyengar, MD

Ultrasound (US) is used as an adjunct to the secondary survey to evaluate for fluid in the pericardium and abdomen. Although this imaging method is used routinely to guide further work-up, it does not preclude further imaging in patients with concerning findings.

I. BASICS OF ULTRASOUND

A. Essential principles
1. **Piezoelectric effect**: Piezoelectric crystals expand and contract to interconvert electrical and mechanical energy.
2. **Pulse-echo principle:** When US waves contact an organ, some waves are reflected and some are transmitted through the tissue. Reflected waves return to the transducer and generate electrical impulses that are converted to the images seen on the monitor.

B. Basic definitions
1. **Frequency:** Number of cycles per second. Increasing frequency improves resolution. High-frequency transducers (≥5 MHz) are good for visualizing superficial structures, whereas lower-frequency transducers penetrate deeper into tissues.
2. **Echogenicity**: The degree to which tissues echo the ultrasonic waves. Anechoic substances show no echoes and therefore appear dark (e.g., fluid or blood). Hyperechoic substances appear brighter than surounding tissue (e.g., gallstones).
3. **Attenuation:** Describes the decrease in amplitude and intensity of a wave as it travels through a medium. It is affected by absorption, scattering, and reflection.
4. **Artifact:** Error in imaging. Shadowing and reverberation are examples of artifact.

C. Advantages and disadvantages of ultrasound
1. **Advantages**
   a. Noninvasive
   b. Rapid
   c. Portable
   d. Provides real-time data
   e. Can be easily repeated
2. **Disadvantages**
   a. Operator dependent
   b. Can miss small amounts of fluid
   c. Cannot detect small bowel injuries
   d. Technically difficult in obese patients
   e. Subcutaneous emphysema obscures the examination.

II. FOCUSED ASSESSMENT WITH SONOGRAPHY FOR TRAUMA (FAST)

A. Overview
1. It allows systematic evaluation of the pericardium, Morrison's pouch, splenorenal space, and the pouch of Douglas.
2. Can be performed in <1 minute.
3. It is usually performed after completion of the secondary examination and before placement of a Foley catheter.
4. It can be done concurrently with the resuscitation.
5. The 3.5-MHz curvilinear tranducer is used in most adult patients. The 2.7-MHz transducer is used for obese patients, and the 5.0-MHz transducer is used for pediatric patients.

B. Areas of evaluation (see Fig. 12-1)
1. **Pericardium.** This area is visualized first so that blood within the heart can be used as a standard by which to set the gain. The probe is placed in a sagittal orientation in the subxiphoid position. Sometimes a subxiphoid view may be difficult to obtain (in obese or very tall patients) and in such cases a left parasternal view with the probe oriented in a transverse plane can be helpful in evaluating the pericardium.
2. **Right upper quadrant**. This area is visualized next. It is used to evaluate the hepatorenal space or Morrison's pouch. The transducer is placed in the right midaxillary line between the 11th and 12th ribs in a sagittal orientation. Often, the probe needs to be swept in a transverse plane in order to achieve a good window. This is the location that most often accumulates fluid that can be detected with ultrasound regardless of source.
3. **Left upper quadrant**. Evaluates the splenorenal space. The transducer is oriented sagittally and placed between the 9th and 11th ribs in the left posterior axillary line. Often, the probe needs to be swept in a transverse, anterior to posterior plane in order to achieve a good window. If the shadowing from the ribs precludes good imaging, the patient can be asked to take a slow deep breath, allowing the spleen to come into better view as the diaphragm moves inferiorly.
4. **Pelvis.** Evaluates the rectovesical/rectouterine space. The transducer is placed in a transverse orientation 2 to 4 cm above the pubic symphysis and swept inferiorly. The bladder should be full for optimal imaging and thus Foley catheter placement should be reserved until the pelvic view has been obtained.

C. Interpreting the results. A positive test reflects fluid in the space.
1. A positive pericardial view in blunt trauma should prompt further evaluation with a pericardial window in the operating room.
2. A positive pericardial view in penetrating trauma should prompt immediate operative intervention with a median sternotomy in the operating room before the patient decompensates.

II. Focused Assessment with Sonography for Trauma (FAST)

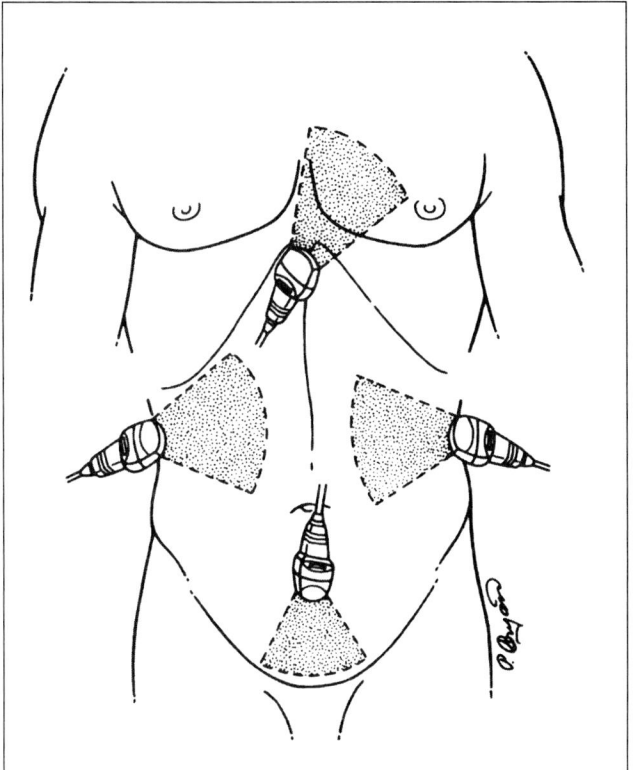

FIGURE 12-1
The four transducer positions for the focused assessment with sonography for trauma evaluation: pericardial, right and left upper quadrants, and pelvis. *(From Cameron JL: Current Surgical Therapy, 8th ed. Philadelphia, Mosby, 2004.)*

3. A positive intra-abdominal view in a hemodynamically unstable patient should prompt a DPL. If there is a large amount of intra-abdominal fluid, exploration in the operating room is warranted.
4. A positive intra-abdominal view in a hemodynamically normal patient should prompt further evaluation by CT scan.
5. Any patient with peritonitis, regardless of FAST results, should be taken to the operating room for exploration.
6. A negative FAST does not "clear" the abdomen of injuries. In this circumstance, clinical judgment should guide the need for further work-up.

D. Other uses for ultrasound

1. **Traumatic hemothorax**. A 3.5-MHz curvilinear transducer is applied to the right or left lower thoracic areas (9th to 10th rib spaces) in the mid to posterior axillary line. The transducer is positioned in a coronal orientation and moved cephalad until the hyperechoic diaphragm is visualized. If there is fluid in the pleural space, the lung can be seen "floating" within the fluid.
2. **Pneumothorax**. A 5.0- to 7.5-MHz linear-array transducer is applied to the right or left upper thoracic areas (3rd to 4th intercostal space) in the mid-clavicular line. The transducer is placed in a transverse orientation, parallel to the ribs. The probe is moved medially and laterally to visualize the pleural space and movement of the lung within. Normal findings are pleural sliding and a comet-tail artifact. Pneumothorax is detected by the absence of the above findings.
3. **Sternal fracture.** A 5.0- to 8.0-MHz linear array transducer is used in sagittal and transverse orientations. Beginning at the suprasternal notch, the probe is moved inferiorly. A sternal fracture can be diagnosed by observing a disruption of the cortical alignment.

III. SUGGESTED READINGS

Dolich MO, et al: 2576 Ultrasounds for blunt trauma. J Trauma. 50:108, 2001.

Hai SA: The surgeon's use of ultrasound in thoracoabdominal trauma. In Cameron JL: Current Surgical Therapy, 8th ed. Philadelphia, Mosby, 2004, pp 925-930.

Rozycki GS: Surgeon-performed ultrasound in trauma and surgical critical care. In Moore Trauma, 5th ed. Norwalk, CT, Appleton & Lange, 2004, pp 311-325.

Rozycki GS, Feliciano DV, Davis TP: Ultrasound as used in thoracoabdominal trauma. Surg Clin North Am 78:295, 1998.

Sisley AC, et al: Rapid detection of traumatic effusion using surgeon-performed ultrasound. J Trauma 48:291, 1998.

Catheters and Tubes

Lauren Kane, MD

I. ARTERIAL CATHETERS

A. Indications
1. **Hemodynamic monitoring** in unstable patients (mean arterial blood pressure < 80 mm Hg)
2. **Arterial blood sampling** in patients requiring frequent evaluation of blood gases (mechanical ventilation, acute trauma resuscitation)

B. Insertion sites
1. **The radial artery** is the most common site because of relative safety, ease of insertion, dual blood supply, and optimal patient comfort. Its disadvantage is that it is unreliable in low flow states.
2. **A femoral arterial line** may be difficult to cannulate in patients without a palpable pulse. Generally it is easy to insert and allows reliable pressure readings. Its disadvantages include patient discomfort and increased risk of infection. Femoral arterial lines are rarely used at Parkland Memorial Hospital.
3. **Brachial arterial access** is not used because of the incidence of upper extremity ischemic complications.

C. Contraindications
1. **Positive Allen's test**. The radial and ulnar arteries are occluded simultaneously. The patient is then asked to clench and unclench the fist until the palm becomes pale. The ulnar artery is then released. If palmar blushing does not occur within 7 seconds, the Allen's test is positive. This indicates inadequate ulnar collateral circulation. Radial or brachial artery catheterization is contraindicated in this instance because of increased risk of distal ischemia.
2. **Lower extremity occlusive arterial disease**. The high rate of ischemic complications is a relative contraindication for dorsalis pedis catheterization in patients with known lower extremity arterial disease.
3. **Anticoagulation**. Increased bleeding and hematoma formation may complicate catheterization, especially in the brachial and femoral arteries.

D. Insertion technique
1. **Radial artery**
   a. Dorsiflex the wrist at 60°.
   b. Palpate the radial artery pulse just proximal to the radial head.
   c. Cleanse and drape the site using sterile technique.
   d. Anesthetize the overlying skin with 1% lidocaine.
   e. It is helpful to break the skin at the site of insertion with an 18-gauge needle to avoid the catheter kinking as it passes through the dermis (optional).
   f. Insert a 20-gauge catheter at a 30° angle to the skin.

g. Advance the needle until blood flows into the hub, advance the wire into the artery, and then advance the catheter into the artery over the wire.
h. Secure the catheter with 3-0 silk suture and apply a sterile dressing.

E. Complications

1. **Thrombosis** is the most common complication, with an incidence of 5% to 8%, although 4% of these result in distal limb ischemia. Thrombosis is more common with larger catheters (20-gauge), catheters left in place for more than 4 days, those placed by surgical cutdown, and intermittent flushing. Treatment is simply removal of the catheter.
2. **Infection** is the second most common complication and is associated with systemic infection, most common in catheters left in place for at least 4 days and those placed by surgical cutdown. Gram-negative rods, Enterococcus spp., and Candida are the most common causes of infection.
3. **Embolism**. Emboli may migrate distally, causing limb ischemia, or proximally, seen with forceful flushing, leading to central nervous system defects. Ischemic symptoms will usually resolve with short-term anticoagulation. If this fails, embolectomy may be indicated for large vessel occlusion.
4. **Ischemic necrosis of overlying** skin occurs in 3% of catheterizations and necessitates catheter removal.

II. SAPHENOUS VEIN CUTDOWN

A. Indications:

1. The major indication is failure to obtain upper extremity venous access.
2. **Obtaining saphenous vein access** avoids delay in resuscitation that occurs while searching for a suitable upper extremity vein. This technique can be done with relative ease by the experienced physician.

B. Anatomy:

1. As a result of its reliable location and subcutaneous course, the saphenous vein is ideally suited for rapid vascular access via the cutdown technique. It is most accessible in the ankle 1.5 cm anterior and cephalad to the medial malleolus. At this level, it can be exposed with minimal dissection. It is the classic pediatric cutdown site (Fig. 13-1).

C. Equipment:

1. Curved hemostat
2. Curved iris scissors
3. Self-retaining tissue retractor
4. Scalpel with No. 11 and 15 blades
5. Small smooth forceps
6. Needle holder
7. Silk suture ties (4-0 and 3-0)

8. Nylon suture on a cutting needle (4-0)
   9. Short large-bore catheter
  10. Plastic venous introducer

D. Technique

1. **The area of skin** to be incised should be prepared widely with an antiseptic solution and draped with sterile towels.
2. **In the conscious patient** the site should be infiltrated with 1% lidocaine solution.
3. **A transverse incision** is made perpendicular to the course of the vessel at this level, extending through the dermis into the subcutaneous tissue (Fig. 13-1A).
4. **Bluntly dissect** the subcutaneous tissue by spreading with a curved hemostat in a direction parallel to the course of the vein. A 1- to 3-cm area of exposed vein is usually adequate for canalization. A self-retaining tissue retractor may be used at this time to facilitate exposure.
5. **Mobilize the vein** from the surrounding tissue by passing a hemostat under it and pass two silk ligatures around the vein, one proximal and one distal (Fig. 13-1B).
6. **With gentle traction** on the proximal ligature, incise the vessel at the 45° angle through one-third to one-half of its diameter using either the No. 11 blade or the iris scissors (Fig.13-1C).
7. **The large-bore catheter** may now be introduced into the lumen of the vein using either the forceps or the Seldinger technique (Fig. 13-1D).
8. **Alternatively**, an intravenous catheter and introducer needle complex may be entered through a separate puncture site (Fig. 13-1E).
9. **Once the catheter is advanced**, the blood is allowed to back-bleed from the cannula, which is then connected to the intravenous tubing.

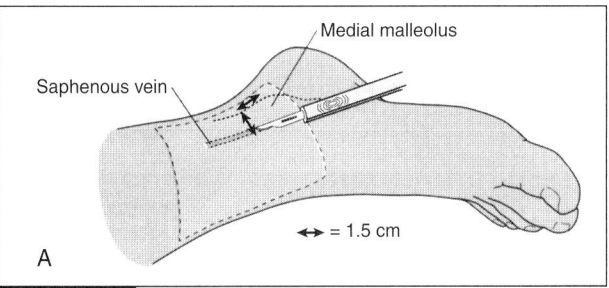

FIGURE 13-1A

Saphenous vein cutdown procedure. See text for details.

II. Saphenous Vein Cutdown

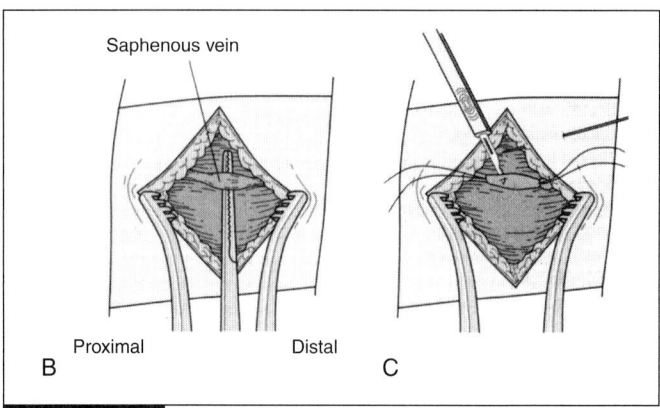

FIGURE 13-1B&C
Saphenous vein cutdown procedure. See text for details.

10. **The proximal ligature** is then tied around the vessel and cannula, and the distal ligature is tied down as well.
11. **The skin is then closed** with nylon suture and the catheter is secured to the skin. A sterile dressing is placed over the catheter site (Fig. 13-1F).

E. Complications and treatment

1. **Wound infection**. Remove the catheter, and give/apply appropriate antimicrobial agents.

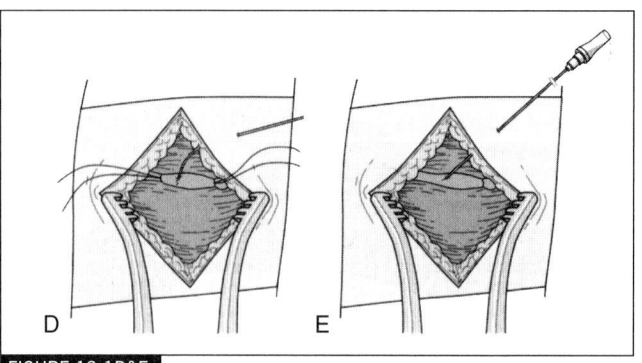

FIGURE 13-1D&E
Saphenous vein cutdown procedure. See text for details.

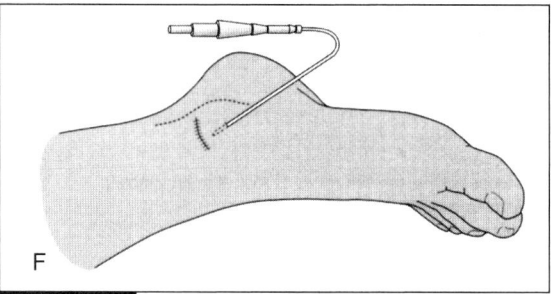

FIGURE 13-1F

Completed saphenous vein cutdown procedure.

2. **Thrombophlebitis.** Remove the catheter. Apply a warm compress and elevate the leg. Antimicrobial agents may be indicated in select circumstances. Vein excision is indicated with suppuration.
3. **Hematoma.** The hematoma is incised and drained.
4. **Failure of wound healing.** This is common in diabetic patients with vascular compromise and is treated with topical dressings. Angiography and revascularization procedures are occasionally indicated.

III. CENTRAL VENOUS CATHETERIZATION

A. Indications
1. Monitoring of resuscitation and central venous pressures
2. Occasionally used for volume resuscitation

B. Anatomy
1. **Subclavian vein**
   a. The subclavian vein begins as a continuation of the axillary vein at the outer edge of the first rib and subsequently joins the internal jugular vein to become the innominate vein.
   b. The subclavian vein lies in close approximation to the posterior border of the medial third of the clavicle.
   c. It is at this point that access to the subclavian vein is simplest and safest via the supraclavicular or infraclavicular approaches (Fig. 13-2).
   d. The advantages of accessing the subclavian vein are catheter stability, patient comfort, and ease of care of the catheter.
2. **Internal jugular vein**
   a. The internal jugular vein emerges from beneath the apex of the two heads of the sternocleidomastoid muscle high in the lateral aspect of the neck.

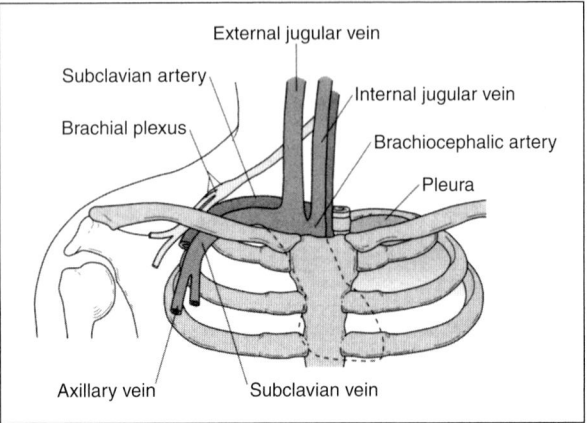

FIGURE 13-2

Subclavian vein and local anatomy.

  b. It proceeds inferiorly to join the subclavian vein behind the medial third of the clavicle.
  c. In the lower cervical region, where access is to be gained, the common carotid artery lies medial and deep to the internal jugular vein in a paratracheal location.
  d. The advantages of accessing the internal jugular vein are that this does not impede cardiopulmonary resusciation and it has a direct route to the heart.
3. **Femoral vein**
  a. The femoral vein is located 1 cm medial to the arterial pulsations. If no palpable pulse is present, locate the femoral vein at the point midway between the anterior spine of the ilium and the pubic tubercule.
C. Central venous catheters. There are three main types of intravenous access systems.
1. **Catheter-over-the-needle technique**. There are two disadvantages to this technique.
  a. First, once blood return is achieved, the catheter itself may still be outside the vessel. This will result in the catheter pushing the vein in front of it and never entering the lumen.
  b. Second, a 14-gauge catheter requires a 14-gauge needle introducer, which is less than ideal when accessing vessels in the chest and neck region.
2. **Catheter-through-the-needle technique**. The main disadvantage of this technique is the risk of catheter shearing and embolism if attempts are made to withdraw it through the needle.

III. Central Venous Catheterization

3. **Seldinger guide-wire technique**, described here, offers rapid access without the aforementioned risks.

D. Technique

1. **Subclavian access:** infraclavicular approach
   a. Prepare the area widely with antiseptic solution and drape the neck and shoulder region with sterile towels. Place the patient in the Trendelenburg position, with the head down 10° to 15°. Some people find it helpful to place a shoulder roll under the patient, but this is optional.
   b. The point of entry is generally the junction of the middle and medial thirds of the clavicle. In the conscious patient, the point of entry is anesthetized with 1% lidocaine along with subcutaneous infiltration of the tissue to the periosteum of the clavicle.
   c. Align the bevel of the needle inferiorly to direct the guide wire toward the innominate vein.
   d. Place the left index finger on the suprasternal notch to facilitate as a reference point for the direction of needle (Fig. 13-3).
   e. Insert the introducer needle at the entry site approximately 2 cm inferior to the clavicle and aim for the superior aspect of the left index finger. A backflash of blood usually occurs at a depth of 3 to 4 cm. At this point detach the syringe and cover the needle hub with the thumb to prevent an air embolus.

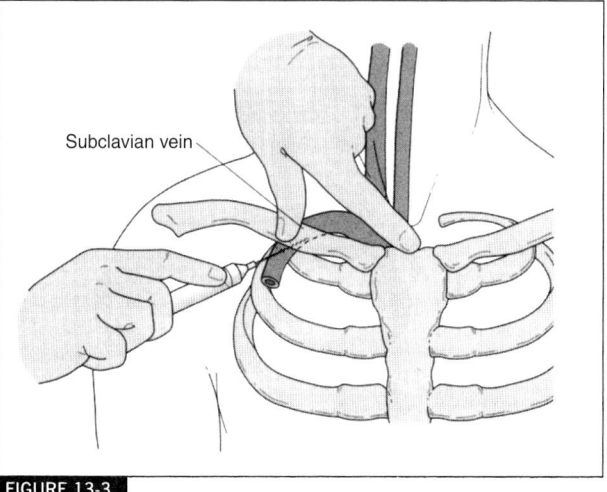

FIGURE 13-3

Hand position during subclavian venipuncture.

f. The J-wire is then advanced into the needle, using the introducer sleeve. The wire should thread smoothly until at least one-fourth of the wire is within the subclavian vein.
   g. The sleeve and introducer needle are subsequently removed, leaving only the guide wire in the vessel.
   h. A small incision is made at the entry site of the wire, approximately the size of the catheter to be introduced. When a standard central venous catheter is used, a dilator may be used first to introduce the catheter into the vessel over the guide wire.
   i. The catheter is secured in place using either 2-0 silk or nylon suture to prevent dislodgement. Antibacterial ointment is placed over the entrance site and the wound is dressed.
2. **Subclavian access–supraclavicular approach**. The main advantage to the supraclavicular approach is evident during cardiac arrest situations, because the operator is located away from the area of sternal compression (Fig. 13-4).
   a. Prepare, drape, and infiltrate the site of entry over the lower neck region.
   b. The point of entry is identified 1 cm lateral to the clavicular head of the sternocleidomastoid and 1 cm posterior to the clavicle.
   c. The introducer needle is held 10 to 15° above the horizontal, pointing toward the contralateral nipple.
   d. Successful access into the vessel occurs at a depth of 2 to 3 cm.
   e. The remainder of the supraclavicular access using the Seldinger technique is the same as described for the infraclavicular approach.
3. **Internal jugular access–central approach**
   a. In this approach, as in all three methods of internal jugular cannulation, the patient is placed in the Trendelenburg position with the head turned away from the side of access.
   b. The patient's neck is prepared with an antiseptic solution and draped with sterile towels, as with all vascular access techniques.
   c. The point of entry is identified by locating the apex of the triangle formed by the two heads of the sternocleidomastoid muscle and the clavicle (Fig. 13-5). In the conscious patient, this area is infiltrated with 1% lidocaine solution.
   d. The carotid pulse is then palpated with the left hand when attempting a right-sided approach, and the needle is retracted medially away from the point of entry.
   e. The needle is directed 30° to 40° off the spine plane, aiming for the ipsilateral nipple. The internal jugular vein is usually found at a depth of 1 to 1.5 cm. A depth of 4 cm should not be exceeded, as this increases the risk for pneumothorax.
   f. Once access to the vein is achieved, the Seldinger wire technique is carried out as noted in the section on infraclavicular access (see above).
4. **Internal jugular access–anterior approach**
   a. The anterior approach to internal jugular cannulation is very similar to the central approach with the exception of the location of entry and direction of the needle travel.

III. Central Venous Catheterization

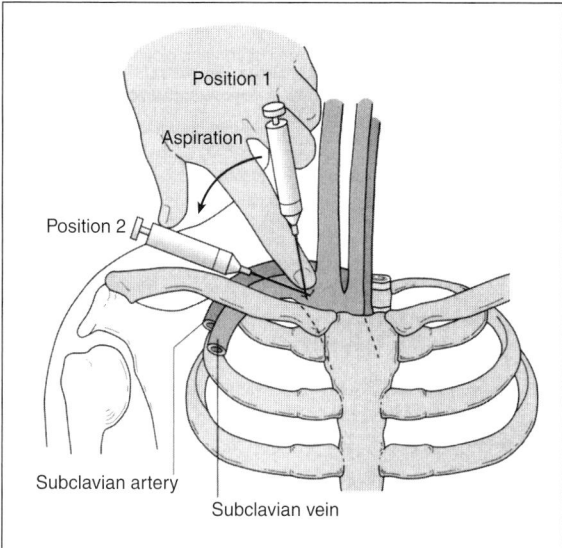

FIGURE 13-4
The junction of subclavian vein and internal jugular vein can be punctured supraclavicularly by advancing the needle medial to the inner edge of the first rib. This junction is larger than either vein and it can be distended further by asking the patient to do a Valsalva maneuver in a forced-expiration phase. The needle is advanced gradually with a constant negative pressure in the syringe. Once a blood flow is obtained, the needle is stabilized to prevent further advancement and entry into the pleural space. The catheter is then inserted. This technique should be avoided on the left side in cirrhotic patients.

    b. The carotid artery is palpated with the left hand with a right-handed attempt, and it is retracted medially.
    c. The needle entry point is along the medial border of the sternocleidomastoid at its midpoint.
    d. The needle is held 30° to 45° off the spine plane, aiming toward the ipsilateral nipple.
    e. After blood return is established, the remainder of the procedure is the same as described previously.
5. **Internal jugular access–posterior approach**
    a. The posterior approach differs primarily in the location of entry and the direction at which the needle travels.
    b. The skin is entered along the lateral aspect of the sternocleidomastoid approximately one third of the distance from the clavicle to the mastoid

III. Central Venous Catheterization

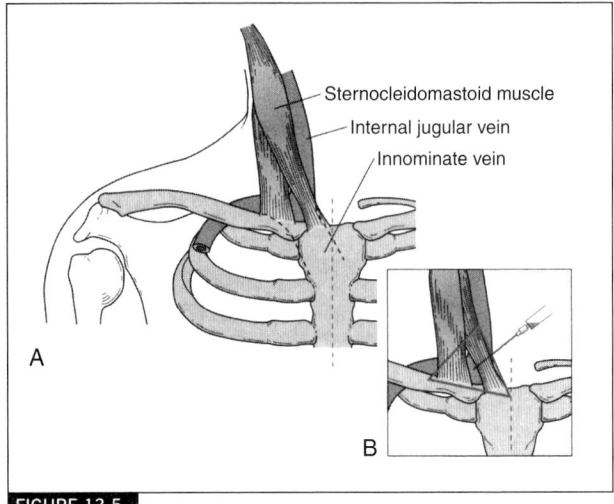

FIGURE 13-5

Central approach to internal jugular vein. (A) Relationship of sternocleidomastoid muscle to chest. (B) Course of internal jugular vein; note its sagittal course.

   process, or at the level of the two heads of the sternocleidomastoid, aiming toward the sternal notch until blood return is obtained.
   c. After this is performed, simply follow the steps in the Seldinger wire technique described previously (Fig. 13-6).
6. **Femoral vein access–Seldinger technique**
   a. Prepare the entire groin area with povidone-iodine (Betadine) antiseptic solution and drape with either sterile towels or a prepackaged sterile paper drape.
   b. Palpate the femoral artery 1 cm below the inguinal ligament. The femoral vein is located 1 cm medial to the arterial pulsations. If no palpable pulse is present, locate the femoral vein at the point midway between the anterior spine of the ilium and the pubic tubercule.
   c. Anesthetize the skin and subcutaneous tissue over the femoral vein using 1% lidocaine.
   d. With the 16-gauge introducer needle held at a 45° angle, advance the needle cephalad until a flash of blood is obtained at a depth of 1.5 to 2 cm.
   e. The syringe is removed from the needle hub and the guide wire is threaded into the vein for at least one third to half its length.
   f. A No. 11 blade is then used to incise the skin; subsequently, a dilator is used to dilate the subcutaneous tissue. The guide

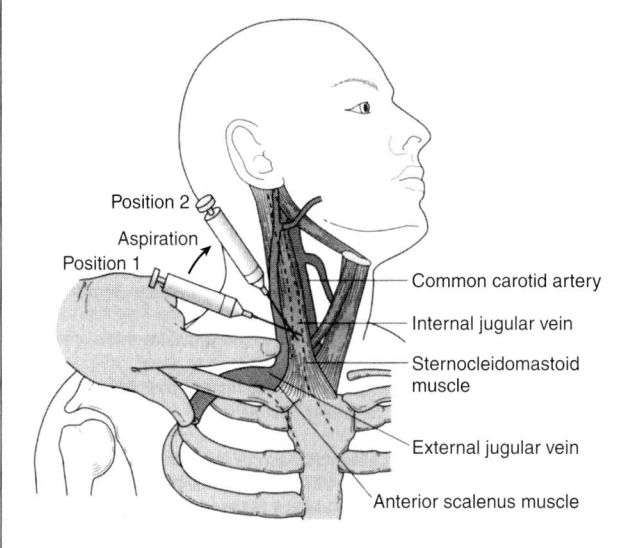

FIGURE 13-6

Illustration of the internal jugular puncture from the posterior border of the sternocleidomastoid muscle. The neck is turned 45° to the opposite side. The needle is inserted at the posterior border of the sternocleidomastoid muscle and advanced at a 45° angle to this border and 45° to the surface of the body. A gentle and constant negative pressure created by a syringe attached to the needle reveals the vein entry (position 1).

wire should be visualized and controlled at all times to prevent embolization.

g. The 16-gauge catheter is then threaded into the femoral vein over the guide wire, which is then removed. Blood is allowed to back bleed through the catheter prior to connecting the catheter to the intravenous tubing.

h. The catheter is secured in place using either 2-0 silk or nylon suture to prevent dislodgement. Antibacterial ointment is placed over the entrance site and the is wound dressed.

E. Pulmonary artery catheter

1. **Indications.** The American Society of Anesthesiologists practice guidelines published in 2003 indicate pulmonary artery catheter monitoring is appropriate or necessary, or both, in the following:

    a. Selected surgical patients undergoing procedures associated with a high risk of complications from hemodynamic changes (e.g., cardiac surgery)

b. In those with advanced cardiopulmonary diseases who would be at increased risk for adverse perioperative events because of their preoperative medical condition

2. **Complications**
    a. Arrhythmias, ventricular fibrillation, right bundle branch block, complete heart block
    b. Catheter insertion-related complications; mechanical complications such as catheter knots
    c. Thromboembolism
    d. Pulmonary infarction
    e. Infection, endocarditis
    f. Endocardial damage, cardiac valve injury
    g. Pulmonary artery rupture, pulmonary artery pseudoaneurysm
    h. Misinterpretation of data, misuse of equipment

F. Ultrasound guidance. The use of ultrasound to locate the vein for access is becoming a common approach to central line placement in difficult to access patients.

1. There are several commonly accepted variations of US guidance: indirect, direct or real-time, and mechanical guide.
    a. Indirect simply uses the ultrasound guidance to locate and mark the vein to be cannulated. However, the indirect method has not had an effect on the rate of complications or failures.
    b. Direct, or real-time, ultrasound guidance involves continuous visualization during the entire procedure. The transducer is placed on the skin and the target vessel is identified and centered on the viewing screen. With the other hand, the cannulation needle is advanced through the skin. There is improved success rate with this technique.
    c. A mechanical guide is an attachment to the ultrasound transducer that controls the depth, angle, and trajectory of the needle during cannulation. Otherwise, this method is the same as the direct method. The use of mechanical guides has some notable disadvantages, such as the need for investing in an additional piece of equipment, bulkier equipment, restriction off the angle of the needle, and lastly, the fixed angle of entry may make some superficial structures difficult to access. Studies claim 100% accuracy.

2. **Ultrasound-guided central line placement** is easiest to perform in the internal jugular vein and femoral vein. The subclavian vein is noted to have an increased level of difficulty and has a greater variability of success, depending on operator experience.

G. Complications and treatment

1. **Overview**
    a. The complication rate of subclavian vein catheterization has generally ranged from 0.3% to 18.8% in most series, depending on the site of insertion, patient population, and definition of complications.

b. The main complications are related to the structures that surround the subclavian vein.
   c. Pneumothorax is reported as the most frequent complication of both subclavian and internal jugular cannulation.
   d. This highlights the importance of obtaining a chest radiograph following all attempts at vascular access because up to 20% of pneumothoraces may not be clinically detectable.
   e. The remainder of the complications associated with internal jugular catheterizations are similar to those with subclavian access.
2. **Pulmonary complications**
   a. For pneumothorax, hemothorax, hydrothorax, or chylothorax, a chest tube needs to be inserted for drainage or evacuation.
   b. For hemomediastinum or hydromediastinum, observation, angiography, or exploration may be indicated for progressive hemomediastinum. Most cases will resolve spontaneously without intervention.
   c. Tracheal perforation–observation in the absence of airway compromise.
   d. Endotracheal cuff perforation–exchange endotracheal tube if air leak compromises adequate ventilation.
   e. Intrathoracic catheter fragmentation–requires retrieval of fragment by fluoroscopy.
3. **Infectious complications**
   a. Generalized sepsis and local cellulitis–requires catheter removal and treatment with appropriate antimicrobial agents.
   b. Osteomyelitis and septic arthritis–requires debridement, drainage, and adequate antimicrobial therapy.
   c. Catheter sepsis is the most common complication of long-term catheter use. The incidence varies depending on the definition of catheter infection. Routine catheter changes every 72 hours can reduce the incidence of catheter infection when combined with a protocol for catheter care. However, this must be balanced against the risks of mechanical complications during multiple catheter insertions. At Parkland Memorial Hospital, catheters are not routinely changed every 72 hours in the intensive care unit, except in the burn unit.
4. **Neurologic complications**. These complications usually resolve with observation but occasionally will require nerve repair.
   a. Phrenic nerve injury
   b. Brachial plexus injury
5. **Vascular complications**
   a. Air embolus usually occurs during insertion of central lines. These patients undergo acute hemodynamic compromise and exhibit signs of acute heart failure. A continuous murmur is sometimes audible over the heart. Treatment is commenced by administering 100% oxygen, placing the patient in the left lateral decubitus position (right side up), and attempting to aspirate the air out of the right atrium using the same central line.

b. Subclavian artery puncture responds to manual compression in the supraclavicular region. If this is unsuccessful, or if the hematoma is expanding, exploration and repair of the arteriotomy are indicated. Pulse or pressure deficits in the arms are also an indication for vascular exploration.
c. Pericardial tamponade is treated expediently by pericardiocentesis and emergency sternotomy with repair of the vascular injury.
d. Septic thrombophlebitis is frequently fatal and associated with generalized sepsis. These patients are initially treated with antimicrobial agents. In severe cases, excision of the vein may be necessary.
e. Catheter embolus is a potentially fatal complication. Fortunately, most catheter fragments can be retrieved using fluoroscopy.
f. Arteriovenous fistula is treated by coil embolization or surgical ligation of the fistula. Distal emboli, high-output cardiac failure, or distal ischemic symptoms are all indications for intervention.
g. Superior vena cava thrombosis is managed by heparinization and ambulatory anticoagulation for 3 to 6 months. Serial duplex examinations will confirm recanalization of these vessels, which is the norm.
h. Advancement of the guide wire too far can lead to the wire catching on intravascular hardware (e.g., IVC filter), requiring fluoroscopic assisted retrieval. When meeting resistance and unsure of the diagnosis, a chest radiograph and abdominal flat plate film can aid in diagnosis.

6. **Miscellaneous complications**
   a. **Dysrhythmias** (atrial and ventricular) are treated by removal of the offending catheter. Hemodynamic instability will require antiarrhymic agents or electric cardioversion.
   b. **Ascites** is managed nonoperatively with diuretics and sodium restriction.
   c. **Catheter knotting** may be managed by untying the knot under fluoroscopy. Rarely is surgery required to remove the knot.
   d. **Catheter malposition** is treated by removing and replacing the catheter. Never advance a catheter after initial placement and securing in place.

H. Pearls and pitfalls

1. **Central access does not guarantee adequate flow**. Flow rates through a peripheral 2-inch, 14-gauge catheter are approximately twice that of a centrally located 8-inch, 16-gauge catheter under identical pressure situations.
2. **The 8 French introducer (cordis)** is a useful tool for rapid infusion.
3. **The guide wire must be controlled at all times** while introducing the dilator, intravenous catheter, or dilator-introducer sheath combination. This is performed by always controlling the distal end of the wire before introducing these into the vessel. Once the vessel is dilated, either the catheter or the introducer sheath may be advanced over the wire into the vessel.
4. **Connect to the infusion port** once blood is allowed to back bleed from the catheter or introducer sheath.
5. **Always obtain a chest radiograph** even after unsuccessful attempts to cannulate a central vein.

IV. URINARY CATHETERS

A. Indications
1. Frequent monitoring of urine output
2. Decompression of the bladder prior to peritoneal lavage
3. Neurogenic injury resulting in inability to void spontaneously
4. Urine collection facilitating diagnosis of hematuria (see, Contraindications)

B. Types of catheters
1. The **Foley catheter** is the most common. Sizes 16 French or 18 French are those most commonly used in adults. The higher the number, the larger the size (1 French is equal to 0.33 mm).
2. **Coude-tip catheter** is used primarily to negotiate the difficult male prostatic urethra when a round-tip Foley catheter will not pass and prostatic hypertrophy is suspected.

C. Contraindications to urethral catheterization in trauma patients
1. **Signs of suspected urethral injury**, such as scrotal hematoma, blood at the male urethral meatus, or a high-riding or free-floating prostate on rectal examination
2. **Known or suspected fracture** of the inferior pelvic ring
3. **Perineal hematomas**. A rectal examination must always be performed prior to insertion of a urinary catheter in patients with any possibility of urethral injury.

D. Pitfalls
1. **Urine must be visualized** in tubing prior to balloon inflation.
2. **Insertion of the full length of the catheter** is recommended to ensure placement into the bladder and to avoid inflation of the balloon in the prostatomembranous urethra.
3. **If the patient is uncircumcised**, replace the foreskin to prevent paraphimosis.
4. **Tape the catheter loosely** to medial aspect of the thigh to avoid dislodgment.

V. NASOGASTRIC TUBES

A. Indications
1. Gastrointestinal decompression to prevent aspiration
2. Identification of injury to the upper gastrointestinal tract
3. Decompression of the stomach prior to peritoneal lavage

B. Contraindications
1. **Known or suspected midface fractures**. The nasogastric tube may be inserted through a disrupted cribiform plate into the cranium.
2. **Suspected vascular neck injuries**. The coughing and retching caused by the nasogastric tube insertion may cause hemorrhage from a previously nonbleeding arterial injury.

C. Types of nasogastric tubes

1. **Levin**. Single-lumen tube with perforated tip and side-holes. This tube enables aspiration of gastric contents.
2. **Salem sump**. Double-lumen tube with irrigation and air-intake ports, allowing continuous tube decompression. This tube is superior for gastric lavage.
3. **Dobhoff**. Single-lumen duodenal feeding tube. Placing the tube distal to the pylorus decreases the risk of aspiration of food in obtunded patients.

VI. CLOSED-TUBE THORACOSTOMY DRAINAGE

A. Indications

1. **Pneumothorax**. If a chest radiograph is not immediately available, trauma to one side of the chest associated with decreased or absent breath sounds or hypotension should be treated urgently with either needle thoracentesis or a chest tube.
2. **Hemothorax**
3. **Empyema**
4. **Chylothorax**

B. Technique for insertion of a chest tube

1. **Site of insertion**. Identify the fifth or sixth intercostal space in the midaxillary line. Feel for the space between the pectoralis and the latissimus muscles. This can be done quickly and will consistently place the chest tube above the diaphragm.
2. **Prepare the skin** with iodine solution and drape in a sterile fashion.
3. **Anesthetize** with 1% to 2% lidocaine with epinephrine. Create a skin weal to mark the site, and then fan out over subcutaneous tissue and to the top of the target rib.
4. **Use a scalpel** to create an incision large enough for fingers and chest tube (Fig. 13-7A).
5. **Tunnel up one to two ribs** from the margin (especially important in thin patients) to create a soft tissue cover that will occlude the hole when the chest tube is removed.
6. **Dissect over the top of the selected rib** with a large Kelly clamp (Fig. 13-7B). Open it widely after it has penetrated the intercostal muscles and pleural space. This can require significant pressure to be applied. In the case of a flail chest or multiple rib fractures, curved heavy Mayo scissors may be used in place of the Kelly clamp to enter the pleural space. The index finger should be inserted to confirm entry into the pleural space, to break up loculations or adhesions, and to demonstrate proper path of the tract.
7. **The chest tube** can then be placed in the Kelly clamp and guided into the pleural space (Fig. 13-7C). Clamp the distal end of the tube to prevent spill of fluid.

VI. Closed-Tube Thoracostomy Drainage

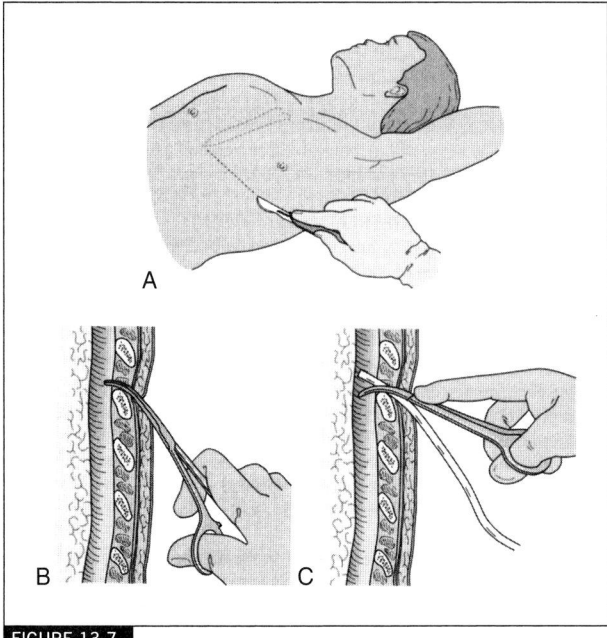

FIGURE 13-7

Technique for closed-tube thoracostomy. See text for details.

8. **Movement of fluid and air** in the tube with respiration should be noted.
9. **Position the tube posteriorly** and attach tubing to suction and drainage device. Unclamp the tube.
10. **Close the incision** and secure the tube to the chest wall with a 2-0 silk or nylon suture. Apply sterile dressing.
11. **Each day the system should be monitored** for volume of drainage, air leak, presence of respiratory fluctuations, and need for continued suction.

C. Removal of chest tube

1. **Materials**. Suture removal kit, 4×4 gauze, petrolatum gauze, and wide tape
2. **Technique**. Prepare a dressing with tape, 4×4 gauze with petrolatum gauze prior to pulling out the chest tube. Cut all suture holding the chest tube to the patient. Instruct the patient to take a deep breath and hold it as the tube is quickly removed. Quickly cover the entrance site with the prepared dressing to avoid creating a new pneumothorax. Obtain a chest radiograph following tube removal.

D. Complications and treatments
1. **Lung injury** is treated by tube removal and replacement.
2. **Diaphragm injury** is an indication for operative therapy and repair.
3. **Intraabdominal solid organ injury** (e.g., liver, spleen) is treated by tube removal. Continuing hemorrhage from the injured organ is treated by operation and repair.
4. **Retained hemothorax or empyema** is a common complication of inadequate chest tube drainage. If the retained fluid is accessible, a second chest tube might provide complete drainage. However, most of these fluid collections are loculated or clotted, in which case thoracoscopy or thoracotomy and decortication will be necessary. The presence of fever and leukocytosis associated with an undrained thoracic collection is an indication for thoracoscopy or thoracotomy.
5. **Persistent pneumothorax or air leak**. In the absence of any leaks in the tubing and connection system, this is most likely due to an inadequately evacuated pneumothorax, parenchymal leaks from pulmonary lacerations, or large airway injuries. Air leaks can be managed with additional chest tubes; however, failure of these leaks to seal will require thoracoscopy and repair of parenchymal injuries.
6. **Rib fractures** will heal with adequate pain control.

VII. SUGGESTED READINGS

Abboud PA, Kendall JL: Ultrasound guidance for vascular access. Emergency Med Clin North Am 22(3), 2004.

Bund J, Maki D: Infections caused by arterial catheters used for hemodynamic monitoring. Am J Med 67:735, 1979.

Deitch EA: Tools of the Trade and Rules of the Road: A Surgical Guide. Philadelphia, Lippincott Williams & Wilkins, 1997.

Etheredge E: Management and Techniques in Surgery. New York, Wiley, 1986, pp 399-402.

Gomella LG, Braen GR, Olding M: Clinician's Pocket Reference. Garden Grove, Prentice-Hall; 1981.

Lawrence PF: Essentials of General Surgery. Philadelphia, Lippincott Williams & Wilkins, 1999.

Miller RD: Miller's Anesthesia, 6th ed. Philadelphia, Churchill Livingstone, 2005

Orland MJ, Saltman RJ: Manual of Medical Therapeutics. Boston, Little, Brown, 1981.

Parks SN: Initial assessment of the trauma patient. In Moore EE, Mattox KL, Feliciano DV (eds): Trauma, 5th ed. East Norwalk, Appleton & Lange, 2004.

Damage Control Surgery

Craig Olson, MD, and
Alexander L. Eastman, MD

I. INTRODUCTION

Poor outcomes with immediate, definitive, operative management of massive multisystem trauma have led to the search for a more effective treatment strategy. At Parkland Memorial Hospital, the principle of damage control surgery (DCS) has been adopted in settings of massive injury requiring surgical intervention and significant physiologic derangement.

II. FUNDAMENTALS OF DAMAGE CONTROL SURGERY

A. Identification of significant metabolic derangement
B. Immediate, abbreviated laparotomy with the following goals:
1. Control hemorrhage.
2. Control contamination.
3. Perform temporary abdominal closure (TAC).

C. Deliberate delay to allow for resuscitation and correction of metabolic derangements

III. PATHOPHYSIOLOGY

Metabolic derangements in the severely injured patient lead to poor outcomes when associated with significant, long operative interventions. These pathophysiologic alterations include the following:

A. Hypothermia
1. Sympathetic surge associated with trauma leads to peripheral vasoconstriction, end organ hypoperfusion, and the development of acidosis associated with an anaerobic metabolism.
2. Large intravenous fluid requirements lead to rapid cooling of core body temperature when fluids are not warmed.

B. Coagulopathy
1. Multisystem trauma leads to a consumptive coagulopathy.
2. Clotting factors are diluted through fluid resuscitation.
3. Hypothermia and acidosis reduce the effectiveness of clotting factors.

C. Acidosis
1. Measured by base deficit and lactate levels
2. Secondary to hypoperfusion

IV. STAGES OF DAMAGE CONTROL

Damage control surgery (DCS) is divided into four distinctive stages: the decision to perform DCS, the operation, intensive care unit resuscitation, and second-look/definitive operation.

A. Decision to perform DCS
1. Preoperative decision to perform a DCS procedure is frequently made in patients with multisystem trauma.
2. Absolute indications for DCS:
   a. Base deficit >8 mEq/L or worsening base deficit
   b. pH < 7.2
   c. Hypotension < 90 mm Hg systolic
   d. Hypothermia < 34° C
   e. PTT > 60 seconds
   f. Operative "clinical" coagulopathy
3. Early recognition of significant physiologic derangement and the need for DCS are critical as inability to correct pH >7.21 and PTT >70 is associated with near certain mortality.
4. Initial resuscitation should begin in the emergency department and continue in the operating room following correction of deficit and using a massive transfusion program as indicated.

B. DCS operative principles
1. The goal of DCS is a short operating time, followed by transport to an intensive care unit.
2. Control of hemorrhage
   a. Ligation of named vascular structures may be necessary and/or temporary vascular clamps may be used.
   b. Vascular shunting may be employed in extremities using surgical shunts, such as a Javid shunt or large-bore IV tubing.
   c. Abdominal packing: packs are inserted into the right upper quadrant, left upper quadrant, and pelvis. The bowel should be separated from laparotomy pads.
3. Control of contamination
   a. Bowel injuries may be quickly closed or resected with stapled ends left in discontinuity.
   b. Delay definitive repair of injury including time-consuming anastomoses and ostomies.
4. Prevent hypothermia.
   a. Warm operating room.
   b. All resuscitation fluids and blood products must be warmed to 38.0° C or higher.
   c. Continuous use of convective warming devices (e.g., Bair huggers)
5. Temporary abdominal closure (TAC)
   a. Allows "easy access" for planned next operative intervention
   b. At Parkland Memorial Hospital, the "Vac-Pack" dressing is employed by packing the abdomen with laparotomy pads separated from the

bowel with a fluid-impervious layer (e.g., a "bogota bag or bowel bag). TAC dressing-specific drains are then placed in the packing, and a seal is created over the wound with the use of loban dressing. These drains are then connected to wall suction. (Note: Commercially available dressings have been made that accomplish the same goal with less "improvisation" but they are not as cost-effective.)
  c. Additional abdominal drains may be used as well.
  d. Because of its ease of application, the Vac-Pack dressing allows bedside changes in the intensive care unit.
6. Angiography/embolization
  a. If pelvic bleeding is suspected, the patient may be transferred to the angiography suite at this time. Significant hepatic parenchymal hemorrhage may also be controlled with angiography.

C. Restoration of homeostasis in the intensive care unit
1. Rewarming
  a. Warm room temperature and other convective measures of warming, such as warming blankets and lamps, are used to maintain body temperature >35° C.
  b. Use of fluid warmer for administration of resuscitative crystalloids and blood products is mandatory.
  c. Continuous arteriovenous rewarming (CAVR) is occasionally performed when body temperature is less than 35° C.
2. Careful fluid resuscitation
  a. Resuscitation may be guided by early use of a pulmonary artery catheter.
  b. If massive bleeding resumes, the patient is returned emergently to the operating room for cessation of likely surgical bleeding.
  c. Avoid over-resuscitation.
  d. Monitor bladder pressure. Bladder pressures >20 mm Hg should raise concern for intra-abdominal hypertension (IAH) and >30 mm Hg for abdominal compartment syndrome (ACS).
3. Ventilatory support
  a. If possible, maintain tidal volumes at 6 mL/kg ideal body weight.
  b. If unable to oxygenate with conventional ventilation, at Parkland Memorial Hospital we use the Volume Diffuse Respirator (VDR) as a salvage therapy.
4. Negative fluid balance
  a. When physiologic balance is restored, natural mobilization of third space fluids may be aided with a continuous furosemide drip, titrated to a net negative balance per hour.
  b. This facilitates abdominal wall closure.

C. Definitive operative intervention
1. Ideally performed at 24 to 36 hours, later if indications of physiologic derangement persist
2. Removal of packs, with replacement if necessary
3. Secondary survey of the abdomen: missed injuries at the time of damage control surgery are not uncommon.

4. Restoration of gastrointestinal and vascular continuity if necessary
5. Performance of other definitive procedures, such as ostomy placement
6. Abdominal closure if possible. If bowel edema prevents this, several techniques (e.g., Wittman patch) can be employed to help reapproximate fascial edges in stages.
7. Multiple "second-looks" may be needed.

V. SUGGESTED READING

Sugrue M, et al: Damage control surgery and the abdomen. Injury 35: 642-648, 2004.

Neurologic Trauma

Kelly Schmidt, MD

I. INTRODUCTION

A. Traumatic brain injury (TBI) is the leading cause of trauma-related death in the United States. Approximately 500,000 new cases of TBI are seen in emergency departments each year.

B. Approximately 5% of patients with severe TBI will have an associated spinal cord injury (SCI). Additionally, there are approximately 10,000 new cases of SCI without TBI per year.

C. Primary brain injury occurs as a direct result of the initial trauma and its incidence can only be impacted by aggressive public health and prevention campaigns.

D. Secondary brain injury occurs as a result of hypoxia, hypotension, cerebral ischemia, cerebral blood flow alterations, cerebral edema, or intracranial hypertension. All treatment modalities (starting in the pre-hospital setting) are aimed at preventing these secondary insults.

E. In 2000, the Brain Trauma Foundation updated the preexisting evidence-based practice guidelines on the management of TBI.

1. Only three recommendations had the Class I supporting evidence necessary to be labeled a practice standard. They are:
   a. Prolonged hyperventilation therapy ($PaCO_2$ <25 mm Hg) should be avoided.
   b. Steroids do not improve outcome or reduce intracranial pressure in patients with severe head injury.
   c. Prophylactic antiseizure medication does not prevent late post-traumatic seizure disorder.

II. INITIAL EVALUATION

All patients, regardless of level of consciousness, should be evaluated with the ATLS algorithm.

A. Primary survey

1. During the disability portion, a rapid determination of the patient's level of consciousness, pupillary size and reactivity, and gross motor function in all extremities is performed.

   a. **Glasgow Coma Scale (GCS)**
      i. The GCS is an objective method of rapidly assessing a patient's level of consciousness (Table 15-1).
      ii. The GCS allows the classification of head injuries as follows:
         (a) Mild = GCS 13 to15
         (b) Moderate = GCS 9 to 12
         (c) Severe = GCS 3 to 8

TABLE 15-1
GLASGOW COMA SCALE

Reaction	Score
Eyes open	
Spontaneously	4
To verbal command	3
To pain	2
No response	1
Best motor response	
To verbal command	
Obeys	6
To painful stimulus	
Localizes pain	5
Flexion withdrawal	4
Flexion abnormal	3
Extension	2
No response	1
Best verbal response	
Oriented and converses	5
Disoriented and converses	4
Inappropriate words	3
Incomprehensible	2
No response	1
Total score	3-15

Patients with a GCS < 8 require both definitive control of their airway and intracranial pressure (ICP) monitoring.

   iii. The GCS motor score is the most reliable and one of the most important prognostic indicators along with age and pupillary reactivity.
      (a) 6 = Obeys verbal commands.
      (b) 5 = Localizes pain. The patient acknowledges a central painful stimulus and moves toward its location in an attempt to remove it, generally crossing midline in so doing.
      (c) 4 = Flexion withdrawal. The patient has a clear response to pain, but it is not directed at removing the stimulus. This is often only apparent when stimulating a distal extremity.
      (d) 3 = Decorticate posturing (abnormal flexion). In response to a painful stimulus the patient strongly flexes the upper extremities and extends the lower extremities symmetrically. This is indicative of a rostral brainstem injury.
      (e) 2 = Decerebrate posturing (also called extending). In response to a painful stimulus the patient extends and internally rotates the arms while flexing the wrists and fingers and extending the lower extremities. This is indicative of a caudal brainstem injury.
      (f) 1 = No motor response. This requires evaluation for spinal cord injury.

iv. Patients who are intubated receive a GCS verbal score of 1 and the overall score is denoted with a "T" (e.g., GCS 10T).

B. Secondary survey

1. A more detailed neurologic examination is performed that includes cranial nerve evaluation and complete motor and sensory examination of the extremities.
   a. **Cranial nerve (CN) examination**
      i. CN I (olfactory) is rarely tested in the acute setting. Anosmia can be associated with occipital trauma as a result of a contrecoup injury.
      ii. CN II (optic) is the most important to evaluate. The classic, unilateral, fixed and dilated pupil is reflective of uncal herniation. Pupils that are slightly asymmetric with the larger pupil reacting sluggishly to light may be an early sign of herniation. This demands immediate investigation.
         (a) Traumatic mydriasis is a purely ocular injury, which yields a fixed and dilated pupil secondary to local trauma to the orbit and globe.
      iii. CN III, IV, and VI (oculomotor, trochlear, and abducens) are the nerves responsible for extraocular movements in the six cardinal fields of gaze. Limitation of movement may suggest extraocular muscle entrapment, particularly in patients with significant facial trauma.
      iv. CN VII (facial) is often at risk for peripheral injury resulting in facial weakness in patients with temporal bone fractures.
      v. CN VIII (vestibular) may also be at risk for peripheral injury in patients with temporal bone or other basilar skull fractures causing tinnitus or hearing loss.
      vi. CN IX, X, XI, and XII (glossopharyngeal, vagus, spinal accessory, and hypoglossal). Patients suffering basilar skull fractures severe enough to affect these lower cranial nerves frequently succumb to their head injuries.
2. Close examination of the scalp, head, and face can help identify open wounds (which can be the source of significant blood loss), depressed skull fractures, and signs of basilar skull fractures.
   a. Clinical diagnosis of basilar skull fractures
      i. CSF otorrhea or rhinorrhea
      ii. Hemotympanum or lacerations of the external auditory canal
      iii. Bilateral periorbital ecchymoses (racoon's eyes)
      iv. Postauricular ecchymoses (Battle's sign)
      v. Cranial nerve deficit as described above

III. IMAGING STUDIES

A. Computed tomography (CT)

1. An urgent CT scan of the head is obtained after completion of the secondary survey in any patient with an altered level of consciousness or signs of significant trauma located above the clavicles.

2. CT allows evaluation of the brain parenchyma as well as the bony anatomy of the skull.
3. CT scans allow decisions for operative versus observational management.
4. When the initial CT scan identifies hemorrhage, a repeat scan is performed 6 hours later to evaluate evolution of the intracranial injury. Over 50% of head-injured patients demonstrate new findings on early repeat CT scans.

B. Angiography
1. CT angiography is faster and less invasive than catheter angiography and in our experience has been as effective in identifying traumatic vascular injuries.
2. Delayed catheter angiography may be considered for endovascular treatment of identified vascular injuries.
3. Indications for angiography include:
    a. Extensive basal cistern subarachnoid hemorrhage
    b. Basilar skull fractures
    c. Cervical spine fractures
    d. Unexplained unilateral neurologic deficit in the face of a normal head CT
    f. Penetrating brain injuries
    g. Neck hematoma or seatbelt sign
    h. LeFort II and III fractures

C. Plain radiography and magnetic resonance imaging (MRI)
1. Neither of these modalities is indicated in the acute evaluation of a head-injured patient. A delayed MRI may provide prognostic information in patients with diffuse axonal injury (DAI).

IV. INITIAL MANAGEMENT

A. Prevention of secondary brain injury
1. Avoid hypotension.
    a. Cerebral perfusion pressure (CPP) = mean arterial pressure (MAP) − intracranial pressure (ICP).
    b. Maintenance of CPP > 60 mm Hg has been shown to reduce secondary ischemic injury from hypotension.
    c. During initial management with no ICP monitor, strategies to keep MAP > 80 to 90 mm Hg will increase CPP.
2. Avoid hypoxia.
    a. When necessary, early intubation for airway protection and treatment of pulmonary injuries to ensure adequate PaO_2 increases cerebral oxygen delivery and subsequently increases brain tissue oxygenation.
3. Treatment of increased ICP before initiation of ICP monitoring
    a. Head of bed elevation
        i. Elevating the head of the bed 30 to 45 degrees can produce a near 50% decrease in ICP.
        ii. Early clearance of the thoracolumbar spine allows elevation of the head, which is more effective than reverse Trendelenburg positioning.

b. Hyperventilation
  i. $PaCO_2$ of 25 to 30 mm Hg should only be used as a **short-term** temporizing measure while diagnostic or therapeutic interventions are initiated.
  ii. Chronic hyperventilation may worsen cerebral ischemia. Maintenance of a $PaCO_2$ around 35 mm Hg is ideal.
c. Mannitol
  i. Mannitol treats increased ICP by causing cellular dehydration and increasing serum osmolarity. It can contribute to hypotension, so ensure that the patient is adequately fluid resuscitated before administering mannitol.
  ii. High-dose mannitol (1.2 to 1.4 g/kg) can be used for acute neurologic deterioration and as a temporizing measure prior to a neurosurgical procedure.
  iii. Bolus dosing of mannitol (0.25 to 1.0 g/kg) can be used for treatment of refractory increased ICP in the intensive care unit setting.
d. Hypertonic saline
  i. Maintenance of serum sodium = 145 to 155 mmol/L via bolus dosing or continuous infusion of 3% normal saline not only treats elevated ICP, but also prevents hyponatremia, which can cause increased cerebral edema, increased ICP, and seizures.
4. Seizure prophylaxis
  a. Of patients with serious TBI (with or without intracranial hemorrhage), 20% to 25% will have at least one post-traumatic seizure.
  b. Seizures can exacerbate TBI, transiently increase ICP, and confuse the clinical picture with a depressed neurologic examination in the post-ictal period.
  c. The frequency of **early** post-traumatic seizures is significantly reduced by administration of antiepileptic drugs (AEDs).
    i. The most commonly used and studied AED is phenytoin. Levetiracetam is a newer agent that is being used more frequently. It has been shown to be effective and does not require monitoring of serum levels.
  d. Continuation of AEDs beyond 7 days has not been shown to prevent the development of **late** post-traumatic epilepsy.
5. Treatment of coagulopathy
  a. Trauma patients can be coagulopathic for many reasons, and even a mildly prolonged prothrombin or partial thromboplastin time can exacerbate intracranial bleeding.
  b. Serial coagulation profiles should be sent during the first 24 to 48 hours post-injury with aggressive correction of abnormal values via fresh-frozen plasma, prothrombin complex concentrate, or vitamin K.

B. ICP monitoring

1. It is recommended that an ICP monitor be placed in patients with a GCS 3 to 8 and either one of the following:
  a. Abnormal CT scan
  b. Normal CT scan with two of the following at admission:

      i. Age > 40 years
     ii. Systolic blood pressure < 90 mm Hg
    iii. Unilateral or bilateral motor posturing
2. Patients with a GCS >8 usually have a motor examination that can be evaluated with serial neurologic evaluations and thus may not require ICP monitoring.
3. ICP monitoring requires bedside placement of either a ventricular catheter or a transducer wire. The ventricular catheter is preferred as it provides a way to treat increased ICP via drainage of cerebrospinal fluid (CSF).
4. Once a monitoring device is in place, treatment of elevated ICP (>20 mm Hg), as described previously, can be performed. Additional interventions include sedation and analgesia, chemical paralysis, drainage of CSF, induction of barbiturate coma, and decompressive craniectomy.

V. SPECIFIC INJURIES

A. Skull fractures
1. Linear, nondisplaced skull fractures require no treatment.
2. Criteria to elevate depressed skull fractures include:
   a. Depression greater than the thickness of the skull
   b. Neurologic deficit related to underlying brain injury
   c. CSF leak
   d. Open, compound fracture
3. Most basilar skull fractures do not require treatment.
   a. The exception is a persistent CSF leak. This should first be treated with CSF diversion (either by ventricular catheter or lumbar drain). If leak continues, surgical intervention may be necessary.

B. Epidural hematoma
1. Usually associated with a skull fracture and laceration of the middle meningeal artery. It can also be related to venous bone bleeding or laceration of a venous sinus.
2. Its appearance on CT scan has a characteristic lenticular shape that does not cross suture lines.
3. Patients occasionally present after a lucid interval of minutes to hours depending on the rate of hematoma expansion. Delayed development of focal neurologic signs and altered mental status suggests the diagnosis.
4. After confirmation with CT scan, treatment is operative evacuation of the hematoma.

C. Subdural hematoma
1. Often the result of a torn cortical or bridging vein
2. Its appearance on CT scan has a characteristic crescent shape with the clot spread over the convexity of the brain.
3. Subdural hematomas are often associated with significant underlying parenchymal injury, which explains the 50% mortality rate despite early clot evacuation.

4. Operative evacuation of a subdural hematoma is indicated for lesions that are large or associated with significant midline shift or neurologic deficit.

D. Contusions

1. Bruising of the brain parenchyma often occurs over bony prominences (frontal, temporal, and occipital poles) as a result of sudden deceleration of the head during trauma.
   a. **Coup-contrecoup injury** describes contusions directly beneath the point of impact (coup) as well as directly opposite the point of impact (contrecoup).
2. Contusions can often be managed conservatively, but they do tend to evolve on serial CT scans. Lesions in the temporal lobe in particular need to be watched closely to ensure life-threatening mass effect requiring surgical intervention does not develop on repeat imaging.
3. Nonemergent, nonneurosurgical operative procedures carry a high risk of exacerbating hemorrhagic contusions and should be avoided if possible in the acute period.

E. Edema

1. The edema that accompanies severe brain injury is poorly understood. It is likely a result of both cytotoxic and vasogenic mechanisms.
2. Because the cranial vault is a fixed volume, severe edema can drastically increase ICP, particularly within compartments delineated by dural reflections (i.e., falx cerebri between cerebral hemispheres, and tentorium cerebelli between the supra- and infratentorial compartments).

F. Diffuse axonal injury (DAI)

1. Patients with low GCS scores and a poor neurologic examination in the face of minimal to no CT scan findings are presumed to have DAI.
2. DAI is a primary lesion of rotational acceleration/deceleration of the head producing a shearing injury of deep white matter tracts (particularly in the corpus callosum and rostral brain stem).
3. MRI can be used to confirm the diagnosis.

G. Penetrating injuries

1. Gunshot wounds to the head account for the majority of penetrating brain injuries. They are also the most lethal.
   a. Brain injury results from:
      i. Soft tissue injury to scalp and face
      ii. Bony injury with comminuted and depressed fracture fragments
      iii. Direct parenchymal injury from the bullet or bullet fragments
      iv. Blast effect injury
   b. Decision for surgical treatment depends on severity and survivability of the injury.
      i. Level of consciousness is the most important prognostic factor. At a minimum, the patient should be localizing to a painful stimulus and have intact brainstem reflexes.
      ii. On CT scan, a bullet path that crosses the midline or traverses the ventricular system is indicative of an injury with a very poor prognosis.

2. Non-missile penetrating injuries require emergent surgical intervention to safely remove an embedded foreign body. Preoperative angiography is often indicated.

VI. OPERATIVE TREATMENT

The decision to operate on a head-injured patient must take into account the CT scan findings, the patient's neurologic examination, and other associated traumatic injuries.

A. General principles

1. Patients in good neurologic condition with a neurologic examination that can be followed easily can be managed nonoperatively despite the presence of significant contusions and small, stable epidural or subdural hematomas.
2. Patients with severe TBI may have a neurologic examination and CT scan findings that are not compatible with survival even with surgical intervention.
3. The families of patients with any type of TBI should be counseled in a caring and compassionate, yet open and honest way regarding the prognosis for a meaningful and functional recovery. Allowing the family to see the patient early and incorporating trauma nurse clinicians into the health care team greatly facilitate early decision making in these complex situations.

B. Operative pearls

1. Early operative intervention for most epidural hematomas and large subdural hematomas yields the best chance for improving neurologic outcome.
2. Establishing arterial blood pressure monitoring and adequate peripheral or central venous access before starting the surgical procedure is critical for accurate blood pressure management and facilitation of fluid administration and transfusions during the procedure.
3. Review of the patient's cervical spine CT is mandatory prior to positioning the patient. Even if no bony abnormality is identified, ligamentous injury may exist so care should be taken to maintain in-line positioning when able.
4. A large, question mark-shaped incision is made that runs in front of the ear, curving posteriorly and then anteriorly to the midline.
5. A large bone flap utilizing the entire exposure is fashioned. Decision to replace the bone flap at the end of the case depends on the intraoperative appearance of the brain and the potential for delayed edema and increased ICP.
6. Epidural hematomas are evacuated without opening the dura.
7. Subdural hematomas are evacuated by opening the dura in a stellate fashion. Contused, nonviable brain can also be evacuated once the subdural clot is removed. The dura is then loosely reapproximated or grafted with a large piece of pericranium to allow room for anticipated swelling.

VII. SPINAL CORD INJURIES AND EVALUATION OF THE SPINE

A. General principles
1. Spine fractures may be associated with as many as 10% of other traumatic injuries.
2. The cervical spine should always be treated as if it were injured, even if suspicion is low. The consequences of missing a cervical spine injury can result in one of the most devastating iatrogenic injuries possible.
3. Plain films of the spine have essentially been replaced by CT scans as the screening imaging of choice.
    a. All patients who are unresponsive should be treated as though they have a spine fracture. A CT scan of the entire spine is quickly and easily obtained when the patient is getting the initial head CT.
    b. In patients who are awake and responsive, only a CT through regions of the spine where the patient has tenderness or palpable deformity is required.
4. 20% of patients with one identified spine fracture will have a second fracture at another location (which can be noncontiguous).
5. Patients must remain with strict spinal precautions until a full spinal evaluation is complete. The backboard should be removed quickly on arrival to the emergency department, but the axial spine should be maintained in line at all times and a hard cervical collar should be in place. A minimum of three people are required to log roll a patient under full spinal precautions: one to control the head and neck, one to control the shoulders and torso, and one to control the lower extremities.
6. Clearance of the cervical spine (i.e., removal of the cervical collar) requires proof that neither bony nor ligamentous injury exists.
    a. In an awake, responsive patient who is not intoxicated and has no distracting injuries, the cervical spine can be clinically cleared. Palpation of the posterior cervical spine with no associated tenderness and demonstration of neck movement in all axes of motion without pain are required to remove the cervical collar.
    b. In an obtunded, intoxicated, or otherwise injured patient, CT scan can rule out bony injury, but ligamentous injury cannot be fully evaluated until the patient is cooperative during a clinical examination or an MRI is obtained.

B. Examination of patients with suspected spine injury
1. **Motor examination**
    a. Awake, cooperative patients can undergo motor testing of individual muscle groups, which can determine the specific level of spinal cord dysfunction (see Table 15-2).

TABLE 15-2
DETERMINATION OF CERVICAL INJURY LEVELS

Vertebra	Motor	Sensory	Reflex
C5	Deltoid	Region over the deltoid	Biceps
C6	Biceps	Thumb and index finger	Brachioradialis
C7	Triceps and wrist	Middle finger	Triceps and wrist extensors
C8	Finger flexion	Ring and fifth finger	None

    b. Spinal cord injury is described by the lowest functioning level.
2. **Sensory examination**
   a. Testing light touch and pinprick sensation in all extremities can help delineate the level of spinal cord injury, while testing joint position sense can help detect posterior column injury.
3. **Reflexes**
   a. The biceps, brachioradialis, triceps, patellar, and Achilles reflexes are always tested and noted to be absent, normal, or increased.
   b. Attention is paid to the symmetry of reflexes as well as a comparison between upper and lower extremity reflexes.
   c. Causes of absent reflexes:
      i. Lower motor neuron lesion (i.e., cauda equina syndrome or peripheral nerve root compression from a herniated intervertebral disk)
      ii. Spinal cord injury causes flaccid paralysis and areflexia for the first 1 to 2 weeks post-injury before spasticity and hyper-reflexia take over.
   d. Hyper-reflexia and the Babinski reflex are the result of an upper motor neuron lesion (i.e., cervical spinal cord compression or brain injury).
   e. Decreased rectal tone is a critical finding. It is particularly important in an obtunded patient as this may be the first indication of an underlying spinal cord injury.
   f. An **incomplete spinal cord injury** is defined by the presence of residual motor or sensory function more than 3 segments below the level of injury. Any preserved distal sensation (particularly in a sacral distribution) or voluntary movement of the lower extremities indicates an incomplete spinal cord injury.

C. Radiographic studies
1. Plain films have largely been replaced by CT scans as initial spine imaging. In a situation where there is no time to obtain a CT scan, at a minimum, a lateral cervical spine film must be obtained.
2. As described previously, CT scans are obtained in any patient who is obtunded, has an abnormality on plain films, or for whom there is a high clinical suspicion of injury.
3. MRI in the acute setting is reserved for those patients whose neurologic examination is consistent with spinal cord injury. MRI is useful in

identifying traumatic disk herniation and spinal epidural hematoma as well as delineating the extent of abnormal spinal cord signal. Delayed MRI is useful in identifying cervical ligamentous injury to allow clearance of a cervical collar.
4. In patients with identified cervical spine fractures, CT angiography is performed to screen for traumatic vascular injuries.

D. Management
1. To avoid early skin breakdown, patients should be removed from the backboard as quickly as possible (even if a fracture or neurologic deficit is identified).
2. Patients with spinal cord injury are at high risk for developing deep vein thrombosis (DVT). DVT prophylaxis with low-molecular weight heparin should be initiated 24 to 72 hours from injury if no other contraindication exists. In patients who cannot be anticoagulated, inferior vena cava (IVC) filters can be placed, but these are not recommended as first-line DVT prophylaxis.
3. When possible, serial neurologic examinations should be performed by the same provider in order to document stability or change in clinical findings. Worsening neurologic function may be an indication for emergent surgery.
4. High-dose corticosteroid use in acute spinal cord injury is associated with considerable controversy. They are generally used with cervical cord injuries but rarely with thoracic or lumbar injuries.
   a. A 30 mg/kg IV bolus of methylprednisolone is administered over 15 minutes.
5. A methylprednisolone IV drip of 5.4 mg/kg/hour is started 45 minutes later.
6. Patients who arrive within 3 hours of injury are treated for 24 hours.
7. Patients who arrive 3 to 8 hours after injury are treated for 48 hours.

E. Spinal shock
1. The sympathetic nervous system regulates heart rate and blood pressure. Sympathetic motor neurons are located in the thoracic spinal cord.
2. Cervical spinal cord injuries can sever the communication between the brain and these sympathetic motor neurons. This can result in hypotension and bradycardia.
3. Spinal shock must be recognized because the associated hypotension often will not respond to volume resuscitation. Continued fluid boluses can result in volume overload.
4. Pressors should be used early to maintain systolic blood pressure >90 mm Hg and MAP = 75 to 90 mm Hg.

F. Pulmonary function
1. Many factors place patients with spinal cord injuries at risk for pulmonary complications.
   a. Lower cervical and thoracic injuries cause loss of innervation of the intercostal muscles. Higher cervical injuries can cause loss of innervation of the diaphragm, leading to ventilator dependence.

b. Pulmonary embolus is common in this patient population.
c. Aggressive fluid resuscitation can lead to volume overload.
2. Aggressive pulmonary toilet, ventilator management, respiratory therapy, and early DVT prophylaxis are used in conjunction with rotating beds in the acute period to prevent pulmonary complications.

G. Surgery

1. The goals for surgical intervention in spine trauma are decompression of the neural elements and restoration of spinal stability via instrumentation and fusion. Surgery also improves pain and allows earlier mobilization to prevent pulmonary complications and speed the transfer to a rehabilitation unit.
2. Indications for emergent surgery are few:
   a. Incomplete neurologic deficit with epidural hematoma or traumatic soft disk herniation
   b. Progressing neurologic deficit

VIII. SUGGESTED READINGS

The Brain Trauma Foundation: The American Association of Neurological Surgeons, Joint Section on Neurotrauma and Critical Care: Guidelines for the management of severe traumatic brain injury. J Neurotrauma 17, 2000.

Greenberg MS: Handbook of Neurosurgery, 6th ed. New York, Thieme Medical Publishers, 2006.

Valadka AB, Andrews BT: Neurotrauma: Evidence-Based Answers to Common Questions. New York, Thieme Medical Publishers, 2005.

Soft Tissue Injuries of the Face

Hema Thakar, MD, and Jennifer Blumetti, MD

I. ANATOMY

- **A. Surface anatomy of the face** (Fig. 16-1)
- **B. Surface anatomy of the nose** (Fig. 16-2)
- **C. Surface anatomy of the ear** (Fig. 16-3)
- **D. Superficial musculoaponeurotic system (SMAS)**: Multilayer fibromuscular and adipose network located deep to the dermis and superficial to the facial motor nerves
  1. It extends from the temporoparietal (TP) fascia to the platysma.
  2. It is an important landmark for protection of the facial nerve branches.
- **E. Facial nerve distribution** (Fig. 16-4): All facial muscles are innervated from the underside.
  1. The temporal branch innervates the frontalis, corrugator, procerus, and orbicularis oculi (upper lid).
     a. The nerve is most superficial as it crosses the zygomatic arch, where it lies beneath the SMAS/TP fascia.
     b. Injury to this nerve results in paralysis of the forehead and brow.
  2. The zygomatic branch innervates the orbicularis oculi (lower lid), buccinator, and upper lip muscles (orbicularis oris, levator labii muscles, zygomaticus muscles) and the ala muscles.
     a. Injury to this nerve results in paralysis of the upper lip and cheek.
  3. The buccal branch innervates the buccinator and the upper and lower lip muscles (orbicularis oris, risorius, depressor anguli oris).
     a. Injury to this nerve results in paralysis of the upper lip and cheek.
  4. The marginal mandibular branch innervates the lower lip muscles.
     a. Injury results in paralysis to lower lip.

II. PHYSICAL EXAMINATION

- **A.** Inspect the face and scalp for soft tissue injuries.
- **B.** Assess soft touch sensation to the face and neck prior to administration of local anesthesia.
  1. **Trigeminal nerve distributions** (Fig. 16-5):
     a. **Ophthalmic (V1)**: supraorbital, supratrochlear, infratrochlear, external nasal, and lacrimal nerves
     b. **Maxillary (V2)**: infraorbital, zygomaticofacial, zygomaticotemporal nerves
     c. **Mandibular (V3) divisions**: mental, buccal, auriculotemporal nerves
  2. **Terminal cutaneous branches of C2-3** (see Fig. 16-5)
     a. Greater auricular and transverse cervical nerves
  3. Locally explore wounds if a sensory deficit is appreciated.
     a. Repair a severed nerve trunk with microsurgical technique if proximal and distal ends can be found.

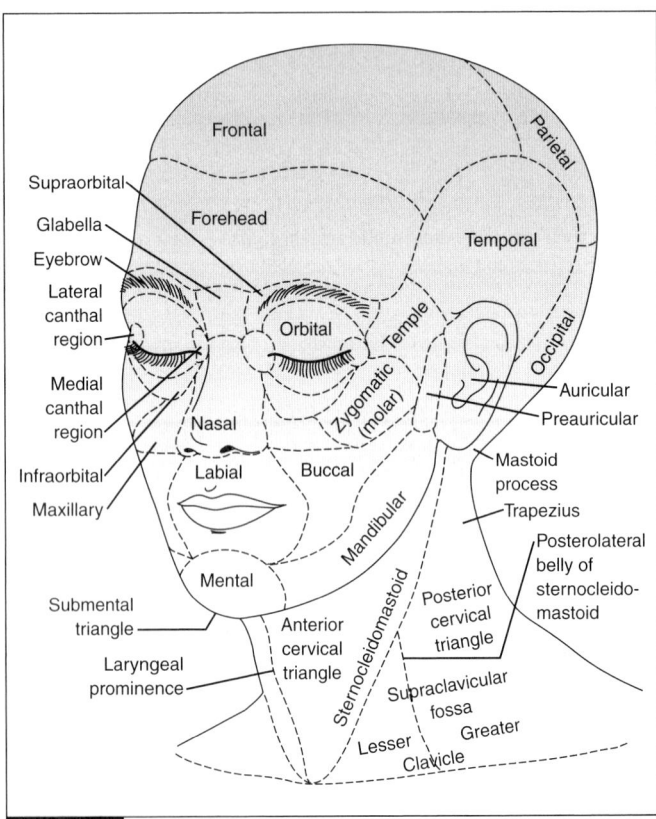

FIGURE 16-1

Surface anatomy of the face and neck.

    b. New nerve endings will grow and renew sensation typically within 6 months if the nerve trunk is intact.

  C. Assess function of the facial nerve distributions prior to administration of local anesthesia.

1. Ask the patient to raise the eyebrows, close both eyes, smile, pucker the lips, and show the lower teeth.
2. Injuries to the facial nerve anterior to the level of the lateral canthus will likely regenerate.
3. Injuries to the facial nerve posterior to the level of the lateral canthus require exploration and microsurgical repair within 2 to 3 days of injury.

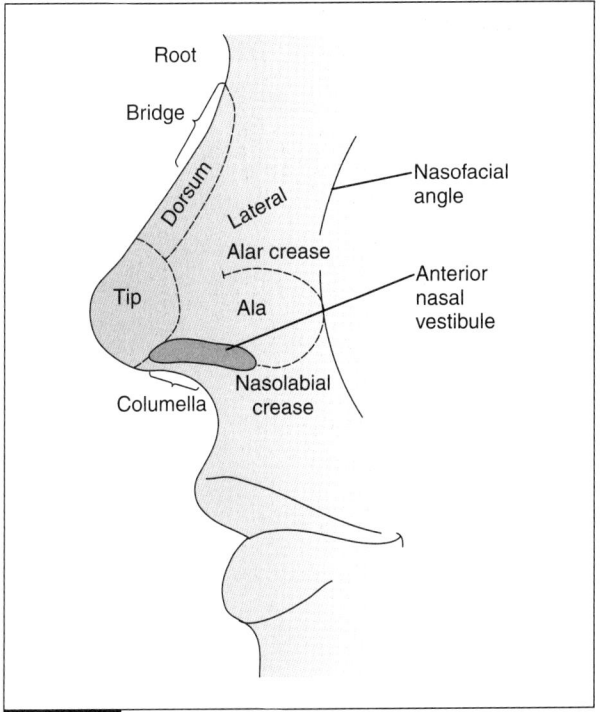

FIGURE 16-2
Surface anatomy of the nose.

4. Obtain an electromyogram if the physical examination is uncertain.
   a. Findings of muscle amplitude in the weak muscles indicate nerve stretch or contusion.
   b. The lack of electrical signal suggests transection of a branch of the facial nerve.

III. WOUND CLASSIFICATION AND BASIC MANAGEMENT

A. Wound types
1. Contusion
   a. Produced by blunt trauma that ruptures subcutaneous vessels without disruption of the overlying skin, resulting in edema, ecchymosis, and hematoma
   b. Drain hematoma if present in eyelid, nasal septum, or ear.

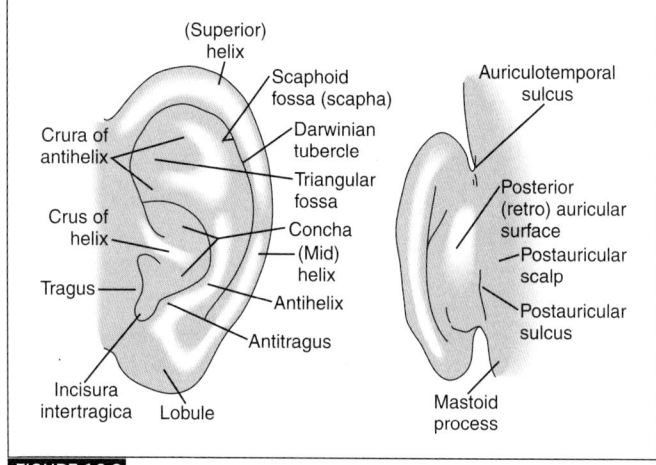

FIGURE 16-3

Surface anatomy of the ear.

2. Abrasion
   a. Avulsion of the epithelium and papillary dermis resulting from shear forces that expose the reticular layer as a raw, bleeding surface
   b. Will re-epithelialize within 7 to 10 days
   c. Irrigate the wound and apply topical antibiotic ointment twice a day for 4 days.
   d. Significant scar may result if the wound depth extends deep into the dermal layer. Debride the wound if it is deep. Closure options include primary closure or full-thickness skin graft.
3. **Laceration**
   a. May be simple, linear, jagged, or stellate. The margins may be abraded, contused, or crushed.
   b. Irrigate and debride the wound. Close in layers. Use 4-0 monocryl for buried deep dermal stitches. Place 6-0 prolene or nylon sutures in skin. Remove skin sutures in 3 to 5 days.
   c. To avoid the need for suture removal, 6-0 fast-absorbing gut can also be used in the skin (appropriate in children or unreliable patients who may not follow up for suture removal).
   d. Apply topical antibiotic ointment twice a day for 4 days.
4. Avulsion
   a. In cases of full-thickness loss of skin, apparent tissue loss is usually found in the form of rolled borders and/or retracted edges.

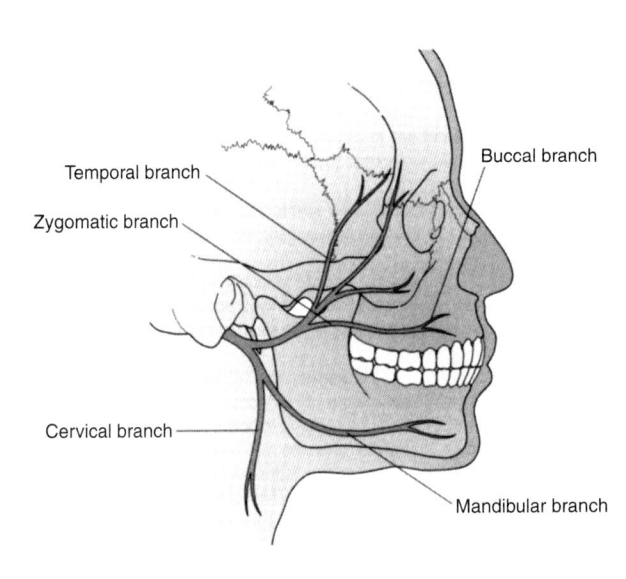

FIGURE 16-4
The branches of the facial nerve.

   b. Small avulsion defects can usually be closed by undermining and local adjacent tissue advancement.
   c. Large avulsion defects can be closed using local flaps or a full-thickness skin graft.
   d. Dermabrasion or scar revision may be performed in the future for poor cosmesis.

IV. ANESTHESIA

Most soft tissue facial injuries can be repaired in the emergency department using local and IV sedation.

A. Sedation may be indicated depending on the extent of injury and length of repair. IV sedation requires supplemental oxygen and monitoring with pulse oximetry, blood pressure, and electrocardiography.
1. Midazolam (Versed) for its amnestic properties
   a. Antagonist: Flumazenil IV bolus at 0.2 mg every 5 minutes up to a total of 1 mg
2. Morphine or fentanyl for analgesia

114 IV. Anesthesia

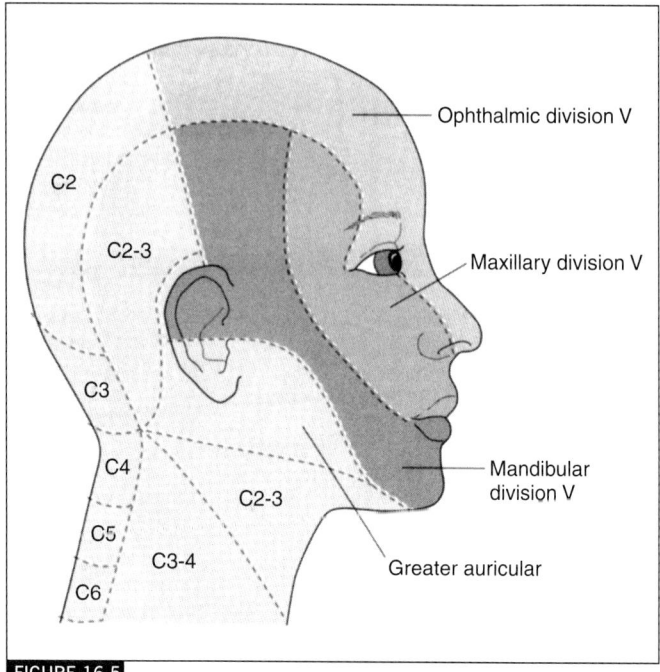

FIGURE 16-5

Sensory anatomy within the face and neck.

    a. Antagonist: Naloxone IV bolus at 0.04 mg every 2 to 3 minutes until desired effect

B. Local anesthesia

1. Lidocaine, 1% to 2%, with 1:100,000 epinephrine is appropriate in any location in the head and neck.
   a. It decreases blood flow to the area of injection.
   b. It provides 3 to 4 hours of soft tissue anesthesia.
2. Local nerve blocks are preferable to infiltration in wound margins.
   a. Local nerve blocks reduce the total dose of anesthetic required.
   b. Avoid distortion of the wound margins from infiltration of local anesthetic.
   c. Decrease edema at the wound edges to promote better healing.
3. **Local blocks in the face**
   a. **Infraorbital block** (transcutaneous nasolabial approach): Blocks the lateral nose, cheek, lip, and lower eylid. Technique: Enter the skin lateral to the alar groove. Advance the needle toward the infraorbital

foramen, which is 4 to 7 mm below the infraorbital rim. Inject 1 to 2 mL of anesthetic.
b. **Mental block**: Blocks the lower lip and chin. Technique: Pull the lower lip out. Enter the mucosa in the sulcus at the base of the second lower bicuspid. Inject 1 mL of anesthetic.
c. **Supraorbital/supratrochlear/infratrochlear block**: Blocks the forehead, frontoparietal scalp, and medial upper eyelid. Technique: Stretch the eyebrow laterally. Enter the skin at the middle third of the eyebrow. Advance the needle toward the supraorbital notch and inject 1 to 2 mL of anesthetic at the notch under the muscle to get the supraorbital nerve. Then advance the needle along the rim in the medial direction and inject with another 1 mL of anesthetic to get the supratrochlear nerve. Continue to advance the needle to the nasal bone and inject another 1 mL of anesthetic to get the infratrochlear nerve.
d. **Dorsal nasal block**: Blocks the cartilaginous dorsum of the nose and nasal tip. Technique: Palpate the junction of the nasal bone and upper lateral cartilages. Insert the needle at the junction along the midline. Inject 1 to 2 mL on each side of the midline.
e. **Zygomaticotemporal block**: Blocks the side of the face from the lateral orbital wall to the hairline. Technique: Insert needle about 1 cm behind the lateral orbital rim. Advance along the bony wall to about 1 cm below the lateral canthus. Inject 1 mL while pulling the needle back.
f. **Zygomaticofacial block**: Blocks the middle and posterior cheek. Technique: Insert the needle just lateral to the confluence of the infraorbital and lateral orbital rims. Inject 1 mL of anesthetic.
g. **Great auricular block**: Blocks the lower third of the ear and the postauricular skin. Technique: Measure 6.5 cm from the lower border of the external acoustic meatus to the middle of the sternocleidomastoid. Inject 1 mL of anesthetic at this location onto the sternocleidomastoid muscle fascia.
h. **Mandibular (V3) block**: Blocks the lower cheek, preauricular and auriculotemporal hair regions. Technique: Insert a 22-gauge spinal needle at the sigmoid notch of the mandible (between the condyle and coronoid). Advance the needle straight to the pterygoid plate. Mark the needle depth at the skin. Then retract the needle and direct it about 1 cm posterior. Advance it only as far as your mark on the needle. Inject 4 to 5 mL of anesthetic.

V. WOUND CLOSURE TECHNIQUES

A. Primary closure
1. Relaxed skin tension lines (RSTL)
    a. The RSTL or Langer lines follow the furrows formed when the skin is relaxed.
    b. They are based on the orientation of the fibers in the reticular layer of the skin.

c. They run parallel to the principal muscle fibers below the skin. Therefore, there is less tension on wound margins when skin closures lie parallel to the RSLT.
d. Lacerations and incisions that fall parallel to these lines produce the most inconspicuous scars. Attempt to place all incisions in the RSTL.

B. Local skin flaps
1. Local skin flaps provide one-stage repair of avulsion defects. They are appropriate to use when unable to close wounds primarily.
2. Local flaps include advancement flaps, rotational flaps, V-Y advancement flap, Z-plasty, and rhomboid flaps.
3. Flap incisions can be hidden in RSTL.
4. Jagged scars are less noticeable on the face relative to single long linear scars.

C. Skin grafts
1. Avoid split-thickness grafts because these lead to poor cosmesis.
2. Split-thickness grafts create color and texture mismatch and therefore are not ideal for repair of facial injuries.
3. Harvest full-thickness grafts from supraclavicular donor sites for best color and texture match.

VI. REPAIR OF FACIAL STRUCTURES

A. Scalp
1. **The layers of the scalp** (Fig. 16-6):
   a. Skin
   b. Subcutaneous tissue
   c. Galea aponeurosis
   d. Loose areolar tissue
   e. Periosteum
2. Scalp lacerations may bleed significantly due to the high vascularity and inelasticity of the subcutaneous layer that prevents blood vessel retraction when lacerated.
3. **Management**
   a. Hemostasis
   b. Debridement and irrigation
   c. Close the galea with 2-0 Vicryl interrupted stitches.
   d. Close the skin with staples, which are less traumatic to hair follicles relative to suture.
   e. Place horizontal mattress 3-0/4-0 prolene suture if hemostasis is inadequate.
4. Large avulsions usually require immediate flap rotation or future skin grafting.

B. Eyebrow
1. Do not shave the eyebrow, as this will distort the anatomy and hinder proper alignment during closure.

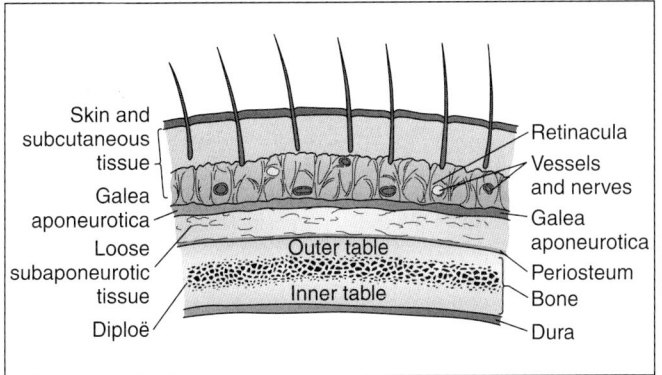

FIGURE 16-6

Anatomic layers of the scalp.

2. Debride only nonvital tissue. Incise or cut parallel to the hair follicles to prevent damage to the follicles.
3. Perform 2-layer closure for full-thickness lacerations. Align the superior and inferior aspects of the eyebrow first.
   a. 4-0 monocryl interrupted sutures for the dermis
   b. 6-0 prolene/nylon/fast-absorbing gut for the skin
4. Avulsion defects may require revision with hair transplantation as a secondary procedure.

C. Eyelids
1. **Anatomy of the upper and lower eyelids** (Fig. 16-7A and B).
2. Any injury of the eyelid should prompt an ophthalmologic examination for associated globe injury.
3. Explore lacerations to the upper lid to rule out damage to the levator aponeurosis.
   a. Ptosis of the eyelid indicates transection of the levator muscle.
   b. Repair the levator muscle with 6-0 monocryl to re-establish the lid fold and function of the eyelid.
4. Simple lacerations to the eyelid can be closed in a single layer.
   a. Use 6-0 prolene/nylon/fast-absorbing gut to approximate the skin.
   b. Avoid placing skin sutures through the septum, which will result in cicatricial ectropion.
5. Marginal lacerations involve the lid margin.
   a. Use 6-0 prolene/nylon to first approximate the lash line, meibomian glands, and gray line (junction of the skin and mucosa). The marginal sutures are left long and taped to the skin surface to prevent corneal abrasion.
   b. Use 6-0 monocryl to approximate the fascia.

6. **Avulsion injuries to the eyelids**
   a. Repair avulsion injuries with full-thickness skin graft from the postauricular area or contralateral eyelid.
   b. Avulsion injuries to the lid margins can be primarily closed if they constitute <25% of the lid length. A lateral canthotomy may be required to achieve tension-free closure. Larger defects may require grafts or rotation flaps.

D. Lacrimal apparatus

1. The lacrimal system is composed of the superior and inferior puncta, canaliculi, lacrimal sac, and duct. More than half of tear drainage is through the inferior canaliculus.
2. Lacerations or fractures to the medial orbital area may result in transection of the canaliculi or lacrimal sac. Damage to this system is usually apparent as epiphora (excessive tearing of the eye).
3. **Laceration through the canaliculus**
   a. Place Silastic canalicular tubing into severed canaliculi. Repair with microsurgical techniques.

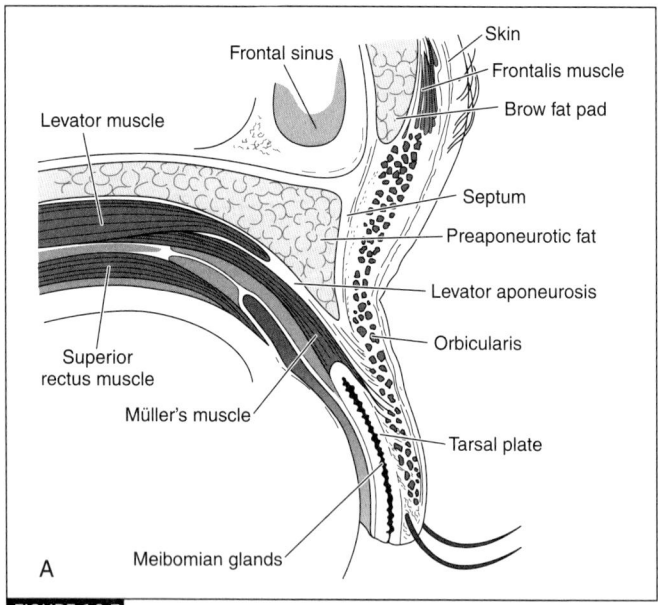

FIGURE 16-7

Anatomic layers of the eyelids. A. Upper eyelid.

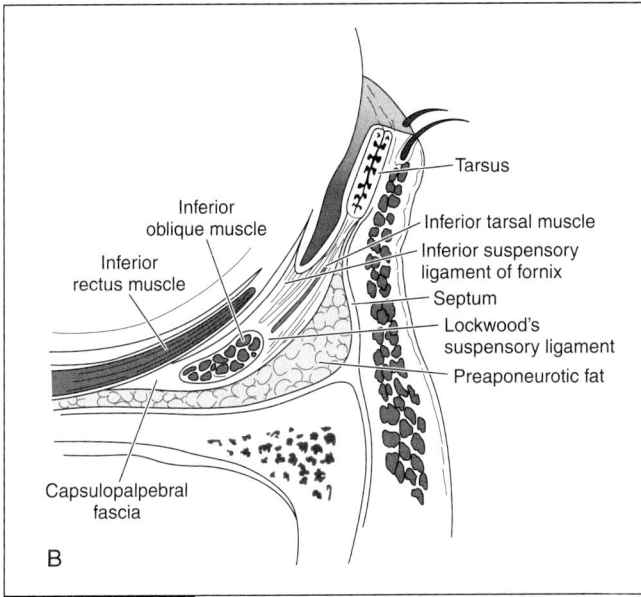

FIGURE 16-7—cont'd
B. Lower eyelid.

E. Nose
1. Inspect the septum for septal hematoma or presence of mucoperichondrial laceration.
   a. Incise and drain hematoma if present.
2. **Through-and-through lacerations**
   a. Repair the mucosa with 4-0 chromic interrupted stitches.
   b. Reapproximate cartilage with 4-0 monocryl interrupted sutures.
   c. Close skin with 6-0 prolene/nylon/fast-absorbing gut. Align known landmarks (i.e., alar rim, tip) for proper orientation.
3. **Options for avulsion defects**
   a. Tack down skin flap if present and viable.
   b. Perform immediate reconstruction with a composite graft if injured skin is available or full-thickness skin graft.
   c. Treat with local wound care and allow healing by secondary intention. Secondary reconstructive flap may be needed for scar revision once the area is completely healed.

F. Lips
1. **Lacerations across vermilion border** (Fig. 16-8):
   a. Align the vermilion border first with a single 6-0 suture.

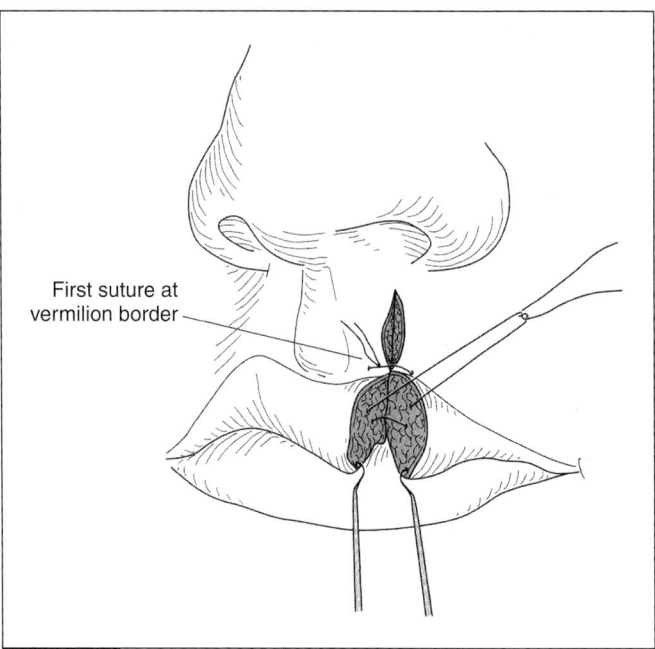

FIGURE 16-8

Repair of laceration involving the lip across the vermilion border.

  b. Approximate orbicularis oris fibers with 4-0 Vicryl.
  c. Close skin with 6-0 prolene/nylon/fast-absorbing gut.
 2. **Through-and-through lacerations**
  a. Close inside-out starting with the mucosa. Repair the mucosa with 3-0 chromic gut.
  b. Irrigate the subcutaneous tissue.
  c. Close remaining layers as above.
 3. **Avulsion defects**
  a. Close avulsion defects primarily if less than 25% of lip tissue is lost.
  b. More extensive tissue loss will require regional advancement flap.
G. **Parotid duct**
 1. **Anatomy**
  a. The parotid duct (Stensen's duct) exits the anterior aspect of the parotid gland.
  b. It courses across the middle third of the cheek along a line from the tragus of the ear to the middle of the upper lip.

c. The duct crosses superficial to the masseter, then pierces the buccinator to enter the oral cavity at the level of the maxillary second molar.

2. **Identification of a duct injury**
   a. Direct inspection of the wound may be insufficient.
   b. Dry the buccal mucosa and then massage the parotid gland and duct. Smooth flow of secretions into the oral cavity indicates a patent duct.
   c. Cannulate the duct orifice with No. 22 angiocath and irrigate. Saline flush in the wound indicates an injury.
   d. Cannulate the duct orifice with a probe. Then inspect the wound for visibility of the probe and laceration.
   e. Obtain sialography if the results of the examination are indeterminate.

3. **Repair of duct injury**
   a. Place Silastic tubing through the intraoral orifice across the laceration.
   b. Repair the duct primarily over the tubing with 6-0 monocryl or PDS.
   c. Maintain the Silastic tubing in place for 5 to 7 days.

H. Ear

1. The ear has an excellent blood supply and can maintain large areas of skin on relatively small pedicles. Therefore, perform minimal debridement.
2. **Skin lacerations with exposed cartilage**
   a. Close the skin over exposed cartilage. Do not leave the cartilage uncovered.
   b. Trim cartilage to skin edges if skin loss is present.
   c. Antibiotics: Give a fluoroquinolone for 7 days for cartilage protection.
   d. Close skin with 6-0 prolene/nylon/fast-absorbing gut.
3. **Lacerations through cartilage**
   a. Repair cartilage with 4-0 monocryl interrupted suture.
   b. Close skin as described above.
   c. Give antibiotics as above for cartilage protection.
4. Place a light pressure dressing on ear repairs to prevent edema, seroma, and sub-perichondrial hematoma. These complications may lead to fibrosis and formation of a "cauliflower ear."
   a. Aspirate a hematoma or seroma under sterile conditions with an 18-gauge needle.
   b. May require daily drainage until the fluid collection stops
5. **Avulsion defects**
   a. Small avulsion defects may be replaced as a composite graft if injured skin is available.
   b. Utilize postauricular skin with advancement flap to cover posterior ear defects.
   c. Provide local wound care for areas without cartilage exposure to heal by secondary intention.
   d. Secondary reconstruction may be done in the future once the wound has healed.

I. Oral mucosa and tongue

1. **Mucosal lacerations**

a. Close the wound with 3-0 chromic suture in interrupted, running, or running locking fashion.
   b. The running locking method will give the tightest, water-sealed closure.
2. **Tongue lacerations**
   a. Perform lingual nerve block to prevent tissue distortion around wound edges.
   b. Close with 3-0 chromic suture.
3. **Submandibular ducts (Wharton's ducts)**
   a. Located in the anterior floor of the mouth
   b. Cannulate to evaluate for injury similar to parotid duct evaluation.
   c. Perform sialography if examination results are indeterminate.
   d. Repair the duct over silastic tubing similarly to the technique described for the parotid duct, above. Keep the tubing in place for 5 to 7 days.
   e. Perform proximal duct diversion if unable to repair injury primarily.

VII. ANIMAL BITES

A. Irrigate and debride to convert wound from contaminated to clean.
B. Close wounds primarily if possible.
C. Close large defects with local advancement flap or allow healing by secondary intention with future scar revision.
D. Prophylactic antibiotics with ampicillin-sulbactam for 7 days are indicated to cover dog and cat flora (gram-positive cocci and *Pasteurella multocida*).
E. Administer tetanus prophylactic.

VIII. SUGGESTED READINGS

Bennett RG: Fundamentals of Cutaneous Surgery. St. Louis, CV Mosby, 1988.

LaTrenta GS: Atlas of Aesthetic Face and Neck Surgery. Philadelphia, Saunders, 2004.

McCarthy JG: Plastic Surgery, Vol 2. Philadelphia, Saunders, 1990.

Nerad JA: Oculoplastic Surgery: The Requisites in Ophthalmology. St. Louis, Mosby, 2001.

Rohrich RJ, Robinson JB: Wound Healing. Selected Readings in Plastic Surgery, Vol 9, No. 3. Dallas, University of Texas Southwestern Medical Center and Baylor University Medical Center; 1999.

Seckel BR: Facial Danger Zones, Avoiding Nerve Injury in Facial Plastic Surgery. St. Louis, Quality Medical Publishing, 1994.

Thal ER., Weigelt JA, Carrico CJ: Operative Trauma Management: An Atlas, 2nd ed. New York, McGraw-Hill, 2002.

Zide BM, Swift R: How to block and tackle the face. Plast Reconstr Surg 101:840-851, 1998.

Facial Fractures I—Upper Facial Skeleton

Avron Lipschitz, MD, and Brian Oleksy, DDS, MD

I. HISTORICAL PERSPECTIVE

A. Until the 1970s, approaches to facial fractures involved closed reductions, minimal incisions, and delayed reconstruction after resolution of swelling.
B. It is now understood that functional and cosmetic results are improved with early definitive treatment, wide exposure, mobilization, and rigid stabilization of fracture fragments.
C. Improved care of facial fractures has been facilitated by advances in miniplate and screw technology and early bone grafting of significant skeletal defects.

II. FRONTAL SINUS FRACTURES

A. Anatomy
1. Paired pneumatized cavities in frontal bone
2. Borders: Anterior and posterior walls (tables), the orbital roof inferiorly, and a bony intersinus septum medially (variable location)
3. Nasofrontal duct: located posteromedially in sinus floor; drains into the middle meatus of the nose
4. Respiratory epithelium lines the sinus and the duct. Disruption leads to stasis of secretions, infections, and mucoceles.
5. Anterior cortical bone wall is much stronger than the other facial bones.
6. Arterial supply is from the supraorbital, supratrochlear, and anterior ethmoidal arteries.
7. The superficial venous system drains to the angular vein, and deep drainage is to the subdural venous system through the foramina of Breschet.
8. Lymphatic drainage follows meningeal and nasal cavity lymphatics so there is a risk of meningitis and brain abscess after fracture.
9. Sensory innervation to the soft tissues of the frontal region is from the supraorbital and supratrochlear nerves (CN V).

B. Clinical presentation
1. A thorough neurological examination is imperative.
2. There is a high likelihood of accompanying facial fractures; the entire maxillofacial region should be examined thoroughly.
3. Forehead and superior orbital rim depressions (can be masked by swelling)
4. Forehead skin lacerations, hematomas, and ecchymoses
5. Glabellar and forehead numbness from damage to supratrochlear and supraorbital nerves
6. Cerebrospinal fluid (CSF) rhinorrhea
   a. Indicates dural tear from fracture of posterior table or cribiform plate

b. Halo test (i.e., done by placing a drop of blood on gauze and examining for a ring of CSF) or laboratory confirmation of beta-2 transferrin
c. Neurosurgery consultation

C. Radiographic evaluation
1. Traditional plain film radiographs have largely been replaced by fine cut (1.5 to 3 mm) axial and coronal CT scans.
2. Used to evaluate involvement of the anterior and/or posterior table
3. Associated intracranial injury
4. Evaluate damage to the nasofrontal duct (posteromedial floor).

D. Management (Fig.17-1)
1. **Goals of treatment:**
   a. Elimination of any factors that predispose toward development of infection or mucocele formation
   b. Restoration of normal sinus function, or complete obliteration if indicated
   c. Repair of cosmetic defects
2. **Timing of treatment**
   a. Early surgical exploration and treatment, as soon as the systemic conditions are stabilized (usually within the first week of injury)
   b. IV antibiotics for 7 to 14 days in those with CSF leak
3. **Nonoperative management** for
   a. Isolated anterior wall fractures without depression
   b. Posterior wall fractures without displacement, CSF leakage, or nasofrontal duct injury
   c. Follow up in 6 to 12 months with imaging.
   d. Antibiotic administration is controversial among the faculty at Parkland Memorial Hospital.
4. **Operative intervention** for
   a. *Depressed anterior wall with cosmetic deformity*: Coronal incision, reposition fracture fragments, remove damaged lining, evaluate posterior wall.
   b. *Nasofrontal duct injury*: Sinus mucosa is removed to prevent future mucocele and the cavity is obliterated using autogenous material (e.g., fat, bone, fascia, muscle).
   c. *Posterior wall fractures without displacement but with CSF leakage*: Head elevation and spinal drainage when necessary for up to 10 days. If drainage is needed for longer than 10 days craniotomy, dural repair, and sinus obliteration are needed. Antibiotics are given at the discretion of the neurosurgeon.
   d. *Displaced posterior wall fractures with nasofrontal duct injury or dural tear*: Mucosa removal, sinus obliteration, or, rarely, cranialization (Fig. 17-2).

E. Postoperative care
1. Systemic decongestants
2. The head of the bed is elevated 30 to 40 degrees.
3. Monitor CSF rhinorrhea.

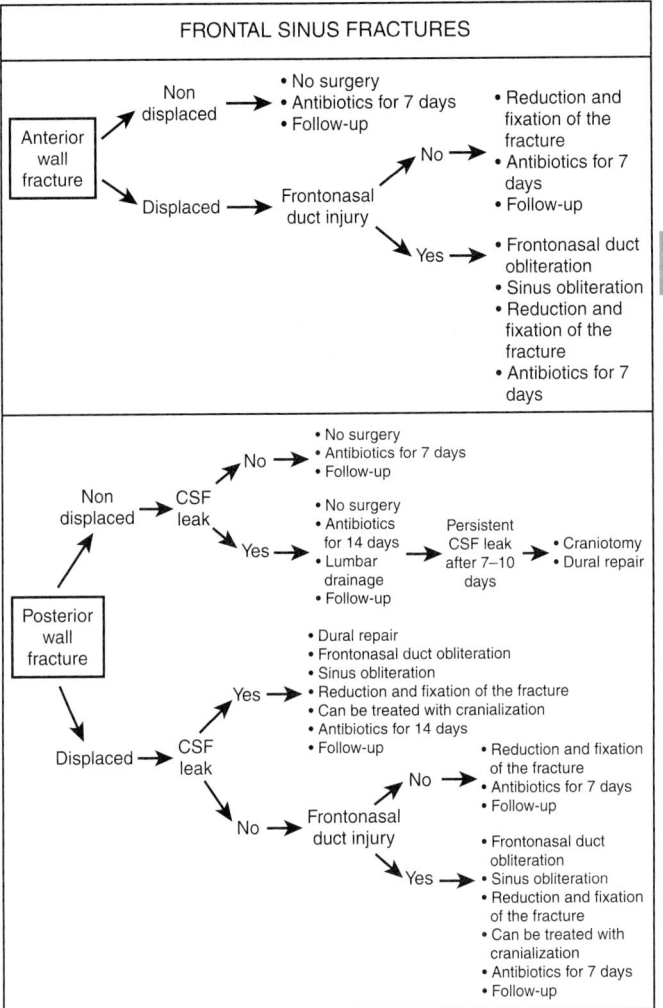

FIGURE 17-1

Treatment algorithm for frontal sinus fractures. (Adapted from Yavuzer R, Sari A, Jackson IT, et al: Management of frontal sinus fractures. *Plast Reconstr Surg* 115(6), 2005.)

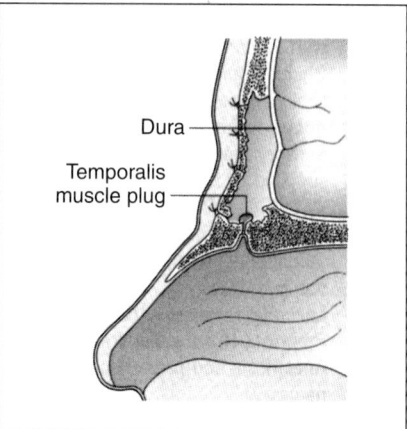

FIGURE 17-2

Cranialization of frontal sinus fracture with comminution of the posterior wall. The posterior table is excised, the nasofrontal duct is plugged with temporalis muscle, and the anterior wall is reduced and stabilized with rigid fixation, supplemented with bone graft as necessary. (From Luce EA: Frontal sinus fractures: Guidelines to management. Plast Reconstr Surg 80:500, 1987.)

4. The patient is cautioned against nose blowing and sneezing.
5. If nasofrontal stents are in place, daily irrigation with sterile saline decreases the incidence of infection and maintains stent patency.
6. Routine postoperative antibiotic use is controversial. The decision to give postoperative antibiotics should be left to the surgeon.

III. NASAL FRACTURES

A. Anatomy
1. **Three vaults**
   a. The upper vault consists of the paired nasal bones and the frontal process of the maxilla.
   b. The middle vault comprises the upper lateral cartilages, the majority of the septum, and the frontal process of the maxilla.
   c. The lower vault contains the lower lateral cartilages and the inferior edge of the septum.
2. **Blood supply**
   a. Internal carotid artery (through the ophthalmic artery)
   b. External carotid artery (through the facial and internal maxillary artery)
3. **Innervation**
   a. Sensory via the first and second divisions of the trigeminal nerve (CN V)

b. Sensory to the external nose is from the infraorbital, anterior ethmoidal, and infratrochlear nerves.
   c. Internal nasal innervation is from the ethmoidal, sphenoidal, and nasopalatine nerves.
B. Clinical presentation
1. Swelling and ecchymosis with possible laceration of the external nose
2. Pain on palpation
3. Epistaxis
4. Nasal deviation/deformity with or without step deformity
5. Septal hematoma
6. Nasal obstruction
7. Epiphora indicating nasolacrimal damage or obstruction
8. Palpation of the nasal bones for mobility/crepitus
9. Presence or absence of CSF (ring test or checking for beta-2 transferrin in nasal discharge)
10. Measurement of intercanthal distance (rule out possible naso-orbital-ethmoid fractures)
11. Intranasal exploration after shrinking the mucosa with topical agents is essential to evaluate the septum.

C. Radiographic evaluation
1. CT scanning is rarely indicated for isolated nasal fractures.
2. CT scan may be useful to rule out associated facial fractures.

D. Management
1. **Epistaxis**
   a. Direct pressure
   b. Insertion of a Foley catheter with inflation of the balloon at the level of the nasopharynx, then pulled forward, or formal anterior and posterior nasal packing
   c. Topical agents such as Afrin nasal spray (oxymetazoline) can be quite useful.
   d. Bleeding can originate from less accessible branches of the external carotid system, such as the maxillary artery, secondary to shearing or laceration. This is usually controlled with reduction of the fracture.
   e. May require selective embolization or ligation of the external carotid system proximal to the site of hemorrhage
2. **Septal hematoma**
   a. Septal hematomas contained beneath the mucoperichondrium should be drained immediately due to the risk of long-term cartilage resorption, loss of nasal support, and saddle deformity.
3. **Fracture management**
   a. **Timing**
      i. Ideally, nasal fractures are reduced in the first 2 hours after trauma, before nasal swelling becomes severe.
      ii. Reduction can be successfully performed any time within the first 2 weeks of injury.

b. **Procedure**
  i. Local anesthetic plus some degree of intravenous sedation is helpful.
  ii. The nose is packed with pledgets containing 4% cocaine, both for hemostasis and anesthetic effect (or Afrin).
  iii. 1% to 2% lidocaine with 1:100,000 epinephrine to block infraorbital, infratrochlear, and intranasal nerves
  iv. A blunt-tipped elevator (Boise) or Asch forceps are used to reduce bones (Fig. 17-3).

E. Postoperative care
1. To maintain stability of the fragments: postreduction packing of the nose is left in place for several days with antibiotic-impregnated gauze.
2. An external nasal splint should be placed to help protect the nose from further trauma and left in place for approximately 1 week.
3. Intranasal splints should also be considered if extensive septal manipulation has been performed.
4. Patients undergoing closed reduction for nasal injuries should always be counseled that subsequent open rhinoplasty may be necessary.

F. Complications
1. Include gross deviation in up to 70%
2. Difficulty breathing in up to 50%
3. May require secondary revision

IV. NASO-ORBITO-ETHMOID (NOE) COMPLEX FRACTURES

A. Introduction
1. Fractures involving the nasal bones, as well as the nasal processes of the frontal bone, and the frontal process of the maxilla.

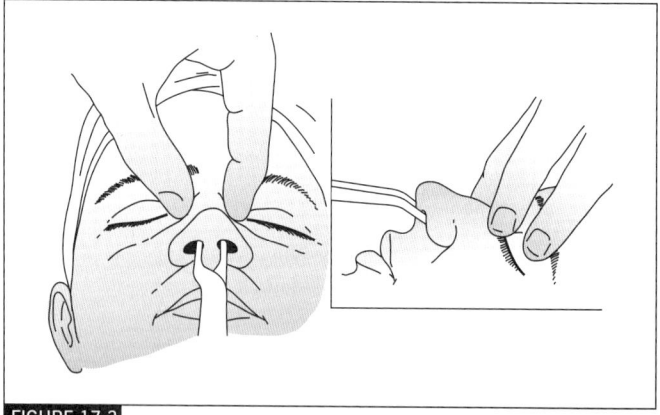

FIGURE 17-3
Reduction of nasal fracture.

IV. Naso-Orbito-Ethmoid (NOE) Complex Fractures

2. Diagnostically and therapeutically complex
3. Commonly occur in association with other facial fractures
4. Result from blunt force, for example, in a steering wheel to face injury during a motor vehicle collision.
5. Vulnerable to injury because fragile framework beneath resists a maximum compressive force of 30 G whereas the rest of the face can resist a force of 50 to 200 G.

B. Anatomy

1. **Medial orbital structures** bordered anteriorly by the frontal process of the maxilla, the nasal processes, and the nasal process of the frontal bone
2. Laterally it consists of the lamina papyraceae and lacrimal fossae.
3. It is inferiorly bound by the lower border of the ethmoidal labyrinths.
4. Posteriorly it is formed by the body of the sphenoid immediately in front of the optic foramen.
5. The nasolacrimal system is part of the NOE complex because it rests in the fossa between the anterior and posterior lacrimal crests of the medial orbital wall.
6. Key structure is the **central segment** of bone to which the medial canthal tendon (insertion of the orbicularis oculi) attaches.
7. **Blood supply** consists of
   a. Ethmoidal branches of the ophthalmic artery
   b. Facial
   c. Maxillary branches of the external carotid
8. Sensory and motor via 5th and 7th cranial nerves. Olfactory function via 1st cranial nerve through the cribiform plate; damage causes partial or complete loss of sense of smell (anosmia).

C. Clinical presentation

1. There is a high likelihood of accompanying head injury, facial fractures, and ocular injury.
2. Retruded nasal bridge, enophthalmos, shortened palpebral fissure, a flat nose, and swollen medial canthal region
3. Edema may mask findings.
4. Palpation of the dorsum of the nose may indicate loss of nasal support.
5. Instability of the central segment causes lateral displacement of the medial canthus (telecanthus). Intercanthal distance of > 35 mm is suggestive of NOE fracture; a distance of > 40 mm is usually diagnostic.
6. Involvement of the medial canthal tendon is demonstrated by the "eyelid traction test," which is done by grasping the lower eyelid with forceps and displacing it laterally: Inability to pull the lower lid taut indicates the likely presence of medial canthal tendon disruption.
7. Under general anesthesia, a surgical instrument is inserted intranasally to the region of the medial canthus, and the medial canthal region is palpated externally while pushing out.
8. Intranasal septal fractures and hematomas should be ruled out.

9. Clear nasal drainage suspected of being CSF from a dural tear and base of skull fracture in the region of the cribiform plate
10. Halo test or laboratory confirmation of beta-2 transferrin

D. Radiographic evaluation
1. Fine cut CT imaging (1.5 to 3.0 mm) is the modality of choice.
2. **Fracture classification**
   a. Type I: single central segment without disruption of medial canthal tendon
   b. Type II: comminuted central segment but medial canthal tendon is attached to large piece of bone
   c. Type III: comminuted central segment with disruption of medial canthal tendon insertion

E. Management
1. **Goals**
   a. Early surgical exploration and treatment, as soon as the systemic conditions are stabilized
   b. Identify, anatomically reduce, and fixate the fractured fragments.
   c. Repair and prevent postoperative telecanthus.
   d. Normal nasolacrimal drainage
   e. Restore cosmesis by re-establishing dorsal nasal height and projection.
   f. Eliminating CSF leakage
2. **Technique**
   a. Coronal incision and direct visualization of bony fragments
   b. Rigid fixation of the fracture segments with titanium microplating systems or wires allows accurate and stable fixation in a one-stage surgical repair.
   c. Closed intranasal reduction is done if the medial canthal ligament is not avulsed.
   d. Primary reconstruction of the dorsal nasal and medial orbital wall areas is indicated if severe comminution prevents stable anatomic reduction.
   e. Autogenous or allogeneic bone grafts
   f. Straighten and repair nasal septum.
   g. External nasal splints and nasal packing further stabilize the segments if severe comminution exists.

F. Postoperative care
1. Elevate head of bed >30 degrees to decrease edema.
2. Caution against nose blowing and sneezing to prevent subcutaneous emphysema.
3. Frequent ophthalmic examination to detect ocular complications

G. Complications
1. CSF rhinorrhea
   a. Usually self-limiting and ceases in 24 to 48 hours
   b. May require surgical intervention if persistent
2. Meningitis (incidence, 4% to 10%)—cover with antibiotics
3. Postoperative proptosis of the globe can be expected if primary grafting of the orbital wall was performed.

4. Postoperative epiphora
   a. Should cease as edema resolves
   b. Dacrocystorhinostomy may be necessary if there is trauma to the lacrimal sac or duct with persistent dacryocystitis or obstruction.
5. Posttraumatic telecanthus or canthal asymmetry
   a. Difficult to repair secondarily
   b. Treated early in the postoperative course if identified
6. Persistent nasal problems
   a. Loss of dorsal support
   b. Airway obstruction
   c. Secondary rhinoplasty may be required.

V. ORBITAL FRACTURES

A. Anatomy
1. 7 orbital bones: frontal, lacrimal, ethmoid, maxilla, zygoma, sphenoid, and palatine
2. Optic canal contents: CNII optic nerve, ophthalmic artery
3. Superior orbital fissure contents: oculomotor (CN III), abducens (CN VI), and trochlear (CN IV) nerves; lacrimal, nasociliary, and frontal divisions of the trigeminal nerve (V); and superior ophthalmic vein
4. Inferior orbital fissure contents: zygomaticofacial and zygomaticotemporal divisions of the trigeminal nerve (V) and inferior ophthalmic vein
5. Infraorbital canal/groove contents: infraorbital nerve (V2) and artery

B. Clinical presentation
1. Subconjunctival and periorbital ecchymosis
2. Periorbital edema and/or proptosis
3. Epistaxis
4. Cheek hypesthesia with orbital floor fracture
5. Binocular diplopia
6. Enophthalmos
7. Entrapment of extraocular muscles causing decreased range of motion

C. Pathomechanics of orbital fractures
1. Roof fractures are rare in adults but more common in children because the child's cranium is proportionately larger than that of adults and the frontal sinus is not completely pneumatized.
2. Lateral orbital wall fractures are usually secondary to zygomatic fractures.
3. Floor and medial wall fractures are caused by either an indirect transmission of force through the orbital rim or direct transmission of pressure from the globe or intraorbital contents to the floor, producing orbital blowout fractures.
4. **Blowout fractures** (*isolated* internal orbital fractures without fracture of the orbital rims) (Fig. 17-4).
   Clinical Findings
   a. Diplopia on upward gaze

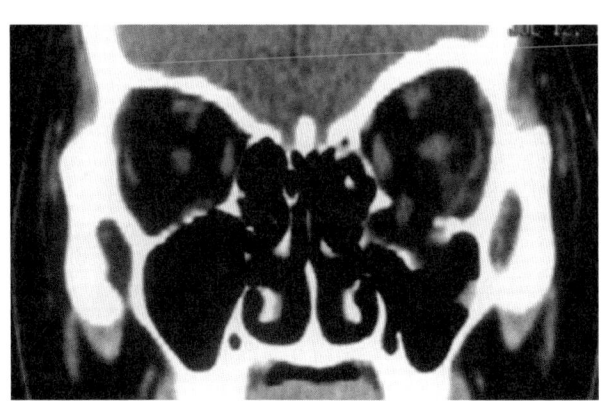

FIGURE 17-4

Blowout fracture. Coronal image of the orbit demonstrates depressed fracture of the inferior wall of the left orbit with herniation of intraorbital fat tissue and inferior rectus muscle.

  b. Enophthalmos
  c. Orbital emphysema
  d. Oculocardiac reflex—bradycardia, hypotension
  e. Potential ischemia of the inferior rectus if entrapment exists so treatment is relatively emergent (more common in children)
  f. **Superior orbital fissure and orbital apex syndrome**: fracture into the superior orbital fissure, injuring cranial nerves III, IV, V1, and VI and producing ophthalmologic, upper lid ptosis, proptosis, a fixed and dilated pupil, and a sensory disturbance over the distribution of the ophthalmic division of the trigeminal nerve, including loss of the corneal reflex
5. Orbital blow-in fracture (Fig. 17-5)
  a. Decreased intraorbital volume and exophthalmos
  b. Pure blow-in fractures involve the roof, walls, or floor of the orbit but not the orbital rim (extremely rare).
  c. Impure blow-in fractures include the rim itself. Early recognition and reconstruction are essential to prevent serious permanent complications.
6. **Traumatic optic neuropathy**
  a. Direct trauma to the optic nerve.
  b. Ischemia of the nerve from increased pressure secondary to edema or hemorrhage

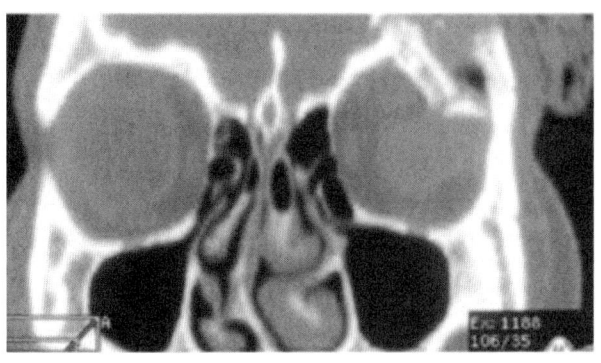

FIGURE 17-5

Blow-in fracture. Coronal image of the orbit in bone window shows a fracture in the roof of the left orbit with the fracture fragment depressed inferiorly into the orbit.

    c. Operative reduction itself may cause damage to vision.
    d. High-dose steroids, mannitol, and possible surgical decompression of the optic nerve if CT shows impingement

D. Radiographic evaluation
1. CT scan with 1.5-mm cuts in both the axial and coronal planes

E. Treatment
1. **Indications for exploration**
   a. Enophthalmos >2 mm
   b. If diplopia in the primary fields of gaze does not clear within 2 weeks
   c. Positive forced duction test due to entrapment
   d. Large orbital floor defect (>1 cm^2)
   e. Significant hypoglobus (an abnormally low vertical position of the globe)
2. **Surgical technique**
   a. Incisional approaches to the orbit include subtarsal, subciliary, and transconjunctival incisions. Relative pros, cons, and technical prerequisites of each approach are beyond the scope of this chapter. See Suggested Readings at the end of this chapter for further details.
   b. Orbital floor fractures require reconstruction of the orbital floor defect with:
      i. Autogenous tissue (commonly autologous membranous bone and cartilage, fascia lata, rib, or iliac bone).
      ii. Alloplast (commonly titanium mesh, MedPor, Teflon, supramyd, Silastic, or Gelfilm)

F. Complications
1. Infection of alloplastic material including implant extrusion

2. Diplopia due to inadequate release of the original incarceration, reincarceration, or adhesions to the reconstruction
3. Enophthalmos secondary to fat atrophy, scar contracture, or loss of the supporting ligaments
4. Ectropion/ retraction of the lower lid are due to scarring.
5. Prevention with Frost suture in the lower lid for 24 to 48 hours postoperatively
6. Postoperative blindness has multiple causes, including impingement on the nerve by the implant reconstruction, hematoma, or damage to the optic nerve from fracture reduction.
   a. Evaluate by urgent CT scanning and return the patient to the operating room.

VI. ZYGOMATICOMAXILLARY COMPLEX (ZMC) FRACTURES

A. Introduction
1. High-energy blunt force to the side of the face typically inflicted during a motor vehicle collision, fall, or interpersonal violence
2. The prominent convex shape of the zygoma makes it particularly vulnerable to injury.
3. The zygomatic arch is thin and easily fractured alone or in concert with the complex.

B. Anatomy
1. The zygoma is a tetrapod (Fig. 17-6).
2. It articulates with the greater wing of the **sphenoid, frontal bone, temporal bone, and maxilla**.

C. Clinical presentation
1. Subconjunctival ecchymosis
2. Periorbital ecchymosis and edema
3. Cheek hypesthesia from damage to infraorbital nerve
4. Diplopia, hypophthalmos
5. Enophthalmos
6. Trismus
7. Loss of cheek (malar) prominence
8. Step defects of the bony lateral and infraorbital rim regions

D. Radiographic evaluation
1. Computed tomography is the gold standard.
2. Plain x-rays are inadequate evaluation in the modern trauma setting.

E. Management
1. **Goals**
   a. Stabilization of the zygomatic arch
   b. Restoration of normal contour and projection of the malar prominence
2. **Technique**
   a. Closed reduction for simple noncomminuted fractures
   b. Open reduction for trismus, orbital complications, facial asymmetry

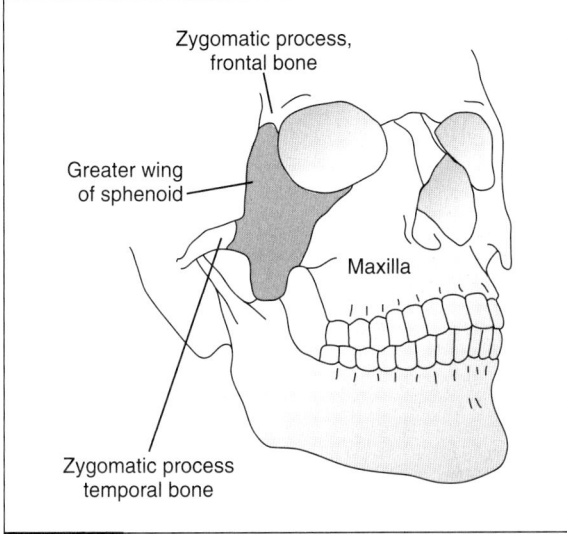

FIGURE 17-6

Articulations of zygoma with midfacial bones. The zygoma makes up the anterior lateral portion of the inferior orbit.

3. **Surgical approaches include**
   a. Coronal, hemicoronal, or pretragal approaches–indicated for multiple or complex fractures
   b. Periorbital incisions (transconjunctival, subciliary, subtarsal; visualize the orbital rim and floor)
   c. Lateral brow approach: visualize zygomaticofrontal suture–reduces zygomatic arch
   d. Maxillary vestibular incision to visualize the zygomaticomaxillary buttress
   e. **Gillies approach**
      i. For isolated arch fracture
      ii. Incision behind temporal hairline that is carried through temporalis fascia
      iii. Approach the zygoma by placing an elevator below the temporalis fascia and above the temporalis muscle to avoid injury to the temporal branch of the facial nerve.

F. Postoperative care
1. Intraoral topical antibiotic (chlorhexidine) if intraoral incision used
2. Topical ophthalmic antibiotic ointment on periorbital incisions
3. Soft diet to decrease trismus and pain
4. Daily ophthalmologic examination

5. Decongestants if maxillary congestion persists
6. Avoid sleeping on the injured cheek.

VII. SUGGESTED READINGS

Converse JM, Smith B: Naso-orbital fractures and traumatic deformities of the medial canthus. Plast Reconstr Surg 38:147, 1966.

Ellis E, Kittidumkerng W: Analysis of treatment for isolated zygomaticomaxillary complex fractures. J Oral Maxillofac Surg 54:386, 1996.

Ellis E III, El-Attar A, Moos KF: An analysis of 2,067 cases of zygomatico-orbital fracture. J Oral Maxillofac Surg 43:417, 1985.

Gruss JS: Naso-ethmoid-orbital fracture: Classification and role of primary bone grafting. Plast Reconstr Surg 75:303, 1985.

Hollier L, Thornton J: Facial fractures upper two thirds. In Selected Readings in Plastic Surgery, vol 9, no. 26, 2002.

Luce EA, Tubb TD, Moore AM: Review of 1,000 major facial fractures and associated injuries. Plast Reconstr Surg 63:26,1979.

Markowitz BL, et al: Management of the medial canthal tendon in nasoethmoid orbital fractures: The importance of the central fragment in classification and treatment. Plast Reconstr Surg 87:843, 1991.

McCarthy JG: Plastic Surgery, vol 2, part 1. Philiadelphia, Saunders, 1990.

Potter JK, Muzaffar AR, Ellis E: Aesthetic management of the nasal component of naso-orbital ethmoid fractures. Plast Reconstr Surg 117:10, 2006.

Rohrich RJ, Hollier LH: Management of frontal sinus fractures: Changing concepts. Clin Plast Surg 19:219, 1992.

Rohrich RJ, Mickel TJ: Frontal sinus obliteration: In search of the ideal autogenous material. Plast Reconstr Surg 95(3), 1995.

Watumull D, Rohrich RJ: Zygoma fracture fixation: A graduated anatomic approach to management based on recent clinical and biomechanical studies. Probl Plast Reconstr Surg 1(2):350, 1991.

Yavuzer R, Sari A, Jackson IT, et al. Management of frontal sinus fractures. *Plast Reconstr Surg* 115(6), 2005.

Zingg M, et al: Classification and treatment of zygomatic fractures: A review of 1,025 cases. J Oral Maxillofac Surg 50:778, 1992.

Facial Fractures II—Maxillary, Midfacial, and Mandibular Fractures

Avron Lipschitz, MD, and Brian Oleksy, DDS, MD

I. MAXILLARY AND MIDFACE FRACTURES

A. Introduction
1. **Causes**: motor vehicle collisions, sports, gunshot wounds
2. Maxilla absorbs energy, protecting the orbit, nose, and intracranial contents.
3. High incidence of associated intracranial, facial, orbital, major thoracic, abdominal, and extremity injuries

B. Anatomy
1. The midface has nine bones: maxilla, zygoma, lacrimal, nasal, ethmoid, sphenoid, palate, vomer, and inferior turbinates (Fig. 18-1).
2. **Buttress system**. Three main **vertical buttresses** (Fig. 18-2A) give strength:
   a. **Nasomaxillary (nasofrontal)**: from the canine eminence to the frontal process of the maxilla
   b. **Zygomaticomaxillary:** bears strongest load–from the first molar to the zygomatic process of the frontal bone
   c. **Pterygomaxillary buttress** projects into the skull base–from the posterior maxilla through the pterygoid plates of the sphenoid
3. **Horizontal buttresses** (Fig. 18-2B) are weaker, reinforce the vertical buttresses, and provide width and projection of the face. These include:
   a. Frontal bar–superior orbital rim and glabellar area
   b. Infraorbital rims
   c. Zygomatic arch
   d. Maxillary arch and palate
4. **Blood supply**
   a. **Upper portion of the midface**: ethmoid artery, a branch of the internal carotid artery
   b. **Lower midface**: facial artery and internal maxillary arteries (two branches from the external carotid artery)
5. **Innervation**
   a. **Sensory**: supplied by three branches of the second (maxillary) division of the trigeminal nerve (CNV)
   b. **Motor**: facial nerve (CNVII) innervates muscles of facial expression.

C. Classification of maxillary/midface fractures (Fig. 18-3):
1. Fracture pattern is classified according to the level of energy required to cause injury.
2. Le Fort classification is often inadequate to fully describe fracture pattern.

I. Maxillary and Midface Fractures

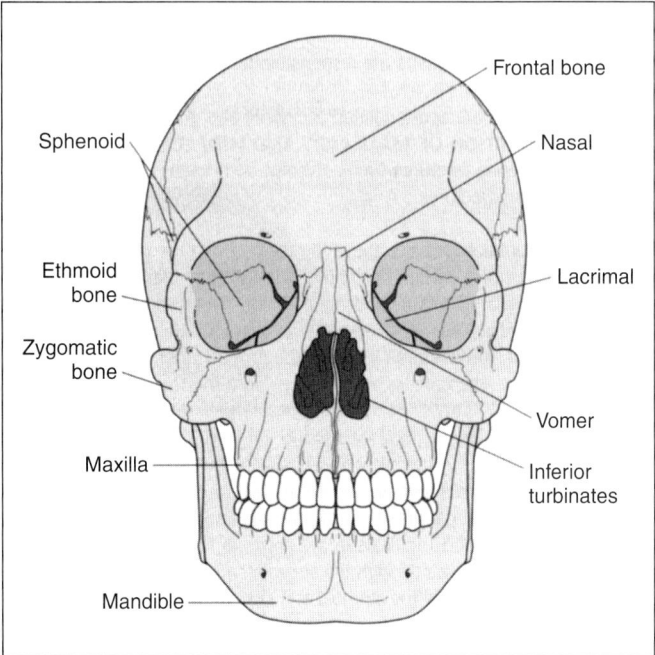

FIGURE 18-1

Frontal view of the skull.

3. A fracture may be a combination of types of Le Fort fractures (e.g., left hemi Le Fort III, right hemi Le Fort I).
   a. **Dentoalveolar fractures**: fracture of teeth and bony segment containing the teeth
   b. **Le Fort I** (low maxillary)
      (i) Transverse maxillary fracture; result of low anterior to posterior force
      (ii) A horizontal fracture above the roots of the teeth, maxillary tuberosity from the pterygoid plates extending from the piriform aperture of the nose to the pterygomaxillary fissure
   c. **Le Fort II** (pyramidal)
      (i) Result of a force delivered at the level of the nasal bones
      (ii) The maxilla and its approximating nasal complex together are separated from the orbital and zygomatic structures.
      (iii) It courses from the pterygomaxillary fissure anteriorly and upward through the infraorbital rim, over the medial orbit and nasal bones.

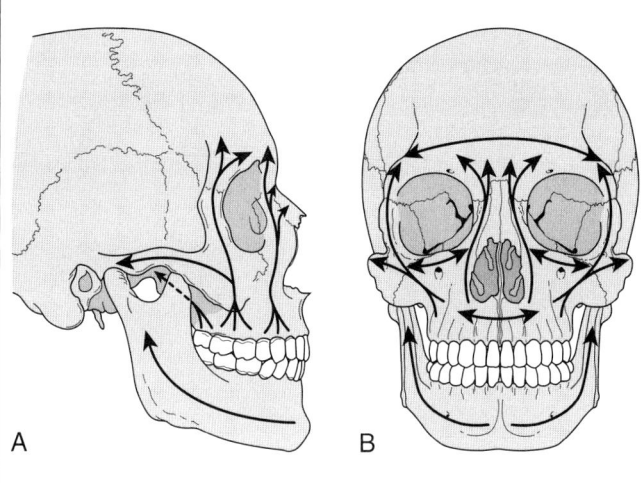

FIGURE 18-2

A, Division of midface reconstruction into upper and lower units and their relationship to cranial base and frontal cranial attachments. B, Horizontal pillars of the face.

   d. Le Fort III (craniofacial dysjunction)
      (i) Maxilla, NOE complex, and zygomas are separated from cranial base.
      (ii) Occurs as a result of high force impact at the orbital level (e.g., motor vehicle collision)
      (iii) Fracture at the nasofrontal and frontomaxillary sutures extending through medial and lateral orbital walls and floor

D. Clinical presentation

1. Facial distortion, elongated face, a mobile maxilla or midface, instability, and malocclusion
2. One hand is held on the anterior maxilla and the other on the nasal root. In general, Le Fort I fractures show movement of the lower maxilla but none at the nasal root, whereas both Le Fort II and III fractures display motion at the nasal root.
3. A step deformity at the infraorbital rim can be felt in Le Fort II fractures. Le Fort III fractures show movement at the lateral orbital rim.
4. The stability of the palate should be checked when a fracture of the midface is suspected.
5. Le Fort II and III fractures have the so-called panda facies: (1) bilateral periorbital and subconjunctival ecchymosis; (2) gross bilateral edema of the middle third of the face; (3) lengthening of the face; and (4) malocclusion.

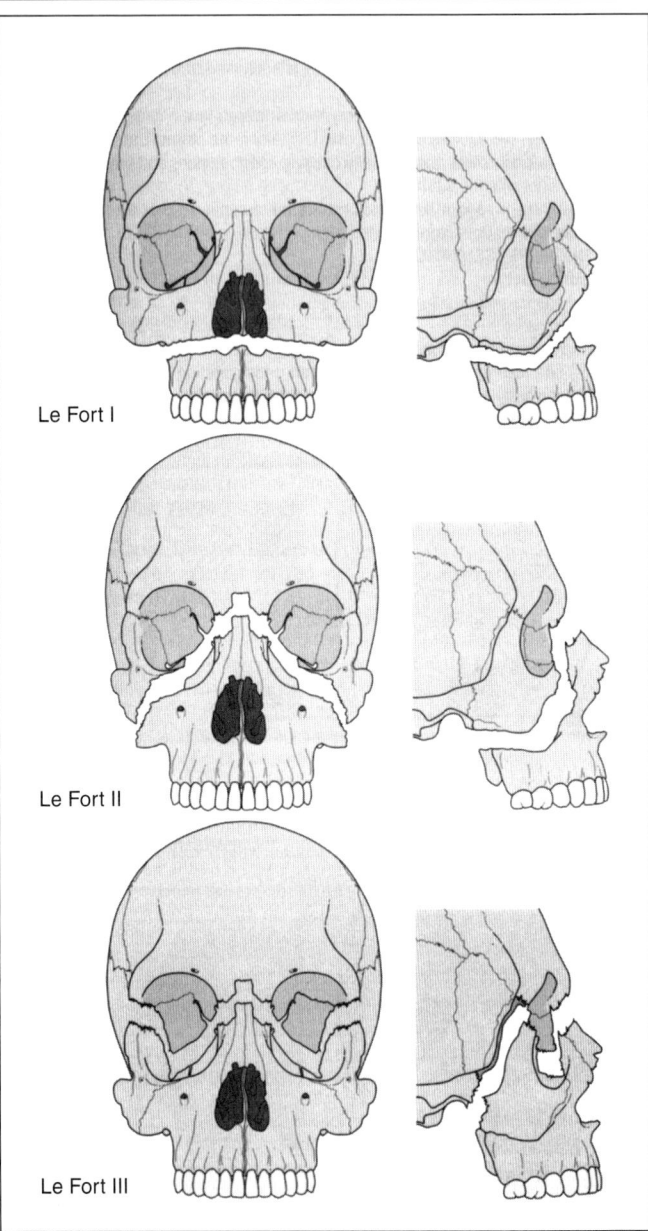

FIGURE 18-3

Common patterns of midface fractures. Several variations of the classic patterns exist. Isolated Le Fort I, II, and III level fractures are the exception rather than the rule.

I. Maxillary and Midface Fractures

6. Associated injuries may present with:
   a. Superior orbital fissure syndrome: ophthalmoplegia, fixed and dilated pupil, increased consensual response in uninvolved eye, ptosis, and loss of corneal reflex
   b. Base of skull fracture: CSF otorrhea, CSF rhinorrhea, and postauricular ecchymosis (Battle's sign)

E. Radiographic evaluation
High-resolution facial CT scanning with coronal and axial cuts is the criterion standard.

F. Management:
The treatment of any serious concurrent injuries takes precedence over the facial fractures and should include maintenance of the airway.

1. Principles of midface fracture management include the following:
   a. Early one-stage repair
   b. Wide exposure of all fracture fragments
   c. Placement into maxillomandibular fixation to re-establish the occlusion
   d. Precise anatomic reduction
   e. Rigid fixation
   f. Immediate autogenous bone grafting
   g. Simultaneous definitive soft-tissue management

2. **Goals**
   a. Restore form (normal facial height, width, and projection) and function (re-establish skeletal buttresses and preoperative occlusion).

3. **Timing**
   a. Most favorable within 24 to 48 hours once patient's condition is stable
   b. Direct fixation allows repair within 2 weeks prior to onset of scar formation, fibrosis, and bone resorption.
   c. If significant delays in treatment are expected, simple maxillomandibular fixation (MMF) should be considered as an interim treatment in order to avoid scar contracture over a malformed facial skeleton.

4. **Technique**
   a. The "inside-out, bottom-to-top" approach is generally the guiding principle in the management of panfacial trauma.
   b. Begin with MMF and mandible fracture reduction, work laterally (zygoma and zygomaticomaxillary [ZM] buttress to establish AP projection), then medial to restore buttress system.
   c. It is also possible to restore smaller components (e.g., NOE first, then assemble each component together).
   d. Closed reduction and immobilization for 4 to 6 weeks is often adequate treatment for isolated dentoalveolar fractures.
   e. Intraoral splints can be useful adjuncts to midfacial fracture reduction and immobilization.

5. **Incisions**
   a. Maxillary vestibular approach
   b. Coronal flap
   c. Periorbital (transconjunctival, subciliary, subtarsal)

6. **Miniplate fixation**
   a. Allows early removal of MMF, early return to function; biomechanical advantage over wire techniques
   b. More sensitive to technical errors than wire technique
   c. Le Fort I: complete mobilization of the maxilla, often with use of disimpaction forceps; then placed in MMF, and bone plates applied at the ZM buttress and piriform apertures
   d. Le Fort II: ZM buttress fixation usually adequate after mobilization and placing into MMF; not usually necessary to perform fixation of nasofrontal process and/or inferior orbital rim
   e. Le Fort III: coronal flap for adequate exposure, exploration, and miniplate fixation at the frontozygomatic and nasofrontal sutures
   f. Bone graft: use for significant bone loss. Harvest from anterior or posterior iliac crest or cranium.
7. **Postoperative care**
   a. Airway patency: consider tracheostomy if prolonged intubation >14 days anticipated (performed at beginning of case).
   b. Nasogastric suction: maintained until the patient is awake and alert and clinical evidence of gastrointestinal function has returned
   c. Routine nasal vasoconstriction and topical steroids can be ordered to help maintain a patent nasal airway.
   d. Elevate the head of the bed at least 30 degrees or more to decrease postoperative edema.
   e. Perioperative systemic antibiotics should be given as indicated. A topical antibiotic rinse (Chlorhexidine) is used with intraoral incisions or injuries.
   f. Analgesia: morphine PCA
   g. Soft diet for 6 weeks
G. **Complications**
1. Malunion, nonunion, plate exposure: address similar to mandible fractures
2. Palpable or observable plate: avoid with thinner plates, may remove after healing
3. Forehead or cheek hyperesthesia: caused by injury to supraorbital and infraorbital nerves; spontaneous regeneration in majority of cases
4. Osteomyelitis: treat similar to mandible fractures
5. Dental injury: may be secondary to trauma, improper reduction technique, improper placement of arch bars, or MMF

II. MANDIBLE FRACTURES

A. **Introduction**
1. The mandible plays an important role in the process of eating, speaking, and breathing. Because of its location in the face it is highly susceptible to fractures, accounting for 10% to 25% of all facial fractures.
2. The most common mechanisms of mandible fractures are assaults, motor vehicle collisions, sports injuries, falls, and gunshot wounds.

3. Most mandibular fractures occur bilaterally (two fractures).
B. Anatomy (Fig. 18-4):
1. The mandible is a U-shaped bone consisting of tooth-bearing and non-tooth-bearing portions.
2. The ascending ramus terminates in the coronoid process and mandibular condyle.
3. The mandibular angle, ramus, coronoid process, and condyle are points of attachment for the muscles of mastication.
4. The condyle articulates with the cranium to form the temporomandibular joint (TMJ).
5. The TMJ is a compressed fibrous disk interposed between the mandibular condyle and the articular fossa, allowing rotational and translational movements.
6. The blood supply of the mandible is from two primary sources:
   a. The inferior alveolar artery, a branch of the maxillary artery
   b. The major muscle groups of the lower face supply blood to the mandible through the perforating periosteal arterioles.
7. **Innervation**
   a. The inferior alveolar nerve, from the 3rd division of the trigeminal nerve, innervates the mandible, mandibular teeth, gingiva, and lower lip.
   b. The nerve parallels the course of the inferior alveolar artery within the bone, both exiting through the mental foramen.

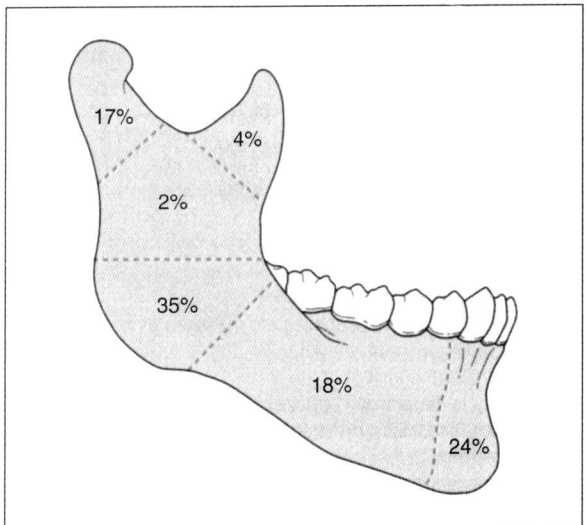

FIGURE 18-4

Anatomic classification of mandible fractures (relative incidence):

8. Normally the mandible contains 16 teeth: six molars, four premolars, two canines, and four incisors.
9. The mandible is thinnest at the angle, with a relatively high incidence of fracture in this region. This may be further compromised by the presence of an impacted third molar (wisdom tooth).
10. Fracture stability is related to the direction of the fracture line and the force of the masticatory muscles acting on the fractured segments. Favorable fractures are reduced with muscle contraction.
11. In at least half of the cases of mandible fracture, there are two fractures. There are indirect and direct fractures. If the blow is to the chin, there will be a symphysis fracture and an indirect condyle fracture usually on the opposite side.

C. Clinical presentation

1. Palpation of the mandible elicits tenderness and may define fracture edges or cause movement of the segments.
2. Pain, malocclusion, trismus, swelling, anesthesia, paresthesia, hemorrhage, and ecchymosis are frequently elicited.
3. Intraoral evaluation may reveal ecchymosis in the floor of the mouth; avulsed, loose, or fractured teeth; and mucosal or gingival lacerations.
4. Multiple crowded, rotated, or missing teeth make fracture reduction more difficult.
5. Protrusion and deviation of the jaw on opening are indicative of ipsilateral condylar fracture.
6. The TMJ is palpated indirectly via the external auditory canal and directly in the preauricular area.
7. The patient's ability to grasp and hold a tongue blade against attempts to remove it (tongue blade test) is useful in excluding mandibular fracture (95% negative predictive value).

D. Radiographic evaluation

1. Mandibular series radiographs (5 views): posteroanterior, Towne's, right and left lateral oblique, submentovertex
2. Panoramic radiographs
3. CT scans are necessary only if other facial fractures are suspected.

E. Management

1. **Goals**
   a. To achieve anatomic reduction and stabilization
   b. To restore pretraumatic occlusion
   c. To restore facial contour and symmetry
   d. To balance facial height and projection
2. **Timing**
   a. Mandibular fractures should be reduced as soon as possible to minimize pain, prevent progression of the soft tissue injury, and reduce the risk of infection.
   b. If treatment must be delayed, the fracture should be stabilized temporarily with bridle wires around the teeth adjacent to the fracture.

c. Antibiotics (penicillin or clindamycin) should be started immediately for all fractures that involve the tooth-bearing area, as they are open fractures.
3. Technique
   a. **Conservative treatment**
      (i) May be indicated when there is radiographic evidence of minimal or no displacement, normal occlusion, and normal mandibular range of motion
      (ii) Diet: soft-food or liquid-only diet for at least 6 weeks
      (iii) Physiotherapy (jaw exercises)
      (iv) Maintain good oral hygiene.
   b. **Closed reduction**
      (i) The fracture is either nondisplaced or minimally displaced.
      (ii) Arch bars and wires are applied to the teeth.
      (iii) Followed by MMF or elastics for 2 to 6 weeks to ensure a stable reduction
      (iv) May be converted to open reduction at any time
   c. **Open reduction**
      (i) Displaced fractures typically presenting with malocclusion or moderate to severe fracture mobility usually require open reduction with or without internal fixation by plating.
      (ii) Specific treatment by fracture site is beyond the scope of this chapter. See references for further reading.
      (iii) Generally, teeth in the line of fracture are extracted if grossly mobile.
      (iv) Minimally mobile and nonrestorable teeth may be retained if they play a key role in reduction of the fracture.

F. Pediatric mandible fractures
1. Mandibular fractures in children are best treated by closed reduction.
2. In children aged 2 to 6 years, sufficient primary dentition is usually present to facilitate arch bars and MMF with wires or elastics.
3. Children aged 9 to 12 years enter the stage of mixed dentition. There may be insufficient numbers of stable teeth present to facilitate placement of arch bars. Therefore, skeletal fixation with the aid of plastic splints may be required.
4. Because of the rapid healing in children, immobilization of pediatric mandibular fractures is usually limited to 1 to 2 weeks.
5. Open reduction of pediatric mandibular fractures is infrequently indicated.

G. Edentulous patients
1. Typically have atrophic mandibles from decreased loading effects from loss of dental support
2. ORIF with plates should be the procedure of choice

H. Postoperative care
1. The primary concern is the maintenance of a patent airway.
2. If significant postoperative edema is present in the floor of the mouth or pharynx, prolonged endotracheal intubation may be necessary if the patient is in MMF.

3. Aggressive postoperative physiotherapy (jaw exercises) is essential to successful rehabilitation, whether open or closed reduction is utilized or whether the patient is an adult or a child.
4. Oral hygiene is essential to reduce the risk of postoperative infection.
5. Nutritional assessment should be made to address diet concerns for adequate caloric intake.
6. Maintain on full liquid diets if MMF is used or soft mechanical diets for the patient treated by ORIF.

I. Surgical complications

1. Chin and lip hypesthesia: inferior alveolar or mental nerve injury. Spontaneous regeneration occurs in most cases.
2. Osteomyelitis: increased risk from poor oral hygiene, devitalized teeth, infected teeth in fracture line, or loose hardware. Treatment consists of removal of unstable hardware, long-term IV antibiotics, removal of infected teeth, surgical debridement of nonviable bone, and late bone grafting.
3. Malunion: Healing of bone in misalignment caused by inadequate immobilization, inaccurate reduction, infection, gross loss of bone, compromised blood supply, malnutrition, or osteopetrosis. Treatment is directed at the underlying cause; consider orthodontic realignment or osteotomy with repositioning and refixation.
4. Non-union: Failure of bone to produce osteogenic tissue; nonosteogenic (fibrous) matrix produced. Treatment is to excise fibrous tissue and nonviable bone and refixation; may require bone grafting.
5. Plate exposure: its etiology is similar to malunion: treat underlying cause; give oral and topical antibiotics; plate should be retained as long as possible; remove the plate when completely healed.
6. Marginal mandibular nerve injury: increased risk with external approach to ORIF; consider repair if noted intraoperatively; usually a temporary neurapraxia from retraction of the nerve during surgery
7. Condylar head necrosis: secondary to vascular compromise; treat with debridement of necrotic bone and reconstruction.
8. TMJ ankylosis: inability to open jaw > 5 mm between incisors; may cause facial deformities from growth disorders at the joint. Fibrous ankylosis: passive jaw opening exercises; bony ankylosis requires reconstruction.
9. Dental injury may be caused by improperly placed arch bars and MMF.

III. SUGGESTED READINGS

Bruce RA, Ellis E III: The second Chalmers J Lyons Academy study of fractures of the edentulous mandible. J Oral Maxillofac Surg 51:904, 1993.

Ellis E III, Scott K: Assessment of patients with facial fractures. Emerg Med Clin North Am 18:411, 2000.

Forrest CR, Antonyshyn OM: Acute management of complex midface fractures. Oper Tech Plast Reconstr Surg 5(3):188, 1998.

Gruss JS, Phillips JH: Complex facial trauma: The evolving role of rigid fixation and immediate bone graft reconstruction. Clin Plast Surg 16(1):93, 1989.

Manson PN, Clark N, Robertson B, et al: Subunit principles in midface fractures: The importance of sagittal buttresses, soft-tissue reductions, and sequencing treatment of segmental fractures. Plast Reconstr Surg 103:1287, 1999.

Manson PN, Crawley WA, Yaremchuk MJ, et al: Advantages of immediate extended open reduction and bone grafting. Plast Reconstr Surg 76:1, 1985.

Manson PN, Glassman D, Vander Kolk C, et al: Rigid stabilization of sagittal fractures of the maxilla and palate. Plast Reconstr Surg 85:711, 1990.

Marchena JM, Padwa BL, Kaban LB: Sensory abnormalities associated with mandibular fractures: Incidence and natural history. J Oral Maxillofac Surg 56:822, 1998.

Markowitz BL, Manson PN: Panfacial fractures: Organization of treatment. Clin Plast Surg 16(1):105, 1989.

Posnick JC, Wells M, Pron GE: Pediatric facial fractures: Evolving patterns of treatment. J Oral Maxillofac Surg 51:836, 1993.

Walker RV, Fonseca RJ: Oral and Maxillofacial Trauma, ed 2, vol 1. Philadelphia, Saunders, 1997.

Zide MF, Kent JN: Indications of open reduction of mandibular condyle fractures. J Oral Maxillofac Surg 41:89, 1983.

Ophthalmic Injuries

Fiemu E. Nwariaku, MD

I. OVERVIEW

1. **Ocular trauma** is often associated with intracranial injuries.
2. **The examiner** should be familiar with the anatomy of the eye (Fig. 19-1). and use of a slit lamp.
3. **An ophthalmologic consultation** must be obtained when the diagnosis or management is in question.

II. EXAMINATION

1. **Examination of the patient with multiple injuries** performed at the bedside is quite different from that of the medically stable patient who should be examined with the slit lamp.
2. **The functional state of the eye** must be determined prior to a detailed anatomical examination.
3. **The use of mydriatic agents** should be postponed until the patient is neurologically stable.
4. **Topical anesthetics** may be utilized to facilitate the examination. However, under no circumstance should the patient be allowed to use the medication for pain control, since repeated usage will lead to corneal decompensation.
A. Visual acuity
1. **Always check visual acuity first** (with the exception of a chemical burn).
2. **Assess each eye individually.**
3. **Assess with a Snellen chart.**
4. **When evaluating distance vision,** a pinhole occluder is able to eliminate refractive error from patients who do not have their glasses.
5. **A near card is useful** when examining at the bedside.
6. **Document appropriately,** such as "patient can read small print at 14 inches (35 cm)."
7. **The elderly presbyope** may be unable to perform a near-vision test without corrective lenses.
8. **If patients cannot read the eye chart,** see if they can count fingers, recognize hand motion, or perceive light.
B. **Visual fields.** Each eye is tested individually as the patient is instructed to fixate on the examiner's nose as follows:
1. **To test the patient's right eye,** the left eye should be occluded.
2. **The patient opens his or her left eye** while closing the right eye.
3. **Fingers are flashed in each quadrant** at a point halfway between the patient and the examiner.
4. Visual field defects commonly seen in trauma patients include:
    a. Retinal detachment

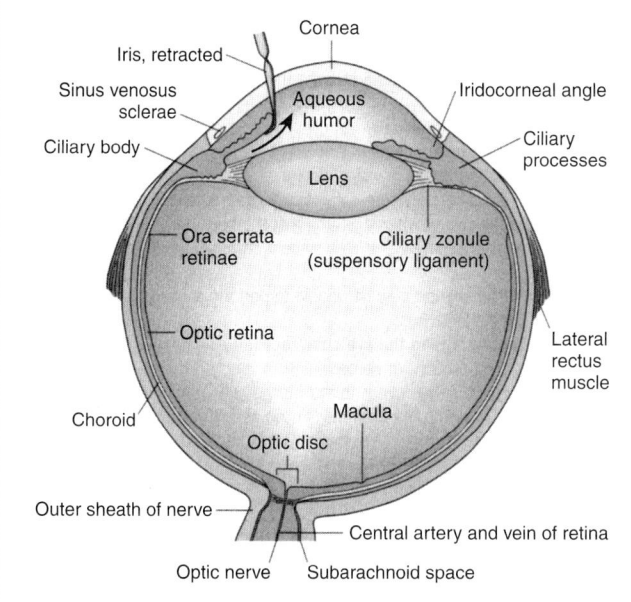

FIGURE 19-1

Horizontal section of eyeball. Observe its three coats: external or fibrous coat (sclera and cornea), middle or vascular coat (choroid, ciliary body, and iris), and internal or retinal layer. The four refractive media are the cornea, aqueous humor, lens, and vitreous body. Arrow indicates flow of aqueous humor from the posterior chamber to the anterior chamber. Aqueous humor is a thin, watery medium formed in the posterior chamber by the ciliary process. (From Moore K: Clinically Oriented Anatomy, 3rd ed. Baltimore, Williams & Wilkins, 1992.)

   b. Vitreous hemorrhage
   c. Cerebral injuries
C. Extraocular movements
1. **The six positions of cardinal gaze** need to be carefully evaluated.
2. **The oculomotor nerve** (CN III) innervates the superior rectus (SR), medial rectus (MR), inferior rectus (IR), inferior oblique (IO), and the levator muscle.
3. **The trochlear nerve** (CN IV) innervates the superior oblique (SO).
4. **The lateral rectus** (LR) is innervated by the abducens nerve (CN VII).
5. **Findings suggestive of injury:**
   a. Double vision
   b. Pain when gaze is directed away from the trapped muscle.

c. Entrapment Limiting mobility

D. Pupils

1. **Pupillary reaction:** brisk, sluggish, or absent?
2. **Shape.** Is the pupil round or irregular?
3. **Determine if an afferent pupillary defect** (APD or Marcus Gunn pupil) is present.
   a. This is accomplished by shining the light in one eye, then quickly shining the light in the opposite eye. Repeat this as many times as it takes to obtain a consistent response.
   b. In the normal patient, the direct response should cause the initial pupil to constrict; the response in the opposite eye will be to constrict.
   c. When the light is quickly moved to the opposite eye, the pupil should remain constricted if light is being perceived equally in both eyes.
   d. In the trauma patient with an APD, one would expect to see a sluggish reaction in the affected eye, a brisk reaction in a normal eye.
   e. When light is moved from the sluggish pupil to the normal eye, constriction will occur, indicating presence of an APD.
4. **Causes of APD include:**
   a. Traumatic optic neuropathy
   b. Retinal detachment
   c. Vitreous hemorrhage
   d. Retrobulbar hemorrhage
   e. Traumatic iritis
   f. Incarceration of iris in wound

E. Orbital rim

1. Examination
   a. Feel for step-off deformity.
   b. Evaluate for dystopia.
   c. Determine if hypesthesia is present in V1, V2, and V3.
2. **Management**
   a. CT scan (see Section III, Imaging)
   b. Blowout fractures can be associated with numerous injuries including extraocular muscle (EOM) entrapment, hyphema, ruptured globe, and traumatic optic neuropathy.
   c. When superior roof fracture exists, combined operative repair with a neurosurgeon is necessary.
   d. Surgical repair is often performed 2 weeks after injury when soft tissue swelling is minimized.
   e. A medial wall blowout fracture may not require surgery unless entrapment or other complications exist.

F. Eyelid

1. **Examination**
   a. Inability to open lid may indicate a CN III palsy or more commonly levator dehiscence (Fig. 19-2).
   b. Inability to close the lid may indicate facial nerve involvement.
   c. Identify foreign bodies and lacerations.

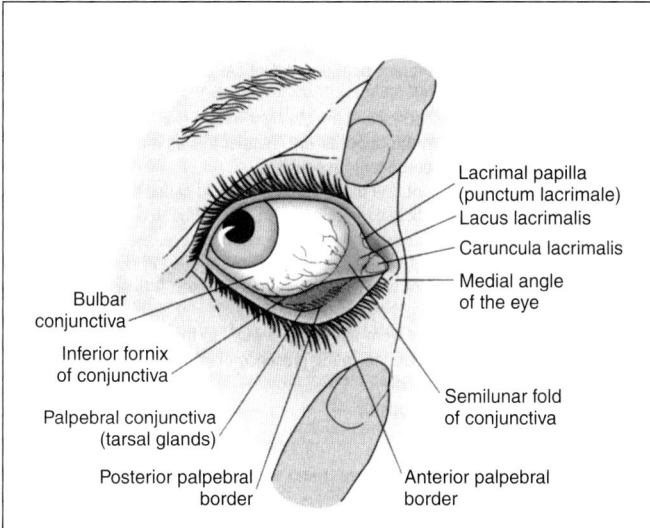

FIGURE 19-2

Right lower eyelid and medial angle. (From Clemente CD. Anatomy: A Regional Atlas of the Human Body, 3rd ed. Philadelphia, Lea & Febiger, 1967.)

   d. Examine under eyelids until cul-de-sacs are visualized, using a bent paper clip to evert the lid.
   e. Avoid pressure on the globe.
2. **Management**
   a. Remove all foreign bodies and irrigate the cul-de-sacs with saline.
   b. Lacerations involving the lacrimal sac should be repaired in the operating room.
   c. Uncomplicated lacerations may be repaired with 6-0 nylon.
   d. Care should be taken to prevent sutures from having contact with the cornea.
   e. The tarsal plate must be appropriately realigned to prevent lid notching.
   f. Excess tension can create an entropion, or an ectropion, or may induce lagophthalmos (inability to close upper eyelid).
   g. If fat is visualized at a laceration site, the orbital septum has been violated and closure of these wounds in the emergency room is ill-advised. Consultation with an ophthalmologist is essential since a large percentage of these patients will develop ptosis.

G. Conjunctiva and sclera
1. Examination
  a. Evaluate for subconjunctival hemorrhage, injection, laceration, abrasion, foreign body.
  b. Fluorescein. Wet a fluorescein strip, apply liberally, and place on conjunctival surface. A Wood's lamp or slit lamp will clearly show areas devoid of corneal epithelium. The entire surface of the globe should be evaluated. If aqueous humor is seen percolating through the fluorescein, a ruptured globe exists (see Section IV, C, Ruptured globe).

2. Management
  a. Subconjunctival hemorrhage, which can exist without additional pathology, will resolve in approximately 2 weeks. If it is present and extends posteriorly, or is present in 360°, a retrobulbar hemorrhage must be ruled out (see Section IV, Retrobulbar hemorrhage).
  b. An injected eye may indicate venous congestion secondary to an obstructive phenomenon.
  c. Conjunctival lacerations need to be evaluated with the slit lamp, if possible, to rule out scleral involvement. Small lacerations are frequently left unrepaired although antibiotic coverage is necessary.

H. Cornea
1. Examination
  a. Evaluate for clarity, foreign body, laceration, or abrasion.
  b. Clarity. A cloudy cornea is usually the result of acute stromal edema often seen with elevated intraocular pressure.
  c. Fluorescein (see Section II, Conjunctiva and sclera).

2. Management
  a. A superficial foreign body embedded in the cornea can be removed with a cotton-tip applicator, a foreign body spud (a blunt needle), or a 25-gauge needle after instillation of topical anesthetic.
  b. Bacitracin ointment (or other nonsteroidal ointments) can be applied 4 times a day.
  c. Pressure patching is best avoided when abrasion is at high risk of infection.
  d. Cycloplegic drops (cyclopentolate 2%) can be applied. The patient should be seen the next day by an ophthalmologist.
  e. Laceration (see Section IV, C, Ruptured globe).

I. Anterior chamber
1. Examination
  a. Evaluate for hyphema, cell and flare, and depth. A flat anterior chamber is often seen with a ruptured globe.
  b. The anterior chamber is difficult to evaluate without the use of the slit lamp.

2. Management
  a. If layered blood (hyphema) is present in the anterior chamber (AC) an ophthalmologist should be contacted regarding management. This would often include:
     i. Bed rest

ii. Atropine
iii. Topical steroids
iv. Medications to control intraocular pressure
b. Surgery may be necessary if the hyphema is large, slow to resolve, or if it creates corneal endothelial staining.
c. All dark-skinned patients should have a sickle cell prep performed.

J. Iris
1. **Examination**
   a. Traumatic iritis will show evidence of cells in the AC.
   b. The patient will usually be extremely photophobic.
   c. Irregularity may be present with a penetrating injury (see Section II, Pupil).
2. **Management**
   a. If there is no evidence of additional pathology the patient may be started on cyclopentolate 2% 4 times a day.
   b. Consult an ophthalmologist prior to initiating topical steroids.

K. Lens
1. **Disruption of lens material** will often produce a traumatic cataract.
2. **Occasionally the lens can dislocate.**
3. **Patients with trauma involving the lens** are at higher risk of endophthalmitis.

L. Vitreous and retina
1. **Examination**
   a. The dilated examination must be deferred untill the patient is neurologically stable.
   b. When a vitreous hemorrhage is present the red reflex may appear darkened.
   c. In patients with suspected traumatic optic neuropathy, it is imperative to examine the fundus to exclude a vitreous hemorrhage which can produce an APD and a decrease in visual acuity.
   d. Most retinal detachments will not be visible by direct (and undilated) ophthalmoscopy although they can certainly cause an APD.
   e. The patient who complains of recent onset of floaters and flashes of light is at risk of a retinal detachment.
   f. Some patients will report a black spot in the affected region.
   g. "Tobacco dust" (pigment seen floating in the posterior chamber) can be seen with a retinal detachment.
2. **Management**
   a. Patients with a vitreous hemorrhage will often need constant bed rest with the head of the bed elevated to 30°.
   b. Activity must be limited (no bending over, no heavy lifting), and close follow-up with ophthalmology is necessary.
   c. Ultrasonography may need to be performed to determine if a coexisting retinal detachment is present.
   d. If a retinal detachment is present it may or may not require immediate surgery.

e. Factors include location of the detachment, vision, and duration of detachment. Immediate consultation with an ophthalmologist is mandatory.

III. IMAGING

A. CT Scan. This is the study of choice for patients with ocular trauma.
1. **Coronal axial views** (1.5-mm sections) should be obtained on all patients with ocular trauma.
2. **Thin 1.5-mm sections** will facilitate identification of foreign bodies, which may be missed on a standard head CT with 5-mm sections.

B. Evaluation
1. Foreign bodies
2. Orbital wall fracture
3. Tenting of the optic nerve
4. Retrobulbar hemorrhage
5. Penetration of cornea, lens, or sclera

IV. RECOGNITION OF VISION-THREATENING EMERGENCIES

The following instances require immediate recognition and intervention, including an urgent consultation with an ophthalmologist.

A. Chemical burn
1. **Perform irrigation immediately**
2. **Apply anesthetic drops**
3. **Irrigation with saline** should be instituted and performed for at least 30 minutes.
4. **Application of a lid speculum** will allow effective cul-de-sac irrigation.
5. **The pH should be checked**, preferably 3 to 5 minutes after irrigation is complete. Irrigation should be reinstituted if pH is not between 7.3 and 7.6
6. **Alkali burns are much more serious than acid burns** since they can directly penetrate the sclera and may take longer to neutralize.
7. **Once the pH is neural, fluorescein should be instilled in the eye** to evaluate if there are epithelial defects present. Cycloplegic drops (scopolamine 0.25%), antibiotic ointment, and an eye patch should be applied.

B. Traumatic optic neuropathy
1. **Evalution**
   a. In patients with orbital blowout fractures, traumatic optic neuropathy must be excluded.
   b. The swinging flashlight test is essential in determining the presence of an APD.
   c. A decrease in visual acuity and poor color vision are other associated findings.

2. **Management**
   a. Use of high-dose steroids for traumatic optic neuropathy is controversial.
   b. In many trauma cases with dirty wounds and open fractures high-dose steroids are relatively contraindicated.
   c. These cases should be handled on an individual basis with ophthalmologic consultation.

C. Ruptured globe

1. **Corneal and scleral lacerations** are often visualized with the penlight examination.
2. **If an obvious lacerations exists**, the examination is terminated; the wound is covered with sterile gauze pending repair in the operating room.
3. **Additional findings on slit-lamp examination include:**
   a. Subconjunctival hemorrhage
   b. Flat anterior chamber
   c. Hyphema
   d. Iris protrusion through cornea
   e. Irregular pupil
4. **Blunt injuries may produce lacerations,** which can occur under or adjacent to the rectus muscles.
5. **Liberal application of fluorescein** will aid in the diagnosis.
6. **Fluorescein should be applied over the suspicious area**. If a subtle laceration exists aqueous humor can be seen percolating through the fluorescein dye.
7. **If an impaled object is present, do not remove.**

D. Retrobulbar hemorrhage

1. **Two signs should always alert the examiner** to the possibility of a retrobulbar hemorrhage.
   a. **Proptosis**
   b. **Subconjunctival hemorrhage**
2. **Proptosis that shows resistance to retropulsion** (retropulsion should not be attempted until a ruptured globe has been conclusively ruled out) may be associated with retrobulbar hemorrhage.
3. **Other signs include increased intraocular pressure and venous congestion.**
   a. In some cases the pressure can become so high that it can occlude the central retinal artery.
   b. If the fundoscopic examination shows a pulsating arterial flow, a central retinal artery occlusion (CRAO) may be imminent.
   c. A lateral canthotomy with cantholysis may be required to alleviate the pressure.

E. Other emergent ophthalmologic conditions

1. **Uncal herniation and aneurysm**—may see pupil involved and CN III palsy
2. **Carotid–cavernous fistula**—congested eye with an ocular bruit
3. **Cavernous sinus pathology**—EOM abnormalities with associated CN V involvement

V. PEARLS AND PITFALLS

1. **Isolated cranial nerve injuries** can occur with closed head trauma.
2. **When an oculomotor nerve palsy is present** with a pupil abnormality, an aneurysm or uncal herniation must be considered.
3. **Pathology involving the cavernous sinus** should be considered, particularly if there is trigeminal nerve involvement.
4. **When EOM abnormalities exist**, in the presence of dilated conjunctival vessels the eye should be auscultated to see if a bruit exists—which may be heard when an arteriovenous fistula is present.
5. **An APD in a trauma patient** can be difficult to identify in a patient with swollen lids. Unless an equal amount of light can be presented in each eye, an accurate determination of an APD cannot be made. Lids can be manually separated. It is imperative to avoid putting pressure on the globe and this is best done using a lid speculum.

VI. SUGGESTED READINGS

American Academy of Ophthalmology, Vol. I-XII, San Francisco, 1994.

Spoor TC, Hartel WC, Lensink DB, *et al:* Treatment of traumatic optic neuropathy with corticosteroids. Am J Ophthalmol 110(6):665–669, 1990.

Steinsapir KD, Goldberg RA: Traumatic optic neuropathy. Surv Ophthalmol 38:487–518, 1994.

Neck Injuries

Jennifer L. McDougal, MD

I. INTRODUCTION

A. Mechanism of injury and anatomic location dictate the priorities in the evaluation and treatment of neck injuries.
B. Penetrating injuries constitute the vast majority and are more likely to injure the soft tissue, vascular structures, and aerodigestive organs.
C. Blunt trauma has a greater predilection for musculoskeletal and neurological injuries.
D. Airway compromise from laryngotracheal injuries, along with sustained hemorrhage from injuries to the major vessels, causes most of the mortalities from neck injuries.

II. INITIAL ASSESSMENT

A. Life-threatening airway obstruction or exsanguinating hemorrhage is addressed emergently.
B. Endotracheal intubation is preferred, although a surgical airway may be necessary.
C. Upon completion of the primary survey, the stable patient is assessed for evidence of neck injury in the secondary survey.
1. The rigid cervical collar must be removed in order to perform an adequate examination. The neck should be stabilized by an assistant during this procedure.
2. Signs and symptoms include expanding hematoma, pulsatile bleeding, airway obstruction, sucking or bubbling neck wounds, instability of the laryngeal cartilage, thrills suggesting arteriovenous fistula, crepitus in patients with aerodigestive injury, and bruits. Assessment is made for skeletal stability by examining the neck for pain and step-offs.
3. In patients with low-velocity penetrating injuries, such as stab wounds or shotgun wounds, determination of platysma muscle penetration is a crucial part of the initial evaluation
   a. Penetrating injuries that violate the platysma have a high incidence of involvement of deeper structures.
   b. Platysma penetration requires further evaluation or therapy, whereas superficial wounds may be managed in an ambulatory setting.
   c. The wound should NOT be probed, as this may dislodge clots and aggravate further bleeding.
   d. Foreign bodies that are lodged in this area should be left in place and removed in the operating room where hemorrhage and airway compromise can be safely managed.
   e. Insertion of a nasogastric tube is deferred in patients with suspected vascular injury in order to avoid the possibility of dislodging clot or stimulating bleeding.

f. Plain radiographs should be obtained to locate missiles or rule out retained foreign bodies.

III. ZONES OF THE NECK

A. The neck is divided into 3 zones (Fig. 20-1) for the purpose of determining priorities, obtaining diagnostic studies, and preoperative planning of surgical procedures.
1. Zone I is the horizontal area between the clavicles and cricoid cartilage that includes the great vessels, trachea, esophagus, innominate vein at the thoracic outlet, and apices of both lungs.
   a. Penetrating injuries to this area usually require significant preoperative planning.
   b. At Parkland Memorial Hospital, multiple diagnostic studies are performed in these patients to help identify injuries and appropriately plan surgical approaches.
      i. A hemodynamically stable patient with a zone 1 injury will undergo aortic arch and great vessel visualization with computed tomographic angiography (CTA), bronchoscopy, and rigid esophagoscopy
      ii. In patients with a low suspicion for esophageal injury, cine-esophagography can be substituted for rigid esophagoscopy to avoid general anesthesia.

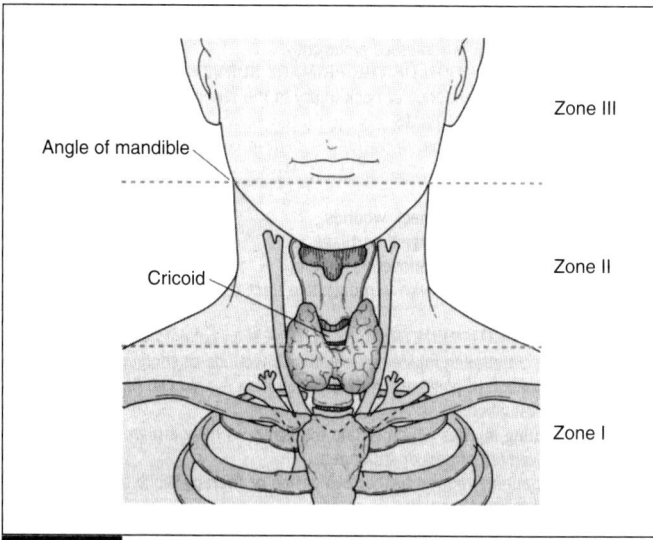

FIGURE 20-1

Anatomic zones of the neck. *(From Moore EE, Mattox KL, Feliciano DV (eds): Trauma. East Norwalk, CT, Appleton & Lange, 1987, p306.)*

c. Most injuries to zone 1 can be approached through a median sternotomy.
   d. Proximal left subclavian artery injuries will require a left anterolateral thoracotomy for proximal control.
   e. A right thoracotomy may be required for high esophageal injuries.
2. Zone II extends from the cricoid cartilage to the angle of the mandible and contains the trachea, carotid artery, jugular vein, vertebral vessels, esophagus, and cervical spine.
   a. Anatomic structures in zone II are easily accessible through an oblique neck incision along the sternocleidomastoid muscle with minimal morbidity.
   b. There are no significant differences in missed injuries between surgical exploration and nonoperative evaluation by angiography, bronchoscopy, and esophagography.
      i. Operative management has cost advantages and low morbidity, and thus operative exploration of zone II injuries is favored at Parkland.
3. Zone III extends from the angle of the mandible to the base of the skull and contains vascular structures including the internal carotid and vertebral arteries.
   a. Operative exposure is frequently limited and distal control of vascular injuries can be challenging, especially with high carotid lesions.
   b. CT angiography is the preferred method of evaluation for stable patients at Parkland.
   c. Several maneuvers can improve operative exposure, including mandibular subluxation; however, this needs to be achieved prior to making the neck incision.

IV. VASCULAR INJURIES

A. Vascular and airway injuries account for the majority of deaths due to neck trauma.
B. The common carotid artery is the most frequently injured structure in most series, occurring in approximately 5% of all vascular injuries.
C. The internal jugular vein is the most commonly injured vein.
D. A normal vascular examination may be present in 10% to 30% of patients with vascular injuries, thus allowing for the possibility of missed injuries when relying solely on physical examination.
E. Radiologic examination is essential to the identification and localization of carotid injuries.
1. Arteriography has been the "gold standard" for assessing the carotid.
2. A study at Parkland Memorial Hospital has demonstrated that CT angiography with at least a 16-channel detector is an acceptable, less invasive method of screening for blunt carotid and vertebral injuries. The use of 0.5-mm-thick images and 3-dimensional reconstructions provide a definite advantage over catheter angiography. This has become the procedure of choice at Parkland Memorial Hospital.

3. Radiologic examinations also provide useful information regarding the collateral circulation and presence of vascular anomalies, which may affect the surgical management.
   a. Only 20% of all individuals have a complete circle of Willis, an important factor when contemplating ligation of the carotid artery.
   b. Approximately 3% of patients obtain blood supply to their spinal cord from the vertebral artery, thus rendering vertebral artery ligation a disastrous complication in this group of patients.

F. Operative management

1. Indications for neck exploration include expanding hematoma, pulsatile hemorrhage, neurologic deficit, presence of a thrill or bruit, and/or airway compromise.
2. All carotid artery or internal jugular venous injuries are repaired, when possible, with lateral arteriorrhaphy or venorrhaphy.
3. Patients with severe venous injuries who have a patent contralateral jugular vein can undergo ligation of the injured jugular vein.
4. It is important to remember that air emboli occur frequently after major venous injuries, and that irrespective of the type of repair used, subsequent thrombosis is common.
5. Major carotid artery injuries may require a vein patch or interposition graft; thus, the contralateral groin should be prepared and draped to allow simultaneous vein harvest.
6. At Parkland, patients requiring prolonged reconstruction or additional repair of concomitant aerodigestive tract injuries undergo routine vascular shunting.
7. Ligation of the external carotid artery may be considered in the unstable patient with multiple injuries.
8. Ligation of the internal carotid artery may be fraught with severe neurologic complications and is avoided.
   a. Internal carotid artery ligation may be considered in the patient with carotid occlusion without distal flow and a dense neurologic deficit.
9. A decision must be made regarding the safety of repair and restoration of flow in patients with a severe neurologic deficit.
   a. This is made more difficult in the patient with a concomitant head injury.
   b. Parkland recommends repair of carotid artery injuries if technically possible in all patients who are not comatose and are hemodynamically stable.
      i. If the patient has evidence of a dense stroke and no antegrade flow, the risk of death may be increased; therefore, ligation without repair may be a satisfactory alternative.
10. Distal carotid injuries located near the base of the skull are often difficult to control operatively due to limited exposure.
    a. These may require embolization or ligation if collateral circulation is adequate.

b. Insertion of a small balloon catheter will facilitate temporary hemostasis in a high, distal lesion.
c. In situations with poor collateral flow, an extracranial-intracranial bypass procedure may be necessary in order to prevent neurologic sequelae.
11. At Parkland Memorial Hospital, intraoperative completion angiography is performed to confirm a patent vascular repair without narrowing, as failure to do so may result in postoperative thrombosis.

G. For blunt cerebrovascular injuries and small intimal flap injuries from penetrating trauma, anticoagulation is advocated when there are no existing contraindications for heparinization.
1. Although open surgical repair remains the gold standard, minimally invasive therapies including endovascular stenting are now being used at Parkland.

H. The majority of vertebral artery injuries are not life threatening and can be managed nonoperatively.
1. Many of these injuries, especially high distal arteriovenous fistulae, are treated with embolization in the presence of adequate collateral circulation.
2. Proximal vertebral artery injuries can be managed by operative proximal and distal ligation.

V. PHARYNGEAL INJURIES

A. Pharyngeal injuries generally occur as a result of penetrating trauma.
B. These injuries may produce minimal signs and symptoms; hence they are frequently missed, resulting in postinjury infections.
C. When identified during exploration, these injuries are repaired with at least two layers of absorbable suture and drained adequately.
1. Proper mucosal apposition will reduce the incidence of postoperative leaks.

D. An isolated hypopharyngeal wound can be managed conservatively with nasogastric tube feeding and antibiotics.
E. Cervical osteomyelitis is a disastrous complication occasionally associated with pharyngo-esophageal injuries that occur in combination with penetrating cervical spine wounds.
1. Contamination with pharyngeal flora is a contributing factor.
2. This complication can be reduced by aggressive debridement, including distal and ligamentous structures, stable spinal fixation, and appropriate antimicrobial therapy.

VI. LARYNGEAL INJURIES

A. Laryngeal injuries are usually mucosal tears, fractures of bony or cartilaginous structures, or avulsions and transections.
B. Laryngeal injuries are classified as supraglottic, transglottic, or cricoid in location.

C. Indications for surgery include significant mucosal disruption or avulsion, arytenoid dislocation, and exposed cartilage.
D. Timing of the operation is important, and studies have shown improved results with early operation.
E. In one series, 87% of injuries repaired within 24 hours had a good airway, compared with 69% in patients treated within 2 to 7 days postoperatively.
F. The preferred method for evaluating the larynx and trachea is by combined use of direct laryngoscopy and bronchoscopy.
G. The most common complications of laryngeal injury are infection, airway stenosis or obstruction, and voice changes.
1. Infection is treated by debridement, drainage, and antibiotics.
2. Airway stenosis is resolved by tracheal or laryngeal reconstruction.
H. A fractured larynx is a contraindication to endotracheal intubation.

VII. TRACHEAL INJURIES

A. Isolated tracheal injuries are rare with both blunt and penetrating trauma.
B. The associated injuries are often more dramatic, and subtle trauma to the trachea may be overlooked.
C. Indicators of possible tracheal injury include sucking neck wounds, crepitus on examination, soft tissue air on plain radiographs, and hemoptysis.
D. Bronchoscopy is accurate in identifying the injury.
E. One-layer repair with absorbable monofilament suture is the preferred method of treatment at Parkland.
1. In the presence of tissue loss, mobilization of the trachea can obtain up to 5 cm of length and provide a tension-free repair.
2. Interposition of vascularized tissue (e.g., omohyoid or sternocleidomastoid muscle) is essential when there is a concomitant esophageal or arterial injury to prevent the development of a fistula.
3. Damage control can be accomplished by the insertion of a T-tube.

VIII. ESOPHAGEAL INJURIES

A. Cervical esophageal injuries occur infrequently.
B. During a 3-year prospective study at Parkland Memorial Hospital, 11 cervical esophageal injuries were identified.
C. Penetrating trauma is the more common etiology, although these injuries may be associated with blunt trauma, such as cervical spine fractures and crush injuries.
D. Missed injuries are not uncommon since they are often masked by trauma to surrounding organs that precludes their identification.
E. Early detection of esophageal injuries is essential as mortality rates have been reported to be as high as 17% following a 12-hour delay.

F. Diagnostic techniques
1. Although diagnostic studies, such as contrast radiography and endoscopy, are fairly reliable, false-negative results do occur.
2. Flexible endoscopy is much less reliable in identifying cervical esophageal injuries.
   a. One series showed that flexible endoscopy had a sensitivity of only 38% compared to 89% for rigid esophagoscopy.

G. Operative issues
1. These injuries may be elusive in the operating room, and a careful search must be performed, including the posterior aspect.
2. Esophageal injuries should be repaired in two layers, and all repairs should have closed-suction drainage and antibiotic prophylaxis.
3. Tenuous repairs are buttressed with a pleural or muscle flap.
4. Massive injuries may require resection or exclusion with distal ligation, gastrostomy tube placement, and proximal diversion in the form of an esophagostomy.

H. Complications
1. Missed injuries can cause infectious complications, such as mediastinitis, cervical abscesses, and sepsis, but the more common problems seen following repair of these injuries are fistula formation and dysphagia.
2. Esophageal leaks are attributed to inadequate debridement, poor surgical technique when repairing the injury, and devascularization of the wall.
3. The incidence of esophagocutaneous fistula is about 10% to 30%.
4. All patients should have a contrast study performed prior to starting an oral diet.

IX. MUSCULOSKELETAL

A. Skeletal and ligamentous injuries are more common following blunt trauma.

B. Evaluation
1. Flexion and extension radiographs, as well as other specialized imaging techniques, may need to be delayed while emergent problems are addressed.
2. When evaluating potential skeletal injuries in the neck, the physician must be compulsive in visualizing the C7-T1 interspace, as well as the odontoid.
3. At Parkland Memorial Hospital, we use CT as the primary modality for evaluating the cervical spine.
4. MRI studies may occasionally be warranted to completely evaluate for ligamentous injury.

C. Specific injuries
1. A stable burst fracture (Jefferson fracture) of the atlas (C1) occurs as a result of impaction of the ring of C1 against the occipital condyles.
   a. It is commonly seen with an axial load imparted to the top of the head.

2. Odontoid fractures are often associated with falls, blows to the head, motor vehicle collisions, and some sports (e.g., gymnastics).
   a. A type 1 fracture extends through the tip of the odontoid.
   b. A type 2 extends through the body.
   c. A type 3 involves the base and the body of C2.
3. Severe extension injuries may cause a hangman's fracture (i.e., a fracture of the pedicle of the axis and a dislocation of C2 on C3).
   a. Owing to the large diameter of the spinal canal at this level, a neurologic deficit may not occur.
D. Treatment of skeletal and ligamentous injuries is by external stabilization or internal fixation, depending on the stability of the fracture.

X. LYMPHATICS

A. The thoracic duct is the most commonly injured lymphatic in the neck.
B. These injuries may be identified during neck exploration but are usually discovered late in the hospital course.
1. Unexplained fever, abscess formation, or abnormal fluid collections should raise the suspicion of a thoracic duct injury.
2. Drainage of milky white fluid from suction drains placed at the time of surgery or aspiration of this material is often the first sign of a lymph fistula, lymphocele, or even a chylothorax.
C. Conservative management is usually adequate as these collections resolve spontaneously.
D. However, if prolonged drainage continues, thoracic duct ligation is preferable to attempts at primary repair.
E. Wide drainage usually results in resolution of these complications.
F. Delayed ligation can be performed if conservative management fails.

XI. PEARLS AND PITFALLS

A. Defer insertion of nasogastric tube in patients with suspected vascular neck injuries.
B. Do not remove impaled foreign bodies in the emergency department, as their removal may precipitate uncontrollable hemorrhage.
C. Use liberal indications for four-vessel angiography in patients with blunt neck injury to identify stretch or intimal flaps.

XII. SUGGESTED READINGS

Britt LD: Neck injuries: Evaluation and management. In Moore EE, Mattox KL, Feliciano DV (eds): Trauma. New York, Mc-Graw Hill, pp 445-457.

Leopold DA: Laryngeal trauma. Arch Otolaryngol 109:106, 1983.

Weigelt JA, Thal ER, Synder WH III, et al: Diagnosis of penetrating cervical esophageal injuries. Am J Surg 154:619, 1987.

Thoracic Trauma

Adam W. Beck, MD

I. INCIDENCE

A. Thoracic trauma accounts for 25% of the approximately 150,000 annual trauma deaths in the United States.

II. ANATOMY

A. Structures at risk include:
1. Vascular – heart, aorta, vena cava, pulmonary vessels and innominate, subclavian, common carotid, jugular, and vertebral vessels
2. Nerves – brachial plexus, vagus, recurrent laryngeal nerves, phrenic nerves, and spinal cord
3. Lungs and tracheobronchial tree
4. Esophagus
5. Thoracic duct
6. Thoracic vertebrae

B. Surface markings
1. Angle of Louis – 2nd intercostal space
2. Nipples – 4th intercostal space
3. Scapular tip – 7th intercostal space
4. "The box" – refers to the area bounded by the nipples laterally, the sternal notch, and the xiphoid process. A penetrating injury in this area mandates either subxiphoid exploration or echocardiography (in the absence of a left hemothorax) to exclude an injury to the heart and great vessels.
5. The plane created by the nipples anteriorly and the scapular tip posteriorly represents the superior excursion of the diaphragm. Penetrating injuries below this level should raise suspicion for intra-abdominal injury.

C. Stab wounds to the thoracoabdominal area
1. If an abdominal injury has been excluded, evaluation of the diaphragm can be performed by video-assisted thoracoscopic surgery (VATS), laparoscopy, or abdominal exploration.

D. Gunshot wounds to the thoracoabdominal area
1. Abdominal exploration is performed in these patients provided that the following criteria are met:
    a. The wound or location of the missile is below the 4th intercostal space anteriorly, 6th intercostal space laterally, or the 7th intercostal space (scapular tip) posteriorly.

III. MECHANISMS OF INJURY

A. Blunt injury
1. Most commonly associated with motor vehicle collisions and falls

2. May result in chest wall contusions, fractures, cardiac or pulmonary contusions, hemo-pneumothorax, major vessel injury, tracheal or esophageal injury

B. Penetrating injury
1. May cause injury to any thoracic structure
2. 80% will not require operative intervention.

C. Iatrogenic injury
1. Pneumothorax from central venous access or barotrauma
2. Esophageal or tracheobronchial perforation from endoscopy
3. Cardiac or vascular perforation from venous access

D. Ingestion. Esophageal burns from the ingestion of corrosives

E. Inhalation. Smoke or other noxious gas inhalation

IV. INITIAL MANAGEMENT

A. ABC
1. The establishment of an adequate airway with ventilation and appropriate volume resuscitation through two large-bore upper extremity lines

B. Chest-tube insertion
1. This is indicated prior to chest radiography in the presence of respiratory distress or diminished breath sounds especially if a tension pneumothorax is suspected.

C. Cardiac ultrasound
1. Patients with precordial penetrating injuries and no indication for an immediate emergency thoracotomy undergo immediate cardiac ultrasound to evaluate for pericardial effusion.

D. Emergency department thoracotomy
1. Generally reserved for patients with penetrating trauma, evidence of cardiac activity or signs of life, and unresponsive
2. Salvage for patients with blunt trauma is dismal and emergency department thoracotomy is generally not used in this patient population.

V. DIAGNOSIS

A. History
1. Obtain the history of the mechanism of injury – deceleration, ejection, seat-belt use, or broken steering wheel.
2. Concerning symptoms include:
   a. Chest pain
   b. Shortness of breath
   c. Hoarseness
   d. Hemoptysis
   e. Stridor
3. Past medical history – especially any cardiorespiratory diseases

B. Physical signs
1. Abrasions
2. Contusions
3. Obvious fractures
4. Seat-belt marks
5. Site of penetrating injury (proximity)
6. **Beck's triad** – jugular vein distention, muffled heart sounds, and hypotension
7. Narrow pulse pressure
8. Pulsus paradoxus
9. Tracheal shift
10. Diminished or absent breath sounds
11. Paradoxical chest motion
12. Point tenderness, crepitus, or deformity
13. Disparate pulses

VI. SPECIFIC STUDIES

A. Chest CT
1. A contrast-enhanced spiral chest CT is obtained when any of the following conditions are present on routine chest film:
   a. Widened mediastinum (either >8 cm or the examiner's perception that the mediastinum is widened or abnormal is relatively sensitive for injury).
   b. First rib fracture
   c. Abnormal aortic knob
   d. Apical capping
   e. Left hemothorax
   f. Widening of the paraspinous stripe
   g. Shift of the trachea toward the right
   h. Deviation of the nasogastric tube
   i. Depression of the left mainstem bronchus
   j. Loss of aortic-pulmonary window
   k. Widening of the paratracheal stripe
   l. Transmediastinal gunshot wounds in order to exclude great vessel injury
2. Improvements in CTA technology have relegated conventional angiography to a solely therapeutic role.

B. Arteriography. Indications:
1. Pulse deficit or upper extremity pulse or blood pressure differential.
2. Stable hematoma (expanding hematoma would warrant operation).
3. New peripheral nerve deficit
4. Penetrating zone I neck injury

C. Barium cine-esophagogram. Indications are as follows:
1. Dysphagia
2. Odynophagia

3. Transmediastinal penetrating injury
4. Penetrating zone I neck injury

D. Echocardiogram
1. Formal echocardiogram is helpful in the stable patient in the evaluation of suspected pericardial effusion on initial focused assessment sonographic evaluation of trauma (FAST) examination.
2. This modality can also be helpful in evaluation for possible blunt aortic injury, but it is logistically difficult to obtain urgently and is usually followed by contrast aortography.

VII. INDICATIONS FOR THORACOTOMY OR STERNOTOMY

A. Thoracic hemorrhage
1. Initial chest tube output of 1000 to 1500 mL of blood
2. 200 mL per hour for ≥2 hours

B. Cardiac tamponade or hemopericardium

C. Transmediastinal wound with hemodynamic instability

D. Large residual hemothorax after two well-placed 36 Fr chest tubes

E. Massive air leak with respiratory distress

F. Severe penetrating parenchymal lung injury

G. Tracheal or bronchial disruption

H. Esophageal perforation or disruption

I. Aortic or great vessel injury

J. Central missile embolus

K. Atrial-caval shunt placement for retrohepatic venous injuries (rare)

L. Chronic chylous fistula

M. Empyema secondary to remote trauma (the alternative is VATS)

VIII. EXPOSURE CONSIDERATIONS

A. Left anterolateral
1. Most versatile incision
2. Easy to perform
3. Expeditious
4. Most cardiac injuries and aortic injuries can be addressed through this incision.

B. Median sternotomy
1. Used for isolated cardiac and certain central vascular injuries (see below)
2. **Cannot expose posterior mediastinum**, thus this technique is not indicated for aortic injury.

C. Standard posterolateral
1. Not used in hemodynamically unstable patients
2. Best exposure for parenchymal injuries

D. Right thoracotomy
1. This procedure is useful for right-sided pulmonary parenchymal and tracheal injury.

E. Left second interspace thoracotomy and "open book" thoracotomy
1. These techniques can be used to control and expose the left subclavian artery.

IX. INTRAOPERATIVE MANAGEMENT

1. Correction of physiologic derangement including acidosis, coagulopathy, hypothermia, hypovolemia, and anemia
2. Autotransfusion of chest tube drainage can be helpful but should usually be stopped after 2 L owing to increased risk of coagulopathy.
3. Cell-saver autotransfuser use may be limited by the potential contamination in traumatic injuries. This is less of a problem with chest injuries than with abdominal injuries.
   a. Autotransfusion is rarely used at Parkland Memorial Hospital.

X. POSTOPERATIVE MANAGEMENT

1. Patients who have undergone median sternotomy or thoracotomy should be monitored in the intensive care unit.
2. Pulmonary artery catheter assists in the volume management with severe cardiac or pulmonary injury.
3. Cardiac arrhythmias are common after thoracotomy.
   a. They may be a manifestation of an underlying cardiac disease.
   b. Supraventricular arrhythmias may occur in conjunction with thoracic trauma.
   c. Supraventricular or ventricular arrhythmias may occur after cardiac surgery.
   d. Calcium channel blockers, β-blockers, or digoxin may be used depending on the etiology of the arrhythmia.
   e. β-Blockers are contraindicated if cardiac dysfunction is present.
   f. Cardioversion for arrhythmias may be indicated for hemodynamic instability (per advanced cardiac life support [ACLS] protocol).
   g. When low cardiac output occurs as a result of injury, inotropes can be used once hypovolemia, arrhythmias, and tamponade are excluded.
4. Adequate analgesia is essential for good pulmonary function.
5. Control of secretions and avoidance of atelectasis are crucial to avoid complications.
6. Patients with penetrating cardiac injuries should be evaluated with transesophageal echocardiography postoperatively as early as possible to evaluate for valvular dysfunction.

XI. INVASIVE PROCEDURES

A. Tube thoracostomy
1. Principles of insertion
   a. Indicated for pneumothorax or hemothorax
   b. Location is usually the 5th or 6th intercostal space, midaxillary line.
   c. Elevate the patient on a rolled sheet.

d. Prepare and drape the patient.
e. Use 1% lidocaine liberally, infiltrating the skin, subcutaneous tissue, fascia, intercostal muscles, superior border of the rib, and pleura. The addition of sodium bicarbonate (1 mL/10 mL of lidocaine) will minimize the discomfort of the lidocaine.
f. In nonemergent situations, rib blocks may be placed prior to insertion.
g. A transverse incision (2 to 3 cm) is made over the 6th or 7th rib.
h. Tunnel superiorly and posteriorly to enter the pleural space on the superior border of the 6th or 7th rib.
i. Digitally explore the wound to ensure the entrance is into the thoracic and not the abdominal cavity.
j. The goal is to place the tube in the posterior apex of the chest cavity.
k. Insert a 36 Fr tube in a superior posterior direction, twisting the tube periodically as you insert (it will not twist easily if the tube is kinked) to ensure that the tube has not entered the lung fissure.
l. Make sure the most proximal hole is within the chest.
m. Place the tube on 20 cm of wall suction in a closed collection system.
n. Suture the tube to the skin.
o. Apply a sterile dressing.
p. An alternate site for a pure pneumothorax is the second intercostal space in the midclavicular line.

2. **Chest tube management**
   a. The chest tube remains on 20 cm of wall suction until the lung has been fully expanded for 24 hours.
   b. Suction is then discontinued and the tube is placed on water seal.
   c. If the lung remains inflated on subsequent radiographic examination, the tube can be removed.
   d. Recurrent pneumothorax can be treated by placing the chest tube back on suction for 24 to 48 hours and repeating the cycle.
   e. Inability to maintain reinflation of the lung suggests a nonhealing parenchymal or bronchial injury.
   f. Commercially available closed suction and collection systems are routinely used and can be connected to autotransfusion chambers (Figure 21-1).
   g. Prophylactic antibiotics for patients with chest tubes in place is a controversial subject. One dose of a first-generation cephalosporin at the time of placement (preferably before the incision) is sufficient.

3. **Chest tube removal**
   a. Any air leak should be sealed and drainage should be <30 mL per 8-hour shift prior to removing the tube.
   b. Cut the securing sutures.
   c. Prepare a dressing of 4 × 4 gauze with petroleum gauze to dress the chest tube entry site.
   d. While holding the dressing over the chest tube entry site, have the patient hold his or her breath and perform a Valsalva maneuver at maximal inspiration, helping to reduce the chance of recurrent pneumothorax.
   e. Quickly pull out the tube in a single motion while applying firm pressure on the dressing.

XI. Invasive Procedures 171

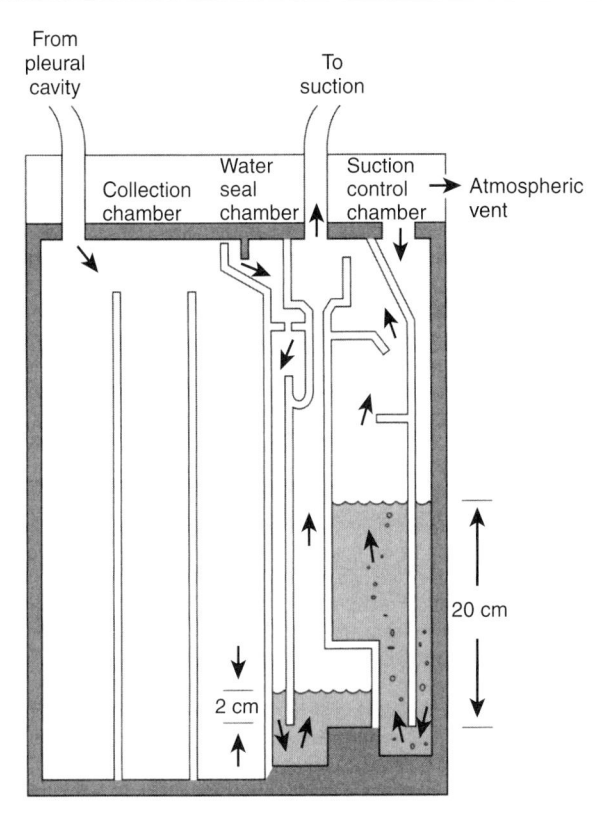

FIGURE 21-1

Commercially available apparatus for chest drainage.

 f. Apply tape to create a completely occlusive dressing, which should remain in place for at least 48 hours.

B. Pericardiocentesis

1. Because we are able to quickly perform emergency department thoracotomy or move the patient to the operating room for management at Parkland Memorial Hospital, we do not perform this procedure.
2. Pericardiocentesis is meant only as a temporizing measure in preparation for operative management.
3. Prepare and drape the xiphoid region.
4. Use a 30-mL syringe and a 1.5-inch 18- or 20-gauge needle (not a spinal needle).

5. Enter the right paraxiphoid region with the needle at 45 degrees to the plane of the anterior chest wall and at 45 degrees to the sagittal plane (angle toward the left shoulder).
6. Advance the catheter while aspirating until blood is encountered.
7. Aspirated blood should be nonclotting, and the patient's hemodynamics should immediately improve.
8. Removal of as little as 20 to 30 mL may relieve tamponade.
9. Repeat as necessary or insert a Silastic pigtail catheter, which can serve as a drain until surgery.

C. Resuscitative thoracotomy

1. Prepare and drape the entire chest.
2. Incise from the sternum to the posterior axillary line in the left inframammary fold toward the axilla (follow the course of the 5th rib).
3. Enter the pleural cavity along the superior margin of the 5th rib, taking care not to lacerate the lung; watch for the internal mammary artery parasternally.
4. Insert a self-retaining rib retractor and retract the lung to expose the pericardium.
5. Extend the thoracotomy across the midline if necessary.
6. Assess the pericardium for tamponade; if present, incise the pericardium widely anteriorly along and above the phrenic nerve.
7. For apparent cardiac injuries, deliver the heart from the pericardium with care, being careful not to impede venous return.
8. Locate the wound and repair it with a pledgetted suture, or digitally control the wound en route to the operating room while continuously volume-resuscitating the patient.
9. Cross-clamping the aorta is indicated if relief of the pericardial tamponade and continuous volume resuscitation do not improve hemodynamics.
10. Palpate the posterior mediastinum and identify the aorta; although the full aorta is 2 cm in diameter, it may be difficult to palpate in a hypotensive patient with little to no cardiac output; a nasogastric tube will help identify the aorta due to its intimate association with the esophagus, which is medial and just anterior to the aorta.
11. Dissect the aorta circumferentially such that a vascular clamp can be placed, and apply pressure.
12. Adjust the pressure so that the patient's systolic pressure is not greater than 120 mm Hg.
13. Once the necessary repairs are completed and the patient is stabilized, **release the clamp slowly**.

D. Subxiphoid exploration

1. Prepare and drape the entire chest and abdomen.
2. Make a midline incision over the xiphoid and upper epigastrium (3 cm above and 5 cm below the xiphoid). This should be made through the linea alba, but not the peritoneum.
3. Divide the xiphoid attachments of the diaphragm with electrocautery.
    a. Hemostasis is **very** important so that there is no question as to the nature of the pericardial fluid once the window is made.

4. The xiphoid may be removed if the costal margin is too narrow for the dissection.
5. Bluntly dissect the pericardium off the posterior sternum, being careful to stay directly under the sternum. Expose the pericardium by sweeping off the prepericardial fat.
6. Grasp the pericardium with Allis clamps.
7. Once the operative field is dry, open the pericardium between the clamps and note the nature of the fluid; if bloody, then proceed to a median sternotomy or left anterior thoracotomy; if clear, the wound may be closed.

E. Intercostal nerve block

1. Used for analgesia for rib fractures or chest tube placement
2. With the patient in the sitting position and leaning slightly forward, the angles of the ribs to be blocked are identified, and this area is prepped and draped (Figure 21-2).

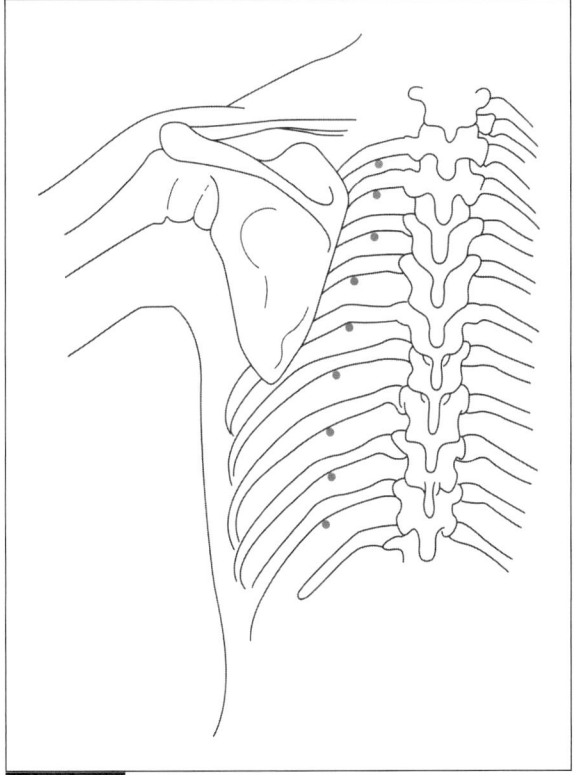

FIGURE 21-2

Preferred site for intercostal block. Injection more medial poses risk of instilling the agent into the dural canal.

3. A 1:1 mixture of 1.0% lidocaine and 0.5% bupiviacaine is used and a skin weal made using a small needle.
4. The periosteum of the rib is then infiltrated and the needle "walked" down to the inferior border of the rib where it is advanced slightly while attempting aspiration.
5. Care should be taken to ensure that the pleural space and the intercostal vessels are not entered.
6. Once the needle is in the notch of the rib, aspiration is again attempted and, if no blood is encountered, 3 to 5 mL of the anesthetic is injected.
7. An intercostal block is done for all fractured ribs at one space superior and inferior to the fractured ribs.
8. When multiple fractured ribs are present, care should be taken not to exceed the maximum recommended dose for either lidocaine or bupivacaine (lidocaine with epinephrine, 7 mg/kg; bupivacaine, 2 mg/kg).

XII. SPECIFIC INJURIES

A. Great vessel injuries
1. Great vessel injury is seen in <5% of patients arriving at trauma centers alive.
2. Risk of death is greatest immediately after transection.
3. As time passes the risk of sudden death decreases but the patient still remains at some finite risk.
4. Of those who survive 10 years without repair 20% will die of pseudoaneurysm rupture within the subsequent 5 years.

B. Ascending aorta
1. Patients usually do not survive injury to the ascending aorta.
2. 80% to 90% of these injuries occur at the aortic isthmus.
3. Patients usually have pericardial tamponade.
4. Treatment is primary aortorrhaphy with polypropylene suture (Prolene).

C. Descending thoracic aorta
1. The majority of patients with injury to the descending thoracic aorta die at the scene, with only 13% to 15% arriving at the emergency department with signs of life.
2. Injuries occur mainly in motor vehicle collisions with front and lateral impact.
3. If an aortic injury is suspected, the patient's blood pressure should be controlled with short-acting β-blockers, keeping the mean arterial pressure (MAP) less than 80. If other injuries preclude immediate repair, blood pressure should be kept below this level during the entire pre-repair period.
4. **Operative technique**
   a. Access is through the left posterolateral thoracotomy (4th intercostal space) using a double-lumen endotracheal tube.
   b. Prepare the femoral area into the operative field, with the patient in the right lateral decubitus position with hips rolled back.

c. Achieve proximal and distal aortic control.
d. Arterial bypass is achieved using a left atrium to femoral artery or atrium to distal aorta bypass using a Biomedicus centrifugal pump.
e. Distal blood pressure should be maintained at 60 to 80 mm Hg under this type of assistance.
f. A proximal clamp may be placed between the left carotid artery and left subclavian artery to provide additional exposure.
g. Encircle the intercostal arteries and temporarily occlude them; do not divide these arteries.
h. A partial tear of the aorta may sometimes be repaired primarily with 3-0 or 4-0 Prolene using pledgets. Otherwise, a short segment of preclotted woven Dacron graft is necessary for repair.
i. Consider use of moderate hypothermia (32°C), but balance this decision with the inherent complications associated with hypothermia-related bleeding.
j. In patients who survive the operating room, mortality is 15% and paraplegia is 5% to 7%.

D. Innominate artery and vein
1. Access is via a **median sternotomy**.
2. **Repair** is as follows:
   a. Open the pericardium first to ensure adequate proximal control.
   b. Suture the bypass graft to the ascending aorta.
   c. Establish vascular control of the distal innominate artery.
   d. Use end-to-end anastomosis with bypass graft.
   e. Use lateral aortorrhaphy at the take-off of the innominate artery.
   f. Remove any clot or debris by back bleeding.
   g. For penetrating injuries, lateral repair will control small injuries but complete transection requires anastomosis.
   h. In cases of associated tracheal and esophageal injuries and vascular repair, interpose sternocleidomastoid muscle or strap muscles between repair of tracheal or esophageal injuries and vascular repair.
   i. The innominate vein rarely requires repair and may be ligated with little consequence (there are anecdotal reports of neurologic deficit after ligation, presumably due to increased cerebral venous pressure).

E. Right carotid and right subclavian artery
1. For proximal control of injuries within 2 cm of the origin of the right common carotid artery and injuries to the right subclavian artery proximal to the vertebral artery, **access is through a median sternotomy**.
2. Requires division of the innominate vein
3. For more distal access to the right common carotid, the incision should be extended into the neck.
4. For distal control of right subclavian injuries:
   a. A supraclavicular approach allows access to the right subclavian at the level of the vertebral artery.
   b. An infraclavicular approach allows access to the more distal artery.

F. Left common carotid artery
1. The proximal portion is well exposed with a **median sternotomy**.
2. Extension along the sternocleidomastoid into the neck provides more distal exposure.

G. Left subclavian artery
1. **Proximal**
   a. Poorly exposed through a median sternotomy due to its posterior origin on the aortic arch and its posterolateral course
   b. An anterior 2nd or 3rd intercostal space thoracotomy provides exposure for proximal control.
   c. In an elective situation, a posterolateral thoracotomy provides good exposure.
2. **Distal**
   a. Initial control can be achieved with a left anterior thoracotomy.
   b. An infra- or supraclavicular incision provides exposure to the distal vessel.

H. Pulmonary artery and vein
1. Access is via a median sternotomy.
2. Penetrating injuries are much more common, and repair of blunt and penetrating injuries is the same. A large vascular clamp is used to control the hilum. This is a useful adjunct to help identify the injury.
3. Repair is by lateral arteriorrhaphy if the anterior main pulmonary artery is injured.
   a. The use of pledgets is important.
   b. Cardiopulmonary bypass is used if the injury is extensive or if the posterior wall of the main artery is involved.
4. The intrapericardial pulmonary vein is very difficult to explore and expose.
   a. Mortality rate for this injury is 70% to 75%.
   b. After controlling hemorrhage (a Foley catheter is often helpful), the patient may require cardiopulmonary bypass to decompress and decrease the size of the heart and expose the area of injury.
5. Hilar control is essential.

I. Thoracic vena cava
1. This is rarely an isolated injury.
2. Both the superior vena cava and inferior vena cava are intrapericardial in the thorax.
3. Access is via a median sternotomy.
4. Repair is with lateral venorrhaphy.
   a. This may require isolation of injuries using intracaval shunt or snares, by way of the right atrial appendage.
5. A large defect may require pericardial patch reconstruction.
6. Posterior injuries of the vena cava may require cardiopulmonary bypass to access the injury through the right atrium.
7. The mortality rate is greater than 50% (there is a high rate of associated injuries).

XIII. SPECIAL SITUATIONS

A. Multiple injuries in patients with a widened mediastinum
1. **Hemodynamically stable**
   a. If the results of a diagnostic peritoneal lavage or sonogram are negative, evaluate the aorta with a chest CT or aortography.
   b. If abdominal evaluation reveals hemorrhage and the patient requires operation, evaluate the aorta after celiotomy.
2. **Hemodynamically unstable**
   a. For positive findings of abdominal hemorrhage, perform a rapid celiotomy followed by chest CT and/or aortography.
   b. Damage-control celiotomy consists of rapid and simple control of hemorrhage and control of contamination followed by temporary closure of the abdominal incision.
   c. Address aortic injury with aortography (if not already performed) or thoracotomy.
   d. After aorta repair is complete, re-open the celiotomy if necessary.
   e. The goal of damage control is to prevent exsanguination from abdominal blood loss while addressing the aortic injury.

B. Rib fracture
1. Chest radiographs and a rib series have false-negative rates up to 30% to 50%.
2. **Inspiratory/expiratory upright chest radiographs** may help reveal an occult pneumothorax.
3. Look carefully for hemothorax or pneumothorax on presentation and during the initial 24 to 48 hours.
4. Treatment is supportive.
   a. Control pain with oral, parenteral, or epidural analgesics or a rib block, depending on the individual patient's needs and associated injuries.
   b. Avoid binding of the chest wall because this contributes to ventilatory abnormality caused by splinting and may contribute to atelectasis and hypoxia.
   c. Focus on analgesia and "pulmonary toilet" (incentive spirometry, deep breaths, and coughing).

C. Sternal fracture
1. Chest radiographs may not show fracture.
   a. A lateral view or sternal view is more helpful but is often not possible to obtain in a patient with multiple injuries.
   b. Look for evidence of associated intrathoracic injuries.
2. Sternal fractures can often be seen using a high-frequency (7.5-MHz) linear array ultrasound probe, which nicely shows the cortical sternal defect.
3. Treatment focuses on associated injuries, but urgent reduction of claviculosternal dislocation by placing a sandbag or rolled towel transversely under the upper thoracic spine may be necessary to relieve

compression of the airway, vessels, or nerves at the thoracic outlet, if present.
   a. Analgesics or local injection may be used.
   b. Early wiring can be beneficial, although it is not routinely performed, if the patient's condition is stable and there is no need for mechanical ventilation.
   c. Sternal, 1st rib, or 2nd rib fractures should alert the physician to the possibility of associated intrathoracic injuries, and appropriate examination and workup should follow.

D. Flail chest
1. Traditionally described as paradoxical movement of a chest wall segment with respiration caused by fractures of 3 or more contiguous ribs, each one broken in more than one place.
2. Indicates significant trauma to the chest, and other injuries should be suspected
3. Morbidity and mortality are related to the underlying pulmonary parenchymal injuries.
4. Treatment is supportive.
   a. Intubation and positive pressure ventilation are undertaken for respiratory failure (progressive fatigue, $Pco_2 \geq 50$ mm Hg, $Po_2 \leq 60$ mm Hg on 100% oxygen by face mask, or negative inspiratory pressure of ≤ 25 mm Hg).
   b. Avoid administration of excess fluid as this may exaggerate edema in an underlying pulmonary contusion.
   c. Analgesia (oral, parenteral, epidural, or intercostal blocks) and pulmonary toilet are the most important factors in preventing further deterioration.
   d. Splinting or binding the chest wall may contribute to ventilatory abnormality and should be avoided.
5. Internal fixation is not routinely done at our institution but may help stabilize the chest wall earlier and should be considered in severe cases or when thoracotomy is performed for another reason.

E. Open chest wound
1. Beware of occulsive dressings in the absence of a chest tube as this may precipitate a tension pneumothorax.
2. A sucking chest wound will lead to ineffectual ventilation of the ipsilateral lung when the cross-sectional area of the wound approaches that of a mainstem bronchus.
3. On plain radiographs, evaluate the extent of the chest wall injury and signs of associated injuries.
4. Treat with occlusive dressing after chest tube placement, followed by debridement and closure of the wound if a large defect is present.
5. Large wounds may ultimately require a flap for coverage.

F. Hemopneumothorax treatment
1. Closed-tube thoracostomy is usually all that is required.
2. If the patient has a stab wound to the upper chest and is asymptomatic and radiographs show no evidence of hemothorax or pneumothorax,

a 6-hour chest film is obtained and, if normal, the patient may be discharged (<1% will become symptomatic or develop delayed hemopneumothorax after a normal chest study 6 hours post-injury).
3. The indications for thoracotomy are listed above.

G. Thoracic duct injuries

1. A history of recent retroperitoneal, posterior mediastinal, or cervical operation or trauma should lead to suspicion of thoracic duct injury.
2. Chylous effusion or chest tube output (a positive fat stain or a high level of triglycerides)
3. Chest radiographs may show pleural effusion.
4. CT may show a mediastinal fluid collection.
5. Lymphangiography may assist with preoperative localization.
6. **Treatment**
   a. Most chyle leaks are self-limited and respond to nonoperative therapy (a low-fat diet, drainage, or total parenteral nutrition).
   b. A fibrothorax may develop if chyle is allowed to collect in the pleural cavity.
   c. Ligation of the thoracic duct should be performed during the initial operative procedure if the injury is recognized and collaterals are plentiful.
   d. If delayed ligation, after failed conservative therapy, is to be performed, administration of a heavy fat (butter or cream) with dye may help with intraoperative identification.
   e. If the injured duct cannot be found via a right posterolateral thoracotomy, then multiple ligations of tissue anterior and to the right of T8-T9 at the level of the diaphragm should be performed.

XIV. SUGGESTED READINGS

Demetriades D, Velmahos GC, Scalea TM, et al. Diagnosis and treatment of blunt thoracic aortic injuries: Changing perspectives. J Trauma 64(6): 1415–1418; discussion, 1418–1419, 2008.

Maturen KE, Adusumilli S, Blane CE, et al. Contrast-enhanced CT accurately detects hemorrhage in torso trauma : Direct comparison with angiograpty. J Trauma 62(3):740–745, 2007.

Phelan HA, Patterson SG, Hassan MO, et al. Thoracic damage-control operation: Principles, techniques, and definitive repair. J Am Coll Surg 203(6):933–941, 2006.

Takagi H, Kawai N, Umemoto T: A meta-analysis of comparative studies of endovascular versus open repair for blunt thoracic aortic injury. J Thorac Cardiovasc Surg 135(6):1392–1394, 2008.

Diaphragmatic Injury

David H. Rosenbaum, MD

I. ANATOMY

A. Attachments
1. Anterior: sternum and posterior aspect of xiphoid process
2. Posterior: 1 to 3 lumbar vertebral bodies
3. Lateral: 6th rib anteriorly, 12th rib posteriorly

B. Excursion
1. **Inspiration:** costal margin
2. **Expiration**
   a. 4th intercostal space anteriorly
   b. 5th intercostal space laterally
   c. 7th intercostal space posteriorly

C. Innervation: phrenic nerve (C3-5)

D. Arterial supply: intercostal arteries

E. Venous return: phrenic veins

II. INCIDENCE

A. 1% of all blunt trauma
B. 10% of all penetrating trauma
C. 3% of all abdominal injuries
D. 5% of all penetrating thoracic trauma

III. MECHANISMS

A. Penetrating trauma
B. Blunt trauma primarily as a result of lateral-impact motor vehicle collisions or falls

C. Theories of mechanism
1. Shearing of a stretched membrane
2. Avulsion from attachments
3. Sudden increase in intra-abdominal pressure

IV. CLINICAL MANIFESTATIONS

A. Half of patients present in shock.
B. Respiratory distress, abdominal pain, and shoulder pain are common.
C. Examination may reveal a scaphoid abdomen or bowel sounds in the affected hemithorax.

V. ASSOCIATED INJURIES

A. Traumatic brain injuries
B. Blunt abdominal injuries (hepatic most common)
C. Blunt thoracic injuries
D. Pelvic fractures

VI. DIAGNOSIS

A. High index of suspicion is required.
1. Penetrating thoracoabdominal trauma
2. Blunt trauma with high-energy transfer
B. Chest radiographs have up to 50% accuracy.
1. Visualization of nasogastric tube within the thoracic cavity is diagnostic.
C. Return of lavage fluid from a thoracostomy tube
D. Diagnostic peritoneal lavage has a false-negative rate of 25%.
E. Computed tomography has 63% sensitivity when there is associated visceral herniation.
F. Thoracoscopy
G. Laparoscopy
1. At Parkland Memorial Hospital, laparoscopy is performed in patients suspected to have diaphragmatic injury without another indication for celiotomy or thoracotomy.
H. American Association for the Surgery of Trauma Organ Injury Scale for Diaphragmatic Injuries (Table 22-1)

VII. MANAGEMENT—ACUTE INJURY

A. Abdominal approach for acute injury—midline incision
B. Transthoracic approach for chronic injury
C. Visualization of the diaphragm
1. **Right hemidiaphragm**: transect the falciform ligament and place downward traction on the liver.
2. **Left hemidiaphragm**: place downward traction on the spleen and greater curvature of the stomach.

TABLE 22-1
AMERICAN ASSOCIATION FOR THE SURGERY OF TRAUMA ORGAN INJURY SCALE FOR DIAPHRAGMANTIC INJURIES

Grade	Injury Description
I	Contusion
II	Laceration ≤2 cm
III	Laceration 2–10 cm
IV	Laceration >10 cm with tisssue loss ≤25 cm^2
V	Laceration with tissue loss >25 cm^2

D. Prior to closure of the defect, the ipsilateral thoracic cavity must be closely evaluated.
E. Place chest tube directly through the wound for irrigation.
1. After irrigating, keep tube on suction and remove once good lung expansion is visualized.
2. Alternatively, place tube thoracostomy under direct visualization.
F. Close the defect with a running or interrupted horizontal mattress stitch with nonabsorbable monofilament suture.
G. Prosthetic mesh may be necessary for a tension-free closure of a large defect.

VIII. POSTOPERATIVE CARE AND PROGNOSIS

A. Patients require an average of 4 to 5 days of ventilatory support.
B. Temporary or permanent paresis of the diaphragm often occurs with large injuries.
C. Diaphragm injury has a mortality of 14% due mostly to associated injuries.
D. A missed injury has a mortality of 40% to 60% if abdominal viscera become incarcerated and strangulated.

IX. SUGGESTED READINGS

Asensio JA, Petrone P, Demetriades D: Injury to the diaphragm. In Moore EE, Feliciano DV, Mattox KL: Trauma, 5th ed. New York, McGraw-Hill, 2004, pp 613-636.

Bergstrom DC, Weigelt JA: Diaphragmatic injury. In Thal ER, Weigelt JA, Carrico CJ: Operative Trauma Management, 2nd ed. New York, McGraw-Hill, 2002, pp 154-167.

Freeman RK, Al-Dossari G, Hutcheson KA, et al: Indications for using video-assisted thoracoscopic surgery to diagnose diaphragmatic injuries after penetrating chest trauma. Ann Thorac Surg 72:342-347, 2001.

Leppaniemi A, Haapiainen R: Occult diaphragmatic injuries caused by stab wounds. J Trauma 55(4):646-650, 2003.

McQuay N, Britt LD: Laparoscopy in the evaluation of penetrating thoracoabdominal trauma. Am Surg 69(9):788-791, 2003.

Shah R, Sabanathan S, Mearns AJ, Choudhury AK: Traumatic rupture of diaphragm. Ann Thorac Surg 60:1444-1449, 1995.

Spann J, Nwariaku F, Wait M: The role of video-assisted thoracoscopic surgery in the evaluation of diaphragmatic injuries. Am J Surg 170(6):628-631, 1995.

Esophageal Trauma

Richard Hershberger, MD, and Stacey Woodruff, MD

Esophageal injury is associated with a high level of morbidity and mortality. Furthermore, the morbidity associated with a missed esophageal injury is severe and unforgiving.

I. ETIOLOGY

A. Incidence—approximately 1% of injured patients
1. The esophagus is injured 10% to 12% of the time if a cervical wound penetrates the platysma.
2. Blunt trauma is an uncommon cause of esophageal trauma.
B. The majority of esophageal injuries are iatrogenic.

II. EVALUATION

A. Signs and symptoms
1. Present in 60% to 80% of injuries
2. Signs and symptoms depend on location of injury, size of the defect, extent of contamination, and length of time from injury.
3. Odynophagia
4. Dysphagia
5. Hematemesis
6. Hemoptysis
7. Cervical crepitus
8. Prevertebral air
9. Widened mediastinum
10. Hoarseness
11. Dyspnea
12. Audible mediastinal crunching (Hamman's sign)

B. Radiologic assessment
1. Plain films aid in discerning trajectory of missiles.
2. Lateral radiograph of the neck
    a. Signs that aid in diagnosis include prevertebral air, subcutaneous emphysema, mediastinal air, and mediastinal widening.
  b. Prevertebral air occurs in 39% of esophageal injuries

C. Esophagography
1. Sensitivity of 93%
2. Gastrografin is used first, unless a tracheoesophageal fistula is suspected.
3. Negative study should prompt further evaluation if clinical suspicion for injury remains high.

D. Esophagoscopy
1. When combined with esophagography a sensitivity of almost 100% is reached.

2. Can be flexible or rigid
   a. Air used for insufflation with flexible scopes can worsen pneumomediastinum or pneumothorax.

III. MANAGEMENT

Time interval between injury and intervention should not exceed 12 hours. Patients undergoing repair after 12 hours experience a twofold increase in morbidity related to the esophageal injury.

A. Options for repair
1. **Primary repair with wide drainage**
   a. Procedure of choice (preserves function and prevents need for further operation)
   b. Resection of the area of injury with single- or double-layer repair
2. **Primary repair with protection**
   a. Benefit of buttressing flaps has not been demonstrated but is associated with fewer complications.
   b. Options for flaps include pleura, muscle, or serosa from a fundal wrap.
   c. Recommended if concurrent tracheal injury exists to prevent tracheoesophageal fistula
   d. Some authors favor the use of a flap in thoracic/abdominal injuries, if there is delay in operative intervention, or after extensive longitudinal dissection of the esophagus.
3. **Esophagectomy with diversion**
   a. Recommended after delay in diagnosis with evidence of severe mediastinal and pleural inflammation
   b. Indicated for extensive injury requiring extensive resection
   c. Options include total esophageal exclusion, esophagectomy, or T-tube drainage.

IV. OUTCOME

Rate of complications is directly related to delay in operative intervention

A. Complications
1. Esophageal leak (most common although <5% with early repair)
2. Wound infections
3. Mediastinitis
4. Sepsis
5. Tracheoesophageal fistula
   a. Can occur with breakdown of repair
   b. Findings can include increasing tidal volume loss from the ventilator, cuff leak, or the presence of a nasogastric tube in the trachea.

B. Mortality
   a. Gunshot wounds have a mortality of 7% to 23%.
   b. Concomitant injuries often determine outcome.

V. CAUSTIC INGESTION

A. Incidence
1. Over 200,000 caustic exposures occur annually in the United States.
2. The majority of accidental ingestions occur in infants and children (80%), whereas the majority of adult ingestions are suicide attempts.

B. Agents
1. **Alkali** (lye)
    a. 95% of cases
    b. Sodium and potassium hydroxide—drain and oven cleaners, bleaches, detergents
    c. Solid form adheres to mucous membranes, resulting in more oropharynx injury.
    d. Liquid form is easier to swallow, resulting in more esophageal and gastric injury.
    e. Rapid penetration and liquefaction necrosis
    f. Regurgitation into the esophagus is common.
    g. Mucosal sloughing in 4 to 7 days; collagen deposition in 2 to 3 weeks; stricture formation common
2. **Acids**
    a. 5% of cases
    b. Sulfuric, hydrochloric, and phosphoric acids—toilet bowl cleaners, antirust compounds, battery fluid, swimming pool cleaners
    c. Rapidly produces coagulation necrosis; eschar limits penetration
    d. 80% of acid burns spare the esophagus.

C. Classification
1. Grade 0—normal mucosa
2. Grade 1—edema, hyperemia of mucosa, desquamation
3. Grade 2—penetration into muscularis, friability, blisters, erosions, ulcerations
4. Grade 3—transmural penetration, extensive necrosis, can lead to mediastinitis or peritonitis

D. Evaluation.
1. **Acute signs and symptoms**
    a. Dysphagia
    b. Odynophagia
    c. Epigastric pain
    d. Perioral pain
    e. Upper gastrointestinal bleeding
    f. Stridor
    g. Fever
    h. Vomiting
    i. Drooling
    j. Burns on lips or oropharynx
2. **Late signs and symptoms**
    a. Dysphagia

b. Early satiety
c. Weight loss
d. Gastric outlet obstruction
e. Stricture formation—at points where caustic agents pool
    i. Cricopharyngeus
    ii. Aortic arch
    iii. Tracheal bifurcation
    iv. Lower esophageal sphincter

E. Diagnostic studies
1. Plain films of chest and abdomen
    a. Pneumomediastinum in esophageal perforation
    b. Pneumoperitoneum in gastric perforation
    c. Confirm perforation with Gastrografin swallow, then barium swallow if negative.
2. Flexible endoscopy
    a. Performed as soon as possible as long as the patient is stable and there is no evidence of perforation
    b. Limit advancement to site of injury to avoid iatrogenic perforation.
    c. Rigid esophagoscopy may lead to perforation.
    d. May underestimate the severity of the injury
    e. Principal utility is to exclude patients without burns.

F. Treatment
1. **Emergency treatment**
    a. Maintain control of airway.
    b. Broad-spectrum antibiotics
    c. Use of steroids is controversial in prevention of stricture formation.
    d. H2 blockers or proton pump inhibitors
    e. Neutralization with water, milk, or acid may release heat and cause further injury after lye ingestion.
    f. Water may dilute acid with minimal heat loss.
    g. Emetics and gastric lavage are not used because of the increased risk of regurgitation and re-exposure of the esophagus to the corrosive agent.
2. **Surgical exploration**
    a. Utilized in the septic patient or patient demonstrating evidence of perforation
    b. May be beneficial in early management of grade-3 burns
    c. Resection for perforation or transmural injury
    d. Esophagectomy and occasional gastrectomy may be necessary.
    e. Formal reconstruction with stomach or colon is delayed for several months until resolution of inflammation and sepsis.
3. **Prevention of stricture**
    a. Barium esophagrams beginning at 2 weeks to evaluate for stricture if asymptomatic, earlier if needed
    b. **Dilatation**
        i. Recommend beginning 2 to 3 weeks after burn if stricture develops
        ii. Early dilatation may cause perforation or accelerated fibrosis.

iii. Pass string or nasogastric tube to maintain lumen for further dilatation.
   c. **Stents**
      i. Removed after 3 weeks if placed during surgery
      ii. May be of some benefit if placed endoscopically after dilatation to maintain patency
G. **Complications**
1. Mediastinitis
2. Pneumonitis
3. Laryngeal edema
4. Perforation
5. Tracheoesophageal fistula
6. Strictures—20% to 30%
7. Antral stenosis appears as early as 5 to 6 weeks. Treatment is vagotomy with gastroenterostomy or pyloroplasty.
8. Esophageal carcinoma
   a. One- to three thousand-fold increase in squamous cell carcinoma
   b. No evidence of increased gastric carcinoma
9. Mortality is 3% to 37%.

VI. SUGGESTED READINGS

Asensio JA, et al: Penetrating esophageal injuries: Multicenter study of the American Association for the Surgery of Trauma. J Trauma 50:289-296, 2001.

Asensio JA, et al: Penetrating esophageal injuries: Time interval of safety for preoperative evaluation—how long is safe? J Trauma 43(2):319-324, 1997.

DePeppo F, Zaccara A, Dall'Oglio L, et al: Stenting for caustic strictures: Esophageal replacement replaced. J Pediatr Surg 33(1):54-57, 1998.

Han Y, Cheng QS, Li XF, Wang XP: Surgical management of esophageal strictures after caustic burns: 30 years of experience. World J Gastroenterol 10(19): 2846-2849, 2004.

Moore E, Feliciano D, Mattox K (eds): Trauma, 5th ed. New York, McGraw-Hill, 2004.

Naude GP, et al: Gunshot injuries to the lower oesophagus. Injury 29(2):95-98, 1998.

Ramaswamy K, Gumaste VV: Corrosive ingestion in adults. J Clin Gastroenterol 37(2):119-124, 2003.

Smakman N: Factors affecting outcome in penetrating oesophageal trauma. Br J Surg 91:1513-1519, 2004.

Weiman DS: Noniatrogenic esophageal trauma. Ann Thorac Surg 59:845-850, 1995.

Westaby S, Adell J (eds): Cardiothoracic Trauma. London, Arnold Publishers, 1999.

Zwischenberger JB, Savage C, Bidani A: Surgical aspects of esophageal disease: Perforation and caustic injury. Am J Respir Crit Care Med 165(8):1037-1040, 2002.

Gastric Trauma

Lance E. Stuke, MD, and Kousta I. Foteh, MD

I. EPIDEMIOLOGY

1. Injuries to the stomach are common in penetrating trauma. They occur in 7% to 20% of cases.
2. Blunt injuries to the stomach are much less common, occurring in only 0.4% to 1.7% of cases.
3. Gastric injury is more common in children than adults.

II. ANATOMY

A. The stomach generally occupies the left upper quadrant
1. Located largely in the intrathoracic abdomen where the lower chest wall offers some protection
B. Layers
1. Serosa
2. Muscularis mucosa
3. Strong, well-vascularized submucosa
4. Thick mucosa
C. Blood supply
1. Right gastric artery – from the splenic artery; provides branches to the duodenum and the pylorus.
2. Left gastric artery – from the celiac axis; supplies the lesser curve of the stomach.
3. Right gastroepiploic artery- from the gastroduodenal artery; supplies the greater curve of the stomach.
4. Left gastroepiploic artery- fromthe splenic artery; supplies the greater curve of the stomach.
5. The arterial supply of the stomach has extensive collateralization such that 3 of the 4 vessels can be ligated without necrosis or significant dysfunction.
6. The venous supply of the stomach for the most part follows the arterial supply.

III. MECHANISM OF INJURY

A. Penetrating injury. Most are the result of gunshot or stab wounds, with mild to moderate tissue damage.
B. Blunt injury
1. Contusions, intramural hematomas, full-thickness hematomas and mesenteric avulsions of the stomach have been reported to occur following blunt abdominal trauma.

2. Blunt gastric trauma is rare. In the EAST blunt hollow-viscus multi-institutional trial, the incidence of stomach injuries was 4.3% of a total 2632 patients identified with any hollow viscus injury.
3. Most blunt injuries occur following motor-vehicle collisions, motor-pedestrian collisions and falls.
4. Gastric perforations caused by blunt forces are generally large and cause significant intraperitoneal contamination.
5. The early onset of peritoneal signs is usually obvious and warrants prompt surgical intervention.
6. The most common sites for blunt gastric injury are along the anterior surface of the stomach or greater curvature.

IV. DIAGNOSIS

A. Penetrating gastric trauma
1. All patients with gunshot wounds to the abdomen undergo celiotomy at Parkland Memorial Hospital.
2. Patients with abdominal stab wounds are managed as follows:
    a. Patients presenting with peritonitis, evisceration or hemodynamic instability are taken emergently to the operating room for exploratory celiotomy without further workup.
    b. In stable patients, local wound exploration is indicated for abdominal wounds located anterior to the axillary line and in whom it cannot be determined if fascial penetration has occurred. If local wound exploration is equivocal or positive (i.e., fascial penetration has been identified or if the end of the tract has not been identified), the patient undergoes a diagnostic peritoneal lavage (DPL) or is taken straight to the operating room, depending on the clinician. If the DPL is positive, then the patient undergoes exploratory celiotomy.
    c. If the wound exploration is negative, then the wound is irrigated thoroughly and then closed.
3. The presence of gross blood in the nasogastric aspirate is suggestive, but not diagnostic, of a gastric injury.
4. Diagnosis of a gastric injury is made at celiotomy.
5. Penetrating gastric injuries are frequently associated with liver, diaphragm and colon injuries.

B. Blunt gastric trauma
1. Requires a high index of suspicion. Many have associated head injuries, distracting injuries or other impairments, making diagnosis difficult.
2. 50% to 80% present with shock and peritonitis.
3. In the unstable patient, after following ATLS protocol (i.e., ABCs) a focused abdominal sonography for trauma (FAST) examination is done first.
    a. If the FAST is negative, a DPL is then performed.
    b. If the DPL is negative, other sources of injury must be investigated.

c. If the FAST is positive, the patient should have an exploratory celiotomy.
4. In stable patients, the FAST is also used early in the evaluation.
   a. If the FAST is negative and the patient remains stable, a CT scan can be obtained.
   b. Whether operative versus non-operative management is undertaken is based on the results of the CT-scan (degree of injury) and clinical suspicion.
   c. If the FAST and CT scan are negative and the patient becomes unstable, a DPL is performed.
   d. If the DPL is positive, then the patient should go to surgery.
   e. If the DPL is negative, then other sources contributing to the patient's instability should be investigated.
5. Associated injuries occur frequently with blunt gastric injury. They are generally severe because of the amount of force required to produce a gastric blowout. The organs most commonly involved include the liver, spleen, bone and thoracic cavity structures.

V. GASTRIC INJURIES

1. Gastric injuries are identified and treated according to their severity.
2. The table below summarizes the type and degree of stomach injury.

Grade	Description of Injury
I	Contusion or hematoma
	Partial-thickness laceration
II	Laceration <2 cm in GE junction or pylorus, <5 cm in proximal 1/3 of stomach, <10 cm in distal 2/3 of stomach
III	Laceration >2 cm in GE junction or pylorus, >5 cm in proximal 1/3 of stomach, >10 cm in distal 2/3 of stomach
IV	Tissue loss or devascularization <2/3 of stomach
V	Tissue loss or devascularization >2/3 of stomach

GE, gastroesophageal

VI. MANAGEMENT

1. Operative management is the rule – there is no role for observation in the treatment of suspected gastric trauma.
2. Control of hemorrhage is the first priority.
3. Control of contamination, especially colonic, is the second priority.
4. Definitive control of specific organ injuries then follows.
   a. Most gastric injuries can be treated with simple debridement and primary repair.
   b. Most intramural hematomas, (grades I-III) are repaired with interrupted silk Lembert sutures and hematoma evacuation.

c. Small grade I and II perforations can be closed primarily in one or two layers. Most surgeons prefer a two layer closure for hemostasis. If a two layer closure is used, the inner layer should be closed with a running absorbable suture, and the outer layer with interrupted silk.
   d. Large (grade III) injuries near the greater curvature can be closed by the same technique or by use of a gastrointestinal anastomsis (GIA) stapler.
   e. A pyloric wound may be converted to a pyloroplasty to prevent stenosis.
   f. Grade IV injuries may be so extensive that a proximal or distal gastrectomy may be required.
   g. Severe injuries (grade V) may require a total gastrectomy with a Roux-en-Y esophagojejunostomy.
   h. If a diaphragmatic injury occurs in conjunction with a gastric injury, care must be taken not to contaminate the pleural space with gastric contents.
5. If a gastroesophageal junction injury is suspected, injuries to the aorta or the celiac plexus should also be anticipated.
   a. If these are identified, vascular isolation should be performed before the gastroesophageal junction is exposed.
   b. Vagus nerve injury should also be considered and, if necessary, a pyloroplasty performed.
6. Distal antral injuries are repaired by simple two-layer closure. If injury is extensive, then a vagotomy with a Billroth I or II procedure should be performed depending on the viability of the proximal duodenum.
7. Care should be taken not to narrow the lumen of the pylorus or the gastroesophageal junction when performing a closure.
8. Antibiotics are given at the time of surgery and continued for 24 hours.
9. Primary closure of the celiotomy incision is acceptable for isolated gastric injuries.
10. Sites of commonly missed gastric injuries include the gastroesophageal junction, the lesser and greater curves, especially at the sites of omental or ligamentous attachments and the posterior wall of the stomach.

VII. POSTOPERATIVE CARE

1. Associated injuries cause the majority of injuries and deaths.
2. Short-term nasogastric suction is generally required in patients with gastric injuries.
3. Routine post-operative prophylaxis for deep vein thrombosis and stress ulceration are employed.

VIII. PEARLS AND PITFALLS

1. In the non-diseased state, the stomach contains few bacteria secondary to its acid environment. Most trauma patients have normal gastric physiology and are, therefore, at very low risk of bacterial contamination from gastric perforation alone. Patients on antacids, or H2-blockers, however, may have increased intraluminal bacterial counts and increased risk of intra-abdominal contamination.
2. The lesser sac should be entered for visualization of the posterior gastric wall. This step is mandatory in cases of anterior gastric wall injuries.
3. When in doubt, operate!

IX. SUGGESTED READINGS

O'Neill PA, Kirton OC, Dresner LS, et al: Analysis of 162 colon injuries in patients with penetrating abdominal trauma: Concomitant stomach injury results in a higher rate of infection. J Trauma-Injury Infection Crit Care 56(2):304–312; discussion 312–313, 2004.

Salim A, Teixeira PG, Inaba K, et al: Analysis of 178 penetrating stomach and small bowel injuries. World Surg 32(3):471–475, 2008.

Watts DD, Fakhry SM. EAST Multi-Institutional Hollow Viscus Injury Research Group. Incidence of hollow viscus injury in blunt trauma: An analysis from 275, 557 trauma admissions from the East multi-institutional trial. [erratum appears in J Trauma 54(4):749, 2003. J Trauma 54(2): 289–294, 2003.

Pancreatic and Duodenal Trauma

Adam W. Beck, MD

I. EPIDEMIOLOGY

A. Pancreatic injuries occur in 3% to 12% of all abdominal trauma.
B. Duodenal injuries occur in 3% to 5% of all abdominal trauma.
C. Penetrating injuries are more common than blunt injuries in both the pancreas and duodenum.

II. ANATOMY OF THE PANCREAS

A. The pancreas is entirely retroperitoneal.
B. There are four nonanatomical divisions:
1. **Head** (including the uncinate process) – lies within the duodenal C-loop
2. **Neck** – portion anterior to the superior mesenteric vessels
3. **Body** – crosses the spine
4. **Tail** – lies within the splenic hilum
5. **There are no distinct anatomical definitions of the four divisions**, but the proximal-distal division is defined by where the superior mesenteric vessels cross the gland posteriorly.

C. Ductal system
1. Main pancreatic duct of **Wirsung**
   a. Usually traverses the length of the entire gland
   b. Shares a common channel into the duodenum with the common bile duct in 35% of patients
2. Accessory duct of **Santorini**
   a. Absent in 10% of patients
   b. May serve as the main duct in 8% to 10% of patients
   c. Empties into the duodenum approximately 2.5 cm superior to the ampulla of Vater.

D. Arterial supply
1. **Gastroduodenal branches**
   a. Anterior superior pancreaticoduodenal artery
   b. Posterior superior pancreaticoduodenal artery
2. **Superior mesenteric artery branches**
   a. Anterior inferior pancreaticoduodenal artery
   b. Posterior inferior pancreaticoduodenal artery
3. **Short branches** from the **splenic** and **left gastroepiploic** arteries
4. **Superior pancreatic artery** – variable origin
5. **Inferior pancreatic artery** – may also supply the spleen

E. Venous drainage
1. Corresponds to arterial supply
2. Empties into the portal vein

III. ANATOMY OF THE DUODENUM

A. Extends from the pylorus to the ligament of Treitz
B. Four portions
1. Superior or 1st portion – **the only intraperitoneal portion**
2. Descending or 2nd portion – **contains the entrance of the common bile duct**
3. Transverse or 3rd portion
4. Ascending or 4th portion

C. Arterial supply
This is essentially the same as for the head of the pancreas.

IV. PANCREATIC INJURIES

A. Mechanism of injury
1. Approximately two thirds of all pancreatic injuries are the result of penetrating trauma.
2. Blunt injuries are usually secondary to direct compression of the pancreas against the spinal column.
3. The following mechanisms of injury are associated with pancreatic trauma:
    a. Direct blows to the upper abdomen – impact with the steering wheel is responsible for 60% of pancreatic injuries following motor vehicle collisions.
    b. Bicycle handlebar injury
    c. High-riding lap restraining belts

B. Associated injuries
1. The majority of early morbidity and mortality is related to exsanguination from associated vascular, liver, or splenic injuries.
2. Major vascular injuries occur in approximately 40% of patients with blunt pancreatic trauma.
3. The most frequently associated organ injuries are the following:
    a. Liver
    b. Stomach
    c. Major arteries and veins

C. Diagnosis
1. Penetrating trauma
   a. If the patient's hemodynamic status is stable, an abdominal radiograph obtained preoperatively for localization of the bullet may provide useful information.
   b. The diagnosis of penetrating pancreatic injury is made at the time of abdominal exploration.
   c. Clues suggesting potential injury include the following:
      i. Central retroperitoneal hematoma
      ii. Peripancreatic or lesser sac hematoma
      iii. Bile staining of the lesser sac, retroperitoneum, or peritoneal cavity

2. **Blunt trauma**
   a. Patients with clear indications for exploratory celiotomy (e.g., peritonitis, positive focused abdominal sonography for trauma (FAST) with hemodynamic instability, or positive diagnostic peritoneal lavage) require no further evaluation.
   b. Physical signs and symptoms related to pancreatic injury include:
      i. Epigastric pain out of proportion to examination findings in a reliable patient
      ii. Contusion or abrasion across the upper abdomen
      iii. Lower rib or costal cartilage separation
   c. Serum amylase, with or without fractionation, **has not proven beneficial in aiding diagnosis.**
   d. Abdominal radiographs are suggestive of pancreatic injury if the following findings are present:
      i. Ground-glass appearance in the mid-abdomen, indicative of fluid or edema in the lesser sac
      ii. Retroperitoneal air
      iii. Obliteration of the psoas shadow
   e. Diagnostic peritoneal lavage is generally a poor modality for diagnosing retroperitoneal injuries.
3. **Abdominal ultrasound** may suggest pancreatic injury if the following findings are present:
   a. Fluid in Morrison's pouch
   b. Fluid in the retroperitoneum
4. **Abdominal CT** scans have a specificity and sensitivity of approximately 80% for pancreatic injuries. The following findings may be seen with pancreatic injury:
   a. Pancreatic parenchyma disruption
   b. Areas of diminished pancreatic enhancement
   c. Peripancreatic fluid
   d. Fluid between the pancreas and splenic vein
   e. Fluid in the lesser sac
   f. Thickening of the left anterior renal fascia (Gerota's fascia)
5. **Endoscopic retrograde cholangiopancreatography** (ERCP) is rarely used for trauma at Parkland Memorial Hospital. It can be performed in stable patients and may be of benefit in the following situations:
   a. When CT has identified a pancreatic injury with questionable ductal integrity and the patient has no other injuries requiring abdominal exploration
   b. If a patient is unstable intraoperatively (hypotensive, hypothermic, coagulopathic) before an evaluation of the ductal system can be completed, ERCP can be performed postoperatively after the patient has been stabilized.

D. Operative evaluation

1. The entire gland must be exposed.
2. The following maneuvers will facilitate exposure:
   a. Opening of the **lesser sac** exposes the anterior pancreatic surface.

b. An extended **Kocher maneuver** (extend medially to the superior mesenteric vessels) exposes the head of the pancreas and the uncinate process.
c. Mobilization of the **hepatic flexure** allows better inspection of the pancreatic head.
d. Mobilization of the **splenocolic** and **gastrolienic ligaments** allows forward and medial rotation of the spleen and facilitates inspection of the pancreatic tail and the posterior surface.
3. Findings indicative of ductal injury include:
   a. Direct visualization of ductal disruption
   b. Complete or near-complete transection of the gland
   c. Laceration involving >50% of the gland diameter
   d. Central pancreatic perforation
   e. Severe maceration of the pancreas
   f. **Blunt trauma may result in ductal injury without transection of the gland**.
   g. **An intact capsule does not ensure integrity of the ductal system**.
4. Intraoperative techniques for pancreatography include:
   a. **Needle cholecystocholangiogram**
      i. A 16- to 18-gauge angiocath is inserted into the gallbladder or cystic duct.
      ii. 20 to 30 mL of water-soluble contrast is injected under fluoroscopy using a C-arm.
      iii. Prevention of contrast reflux and better visualization of the pancreatic duct may be provided by contracture of the sphincter of Oddi by giving IV morphine or by direct finger compression of the proximal common bile duct.
   b. **Duodenotomy** with direct injection (rarely performed at Parkland Memorial Hospital)
      i. The major and minor papillae are directly cannulated.
      ii. 2 to 5 mL of water-soluble contrast is injected.
   c. **Secretin stimulation**
      i. Secretin is given IV at 1μg/kg.
      ii. Injury is confirmed by direct visualization of pancreatic secretions from the site of suspected injury.

E. **Injury classification**
1. **Grade I**
   a. **Hematoma**—minor contusion without ductal injury
   b. **Laceration**—superficial laceration without ductal injury
2. **Grade II**
   a. **Hematoma**—major contusion without ductal injury or tissue loss
   b. **Laceration**—major laceration without ductal injury or tissue loss
3. **Grade III:** distal transection or parenchymal injury with ductal injury
4. **Grade IV:** proximal (medial to the mesenteric vessels) transection or parenchymal injury involving ampulla
5. **Grade V:** massive disruption of the pancreatic head

6. **Advance one grade for multiple injuries to the pancreas**.

F. Treatment

1. Treatment follows five basic principles once the diagnosis of pancreatic injury has been made.
   a. **Control pancreatic bleeding**.
      i. Electrocautery
      ii. Topical hemostatic agents
      iii. Direct suture ligation, with care taken to avoid ligation or injury of the duct
   b. **Debride devitalized pancreas**. The debridement should be minimal to avoid excessive hemorrhage and to allow time for demarcation of necrotic vs. viable pancreas.
   c. **Identify ductal injuries**.
   d. **Preserve at least 20% of functional pancreatic tissue if possible**.
   e. **Provide adequate internal and external drainage of pancreatic injuries or resections**.
      i. Internal drainage is provided by restoration of gastrointestinal and ductal anatomy where applicable.
      ii. External drainage is best provided by closed-suction drainage. Sump drainage may also be used if necessary.
      iii. **The majority of complications result from failure to identify and control ductal injuries—adequate drainage is paramount**.

2. **Grade I and II injuries**
   a. Account for 80% of all pancreatic injuries
   b. Require only hemostasis and adequate external drainage
   c. Drains are generally left in place for 7 to 10 days with the following criteria for removal:
      i. Patient is tolerating oral feedings.
      ii. Drain effluent <200 mL per day
      iii. Drain amylase <serum amylase
   d. Feeding jejunostomy should be considered for any multiply injured trauma patient with even minor pancreatic injuries.

3. **Grade III injuries**
   a. Best treated by distal pancreatectomy
   b. Splenic salvage can be attempted in the **stable** patient.
   c. Distal pancreatic resection may be performed with:
      i. A stapling device (e.g., thoracoabdominal [TA] stapler). The duct should be over-sewn with nonabsorbable monofilament suture.
      ii. Sharp transection and suture control
   d. The duct should be identified and individually ligated with nonabsorbable monofilament suture using a U-shaped or figure-of-8 stitch.
   e. Mattress sutures are used to control the parenchymal hemorrhage.
   f. Omentum may be used to buttress the stump closure.
   g. A closed-suction drain should be left near the suture or staple line and managed as above.
   h. Feeding jejunostomy is performed if the patient is stable.

4. **Grade IV and V injuries**
   a. Evaluation of the pancreatic and common bile ducts is essential.
   b. Injuries to the proximal gland without ductal injury are best managed with external drainage.
   c. Injuries to the proximal gland and duct that spare the ampulla and the duodenum can be treated as follows:
      i. Distal pancreatectomy if there is approximately 20% of the gland that can be salvaged
      ii. Transection of the pancreas at the site of injury, proximal duct ligation, and distal roux-en-Y pancreaticojejunostomy if there is concern about the proximal gland being able to meet the necessary exocrine and endocrine functions (i.e., proximal gland size <20%).

G. **Complications**
1. **Injury to the pancreatic duct** is the single most important determinant of outcome in patients with pancreatic injury.
2. **Multiple organ failure** and **sepsis** result in 30% of deaths in pancreatic trauma.
3. **Fistula**
   a. This is the most common complication, occurring in 10% to 35% of significant pancreatic injuries.
   b. The majority are minor (<200 mL per day) and resolve spontaneously in 2 to 4 weeks.
   c. High-output fistula (>700 mL per day) is rare and may require surgical intervention for resolution.
   d. If a high-output fistula persists for more than a few days, ERCP is indicated to determine if ductal obstruction is the cause.
   e. Somatostatin injected subcutaneously at a dose of 50 µg every 12 hours has a variable response in decreasing the fistula output. However, it is not proven to aid in fistula closure. This should only be used after duct obstruction and infection have been ruled out as possible causes of the persistent fistula.
4. **Abscess**
   a. Occurs in 10% to 25% of pancreatic trauma patients
   b. Early drainage, either surgical or percutaneous, is essential.
   c. Mortality rate for these patients is 25%.
5. **Pancreatitis**
   a. Occurs in 8% to 18% of patients after pancreatic surgery
   b. Treated with nasogastric decompression, bowel rest, and nutritional support
   c. If there is any question that necrotic pancreas remains, repeat exploration and debridement may be necessary.
   d. **Hemorrhagic pancreatitis** may be indicated by bloody drain effluent or a decrease in serum hemoglobin as well as the **Grey-Turner sign** (flank ecchymosis) or **Cullen sign** (periumbilical ecchymosis). The mortality rate of hemorrhagic pancreatitis approaches 80%.
   e. May have secondary hemorrhage requiring transfusion

i. Occurs in 5% to 10% of pancreatic trauma patients
ii. Generally occurs when pancreatic drainage after debridement is inadequate or when infection develops
iii. May require reoperation or angiographic embolization for control

6. **Pseudocysts**
   a. May result from blunt pancreatic injuries that are overlooked or treated nonoperatively
   b. Status of the pancreatic duct dictates the treatment.
   c. ERCP to determine the integrity of the duct should precede any intervention.
   d. If the duct is intact, percutaneous drainage is generally sufficient therapy.
   e. If the duct is injured or stenosed, the treatment options include:
      i. Re-exploration and partial gland resection (preferred)
      ii. Internal roux-en-Y drainage of the pseudocyst
      iii. Endoscopic transpapillary stenting of the injured duct

V. DUODENAL INJURIES

A. Mechanism of injury
1. Approximately 85% of duodenal injuries result from penetrating trauma and 15% from blunt abdominal trauma.
2. Blunt injury to the duodenum occurs by one of the following mechanisms:
   a. **Crush injury** occurs when a direct blow to the upper abdomen crushes the duodenum against the vertebral column.
   b. **Bursting injury** occurs when the intraluminal pressure is greater than the bowel wall strength (e.g., seat belt obstruction of a loop of bowel).
   c. **Shearing injury** occurs when the force of the deceleration exceeds the stabilizing force of the duodenum at the ligament of Treitz.
3. **Blunt duodenal injuries have a higher mortality than penetrating injuries.**

B. Associated injuries
1. The most common cause of early death in patients with duodenal injuries is exsanguinating hemorrhage from associated vascular, liver, or splenic injuries.
2. The most frequently associated injuries are:
   a. Liver
   b. Major arteries and veins
   c. Colon

C. Diagnosis
1. **Penetrating trauma**
   a. The diagnosis of penetrating duodenal injury is generally made at the time of abdominal exploration.
   b. With gunshot injuries, a preoperative abdominal radiograph (if the patient's hemodynamic status allows) may be helpful for localization of the bullet.
2. **Blunt trauma**
   a. Blunt injuries to the duodenum are more difficult to diagnose than penetrating injuries.

b. Presenting symptoms may be vague, poorly localized, and **delayed for up to 72 hours** secondary to retroperitoneal location.
c. Physical findings may also be nonspecific but may include contusions or abrasions across the upper abdomen, steering wheel or seat-belt marks, and midepigastric tenderness.
3. **Serum amylase**
   a. Although often evaluated, **serum amylase is a poor indicator of injury**.
   b. Only 53% of duodenal injuries have abnormal serum amylase values.
4. **Abdominal radiographs** may show the following:
   a. Location of a foreign body
   b. Mild scoliosis of lumbar spine
   c. Obliteration of the right psoas shadow
   d. Retroperitoneal air
   e. Free intraperitoneal air
   d. Air in the biliary tree
5. **Upper gastrointestinal series**
   a. May localize site of injury
   b. Initial study is performed with water-soluble contrast (Gastrografin) and, if negative, may be repeated with barium.
   c. Intramural hematoma is suggested by a "coiled spring" or "stacked coin" appearance of the involved segment of bowel.
6. **Diagnostic peritoneal lavage**
   a. Poor test due to retroperitoneal location of duodenum
   b. Amylase, bile, or food particles in lavage fluid indicate hollow viscus injury.
7. **Computed tomography scan**
   a. When performed with **IV and oral contrast** this is the **diagnostic test of choice** in a stable patient with blunt abdominal trauma and suspected retroperitoneal injury.

D. **Intraoperative evaluation**
1. **Findings suggestive of duodenal injury are:**
   a. Central or right upper quadrant retroperitoneal hematoma
   b. Bile staining of the peritoneal cavity, retroperitoneum, or lesser sac
   c. Retroperitoneal or peripancreatic fluid or edema
   d. Air or crepitus anterior or lateral to duodenum, or in the transverse mesocolon
2. **Injury classification**
   a. **Grade I**:
      i. **Hematoma**—involving single portion of duodenum
      ii. **Laceration**—partial thickness, no perforation
   b. **Grade II**:
      i. **Hematoma**—involving more than one portion
      ii. **Laceration**—disruption of <50% of circumference
   c. **Grade III laceration**:
      i. Disruption of 50% to 75% of circumference of second portion of duodenum (D2)
      ii. Disruption of 50% to 100% of first (D1), third (D3), or fourth (D4) portion of the duodenum

d. **Grade IV laceration**—disruption >75% circumference of D2, involving ampulla or distal common bile duct
e. **Grade V laceration**—massive disruption of duodenopancreatic complex
f. **Grade V vascular**—devascularization of the duodenum

E. Treatment

1. **Duodenorrhaphy** is successful treatment in 70% to 85% of all duodenal wounds.
2. **Grade I laceration**
   a. Primary closure with single-layer closure to avoid narrowing of the lumen
   b. Absorbable monofilament suture is preferred.
3. **Grade II laceration**
   a. Treated by primary closure after minimal debridement of devitalized tissue
   b. If a two-layer closure is used, the inner layer is closed with a running absorbable suture and the outer layer with an interrupted nonabsorbable suture. Note: single-layer closure is acceptable.
   c. **Transverse closure of lacerations is preferred** to prevent narrowing of the duodenal lumen.
   d. If the injury dictates **longitudinal** closure, a **one-layer** closure incorporating serosa, muscularis and submucosa may prevent narrowing. This single-layer closure does not include the mucosa.
4. **Grade I/II hematoma**
   a. If diagnosed preoperatively and if it is an isolated injury, management is nonoperative using the following measures: nasogastric decompression, total parenteral nutrition, and serial Gastrografin studies every 5 to 7 days if there are no signs of resolving the obstruction. A celiotomy with evacuation of the hematoma should be considered if the signs of obstruction persist after 14 to 21 days of conservative therapy. Coagulation disorders are associated with this injury and should be evaluated with the appropriate tests.
   b. If diagnosed intraoperatively, the duodenum must be adequately inspected to rule out perforation. A Kocher maneuver may evacuate the hematoma although controversy exists over the intentional incision of the serosa to facilitate the evacuation. Either a gastrojejunostomy or feeding-tube jejunostomy should be considered at the time of exploration.
5. **Grade III injuries**
   a. Primary end-to-end anastomosis is the procedure of choice.
   b. Two-layer closure is advocated, though one layer is acceptable.
   c. If the duodenum cannot be adequately mobilized for primary repair, a roux-en-Y limb can be anastomosed to the proximal duodenal limb with oversewing of the distal injury.
   d. The use of gastric diversion or duodenal decompression via tube duodenostomy is controversial in these injuries. At Parkland Memorial Hospital, these techniques are reserved for more severe injuries.

6. **Grade IV injuries**
   a. Primary closure is rarely possible, by definition.
   b. If the ampulla and bile duct are intact, a roux-en-Y duodenojejunostomy is the procedure of choice.
   c. When the ampulla is disrupted, the choices for repair include reimplantation of the ducts or pancreaticoduodenectomy.
   d. Reimplantation is performed as follows:
      i. The bile and pancreatic ducts are approximated using interrupted absorbable suture.
      ii. An opening is made in the posterior duodenal wall.
      iii. The joined bile and pancreatic ducts are approximated to the duodenum with interrupted full-thickness absorbable suture.
      iv. The ductal repair should be stented and the duodenal repair diverted or decompressed.
   e. **Most commonly, a pancreaticoduodenectomy is required for these injuries.**
   f. **Reimplantation is rarely used at Parkland Memorial Hospital.**
7. **Grade V injuries**
   a. Require pancreaticoduodenectomy
   b. Drainage of the anastomotic sites and feeding jejunostomy are essential.
8. **Duodenal diversion and decompression**
   a. These are adjunctive procedures designed to protect the duodenal repair.
      i. Pyloric exclusion
      ii. Duodenal diverticularization
      iii. Tube duodenostomy
   b. Pyloric exclusion is performed with absorbable 3-0 suture or, alternatively, a TA stapling device.
      i. The staple line should be just distal to the pylorus to avoid retained gastric antrum within the duodenum.
      ii. Side-to-side gastrojejunostomy is performed at the site of the gastrotomy.
      iii. The pylorus reopens in 90% of patients within 2 to 3 weeks.
   c. **Feeding jejunostomy tubes should be placed in all patients requiring duodenal diversion.**
      i. Grade I and II injuries do not require diversion or decompression.
      ii. Controversy exists over use of these techniques in Grade III injuries, but if deemed necessary, tube duodenostomy is recommended.
      iii. Grade IV and V injuries should have diversion or drainage.

F. Postoperative care
1. Postoperative management follows the same guidelines as for pancreatic injuries.
2. **Prior to resuming oral feeding, the duodenal repair should be studied with an upper gastrointestinal study.**

G. Complications
1. Postoperative complications are **common** in duodenal injuries with **only about one-third having an uncomplicated recovery.**

2. **Duodenal fistula** is one of the two major complications after injury.
   a. **Usually presents after the 5th postoperative day, but also as late as the 9th day**
   b. Signs indicating fistula are the following:
      i. Bilious drainage at drain site
      ii. Deterioration in patient status with fever, hypotension, and increased abdominal tenderness
   c. Diagnosis is made by an upper gastrointestinal series in patients with an intact pylorus or through the drain or duodenostomy tube.
   d. Treatment is nonoperative initially, so long as duodenal drainage has been established, with bowel rest and adequate nutrition.
   e. If surgical intervention is required, the following procedures may be used:
      i. Duodenal exclusion
      ii. Roux-en-Y drainage
      iii. Duodenal diverticularization
3. **Duodenal obstruction** is the other major complication after duodenal injury.
   a. Partial obstruction requires nonoperative treatment for at least 3 to 4 weeks.
   b. Complete obstruction
      i. Nonoperative treatment initially
      ii. If no improvement in 1 week, consider operation.
      iii. Gastrojejunostomy is most commonly used.
4. The overall mortality rate for duodenal injuries is around 20%.
   a. Mortality within the first 72 hours is usually related to associated injuries.
   b. The duodenal injury itself is responsible for only 2% of deaths.

VI. SUGGESTED READINGS

Carrillo EH, Richardson JD, Miller FB: Evolution in the management of duodenal injuries. J Trauma 40(6):1037–1045; dicussion 1045–1046, 1996.

Seamon MJ, Pieri PG, Fisher CA, et al: A ten-year retrospective review: Does pyloric exclusion improve clinical outcome after penetrating duodenal and combined pancreaticoduodenal injuries? J Trauma 62(4):829–833, 2007.

Timaran CH, Martinez O, Ospina JA: Prognostic factors and management of civilian penetrating duodenal trauma. J Trauma 47(2):330–335, 1999.

Small Bowel Trauma

Barbra S. Miller, MD

I. EPIDEMIOLOGY

A. **Blunt small bowel injury is rare** (1.2% of blunt trauma admissions), with perforation seen in 0.3%. The intestine is the third most commonly injured organ in blunt trauma (most common hollow viscus injury).
B. **The incidence of small bowel injury from gunshot wounds** exceeds 80% (mandating celiotomy), while that from stab wounds approaches 30% (use a more selective approach).
C. Together, the stomach and small bowel represent the most commonly injured organs in penetrating trauma.

II. ANATOMY

A. **The small bowel** from the ligament of Treitz to the ileocecal valve has an average length of 5 to 6 meters.
B. The small bowel is vulnerable to injury because it is **protected anteriorly only by the abdominal wall** and occupies most of the abdomen.
C. **The mesentery extends from** the left side of L2 to the right sacroiliac joint and crosses the third portion of the duodenum, aorta, inferior vena cava, right ureter, and gonadal vessels.
D. **The superior mesenteric artery (SMA)** emerges from under the pancreas and travels anterior to the uncinate process of the pancreas. It is the main blood supply to numerous small intestinal branches and the middle, ileocolic, and right colic arteries.
E. **The superior mesenteric vein (SMV)** corresponds to the SMA. It passes under the pancreas and joins with the inferior mesenteric vein and splenic vein to form the portal vein.
F. **The jejunum has a larger diameter and thicker folds** than the ileum and is supplied by single arcades rather than the two or three sets of vascular arcades seen in the ileum.
G. **The ileum is the site of** vitamin B_{12} absorption and is involved in enterohepatic circulation of bile salts.
H. **Bacterial counts increase from proximal to distal**.

III. MECHANISM OF INJURY

A. **Penetrating injury**: most penetrating injuries are secondary to stab wounds or gunshot wounds.
1. Firearms cause damage by direct force and by a lateral blast effect. Projectiles do not travel in straight lines, and therefore organ injury cannot be predicted by mentally constructing a line connecting entrance and exit wounds.

2. Stab wounds are more predictable and usually less severe than gunshot wounds. The mobility of the small bowel allows the intestine to slide away from the offending object. It is important to note or inquire as to the length and width of the weapon.
- **B. Blunt injury:** the mechanism of injury is more varied and sometimes less obvious. Examples include:
1. Shearing forces—with sudden deceleration, avulsion of the small bowel from fixed points of attachment may occur (ligament of Treitz, ileocecal junction).
2. Bursting (blowout) injury—a segment of bowel may rupture due to a sudden increase in intra-abdominal pressure and the occlusion of those segments of bowel both proximal and distal, creating a pseudo-closed loop of bowel.
3. Crushing injury—sudden force to the abdomen can crush the intestine between a firm object such as the lumbosacral spine.
4. Seat belt syndrome
    a. Characterized by injuries to the small bowel
    b. May cause chance-type lumbar fractures (transversely oriented fractures through the vertebrae)
    c. May occasionally cause injuries to the stomach or colon
    d. Presence of ecchymosis on the abdominal wall at the site of the lap belt is known as "seat belt" sign.

IV. DIAGNOSIS

- **A. Penetrating trauma**
1. **All patients with gunshot wounds to the abdomen undergo exploratory celiotomy** after advanced trauma life support (ATLS) evaluation is completed and chest and abdominal films are obtained (to evaluate for hemo/pneumothorax and potentially locate projectile). Radiologic markers are placed at the penetrating wound sites for x-rays.
2. **Local wound exploration is performed for an anterior stab wound** in asymptomatic hemodynamically normal patients. Positive local exploration (penetration of posterior abdominal wall fascia) or equivocal exploration (due to inability to view posterior fascia) is followed by diagnostic peritoneal lavage (DPL). If DPL criteria are positive, the patient undergoes exploratory celiotomy.
3. **Exploratory celiotomy is indicated, without further evaluation, in patients with evisceration, peritonitis, or hemodynamic instability.**
- **B. Blunt trauma**
1. **Evaluation for blunt small bowel injury is difficult.**
2. **In the unstable patient focused abdominal sonography for trauma (FAST) is used** to identify fluid (i.e., blood) in the peritoneal cavity.
3. **For unstable patients**
    a. **Positive FAST**—to the operating room for exploratory celiotomy

b. **Negative FAST**— DPL
   c. **Positive DPL**—to the operating room
   d. **Peritonitis by examination**—to the operating room
4. **Stable patients** can be evaluated for small bowel injury using abdominal ultrasound, abdominal CT, and DPL.
   a. **Perform FAST.**
      i. **Positive FAST:** obtain CT scan.
      ii. **Negative FAST:** if there is no significant abdominal tenderness and the patient has no alteration in mental status or other indications for CT scan, it may be assumed that there is no small bowel injury and evaluation for this type of injury can be stopped.
   b. **If CT is suggestive of small bowel injury,** perform DPL or the patient should be taken to the operating room, depending on the degree of suspicion for injury.
   c. **If CT does not suggest small bowel injury** and there is no other indication for surgery, observe the patient in the hospital with serial abdominal examinations.
5. **Unexplained intra-abdominal free fluid,** bowel wall thickening, pneumoperitoneum, mesenteric fat streaking or hematomas, and extravasation of contrast are worrisome features on CT for blunt small bowel or mesenteric injury. (We do not routinely use oral contrast at Parkland Memorial Hospital for CT evaluation of blunt abdominal trauma.)
6. **Ultrasound and CT considerations:** conventional CT and ultrasound lack adequate sensitivity for identifying hollow viscus injury unless there is a large amount of free intraperitoneal air or fluid without solid organ injury. The use of helical CT scanners is associated with increased sensitivity in detection of small bowel and mesenteric injuries.

V. MANAGEMENT PRINCIPLES

A. **Operative management is the standard of care in our institution.** There is no role for observation in the treatment of suspected intestinal trauma.
B. **The Small Bowel Injury Grading Scale** is used as a guide for repair (Table 26-1).
C. **One dose of an antibiotic** effective against enteric flora is administered prior to operation.
D. **25% of patients with small bowel injury** requiring operative intervention will have multiple small bowel injuries, emphasizing the need to examine the entire small bowel at exploration.
E. **Systematic exploration is** performed through a midline incision. Priorities are listed as follows in descending order:
1. Locate and control hemorrhage.
2. Control enteric contamination with clamps.
3. Identify and repair injuries.

TABLE 26-1
AAST SMALL BOWEL INJURY GRADING SCALE

Grade*	Type of injury	Description of injury	ICD-9	AIS-90
I	Hemotoma	Contusion or hematoma without devascularization	863.20	2
	Laceration	Partial thickness, no perforation	863.20	2
II	Laceration	Laceration <50% of circumference	863.30	3
III	Laceration	Laceration ≥50% of circumference without transection	863.30	3
IV	Laceration	Transection of the small bowel	863.30	4
V	Laceration	Transection of the small bowel with segmental tissue loss	863.30	4
	Vascular	Devascularized segment	863.30	4

*Advance one grade for multiple injuries, up to grade III.

- **F. The bowel is eviscerated** to the right side and carefully inspected in its entirety.
- **G. Repair of injuries should not occur** until the entire small and large bowel have been inspected. These injuries may have to be resected if other injuries are identified in close proximity or within the blood supply for that portion of the bowel.
- **H. Active mesenteric bleeding** should be controlled with careful suture ligation. Hematomas at the root of the mesentery are carefully evaluated due to concern for compromising blood supply to large portions of the bowel. Small nonexpanding hematomas should be reassessed at frequent intervals to ensure stability. Mesenteric hematomas adjacent to the bowel should be carefully opened and the mesenteric aspect of the bowel assessed for injury.
- **I. All but 50 cm of the small bowel may be resected** without compromising bowel function. It is more important to preserve the distal ileum than the jejunum.
- **J. Simple perforations** and small lacerations are closed using interrupted silk suture. Single-layer closures are preferred. If a two-layer closure is used, the inner layer can be either running or interrupted and is solely for hemostasis. The bowel is closed with seromuscular Lembert sutures.
- **K. All wounds are closed transversely** so the bowel lumen is not compromised. Large serosal injuries are repaired with a single layer of interrupted silk Lembert sutures.
- **L. Bowel of questionable viability can be left and reassessed** upon return for second-look celiotomy in 24 hours. This is only done if the area in question would require an extensive resection and there is concern for short-gut syndrome. Doppler signal and fluoroscein staining can be used to assess bowel viability.

M. Resection and primary anastomosis are indicated in the following situations:
1. Through-and-through wounds
2. Devascularized segments
3. Wounds > 50% of the bowel diameter
4. Multiple wounds in close proximity such that primary repair of all wounds would compromise the diameter of the bowel lumen

N. Measure the remaining length of the small bowel and document in the operative note.

VI. POSTOPERATIVE CARE

A. Antibiotics are continued for no more than 24 hours postoperatively. A single postoperative dose is used in most cases.
B. Nasogastric suction is continued until bowel function returns.
C. Enteral feedings are started as soon as possible.
D. Patients are monitored closely for early signs and symptoms of postoperative complications.

VII. COMPLICATIONS

A. Bleeding requires reexploration.
B. Abdominal abscess—CT-guided percutaneous drainage, if possible, is preferred; otherwise celiotomy is performed if there is no improvement in the patient's condition.
C. Fistula is managed nonoperatively in the absence of distal obstruction, generalized peritonitis, signs of systemic sepsis, or high output.
D. Anastomotic dehiscence is rare (0.5% to 1% of all cases), but it is catastrophic if missed.
E. Ischemic bowel may lead to obstruction or may progress to necrosis and perforation. It requires reoperation.
F. Short-gut syndrome
G. Mechanical small bowel obstruction versus prolonged postoperative ileus—nasogastric tube decompression and conservative management for 10 to 14 days. Obtain a CT scan to evaluate for intra-abdominal abscess as a possible cause for ileus. If no resolution after 2 weeks, consider reexploration.

VIII. PEARLS AND PITFALLS

A. Bacterial counts in the proximal small bowel are < 10,000 organisms/mL. Therefore, distal small bowel perforation carries a greater risk of intra-abdominal or wound infection than proximal small bowel perforation.
B. A high index of suspicion with early operation is the key to avoiding serious consequences. The peritoneal cavity can overcome

contamination if the source of contamination is controlled, but it does not tolerate continued contamination. Relatively brief delays in diagnosis (as little as 8 hours) can result in significant increases in morbidity and mortality directly attributable to missed small bowel injuries.

IX. SUGGESTED READINGS

Brasel KJ, et al: Incidence and significance of free fluid on abdominal computed tomographic scan in blunt trauma. J Trauma 44:889-892, 1998.

Brundage S, et al: Stapled versus sutured gastrointestinal anastomoses in the trauma patient: A multicenter trial. J Trauma 51:1054-1061, 2001.

Chandler CF, et al: Seatbelt sign following blunt trauma is associated with increased incidence of abdominal injury. Ann Surg 10:885, 1997.

Cunningham MA, et al: Does free fluid on abdominal computed tomographic scan after blunt trauma require laparotomy? J Trauma 44:599-603, 1998.

Diebel LN: Stomach and small bowel. In Mattox KL, Feliciano DV (eds): Trauma. East Norwalk, CT, Appleton & Lange, 687-706, 1996.

Fakhry SM, et al: Current diagnostic approaches lack sensitivity in the diagnosis of perforated blunt small bowel injury: Analysis from 275,557 trauma admissions from the EAST Multi-Institutional HVI Trial. J Trauma 54:295-306, 2003.

Fakhry SM, et al: Relatively short diagnostic delays (<8 hours) produce morbidity and mortality in blunt small bowel injury (SBI): An analysis of time to operative intervention in 198 patients from a multi-center experience. J Trauma 48:408-415, 2000.

Hackam DJ, et al: Effects of other intra-abdominal injuries on the diagnosis, management, and outcome of small bowel trauma. J Trauma 49:606-610, 2000.

Killeen KL, et al: Helical computed tomography of bowel and mesenteric injuries. J Trauma 51:26-36, 2001.

Ledgerwood AM: Small intestine. In Thal ER, Weigelt JA, Carrico CJ (eds): Operative Trauma Management: An Atlas, 2nd ed. New York, McGraw-Hill, 2002, pp 184-201.

Malhotra AK, et al: Blunt bowel and mesenteric injuries: The role of screening computed tomography. J Trauma 48:991-1000, 2000.

Rodriguez C, et al: Isolated free fluid on computed tomographic scan in blunt abdominal trauma: A systematic review of incidence and management. J Trauma 53:79-85, 2002.

Watts DD, et al: Incidence of hollow viscus injury in blunt trauma: Analysis from 275,557 trauma admissions from the EAST Multi-institutional Trial. J Trauma 54:289-294, 2003.

Witzke JD, et al: Stapled versus hand sewn anastomoses in patients with small bowel injury: A changing perspective. J Trauma 49:660-666, 2000.

Liver and Biliary Tract Trauma

David Curtis, MD

I. OVERVIEW

A. The liver is the most frequently injured soliid organ in the abdomen.
B. Hepatic injury is more common in patients with penetrating injuries (30%) than in patients with blunt abdominal trauma (15% to 20%).
C. The overall mortality of liver trauma is approximately 10%. Blunt injuries are usually more complex and result in mortality approaching 25%.
D. Most deaths occur in the early postoperative period (<48 hours) from shock and transfusion-related coagulopathies.

II. ANATOMY

A. Knowledge of the anatomy of the liver (Fig. 27-1) is critical for the management of hepatic trauma.
B. The right and left lobes of the liver are separated by a plane from the gallbladder fossa to the inferior vena cava (IVC).
C. To adequately mobilize the liver, its numerous ligamentous attachments must be incised. These include the following:
1. The falciform ligament
2. The right and left triangular ligaments
3. The coronary ligament

(Care must be taken when incising these ligaments not to damage the phrenic or hepatic veins.)

D. The right and left hepatic veins are intraparenchymal except for 1 to 2 cm prior to entering the IVC. The middle hepatic vein usually joins the left hepatic vein in the parenchyma of the liver (85%).
E. The retrohepatic IVC is 8 to 10 cm in length and along with the major hepatic veins receives blood directly from numerous small hepatic veins.

III. CLASSIFICATION OF HEPATIC INJURIES

The most recent and comprehensive classification system has been compiled by the Organ Injury Scaling Committee of the American Association for the Surgery of Trauma and includes findings on both the preoperative (CT scan) and intraoperative assessment of hepatic injuries (see Table 27-1).

IV. INITIAL MANAGEMENT

A. In patients with blunt trauma to the upper quadrants of the abdomen or the lower chest (with or without rib fractures), injury to the liver should be suspected.

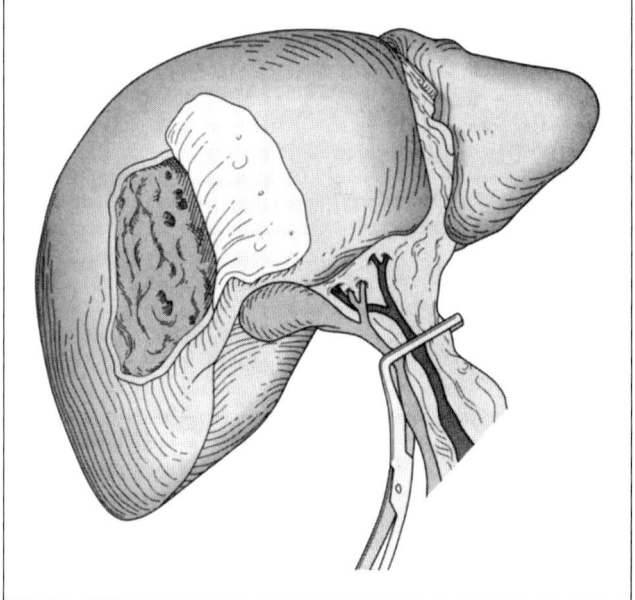

FIGURE 27-1

Pringle maneuver using an atraumatic vascular clamp. (From Walt AJ, Levison MA: Hepatic trauma: Juxtahepatic vena cava injury. In Champion HR, Robbs JV, Trunkey DD (eds): Rob and Smith's Operative Surgery, 4th ed. London, Butterworths, 1983, p 378.)

B. Penetrating (gunshot, shotgun, or stab) wounds below the nipple or in the upper quadrants of the abdomen also are likely to cause hepatic injury.

C. Occasionally patients with severe blunt or penetrating injury present with hypotension and a distended abdomen. They require rapid resuscitation and should be taken immediately to the operating room.

D. The hemodynamically normal patient with an isolated gunshot wound or shotgun wound to the abdomen or chest (below the nipple) requires minimal preoperative studies. Initial resuscitation should include:

1. Intubation and chest tubes as necessary
2. Two large-bore upper extremity IV lines
3. Foley catheter
4. Nasogastric tube

E. After marking the entrance and exit wounds, a scout film may be helpful to locate the presence of the missile(s).

TABLE 27-1
AMERICAN ASSOCIATION FOR THE SURGERY OF TRAUMA CLASSIFICATION SYSTEM

LIVER INJURY SCALE		
Grade*		Description
I	Hematoma	Subcapsular, <10% surface area
	Laceration	Capsular tear, <1 cm parenchymal depth
II	Hematoma	Subcapsular, 10% to 50% surface area
		Intraparenchymal, <10 cm in diameter
	Laceration	Capsular tear, 1 to 3 cm parenchymal depth, <10 cm length
III	Hematoma	Subcapsular, >50% surface area or ruptured subcapsular or parenchymal hematoma
		Intraparenchymal hematoma >10 cm or expanding
	Laceration	>3 cm parenchymal depth
IV	Laceration	Parenchymal disruption involving 25% to 75% of hepatic lobe or 1 to 3 Couinaud's segments
V	Laceration	Parenchymal disruption involving >75% of hepatic lobe or >3 Couinaud's segments within a single lobe
	Vascular	Juxtahepatic venous injuries; i.e., retrohepatic vena cava/central major hepatic veins
VI	Vascular	Hepatic avulsion

*Advance one grade for multiple injuries up to grade III.

F. FAST examination can be used as an adjunct to the physical examination to direct studies and therapy. Pericardial and thoracic images are also useful in cases of penetrating trauma to assist in directed therapy.

V. DIAGNOSIS AND ASSESSMENT

A. After completion of the primary and secondary surveys the decision is made to explore the abdomen or perform further diagnostic studies. If the patient has a gunshot wound to the abdomen, signs of peritonitis, hemodynamic instability, or a distended abdomen, then emergent surgical exploration is required. Further evaluation should address other life-threatening injuries but should not delay operative intervention. The FAST examination can be quickly performed and may assist in decision making in unstable blunt trauma patients.

B. In the *stable* patient with a stab wound to the abdomen and an otherwise normal abdominal examination, further evaluation is undertaken to plan treatment.

C. If the stab wound is *anterior* or on the *flanks (and tracks anteriorly)* initial work-up should include *local exploration*.

of the stab wound to document penetration of the anterior muscle fascia. If lack of penetration is confirmed, the wound may be closed and the patient discharged. If the wound penetrates the muscle fascia or the exploration is equivocal, diagnostic peritoneal lavage (DPL) should be performed. DPL is >95% accurate in detecting intra-abdominal injury when using the following criteria for a positive test.
1. RBC count >100,000 cells/mm^3
2. WBC>500 cells/mm^3
3. Elevated amylase, any bile, bacteria, or foreign material.
4. A positive DPL mandates exploratory celiotomy.
- **D.** If the stab wound is on the *back or tracks posteriorly* from the flank, an abdominal CT scan is recommended. This study is generally performed with IV and oral contrast, and then rectal contrast if needed.
- **E.** Two situations warrant special mention:
1. If the stab wound is thoracoabdominal, i.e., it could have penetrated the diaphragm (on the chest below the nipple), surgical evaluation is indicated to rule out diaphragmatic injury. (CT and DPL have high false negative rates for this injury.) Exploratory laparotomy is largely being replaced as the standard for evaluation for possible diaphragmatic injury by direct visualization using laparoscopy or thoracoscopy, techniques that have been very successful at Parkland Memorial Hospital and documented in the literature.
2. In the patient with a previous operation that precludes DPL, a CT scan can be helpful if it definitely shows the end of the knife track; otherwise, an exploratory celiotomy or serial physical examinations are necessary to rule out intra-abdominal injuries.
- **F.** In stable patients with blunt abdominal trauma the FAST examination is a significant adjunct to the physical examination. It assists in the rapid bedside detection of free fluid in the pericardial and peritoneal cavities. It has largely, but not completely, replaced the use of DPL in the initial evaluation of these patients.
- **G.** CT scans are obtained in stable patients to confirm positive sonographic findings, further evaluate equivocal results, and evaluate patients with injuries that may cause false-positive FAST findings including pelvic and spinal fractures. It is used in patients with hematuria, concern for hollow viscus injury (seat-belt marks), persistent tachycardia, and other significant mechanisms of injury.
- **H.** DPL is an excellent diagnostic test and is still useful in the evaluation of trauma patients. Its past broad application has diminished with the advance of sonography and CT scanning. The principal disadvantages of the DPL include its invasiveness, and in patients with minor injuries the test is positive even in the presence of minimal bleeding (20 mL of blood in the peritoneal cavity). Bleeding may have stopped by the time the celiotomy is performed. DPL remains applicable in the detection of hollow viscus injury and differentiation of the source of free fluid in heavily resuscitated patients.

VI. NONOPERATIVE MANAGEMENT

A. As a result of the significant incidence of nontherapeutic abdominal exploration, isolated blunt hepatic injury is increasingly managed nonoperatively. The criteria for *nonoperative management* include the following:
1. Hemodynamic stability
2. No peritonitis on abdominal examination
3. Ability of the surgeon to follow serial physical examinations (i.e., the patient is neurologically intact)
4. Delineation of hepatic injury and absence of other intraperitoneal injuries by CT scan. However, hemodynamic status is more significant than grade of injury.
5. Minimal transfusion requirements 2 units of packed red blood cells (PRBCs)

B. This approach requires careful observation of the patient, usually *in the intensive care unit with repeat examinations and serial hematocrits*. These injuries may cause slow bleeding, and physical signs may be evident only when the patient becomes hemodynamically unstable.

C. This should be a multidisciplinary approach. Angiography with embolization of bleeding vessels can assist in the success of nonoperative management. Early angiography may be necessary for contrast extravasation found on CT scan and may decrease the transfusion requirements and possibly decrease the infectious complications. Angiography, endoscopic retrograde cholangiopancreatography (ERCP), and interventional radiology may also become necessary in the treatment of complications.

D. Nonoperative management should not be viewed as conservative management. It is clearly more difficult to manage the patients without knowing the full extent of their injuries.

E. Nonoperative management should not lead to excessive blood transfusions or delays in operative intervention should the situation change and/or the above criteria are not met later in the patient's course. From 10% to 15% of these patients may evolve to require an operation less than 8 hours after admission.

F. Nonoperative management is not without morbidity. These patients can develop liver-related complications, including bile leaks, hepatic abscess, hepatic necrosis, and hemobilia, as well as non-liver-related complications, including pneumonia, bacteremia, urinary tract infections, adult respiratory distress syndrome, upper gastrointestinal bleeding, and multiple organ failure.

VII. OPERATIVE MANAGEMENT

A. Initial management
1. Be prepared to combat hypothermia.
   a. Have a *warmed operating room* available.

  b. Give warm IV fluids.
  c. Heating pad on the operating room table
  d. Convection heater prepared for use
2. The patient should be prepared and draped from the neck to the mid thigh to allow access to the chest via a sternotomy or thoracotomy and to allow access to the upper leg for harvesting a saphenous vein for a vascular injury.
3. Prophylactic antibiotics are given and a midline incision from the xiphoid to the pubis is used if maximum exposure is deemed necessary. The incision may be extended to include a sternotomy if retrohepatic vena cava or hepatic vein injury is present and requires control of the IVC within the pericardium.
4. All intraperitoneal blood should be quickly evacuated and bleeding sources controlled with packs and then located by rapid examination of the liver, spleen, mesentery, bowel and retroperitoneum.
5. In patients with blunt trauma, solid organ injuries are usually the source of bleeding and gastrointestinal tract or retroperitoneal vascular injuries are less common.
6. In patients with penetrating trauma, however, injuries to small bowel (60%), colon (40%), liver (30%), vascular structures (25%), and stomach (20%) are all common.

B. Simple injuries (grades I and II)

1. The majority of hepatic injuries (blunt 60% and penetrating 90%) are minor and will have stopped bleeding or, if not, can be managed by simple techniques. These include suture ligatures, electrocautery or argon beam coagulation, and application of topical agents.
2. For 1- to 3-cm deep bleeding lacerations, suture hepatorrhaphy using horizontal mattress sutures of 0 chromic on a large blunt needle are used to loosely approximate liver parenchyma. Care must be taken to first directly ligate all open bile ducts or vessels and to not strangulate (and subsequently necrose) the hepatic tissue.
3. Topical agents (i.e., Surgicel or Avitene) are useful once major hemorrhage is controlled. They are applied to the raw parenchymal surfaces and compressed with laparotomy pads for 5 to 15 minutes and repeated as necessary.
4. Fibrin glue is also used as a topical hemostatic agent, although there are reports of severe adverse reactions when it is injected into injured hepatic parenchyma.

C. Complex hepatic injuries (grade III or greater) occur in approximately 10% of penetrating and 40% of blunt trauma and require advanced hemostatic techniques.

1. In the face of extensive hepatic injury and massive hemorrhage, the initial management of complex hepatic injuries should be the control of the hemorrhage with manual compression of the injury using laparotomy pads. This allows the anesthesiologist time to correct hypovolemia and acidosis. After completion of intraoperative resuscitation, the liver is released and the injury is further addressed.
2. Prior to definitive hemostatic control of the liver injury, the portal triad is occluded with manual compression, a Rummel tourniquet, or an

atraumatic vascular clamp (the **Pringle maneuver**) (Fig. 27-1). This should control most bleeding unless there is a major venous injury. Continued bleeding with this maneuver indicates that a branch of the portal vein or hepatic artery is injured and needs repair.
3. Numerous studies have shown that the normal **liver can tolerate up to 90 minutes of warm ischemia** during elective liver resections without subsequent complication. This experience cannot be extrapolated to the trauma setting, but it does suggest that the upper limit of warm ischemia time is much longer. Intestinal venous congestion can become a problem with uninterrupted application of the Pringle maneuver. We use intermittent clamping for periods of 15 to 20 minutes with 5- to 6-minute breaks to alleviate venous congestion. This appears to extend the tolerable length of time to 120 minutes, through "ischemic preconditioning."
D. Hepatotomy with selective vascular ligation is the most widely used method to control extensive bleeding in the depths of a laceration or in the tract of a penetrating wound.
1. Glisson's capsule is incised.
2. The liver is finger-fractured through the parenchyma in the line of the laceration. One must keep in mind the position of the left and right hepatic ducts to avoid injuring them.
3. Thin Deaver retractors are then inserted into the open laceration and the bile ducts and vessels are selectively clipped or ligated.
4. Large intrahepatic branches of the portal or hepatic veins are repaired using 5-0 or 6-0 monofilament suture.
5. After hemorrhage is controlled and necrotic parenchyma debrided, the resulting hepatotomy site can be filled with a pedicle of omentum based on the right gastroepiploic vessel (Fig. 27-2).
6. The liver edges are then loosely approximated with 0 chromic liver sutures.
7. This omentum will tamponade minor oozing, decrease dead space, and increase absorption of small amounts of blood and bile.
E. Deep liver suturing using mattress or simple sutures through uninjured liver to compress an area of injury may control hemorrhage. This technique is not generally recommended, however, because it fails to control bleeding that is deep to the sutures and may lead to liver necrosis and subsequent abscess.
F. Resectional debridement (do not confuse this with anatomic resection) is indicated when there is partially devascularized tissue on the liver edge or in a laceration. Adequate debridement is essential to decrease the incidence of abscess formation. If resectional debridement is used on the edge of a hepatic lobe it is not necessary (and probably undesirable) to use an omental cover since this tends to trap fluid between it and the raw surface of the liver. **Hepatic resection** refers to anatomic removal of a segment (or lobe) and is reserved for patients with total destruction of a segment (or lobe) or when needed to control

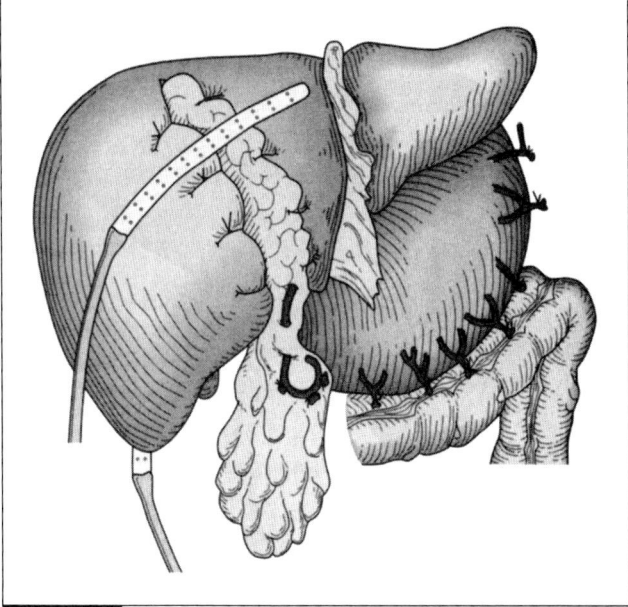

FIGURE 27-2
Omental pedicle based on right gastroepiploic artery packing a hepatotomy. (From Pachter HL, Liang HG, Hofstetter SR: Liver and biliary tract trauma. In Moore EE, Mattox KL, Feliciano DV (eds): Trauma, 2nd ed. East Norwalk, CT, Appleton & Lange, 1991, p 450.)

exsanguinating hemorrhage. Formal resection is rarely used in the trauma setting as it carries a high mortality rate. A small percentage of patients managed nonoperatively will require formal resection for devascularization injuries that are revealed over a period of time.

G. Selective **hepatic artery ligation** can be used to control arterial hemorrhage from the liver parenchyma. This maneuver is usually tolerated because of the high oxygen saturation of the portal blood and can be performed without subsequent hepatic necrosis. However, it is seldom used since more selective intraparenchymal vessel ligation is preferable and it is ineffective in controlling bleeding from portal and hepatic veins. In addition, a few cases of hepatic lobar infarction have been reported. It is indicated in the rare instance when selective clamping of an extrahepatic artery causes cessation of arterial bleeding in a hepatotomy or laceration and the bleeding vessel cannot be seen inside the liver. A **cholecystectomy** is recommended if the right hepatic artery is sacrificed to prevent subsequent gallbladder necrosis.

- **H. Perihepatic packing** is indicated in patients with extensive uncontrolled lacerations, expanding subcapsular hematomas, transfusion-induced coagulopathy, severe hypothermia (<32°C), or acidemia (pH <7.2). This is typically referred to as damage control, where hemorrhage and contamination are controlled rapidly and the operative procedure of definitive repair is truncated due to the patient's development of the triad of coagulopathy, acidosis, and hypothermia.
  1. The packing should be removed after the patient has stabilized hemodynamically and hypothermia, acidemia, and coagulopathy have been corrected. This usually occurs between **24 and 72 hours** after the **initial operation**. Reoperation after stabilization also allows debridement of nonviable hepatic tissue, partial hepatectomy, or formal lobectomy; as well as definitive repairs elsewhere, removal of clots, irrigation of the abdomen, and establishment of new drainage. The survival rate with perihepatic packing approaches 75%, which is excellent in this group of moribund patients. However, one can expect a **10% to 25% incidence of intra-abdominal sepsis** (mainly subphrenic abscess) and other complications.
- **I. Internal tamponade** of through-and-through liver injuries, especially bilobar penetrating injuries, may be employed in patients who would otherwise require extensive hepatotomy and debridement. This is especially true in patients with extensive associated injuries and in a damage control scenario. This is accomplished by passing a red rubber catheter through the missile tract. A pack made of several Penrose drains is tied to the end of the catheter and pulled back through the tract and left within the substance of the liver. The end of the Penrose pack is then brought through the skin. The pack tamponades the bleeding and serves as a drain. A similar situation can be achieved with a sterilized **Sentgstaken-Blakemore** tube passed through the tract and inflated. Finally, a technique of balloon tamponade can be performed using a red rubber catheter and a Penrose drain tied at each end (Fig. 27-3). Radiopaque contrast can be instilled through the red rubber catheter to distend the Penrose drain and tamponade the bleeding.
- **J. Drainage**. If there are no apparent bile leaks, grade I or II injuries (see Table 27-1) usually do not require drainage. A simple method to evaluate the injury is to place a lap pad over the area for several minutes and then examine it for bile staining. Complex hepatic injuries, however, should be widely drained. **Closed suction drainage** (Jackson-Pratt or Blake drains) is preferable for egress of blood and bile.
- **K.** Injuries to the **retrohepatic IVC** or **hepatic veins** are frequently lethal. If patients with these injuries are to survive, it is critical that the injury be recognized early, that is, prior to significant hemorrhage and coagulopathy. Adequate mobilization of the liver is mandatory for successful repair. Techniques for repair of these injuries require methods to decrease blood flow through this area and include total vascular isolation of the liver (clamping the hepatoduodenal ligament,

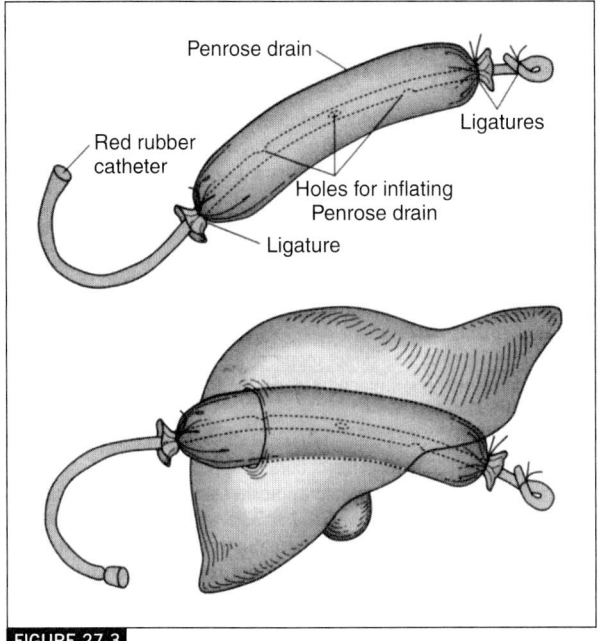

FIGURE 27-3

Internal tamponade of penetraing liver injury using a red rubber cathether and Penrose drain. (From Morimoto RY, Birolini D, Junqueira AR Jr, et al: Balloon tamponade for transfixing lesions of the liver. Surg Gynecol Obstet 164:87-88, 1987.)

suprarenal IVC and suprahepatic IVC sequentially; Heaney technique), the use of a transatrial chest tube or endotracheal tube shunts, and venovenous bypass. Vascular isolation of the liver can result in profound hypotension or cardiac arrest if preload cannot be maintained. Rarely a **transatrial shunt** (atriocaval) is employed (Fig. 27-4). After a median sternotomy is performed, a 36 French chest tube is passed through the right atrial appendage into the IVC, with its distal end and side openings at the renal veins. A side hole made in the proximal end allows blood flow from the shunt into the right atrium. Rummel clamps are then tightened at the suprarenal and intrapericardial IVC. An alternative approach utilizes an endotracheal tube as a shunt with a hole made in the proximal end in the right atrium. This obviates the need to secure the suprarenal IVC since the balloon is inflated for occlusion. An intracaval shunt can also be placed from below, thus obviating the need to encircle the suprahepatic vena cava. After the shunt is in place, the hepatic ligaments are taken down and the repair can be accomplished

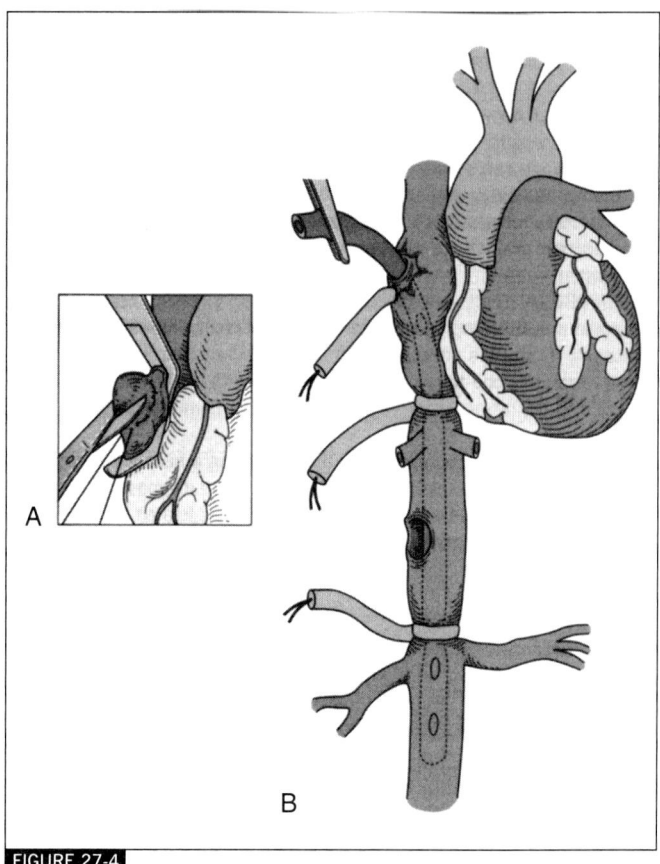

FIGURE 27-4

Atriocaval shunt using a 36 French chest tube. (From Pachter HL, Liang HG, Hofstetter SR: Liver and biliary trauma. In Moore EE, Mattox KL, Feliciano DV (eds): Trauma, 2nd ed. East Norwalk, CT, Appleton & Lange, 1991, p 450.)

using standard vascular techniques. Partial occlusion of the IVC with a Statinsky clamp can isolate certain injuries and facilitate repair without need for shunting or bypass. Last, aortic cross-clamping is seldom used unless there is a concomitant injury to the abdominal aorta.

L. There have been several reports of orthotopic liver transplantation after severe devascularizing injuries to the liver. This rare possibility can benefit the occasional patient with severe hepatic injury.

M. Angiography with embolization of bleeding within the liver has been shown in the literature and our experience at Parkland Memorial Hospital to assist with achieving hemostasis in critically injured trauma patients. Damage control laparotomy with liver packing, followed by hepatic angiography and embolization, has been used in selected cases. It has been shown to be an independent predictor of decreased mortality in severe hepatic injuries (grades IV and V) and must be available in centers caring for severe liver injuries.

VIII. COMPLICATIONS

A. **Recurrent bleeding** occurs in approximately 3% of all hepatic injuries, but this increases to approximately 7% with complex (grade III or greater) injuries. If coagulopathy is excluded and the patient's condition permits, hepatic angiography with embolization is preferred to reoperation alone. Repeat exploration with perihepatic packing can be used if the hemorrhage cannot be otherwise controlled.

B. **Intra-abdominal abscesses occur in 2% to 10% of all hepatic trauma** and are related to the extent of the hepatic injury, other associated injuries (especially colonic), the number of transfusions, and the type of drainage. In general, perihepatic abscesses can be avoided with careful hemostasis, debridement, and adequate drainage. If a perihepatic abscess does occur, percutaneous CT-guided drainage is the treatment of choice and has a success rate of >90%. If reoperation is necessary, exploration through previous incision is used to allow thorough exploration. On occasion, an extraperitoneal approach through the bed of the twelfth rib is used.

C. **Biliary fistula** (as defined by greater than 50 mL of biliary drainage per day for 2 weeks) occurs in a small number of patients following hepatic injury (1% to 10%). They can most often be managed conservatively with continued drainage and only rarely need reoperation for repair. Endoscopic retrograde cholangiopancreatography (ERCP) and endoscopic drainage or stenting may also be utilized in patients with persistent fistulas.

D. **Hemobilia** is another rare complication following hepatic trauma and usually presents after the patient has been released from the hospital. Approximately one third of patients present with the **classic triad of right upper quadrant pain, gastrointestinal tract hemorrhage, and jaundice**. Bleeding may be intermittent, and thus obtaining a history of trauma and a high index of suspicion are key to making the diagnosis. The diagnosis is confirmed by emergent **angiography** and is treated by embolization of the offending artery or pseudoaneurysm. Surgical treatment is very rarely required.

IX. GALLBLADDER INJURIES

A. Injuries to the gallbladder are uncommon and are almost always associated with other intra-abdominal injuries.

B. Gallbladder injuries are classified into five categories:
1. Rupture
2. Avulsion
3. Contusion
4. Cholecystitis (secondary to blood obstructing the cystic duct)
5. Necrosis (secondary to ligation or embolization of the right hepatic artery)

C. The usual treatment for any trauma is **cholecystectomy**; however, lesser procedures such as cholecystostomy may be desirable in the trauma patient with coagulopathy or cirrhosis or in the hemodynamically unstable patient in whom dissection of the gallbladder bed may lead to uncontrolled hemorrhage.

X. EXTRAHEPATIC BILE DUCT INJURY

A. These injuries occur in 3% to 5% of patients with abdominal trauma. There is a high incidence of associated intra-abdominal injury. The common bile duct is injured most frequently, followed by the confluence of hepatic ducts and then the left hepatic duct.

B. Initial management begins as with any intra-abdominal injury. Hemorrhage is controlled first. Then adequate exposure is obtained if a bile duct injury is suspected. This usually involves performing a wide Kocher maneuver. Diagnosis often rests on obtaining a cholangiogram intraoperatively.

C. Injuries are categorized as simple (involving <50% of ductal wall) or complex (>50% of ductal wall or transection)(Table 27-2).
1. Simple injuries are usually treated with primary repair and drainage.

TABLE 27-2
AMERICAN ASSOCIATION FOR THE SURGERY OF TRAUMA CLASSIFICATION SYSTEM

EXTRAHEPATIC BILIARY TREE INJURY SCALE	
Grade*	Description
I	Gallbladder contusion/hematoma
	Portal triad contusion/hematoma
II	Partial gallbladder avulsion from liver bed; cystic duct intact
	Laceration or perforation of the gallbladder
III	Complete gallbladder avulsion from liver bed
	Cystic duct laceration
IV	Partial or complete right hepatic duct laceration
	Partial or complete left hepatic duct laceration
	Partial common hepatic duct laceration (<50%)
	Partial common bile duct laceration (<50%)
V	>50% transaction of common hepatic duct
	>50% transaction of common bile duct
	Combined right and left hepatic duct injuries
	Intraduodenal or intrapancreatic bile duct injuries

*Advance one grade for multiple injuries up to grade III

2. Complex injuries generally require construction of a biliary-enteric anastomosis, usually a Roux-en-Y choledochojejunostomy, since primary repair is more often complicated by stricture formation. Transanastamotic stents remain controversial.
3. Complications include anastomotic leak, stricture formation, and recurrent cholangitis.

XI. PORTA HEPATIS INJURIES

A. Porta hepatis injuries are rare and are usually associated with multiple intra-abdominal injuries as well. They result in a high mortality (50%) and high morbidity (80% require reoperation).
B. The portal vein is the most commonly injured structure in the porta hepatis, followed by the bile ducts and lastly by the hepatic artery. Combined injuries are almost universally fatal.
C. If the hepatic artery is injured (and the portal vein is not injured) the most expedient solution is **ligation**.
D. If the portal vein is also injured, the artery or vein or both should be repaired. Portal vein injuries should be repaired with a lateral venorrhaphy, if possible; however, if this is not possible, then ligation of the vein is the preferred treatment. This will result in splanchnic sequestration of blood, and patients must have their volume status monitored closely.

XII. PEARLS AND PITFALLS

A. On first encountering a rapidly bleeding liver injury, bimanual compression of the surrounding liver parenchyma can stop the hemorrhage and allow the anesthesia team to correct severe hypovolemia and shock.
B. If hemorrhage continues after application of the Pringle maneuver, one must consider the patient to have a significant hepatic venous injury or an anomalous hepatic artery.

XIII. SUGGESTED READINGS

Anderson IB, et al: Liver trauma: Management of devascularizing injuries. J Trauma 57:1099-1104, 2004.

Asensio A, et al: Operative management and outcomes in 103 AAST-OIS Grades IV and V complex hepatic injuries: Trauma surgeons will need to operate, but angioembolization helps. J Trauma 54:647-654, 2002.

Dawson DL, et al: Injuries to the portal triad. Am J Surg 161:545-550, 1991.

Johnson JW, et al: Hepatic angiography in patients undergoing damage control laparotomy. J Trauma 52:1102-1106, 2002.

Kim Y-I: Ischemia-reperfusion injury of the human liver during hepatic resection. J Hepatobiliary Pancreat Surg 10:195-199, 2003.

Leppäniemi A, Haapiainen R: Occult diaphragmatic injuries caused by stab wounds. J Trauma 55:646-650, 2003.

Man K, et al: Tolerance of the liver to intermittent Pringle maneuver in hepatectomy for liver tumors. Arch Surg 134:533-539, 1999.

Miller CM, et al: Intermittent inflow occlusion in living liver donors: Impact on safety and remnant function. Liver Transplantation 10:244-247, 2004.

Mohr AM, et al: Angiographic embolization for liver injuries: Low mortality, high morbidity. J Trauma 55:1077-1082, 2003.

Pachter HL, Liang HG, Hofstetter SR: Liver and biliary trauma. In Moore EE, Mattox KL, Feliciano DV (eds): Trauma, 3rd ed. East Norwalk, CT, Appleton & Longe, 1996, 487-523.

Poggetti RS, et al: Balloon tamponade for bilobar transfixing hepatic gunshot wounds. J Trauma 33:694-697, 1992.

Rodriguez-Montes JA, et al: Complications following repair of extrahepatic bile duct injuries after blunt abdominal trauma. World J Surg 25:1313-1316, 2001.

Seligman JY, Egan M: Balloon tamponade: An alternative in the treatment of liver trauma. Am Surg 63:1022-1023, 1997.

Sriussazdaporn S, et al: A multidisciplinary approach in the management of hepatic injuries. Injury 33:309-315, 2002.

Trunkey DD: Hepatic trauma: Contemporary management. Surg Clin North Am 84:437-450, 2004.

Velmahos GC, et al: High success with nonoperative management of blunt hepatic trauma. Arch Surg 138:475-481, 2003.

Weigelt JA: In Trunkey DD, Lewis FR (eds): Current Therapy of Trauma, 3rd ed. Toronto, BC Decker, 1991, pp 247-250.

Splenic Trauma

Scott Brakenridge, MD, and Christopher Bell, MD

I. HISTORY

- **A.** Anecdotal reports in ancient Greek and Roman texts of splenectomy suggest the spleen is not a critical life-sustaining organ.
- **B.** 1893: first successful total splenectomy performed by Reigner
- **C.** 1919: Morris and Bullock are first to report an increased risk of overwhelming post-splenectomy infections in animal studies.
- **D.** 1900 to 1950: total splenectomy for traumatic injury is the standard of care. Operative mortality was reported to be 30% to 40%. Nonoperative mortality was as high as 90%. (Note: This predates detection of clinically occult but radiographically detectable splenic injuries.)
- **E.** 1950s: first reports of post-splenectomy susceptibility to overwhelming infections in the pediatric population
- **F.** 1970s to 1990s: studies begin to emerge on overwhelming post-splenectomy infection in the adult trauma population.
- **G.** 2005—repairs of splenic salvage using angiographic embolization

II. ANATOMY (Figure 28-1)

- **A. Location/macroscopic**. The spleen is a slightly concave, solid, dark red organ located in the posterior left upper quadrant of the abdomen. The approximate size of the adult spleen is 12 cm in length, 7 cm in width, and 3 to 4 cm in thickness. The average adult splenic weight is 150 g (range, 80 to 300 g). Anatomic relationships include:
  1. Superior/lateral: left hemidiaphragm and left posterolateral ribs 9 to 11
  2. Posterior: left adrenal and kidney as well as the body/tail of the pancreas
  3. Medial: greater curvature of the stomach
  4. Inferior: distal transverse colon and splenic flexure
- **B. Capsule**. Composed of an external layer of thin peritoneum and an internal fibroelastic layer. Completely covers the organ exterior and invests into the splenic parenchyma, forming a branching network of trabeculae, which subdivide the organ into functional compartments. The capsule is thicker and more elastic in children.
- **C. Attachments**. Peritoneal reflections anchoring spleen to surrounding structures. These ligaments require division for mobilization and/or splenectomy.
  1. **Splenophrenic**. Lateral border of spleen to posterior/lateral abdominal wall and left hemidiaphragm; relatively avascular
  2. **Splenocolic**. Lower splenic pole to the transverse colon/splenic flexure; relatively avascular

II. Anatomy

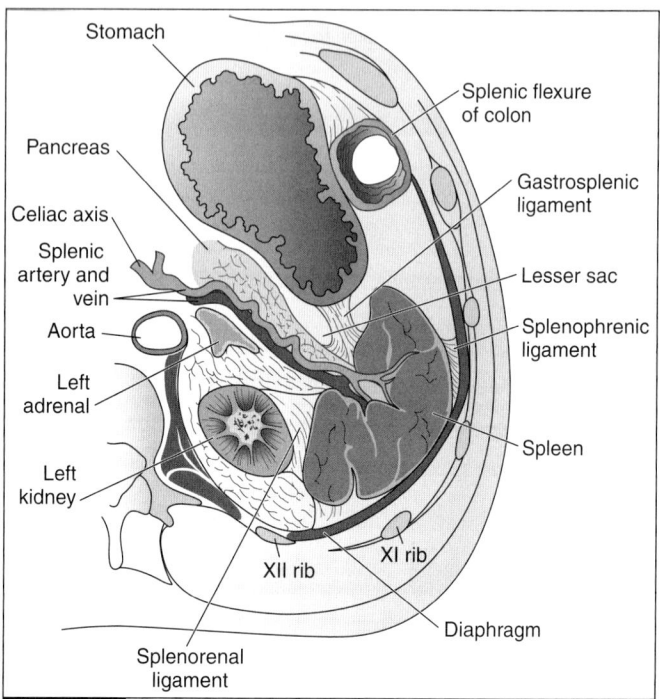

FIGURE 28-1

Location of the spleen and its related structures. (From Thal ER, Weigelt JA, Carrico CJ. In Thal ER, Weigelt JA, Carrico CJ (eds): Operative Trauma Management, 2nd ed. New York, McGraw-Hill, 2002.)

3. **Splenorenal**. Extends from the splenic hilum to the anterior left border of the left kidney. Invested underneath are the splenic vessels and tail of the pancreas. It is relatively avascular.
4. **Gastrosplenic**. Continuation of the splenorenal ligament from the splenic hilum anteriorly and superiorly to the greater curvature of the stomach; **contains the short gastric vessels**

D. Vascular supply. The spleen receives approximately 5% of total cardiac output. Its primary arterial supply is from the celiac axis via the splenic artery.

1. **Splenic artery**. The course of the artery may be tortuous, but it is generally located along the upper border of the body/tail of pancreas. Terminal branching at the splenic hilum is variable, but the artery most commonly (85%) divides into two primary branches supplying the superior and inferior poles.
2. **Short gastric arteries**. These arise from the left gastroepiploic artery along the greater curvature of the stomach. They average in number

from 4 to 6, run within the gastrosplenic ligament to the splenic hilum, and are easily damaged during splenic mobilization.
3. **Venous drainage**. Venous drainage is primarily via the variable splenic vein, which courses inferior to the splenic artery to its confluence with the superior mesenteric vein, where it drains to the portal venous system. Supplemental drainage is via short gastric veins in the gastrosplenic ligament.
E. **Accessory spleens**. These are present in 15% to 30% of patients. Most common locations include within the gastrosplenic or splenocolic ligaments, in the splenic hilum, or surrounding the tail of the pancreas. If present, salvage should be attempted in the face of major splenic trauma necessitating total splenectomy.

III. EPIDEMIOLOGY

A. **Blunt trauma**. The spleen and liver are the most commonly injured organs following blunt abdominal trauma. Mechanisms include motor vehicle collisions, falls, pedestrian vs. automobile incidents, and contact sports injuries. Deceleration forces result in ligament/capsular avulsions and organ fracture. Puncture from rib fractures can also cause splenic injury.
B. **Penetrating trauma**. Splenic fractures, lacerations, and hilar injuries can be caused by penetrating injury to the left upper quadrant, including injuries resulting from firearms, stabbing, and shrapnel.
C. **Intraoperative/iatrogenic**. Excessive traction during mobilization of the spleen, stomach, or colon can lead to vascular avulsion injuries. It can also lead to capsular rupture of an already injured spleen.

IV. DIAGNOSIS

A. Clinical manifestations
1. **The history of the injury** may include trauma to the abdomen or left lower aspect of the chest. Manifestations are nonspecific abdominal pain (30%), left shoulder pain (15%), or syncope.
2. **Physical examination** is accurate 65% of the time and includes peritonitis, left upper quadrant abdominal tenderness, referred pain to the left shoulder (Kehr's sign), fixed dullness to percussion on the left, and shifting dullness on the right (Ballance's sign).
3. **Clinical signs** include hypotension, tachycardia, a reduction in hematocrit, and a moderate increase in the white blood cell count.
B. **Plain radiographs** are not a reliable diagnostic study but they may show left lower rib fractures (associated with splenic injury in 20% of patients), elevated left hemidiaphragm, left pleural effusion, enlarged splenic shadow, or medial displacement of the gastric shadow.
C. Ultrasound or FAST (**F**ocused **A**bdominal **S**onography for **T**rauma)
1. Evaluates for **fluid in the pericardial sac** as well as for **free fluid in the abdomen** and is portable, rapid, and noninvasive, though also nonspecific

2. There are **four views:** pericardial, right upper quadrant (Morrison's pouch), left upper quadrant, and pelvic (pouch of Douglas) that evaluate for fluid in the dependent regions of the peritoneal cavity.
3. Not useful for grading the degree of injury
4. **Patients with positive FAST scans who are hemodynamically normal should undergo computed tomography (CT). Patients with positive FAST scans who demonstrate hemodynamic instability should be treated with immediate operative exploration.**

D. Computed tomography
1. CT is the **procedure of choice** for diagnosis and estimation of the degree of splenic injury in the hemodynamically normal patient.
2. **Contrast blush** (intraparenchymal hyperdense contrast collection) suggests active hemorrhage and is associated with failure of nonoperative management in all solid organ injuries.
3. CT is used for follow-up of the injuries managed nonoperatively but is generally not necessary unless clinically indicated.

E. Diagnostic peritoneal lavage (DPL)
1. DPL is a safe, efficient, rapid, and inexpensive diagnostic study but is not organ specific.
2. It is recommended in the hemodynamically unstable patient to evaluate for hemoperitoneum.
3. The test is considered positive if lavage fluid contains > 100,000 red cells/mm^3 in blunt and penetrating trauma. A positive DPL mandates operative exploration.

F. Angiography may be used in patients demonstrating a contrast blush on CT scan to identify and treat a vascular abnormality, including pseudoaneurysm or arteriovenous malformation. Selective splenic artery embolization may be used in select cases being managed nonoperatively.

G. Exploration is mandatory in patients with gunshot wounds to the abdomen.

V. INJURY GRADING SYSTEM

A. The AAST system (Table 28-1) is the most commonly cited and used splenic injury grading system.
1. Includes grading scales for both splenic hematoma and laceration. Grading scale ranges from 1 to 5. Advance one grade for multiple injuries in different areas of the spleen, up to Grade III.
2. Active bleeding constitutes a grade III or greater injury.
3. There is correlation between grade of splenic injury established from CT scan findings and frequency of necessity for operative intervention. However, this grading tends to underestimate the degree of splenic injury compared to what is found upon operation.

B. Splenic injury scoring is helpful in standardizing description of splenic injuries and may help in guiding treatment. However, **operative vs.**

TABLE 28-1
AMERICAN ASSOCIATION FOR THE SURGERY OF TRAUMA SPLENIC INJURY GRADING SYSTEM

Grade	Injury	Description
I	Hematoma	Subcapsular, <10% surface area
	Laceration	Capsular tear, <1 cm parenchymal depth
II	Hematoma	Subcapsular, 10% to 50% surface area; intraparenchymal hematoma <5 cm in diameter
	Laceration	1-3 cm parenchymal depth, does not involve a trabecular vessel
III	Hematoma	Subcapsular, >50% surface area or expanding; ruptured subcapsular hematoma; intraparenchymal hematoma >5 cm or expanding
	Laceration	>3 cm depth or involving trabecular vessels
IV	Laceration	Laceration involving segmental or hilar vessels producing major devascularization (>25% of spleen)
V	Laceration	Completely shattered spleen
	Vascular	Hilar vascular injury which devascularizes spleen

nonoperative management is ultimately determined by the clinical status of the patient.

VI. TREATMENT OPTIONS

- A. **Operative management** should be performed in those patients demonstrating peritonitis or hemodynamic instability, those failing nonoperative therapy, and those with gunshot wounds to the abdomen.
- 1. **Celiotomy begins with a midline incision** from the xiphoid to below the umbilicus, which will allow adequate exposure to the spleen and other intraabdominal organs. The spleen is retracted gently with the nondominant hand while the ligamentous attachments are incised. The assistant provides countertraction of the left abdominal wall while a plane is developed behind the spleen and tail of pancreas and in front of Gerota's fascia (Figure 28-2).
- 2. Vascular control is obtained after the spleen and tail of the pancreas are mobilized medially. The vessels may be compressed between the thumb and index finger of the nondominant hand. Ligation of the splenic vessels is usually performed in succession from a posterior approach.
- 3. **Splenectomy is indicated with significant blood loss (>1000 mL), significant associated injuries, hilar involvement, coagulopathy, or massive splenic disruption**.
- 4. Splenic salvage includes splenorrhaphy and partial splenectomy (Table 28-2).
  - a. Splenorrhaphy can be performed with absorbable mesh (Dexon) (Figures 28-3 and 28-4). Other strategies include the use of topical hemostatic agents, including Surgicel, Avitene, and topical thrombin, as well as the application of mattress sutures to allow tamponade of hemorrhage.

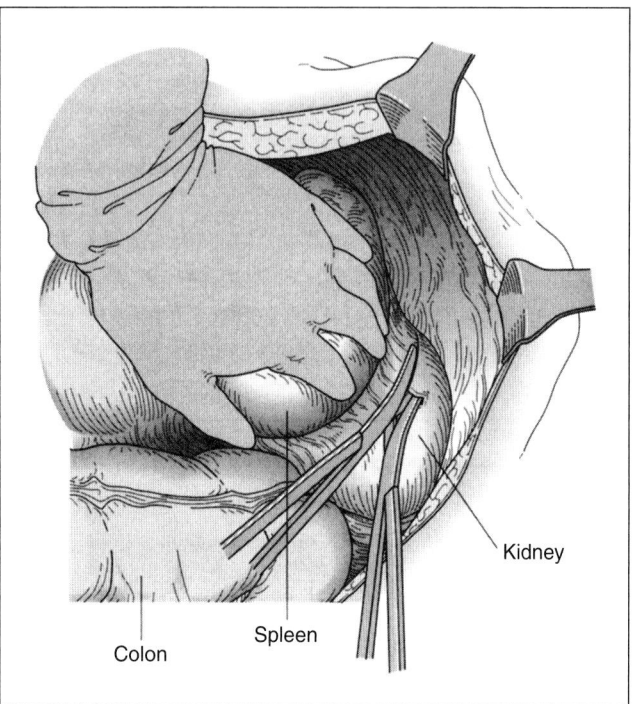

FIGURE 28-2
Mobilization of spleen by incision of ligamentous attachments. (From Moore FA, Moore EE, Abernathy CM: Injury to the spleen. In Moore EE, Mattox KL, Feliciano DV (eds): Trauma, 2nd ed. East Norwalk, CT, Appleton & Lange, 1991.)

TABLE 28-2
FACTORS CONTRIBUTING TO CHOICE OF OPERATIVE MANAGEMENT

Indications for Operative Splenic Salvage	Indications for Splenectomy
Blood loss <500 mL	Blood loss >1000 mL
Minimal associated injuries	Significant associated injuries
No hilar involvement	Hilar involvement
Minimal or moderate degree of splenic injury	Massive splenic disruption
No coagulopathy	Coagulopathy

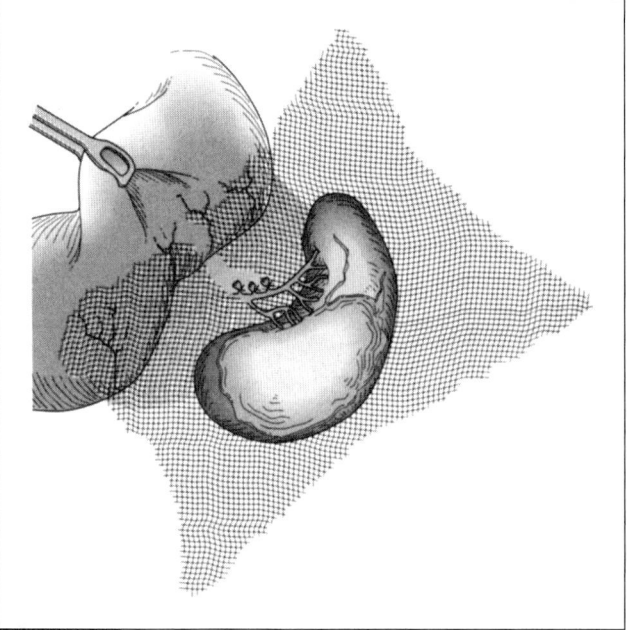

FIGURE 28-3

Mesh splenorrhaphy. With capsular loss, the spleen may be encased in a woven polyglycolic acid mesh. (From Moore FA, Mattox EE, Feliciano DV (eds): Trauma, 2nd ed. East Norwalk, CT, Appleton & Lange, 1991.)

5. Partial splenectomy may be performed for polar injuries. At least 30% of the spleen must be preserved to maintain function.

B. Nonoperative management

1. **Requires ICU monitoring in a dedicated trauma center and immediate ability to convert to operative management should that become necessary**
2. **Indications for nonoperative management:**
   a. Hemodynamic stability
   b. Minimal evidence of blood loss, <2 units packed red blood cells as transfusion requirement
   c. Absence of active contrast extravasation on CT scan

(Note: presence of blush seen on CT is associated with a low chance of success of nonoperative management.)

   d. Absence of other indication for laparotomy

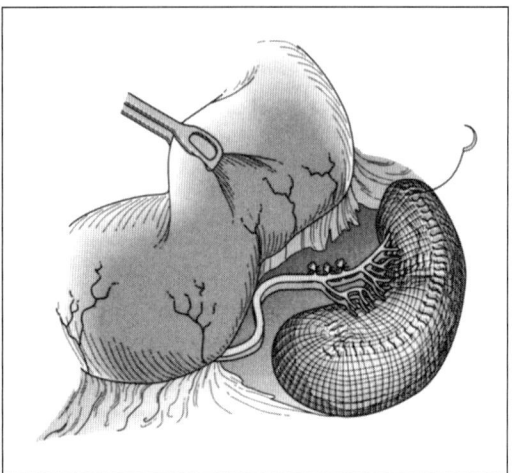

FIGURE 28-4

The mesh is sutured along the anterior surface of the spleen. (From Moore FA, Mattox EE, Feliciano DV (eds): Trauma, 2nd ed. East Norwalk, CT, Appleton & Lange, 1991.)

3. **Length of intensive care unit (ICU) monitoring is generally 24 to 48 hours initially, with serial hematocrit evaluation and continuous hemodynamic monitoring**. Patients are generally transferred to the ward if hemodynamically stable with stable hematocrit levels after this period of ICU monitoring. An operative team must be available at all times should operative intervention become necessary at any point.
4. **Blood transfusion is limited to 2 units of packed red blood cells**. If the patient has an ongoing transfusion requirement of more than 2 units, operative management should be performed.
5. Recovery recommendations include restricted activity in terms of contact sports, running, or similar stresses for 3 months following injury. Repeat CT is obtained in patients engaging in contact sports/physical activity to ensure complete healing.
6. The majority of pediatric splenic trauma is successfully managed nonoperatively.

C. Angiography is performed in patients who are hemodynamically normal and have a blush on initial CT scan. This technique will allow both diagnosis and treatment with various embolization techniques (selective arterial embolization versus proximal arterial embolization).

VII. POSTOPERATIVE COMPLICATIONS

A. Atelectasis is the most common postoperative complication and should be treated with aggressive pulmonary toilet.

B. Patients with postoperative sepsis may have associated pancreatic injury and pancreatic fistula. If there is evidence of pancreatic fistula on CT scan, a percutaneous drain is placed and immediate reoperation should generally be avoided. The presence of elevated amylase levels in the fluid confirms the diagnosis of pancreatic fistula. The routine placement of drains is not done with splenectomy or splenorrhaphy unless there is concern for pancreatic involvement.

C. Subphrenic hematoma or abscess can occur as a result of inadequate hemostasis or associated pancreatic or gastric injury.

D. Thrombocytosis may occur after splenectomy, and aspirin is given to patients whose platelet counts are equal to or greater than 1,000,000/mm^3.

VII. OVERWHELMING POSTSPLENECTOMY INFECTION (OPSI)

A. Incidence. This is a rare complication of splenectomy. Children may be at higher risk. The risk for hematologic/malignant disease after splenectomy is greater than the risk following trauma. Onset can be at any time, but 50% to 70% of OPSI occurs less than 2 years after splenectomy.

B. Syndrome consists of rapid development of severe sepsis with **hypotension, disseminated intravascular coagulation, respiratory distress, and coma** within hours of presentation. It is often preceded by a 1- or 2-day prodromal phase of fever, chills, and other nonspecific symptoms of infection. Pneumonia and meningitis are most common, but >50% of patients have no identifiable foci of infection.

C. Mortaltiy is 50% to 70% for patients presenting with full-blown OPSI, even with aggressive antibiotics and ICU care; over 50% of patients die within the first 48 hours. Morbidity for survivors is significant and includes extended hospital course, gangrene/amputation, deafness, and endocarditis.

D. Organisms. *S. pneumoniae* is responsible for 50% to 90% of infections. Others include *N. meningitides*, *H. influenzae*, and Streptococcus and Salmonella species. *Capnocytophaga canimorsus* (formerly called DF-2) can cause fulminant sepsis following dog bites

E. Treatment. Aggressive empiric antibiotic therapy should be initiated awaiting pan-culture/sensitivities. Lumbar puncture should be included, if indicated, secondary to high rate of meningitis. Start with third-generation cephalosporin +/− gentamycin, Ciprofloxacin, or Vancomycin. Continue aggressive supportive therapy and monitoring/treatment for disseminated intravascular coagulation.

F. Prophylaxis. Presplenectomy immunization (2 weeks before splenectomy) is optimal but most often impossible for traumatic splenectomy. Immunization for Pneumococcus, Meningococcus, and *H. influenzae* type B should be administered prior to discharge. Pneumococcal booster should be considered every 5 to 6 years for high-risk patients.

VIII SUGGESTED READINGS

Bisharat N, Omari H, Lavi I, Raz R: Risk of infection and death among postsplenectomy patients. J Infect 43(3):182-186, 2001.

Bridgen ML, Pattullo AL: Prevention and management of overwhelming postsplenectomy infection—an update. Crit Care Med 27:836-842, 1999.

Dent D, Alsabrook G, Erickson BA, et al: Blunt splenic injuries: High nonoperative management rate can be achieved with selective embolization. J Trauma 56:1063-1067, 2004.

Foster JN Jr, Prey D: Rupture of the spleen: An analysis of twenty cases. Am J Surg 47:487, 1940.

Haan JM, Biffl W, Knudson MM, et al: Splenic embolization revisited: A multicenter review. J Trauma 56:542-547, 2004.

King H, Shumacker HB: Splenic studies: I. Susceptibility to infection after splenectomy performed in infancy. Ann Surg 239, August 1952.

Land-Sudden J: Observation on the surgery of the spleen. Br J Surg 1:157, 1912.

Lynch AM, Kapila R: Overwhelming postsplenectomy infection. Infect Dis Clin North Am 10:693, 1996

Mattox KL, Fleiciano DV, Moore EE: Trauma, 5th ed. New York, McGraw-Hill, 2003.

Moore EE, Cogbill TH, Jurkovich GJ, et al: Organ injury scaling: Spleen and liver (1994 revision). J Trauma 38:323, 1995.

Morris DH, Bullock FD: The importance of the spleen in resistance to infection. Ann Surg 70:153, 1919.

Robinette CD, Fraumeni JF Jr: Splenectomy and subsequent mortality in veterans of the 1939-1945 war. Lancet 2(8029):127-129, 1977.

Shapiro MJ, Krausz C, Durham RM, et al: Overuse of splenic scoring and computed tomographic scans. J Trauma 47:651, 1999.

Sherman R: Perspectives in management of trauma to the spleen: 1979 presidential address, American Association for the Surgery of Trauma. J Trauma 20:1, 1980.

Townsend CM, Beauchamp RD, Evers BM, Mattox KL: Sabiston Textbook of Surgery, 18th ed. Philadelphia, Saunders, 2008.

Colon and Rectal Trauma

Josh Roller, MD

I. INTRODUCTION

A. Colon injuries occur in 15% to 39% of penetrating abdominal wounds and in 1% to 5% of blunt abdominal trauma.
B. Large bowel trauma often occurs in association with injuries to other organs.
C. Colon injuries from gunshot wounds rank second only to small bowel injuries from gunshot wounds. They rank third behind small bowel and liver injuries after abdominal stab wounds.
D. Other intra- and extra-abdominal injuries often coexist with colon injuries from blunt abdominal trauma.
1. The most commonly associated intra-abdominal injuries include:
   a. Liver (37% to 64%)
   b. Spleen (50% to 55%)
   c. Mesentery (13% to 50%)
2. The most commonly associated extra-abdominal injuries include:
   a. Skeletal (53%)
   b. Facial (33%)
   c. Neurologic (32%)
   d. Thoracic (10%)
E. Severe injuries most commonly occur in the sigmoid, right colon, and cecum from frank rupture or devitalization from vascular compromise.
F. Crush injuries are associated with pelvic fractures.
G. Delays in diagnosis may be secondary to perforation of colonic hematomas days or weeks after the initial injury. A large tear in the mesentery can also occur with subsequent bowel necrosis and perforation hours or even days after the initial injury. Patients then present with frank peritoneal signs, acidosis, and sepsis.
H. Rectal injuries represent only 3% to 5% of the total injuries to the colon but are considered to be the most serious of all intestinal injuries due to the extraperitoneal location and easy rapid spread of perirectal infection throughout the retroperitoneal pelvis and abdomen.
I. AAST—organ injury scale for colon injuries (see Table 29-1)

II. MECHANISMS OF INJURY

A. Blunt colon/rectal injury
1. **Compression forces** act by increasing the intraluminal pressure or by compressing fluid-filled bowel against immobile surfaces (e.g., vertebrae, pelvis). This results in a spectrum of injuries that range from stretching the bowel wall to full-thickness perforation.

TABLE 29-1

AAST ORGAN INJURY SCALE FOR COLON INJURIES

Grade	Type of Injury	Injury Description
I	Hematoma	Contusion or hematoma without devascularizaiton
	Laceration	Partial thickness, no perforation
II	Laceration	<50% of circumference
III	Laceration	≥50% of circumference
IV	Laceration	Transection of colon
V	Laceration	Transection of colon with segmental tissue loss

2. **Deceleration forces** cause stretching and tearing of bowel at points of fixation (ligament of Treitz, the ileocecal valve, phrenocolic ligament). Injuries range from tearing of the bowel wall or shearing of the mesentery to loss of vascular supply to the segment of bowel.
B. **Penetrating colon injuries** result from gunshot wounds, stab wounds, impalement by foreign objects, and iatrogenic causes.
C. **Penetrating rectal injuries** may result from surgical procedures (e.g., obstetric, urologic, gynecologic), perforation from proctosigmoidoscopy or barium enemas, ingestion of foreign body, blunt and penetrating trauma to the perineum, sexual assault, autoeroticism, insertion of enema nozzles and thermometers, suicide attempt by rectal administration of corrosives, and impalement by foreign objects (most often due to falls and most commonly in children).

III. EVALUATION AND DIAGNOSIS

A. **Penetrating colorectal trauma**
1. ABCs of resuscitation
2. Mark gunshot wound with radiologic marker or paper clip prior to x-ray of the chest and kidney, ureter, and bladder (KUB).
3. X-rays of the chest and KUB are used only to define missile location and determine the need for a chest tube.
4. Hemodynamically unstable patients with penetrating abdominal trauma proceed directly to the operating room for exploratory celiotomy.
5. At Parkland Memorial Hospital, all gunshot wounds to the lower chest and abdomen undergo exploratory celiotomy.
6. Stab wounds to the abdomen are *initially* evaluated by physical examination. Peritonitis, evisceration, or intra-abdominal bleeding necessitates immediate exploratory celiotomy.
7. If stable and without signs of peritonitis or evisceration, anterior abdominal stab wounds should undergo local wound exploration. Penetration of the posterior fascia or peritoneum is considered positive, and diagnostic peritoneal lavage (DPL) is then performed. If the DPL is negative, the patient is admitted for observation and serial abdominal examinations.

8. If exploration is equivocal, diagnostic laparoscopy may be pursued to identify peritoneal penetration. If peritoneal penetration is detected, exploratory celiotomy is performed.
9. Stab wounds to the flank or back can be are evaluated with a contrast (oral or intravenous) abdominal CT. Extravasation of contrast, hematoma, violation of the peritoneum, and free fluid in the abdomen are indications for exploration celiotomy. Rectal contrast is used in those cases that are highly suspicious for colon injury.
10. Ultrasound is not used in penetrating abdominal trauma at Parkland Memorial Hospital.
11. All penetrating injuries of the trunk, buttocks, perineum, and upper thighs should be assessed for possible rectal injury. A careful digital rectal examination (DRE) should be performed as frequently an injury can be palpated. Blood may indicate a colon and/or rectal injury. If present, proctoscopy is performed to exclude a rectal injury.
12. All gunshot and stab wound victims who are hemodynamically stable and have injuries in proximity to the rectum undergo proctoscopy to 25 cm prior to surgery.
13. Diagnosis of extraperitoneal rectal injuries by proctoscopy is helpful in making intraoperative decisions (diverting colostomy and retrorectal drains if injury is seen below the peritoneal reflection). A vaginal examination in females should be performed to rule out concomitant injuries to the urogenital system.

B. Blunt colorectal trauma

1. ABCs of resuscitation
2. If physical examination reveals intra-abdominal bleeding and/or peritoneal irritation, exploratory celiotomy is performed. Clinical signs of bowel injury (peritonitis) are present in as few as 30% of patients, and thus a high index of suspicion must be maintained to diagnose blunt colon/rectal injuries. The presence of a seatbelt sign should raise the suspicion for enteric and mesenteric injuries.
3. DRE and stool guaiac tests should be performed on all blunt trauma patients. DREs and stool guaiac tests may be positive in 65% to 75% and 70% to 90%, respectively, of patients with colorectal injuries.
4. FAST is performed on all hemodynamically unstable patients with a blunt injury mechanism. A positive ultrasound in the setting of hemodynamic instability warrants exploratory celiotomy.
5. If a patient is hemodynamically unstable with a negative focused abdominal sonography for trauma (FAST) examination, DPL is performed.
6. Plain abdominal radiographs are rarely of value in defining intra-abdominal injury, but air under the diaphragm seen on a chest film warrants celiotomy.
7. FAST or abdominal CT is used to further evaluate hemodynamically stable patients without clinical evidence of intra-abdominal hemorrhage or peritonitis.

8. The sensitivity of abdominal CT scan in defining bowel injuries is poor (50% to 70%). False-negative rates are as high as 15%.
a. CT findings include: bowel wall disruption and oral contrast extravasation, intraperitoneal/retroperitoneal air, intraperitoneal/retroperitoneal fluid, focal areas of bowel wall thickening, abnormal bowel wall enhancement, diffuse bowel wall thickening/enhancement, and mesenteric infiltration/streaking/hematoma.
9. A high index of suspicion for colorectal injury should be present when patients have pelvic fractures, rectal foreign bodies, and crush injuries.
10. The diagnosis of most blunt colorectal injuries is made intraoperatively. There is a 10% to 15% incidence of blunt colon injury among patients undergoing celiotomy after blunt trauma.
11. Serosal tears of the colon occur frequently but are rarely of clinical significance.

IV. NONOPERATIVE MANAGEMENT

A. Iatrogenic or accidental partial-thickness injuries to prepped colon or rectum by endoscopy, enema tips, or thermometers can be cautiously observed.

B. Treatment by NPO, antibiotics, and careful observation with serial abdominal examinations is usually sufficient, but monitoring for signs and symptoms of sepsis for 2 to 3 days is important.

C. If a perforation is caused by biopsy or fulgauration, the lesion is treated surgically as a stab wound and primarily repaired.

V. OPERATIVE MANAGEMENT: COLON INJURIES

A. Initial management
1. **Preoperative**
   a. Fluid resuscitation and stabilization
   b. Administration of intravenous antibiotics to cover aerobic and anaerobic organisms with broad coverage of gram-negative species. Typically, use of a second-generation cephalosporin or beta-lactam penicillin is sufficient.
   c. Attempt to identify any foreign bodies in vivo radiographically.
2. **Intraoperative priorities**
   a. Control of massive hemorrhage
   b. Control spill from any hollow viscus perforations. Fecal spill can be controlled by noncrushing bowel clamps or quick suturing of any perforations.
   c. Systematic inspection of the colon should be performed, usually in a proximal to distal fashion. Retroperitoneal injuries of the large bowel are easily missed unless the colon is fully mobilized.

d. Careful inspection of subserosal, pericolic, and mesenteric hematomas is essential. Division of a few mesenteric vessels at the colonic-mesenteric junction is sometimes necessary for complete evaluation.

B. Specific operative management

1. Colon injuries are classified as destructive or nondestructive and assessed according to the colon injury scale (see Table 29-1). A nondestructive colon injury is one that is amenable to primary suture repair with limited amounts of debridement (CIS I to III). Destructive wounds consist of those injuries that require segmental resection (CIS IV and V).
2. All areas of the colon are amenable to primary repair.
3. Management options include primary repair, primary resection and anastomosis, and repair or resection with formation of a colostomy.
4. Risk factors for increased morbidity and mortality after colon injury include persistent hypotension, delay in treatment of more than 12 hours, major fecal contamination (gross spillage in more than one quadrant of the abdomen, penetrating abdominal trauma index (PATI) and ISS > 25), and blood transfusion of more than 6 units.
5. **Nondestructive colon injury**. Primary repair is safely performed in most patients with a CIS of I to III.
   a. Simple closure is done after adequate debridement of devitalized tissue to ensure a good blood supply to the tension-free repair.
   b. One- or two-layer closure techniques may be used. Absorbable sutures are used for the inner layer (simple, running, or running lock style) and permanent Lembert sutures (silk) are used for the outer layer.
6. **Destructive colon injury**. Although there is widespread debate and no clear consensus, traditionally patients with destructive colon injuries can undergo resection and anastomosis safely if they are:
   a. Hemodynamically normal
   b. Requiring less than 6 units of blood
   c. Have no significant underlying disease (AIDS, cirrhosis, malignancy)
   d. Have only mild to moderate fecal contamination (confined to only one quadrant)
   e. Seen in less than 12 hours following injury and operation
7. **Colostomy**. Although trends are changing, traditionally colostomies have been reserved for patients with evidence of shock, major fecal contamination, transfusion of more than 6 units of blood, operative intervention more than 12 hours following injury, significant underlying comorbidities or associated injuries
   a. The mobile sigmoid or right transverse colon is used to construct the colostomy.
   b. The colostomy can be constructed at the site of the injured bowel. It can also be made proximal to the injury for fecal diversion to protect a distal primary repair.
   c. The right ascending colon and cecum are *not* used to construct colostomies because they are difficult to mobilize, the wall of the colon is thin, the lumen is large and difficult to fashion as a

colostomy, and the liquid stool is not substantially different from that found in the distal small bowel.
  d. Loop colostomies are easily constructed. Stapling of the distal segment prevents fecal spill into the distal limb.
  e. Hartmann's procedure is frequently used (end colostomy with sewn or stapled closure of the distal bowel provides complete fecal diversion).
  f. Double-barrel colostomies may be used when complete fecal diversion is required. (Note: the two ends should be drained in separate bags.)
8. Drains are not routinely used in the management of these injuries.

VI. MANAGEMENT: RECTAL INJURIES

1. Primary repair of rectal injuries depends on the anatomic location of the injury.
   a. Injuries to the areas of the rectum covered by peritoneum (anterior and lateral sidewalls of the upper two-thirds of rectum) can be treated as colon injuries.
   b. Extraperitoneal (circumferential distal one-third and upper two-thirds posteriorly) rectal injuries require diversion and drainage.
      i. Sigmoid colostomy, preferably a loop colostomy with a stapled distal end, is necessary for diversion of the fecal stream.
      ii. Pre-sacral drains are placed. A transverse incision is made midway between the coccyx and anus. Dissection is carried down to the anococcygeal ligament, which is incised. Blunt dissection is then used to open the retrorectal space to allow placement of drains. Drains are sutured into place. Drains are removed if no significant leak has occurred within 5 days postoperatively. Closed-suction or large Penrose drains may be used.
      iii. Repair of the injury is not necessary. It should only be attempted if visualized and performed easily without extensive dissection. Some low rectal injuries can be repaired transanally.

VII. RECTAL FOREIGN BODIES

A. Foreign bodies in the rectum are removed manually or by endoscopic maneuvers if the patient is stable and without abdominal tenderness.
B. Celiotomy is reserved for patients with peritoneal signs and for those patients with foreign bodies that cannot be removed from the rectum.
C. Colotomy with primary repair is usually the preferred operative approach, but colostomy may be necessary if any of the aforementioned risk factors are present.
D. Transrectal removal of foreign bodies may be facilitated by using a Foley balloon, obstetric forceps, or vacuum tractor.

VII. POSTOPERATIVE CARE

A. Wounds are left open with almost all colon injuries having significant spill and left to heal by secondary intention, or they are treated by delayed primary closure at the bedside on the fourth or fifth postoperative day if the wound is clean.

B. Antibiotic administration is continued for 24 hours.

C. Oral feedings are begun as soon as bowel function returns to normal. This is defined clinically as the return of normoactive bowel sounds, flatus, and/or bowel movements.

D. Colostomy closure is timed according to the patient's condition, but not before 8 to 12 weeks postoperative. If the colostomy was done to protect a colon repair, barium enema examination of the distal segment should be performed to ensure there is no leak or stricture at the site of the repair. All patients undergo bowel preparation prior to colostomy closure and are given systemic perioperative antibiotics.

E. In carefully selected cases when an injury has been exteriorized as a colostomy, early colostomy closure has been done successfully in patients recovering satisfactorily with healing wounds and without evidence of sepsis.

VIII. COMPLICATIONS OF COLORECTAL INJURIES

A. Sepsis accounts for the majority of the morbidity in these injuries. An Inovay Severity Score (ISS) or Penetrating Abdominal Trauma Index (PATI) greater than 25 is associated with an increased incidence of sepsis.

B. Intra-abdominal abscess occurs in 5% to 20% of patients. CT- or ultrasound-guided percutaneous drainage is the preferred method of treatment.

C. Wound infection

D. Colocutaneous fistula occurs in 1% to 4% of patients. Most will close with conservative therapy and local wound care.

E. Colorectal injuries associated with multiple organ injuries have an increased mortality rate.

F. Anastomotic leak occurs in 1% to 7% of patients, typically 7 to 9 days postoperatively. It presents as subfascial wound infection and fecal fistula. Percutaneous drainage may be used to control the leak and form a controlled fistula.

G. Colostomy-related complications include stomal prolapse, small bowel obstruction, stomal necrosis, and peristomal abscess.

IX. SUGGESTED READINGS

Demetriades D, Murray JA, Chan L, et al: Penetrating colon injuries requiring resection: Diversion or primary anastomosis? An AAST prospective multicenter study. J Trauma 50:765-775, 2001.

Eastern Association for the Surgery of Trauma (EAST): EAST Practice Parameter Workgroup for Penetrating Colon Injury Management. Practice Management Guidelines for Penetrating Intraperitoneal Colon Injuries. EAST trauma practice guidelines, 1998. Available at: http/www.east.org/tpg.html

Maxwell RA, Fabian TC: Current management of colon trauma. World J Surg 27:632-639, 2003.

Moore EE, et al: Injuries to the colon and rectum. In Trauma, 5th ed. East Norwalk, CT, Appleton & Langer, 2004, pp 735-753.

Nelson R, Singer M: Primary repair for penetrating colon injuries (Cochrane Review). In The Cochrane Library, Issue 3, 2002.

Williams MD, et al: Colon injury after blunt abdominal trauma: Results of the EAST Multi-institutional Hollow Viscus Injury Study. J Trauma 55:906-912, 2003.

Renal Trauma

Lance Walsh, MD, PhD

I. EPIDEMIOLOGY

A. Of patients with abdominal trauma, 10% have injury to the urinary tract. Renal injury occurs in 1% to 5% of all traumas.
B. Blunt trauma accounts for 90% of renal injuries, while penetrating trauma accounts for 10%.
C. Renal injuries due to blunt trauma are associated with other intra-abdominal injuries in 44% of cases (most commonly the spleen, liver, chest, colon, and small bowel). Renal injuries due to stab wounds and gunshot wounds are associated with other intra-abdominal injuries in 30% to 70% and 77% to 100% of cases, respectively.

II. ANATOMY

A. The kidney lies in the retroperitoneum surrounded by perirenal fat, Gerota's fascia, and the major muscle groups: posteriorly, by the psoas and quadratus lumborum; laterally, by the latissimus dorsi and serratus posterior; and superiorly, by the diaphragm.
B. The right kidney lies posterior to the liver, with the colon lying anterior and the duodenum anteromedially.
C. The left kidney lies lateral to the stomach, inferior to the spleen and posterolateral to the jejunum and pancreas. The colon crosses anterior to both kidneys.
D. The tail of the pancreas often lies in the hilar area of the kidney.
E. The following are the five compartments of the retroperitoneum in the area of the kidney:
1. Anterior perirenal space between the posterior peritoneum and Gerota's fascia
2. Posterior perirenal space between Gerota's fascia and transversalis fascia posteriorly
3. Central space, which contains the aorta, vena cava, and their branches
4. Perinephric space
5. Subcapsular space

III. MECHANISM OF INJURY

A. Penetrating trauma
1. Stab wounds and gunshot wounds tend to be less predictable and more severe than blunt trauma.
2. Stab wounds to the anterior abdomen are more likely to injure vital renal structures such as the pelvis, hilum, and pedicle. Flank wounds posterior to the anterior axillary line are more likely to injure peripheral and nonvital renal structures such as parenchyma.

3. Gunshot wounds may cause extensive tissue disruption due to blast effect.

B. Blunt trauma
1. Motor vehicle collisions, falls, and direct blows to the flank lead to renal injuries as the kidney is thrust against the rib cage or vertebral column. Fractured ribs and transverse processes of the lumbar spine can also lacerate the kidney.

C. Sudden deceleration injuries (e.g., a fall or high-speed motor vehicle collision). The kidney is fixed to the body in two places, the pedicle and the ureter. Sudden deceleration may:
1. Stretch the renal artery and produce an intimal tear, producing turbulence, thrombosis, and occlusion with complete or segmental renal ischemia
2. Avulse the ureteropelvic junction (UPJ)

IV. CLASSIFICATION

A. The Committee on Organ Injury Scaling of the American Association for the Surgery of Trauma has classified renal injuries as grade 1 through 5 as shown in Table 30-1.

V. INITIAL EVALUATION

The goal is prompt recognition and appropriate radiographic evaluation of all upper urinary tract injuries. Major blunt renal injury usually occurs with other major injuries of the head, chest, and abdomen.

A. History
1. Mechanism of injury—blunt, penetrating, or deceleration
2. Type of weapon used

TABLE 30-1
AMERICAN ASSOCIATION FOR THE SURGERY OF TRAUMA CLASSIFICATION OF RENAL INJURIES

Grade	Type	Description
I	Contusion	Microscopic or gross hematuria; urologic studies normal
	Hematoma	Subcapsular, nonexpanding, without parenchymal laceration
II	Hematoma	Nonexpanding perirenal hematoma confined to renal retroperitoneum
	Laceration	<1.0 cm parenchymal depth of renal cortex without urinary extravasation
III	Laceration	>1.0 cm parenchymal depth of renal cortex without collecting system rupture or urinary extravasation
IV	Laceration	Parenchymal laceration extending through renal cortex, medulla, and collecting system
	Vascular	Main renal aretery or vein injury with contained hemorrhage
V	Laceration	Completely shattered kidney
V	Vascular	Avulsion of renal hilum that devascularizes kidney

3. History of hypotension in the field

B. Physical examination
1. Flank pain or ecchymosis
2. Lower rib or vertebral body fractures
3. Upper abdominal mass or tenderness
4. Crepitance over lower rib cage or lumbar area
5. Site of gunshot wound entrance or stab wound penetration
6. Abdominal distension or ileus (may be associated with retroperitoneal urinary extravasation)

C. Laboratory studies
1. **Urinalysis**
   a. Gross hematuria or microscopic hematuria (defined as >5 red blood cells per high-power field) associated with hypotension (systolic blood pressure <90 mm Hg) indicates the need for genitourinary tract imaging.
   b. The degree of hematuria does not correlate with the severity of renal injury.
2. Hematocrit is helpful in selective operative versus nonoperative management of renal trauma.
3. Creatinine, if elevated, may suggest preexisting renal disease, which may change the **approach to radiographic evaluation and operative approach.**

D. Radiologic evaluation of renal injury (please refer to uroradiology in Chapter 31). Indications for genitourinary imaging are as follows:
1. Penetrating injury associated with any degree of hematuria or if the wound tract indicates possible genitourinary involvement
2. Blunt trauma associated with:
   a. Gross hematuria
   b. Microscopic hematuria and associated hypotension or history of hypotension (blood pressure <90 systolic)
   c. Injuries in proximity to urogenital structures (lower spine, rib, and transverse process fractures, pelvic fractures)
3. Significant deceleration injury (e.g., fall from height)
4. All pediatric patients with any degree of hematuria

VI. MANAGEMENT

A. Minor renal injuries (grades 1 and 2) account for 70% of all injuries and they do not require intervention.

B. Major renal injuries (grades 3 and 4) account for 10% to 15% of all injuries. Their management depends on the clinical status of the patient and other associated injuries. Renal exploration usually results in renal reconstruction and less likely nephrectomy.
1. Patients who are hemodynamically stable with grade 3 or 4 renal injury may be managed conservatively if celiotomy is not indicated for treatment of associated injuries.
2. When celiotomy is indicated for treatment of associated injuries, renal exploration and reconstruction are recommended. This reduces

the rate of urologic complications but may increase the nephrectomy rate.
3. Grade 4 injuries involving the main renal artery require exploration.
4. At Parkland Memorial Hospital, all penetrating injuries to the kidney are explored.
5. Nonoperative management of stab wounds is more acceptable if the injury can be accurately staged.

C. Grade 5 injuries account for 10% to 15% of all injuries.
1. Grade 5 injuries involving the renal pedicle almost always require immediate surgery to control life-threatening bleeding and typically result in nephrectomy.
2. Renal artery thrombosis 6 hours after injury warrants a conservative approach as renal salvage is unlikely after ischemia of this duration (unless it involves a solitary kidney, bilateral kidneys, or a pediatric patient).
3. Conservative management of multiple parenchymal fractures may be done in select patients who are hemodynamically stable at presentation and do not have a renal pedicle injury.
4. Urologic complications in cases managed nonoperatively may often be approached by minimally invasive endourological techniques such as retrograde stenting for persistent urinoma.

D. Absolute indications for renal exploration
1. Persistent, life-threatening bleeding; expanding, pulsatile, or uncontained retroperitoneal hematoma
2. Renal pedicle avulsion

E. Relative indications for renal exploration
1. Persistent renal bleeding defined as requiring transfusion >3 units of packed red blood cells/24 hours
2. Extracapsular urinary extravasation
3. Nonviable renal tissue
4. Incomplete staging

F. Specific scenarios
1. **Extravasation**
   a. Urinary extravasation indicates at least a grade 4 injury from parenchymal laceration into the collecting system, laceration of the renal pelvis, or avulsion of the ureteropelvic junction.
   b. Most cases of urinary extravasation can be managed expectantly; extensive extravasation may be monitored by serial CT.
   c. Intervention is required if persistent leak, urinoma formation, or sepsis develops.
   d. Persistent urinary extravasation from a viable kidney responds to stent placement or percutaneous drainage.
   e. Immediate exploration is required for ureteropelvic junction avulsion.
   f. If associated with a deep laceration with concomitant bleeding, the bleeding can be managed with angiography with selective embolization; if this fails, the injury should be surgically repaired.

2. **Nonviable tissue**
   a. Expectant management of significant devitalized parenchyma can lead to short-term complications such as abscess formation, delayed hemorrhage, and long-term morbidity (e.g., hypertension).
   b. Grade 3 and 4 injuries with devitalized fragments and concomitant intraperitoneal organ injury should undergo immediate surgical repair. There is a twofold increased incidence of urologic complications when devitalized fragments occur along with other intra-abdominal injuries.
   c. Early renal exploration may be beneficial in patients with large, nonviable fragments and urinary extravasation or retroperitoneal hemorrhage even without intraperitoneal injury.
3. **Incomplete staging**
   a. When a renal injury has not been accurately staged preoperatively, an intraoperative one-shot intravenous pyelogram should be performed. Any abnormality noted may need exploration.
4. **Vascular injury**
   a. Renovascular injuries require immediate operative repair. Exceptions include main renal arterial thombosis with delayed diagnosis, segmental arterial thrombosis, and segmental arterial laceration.
   b. Surgical repair of main renal artery injuries should be performed within 6 hours.
   c. Preservation of significant renal function has been achieved in only 15% to 30% of revascularizations despite early diagnosis and repair of renal artery thrombosis. If found late, nephrectomy is usually necessary but removal is not emergent as atrophy and hypertension will usually follow. When diagnosis of main renal artery thrombosis is delayed, nephrectomy should be performed at the time of exploratory celiotomy for associated injuries.
   d. Cases of isolated renal artery thrombosis without the need for exploration can safely be observed.
   e. Angiography and selective embolization help to control bleeding from segmental arteries. Surgical exploration is indicated only if selective embolization of the segmental artery fails.
G. Nonoperative approach consists of supportive care with bed rest, serial hematocrit assessment, volume repletion, antibiotics, and careful monitoring and imaging follow-up using repeated CT scans.
H. Operative approach to the kidney
1. Midline transabominal incision
2. Major visceral and vascular injuries should be repaired first unless renal hemorrhage is massive and life threatening.
3. Early isolation of the renal vessels
4. Incision of the retroperitoneum over the aorta medial to the inferior mesenteric vein
5. Superior dissection will reveal the left renal vein crossing the aorta anteriorly (12% of patients will have a retroaortic left renal vien).

Both renal arteries should be easily seen at this time. All vessels are encircled with vessel loops.

6. The kidney is now approached by incising the retroperitoneum lateral to the colon.
7. For massive bleeding, the ipsilateral renal artery may be occluded, but warm ischemia time should be limited to less than 30 minutes.

I. Operative techniques

1. Simple lacerations may be closed after sharp debridement with 2-0 to 4-0 chromic suture and drained with posterolaterally placed closed-suction drains.
2. Defects in the collecting system should be closed in a watertight fashion with 4-0 chromic suture and drained as above. Indigo carmine injection into the pelvis with the ureter occluded helps define collecting system defects.
3. When possible, preserve the renal capsule to close over with interrupted sutures. Large capsular defects may be covered with omentum or free grafts of peritoneum and drained.
4. Wounds may be closed over a bolster of Surgicel and Gelfoam placed in the depths of the laceration.
5. Nephrectomy may be necessary if bleeding persists or if the patient becomes unstable secondary to continuing blood loss.
6. Heminephrectomy may be used if polar lacerations have produced greater areas of devitalized parenchyma.
7. In case of renal vascular injury with occlusion, the artery may be reconstructed via end-to-end anastomosis, autotransplantation, or graft. This must be performed within 6 hours.
8. **"Damage control"**—as an alternative to nephrectomy, if the patient is hypothermic, acidotic, or coagulopathic, initial packing of renal fossa is followed by definitive repair after correction of the metabolic derangements.

VII. POSTOPERATIVE CARE

A. Early complications (within 30 days) may include bleeding, infection and perinephric abscess, sepsis, urinary fistula, hypertension, urinary extravasation, and urinoma.

1. Patients should be rescanned if they develop fever, increasing flank pain, or persistent bleeding.
2. Closed-suction drains can be removed when drainage becomes scant. Be aware of the possiblity of delayed urine leak.
3. Follow hematocrits and creatinine in the postoperative period.
4. Follow-up CT is strongly suggested 3 to 4 weeks following discharge.
5. Monitor for bleeding episodes in the month after surgery. Observe for persistent hematuria. Clot formation suggests a large amount of bleeding from the upper urinary tract. Arteriogram is strongly indicated

in these patients. Possible causes are arteriovenous malformations and missed arterial bleeding at the time of celiotomy.

6. Monitor renovascular hypertension intensively for at least a year and then indefinitely. Postoperative hypertension must always be investigated. Renal artery stenosis may accompany vascular repair at the time of the injury. Also, one should consider renal compression due to hematoma. This type of hypertension may necessitate nephrectomy if refractory to medical management.

B. Delayed complications include bleeding, hydronephrosis, calculus formation, chronic pyelonephritis, hypertension, arteriovenous fistula, hydronephrosis, and pseudoaneurysm.

VIII. SUGGESTED READINGS

Knudson MM, Harrison PB, Hoyt DB, et al: Outcome after major renovascular injuries: A Western Trauma Association multicenter report. J Trauma 49(6):1116–1122, 2000.

Santucci RA, Fisher MB: The literature increasingly supports expectant (conservative) management of renal trauma—a systematic review. J Trauma 59(2):493–503, 2005.

Shariat SF, Roehrborn CG, Karakiewicz PI, et al: Evidence-based validation of the predictive value of the American Association for the Surgery of Trauma kidney injury scale. J Trauma 62(4):933–939, 2007.

Shariat SF, Trinh QD, Morey AF, et al: Development of a highly accurate nomogram for prediction of the need for exploration in patients with renal trauma. J Trauma 64(6):1451–1458, 2008.

Radiologic Evaluation of the Genitourinary Tract in Trauma

Lance Walsh, MD, PhD

I. INDICATIONS FOR GENITOURINARY IMAGING

A. Penetrating injuries to the torso, abdomen, or genitalia associated with any degree of hematuria or if the wound track indicates possible genitourinary involvement
B. Blunt trauma associated with:
1. Gross hematuria
2. Microscopic hematuria and associated hypotension or a history of hypotension (systolic blood pressure <90)
3. Injuries in proximity to urogenital structures (lower spine, rib, and transverse process fractures, pelvic fractures)
C. Significant deceleration injury (e.g., fall from height)
D. All pediatric patients with any degree of hematuria
E. Special considerations
1. Degree of hematuria does not correlate with the extent of injury. Ninety-five percent of significant renal injuries are associated with hematuria, but hematuria may be absent with renal vascular injury, ureteropelvic junction (UPJ) avulsion, and ureteral injury.

II. DIAGNOSTIC STUDIES

A. Kidney, ureter, bladder (KUB) radiography
1. Significant findings that may indicate urogenital injury include rib fractures, pelvic fractures, foreign bodies, loss of psoas shadow, and vertebral fractures.
B. CT scan of the abdomen and pelvis
1. The ability to stage abdominal injuries has led to greater nonoperative management.
2. CT provides greater sensitivity and specificity than intravenous pyelography (IVP) in the detection and characterization of renal injuries.
3. It is more sensitive in detecting extravasation from the renal pelvis and ureter.
4. CT cystogram can be performed at same time if indicated to determine intra- or extraperitoneal bladder rupture. Clamping the Foley catheter is not an acceptable alternative.
5. Observe for:
    a. Renal laceration (low attenuation area)
    b. Subcapsular hematoma (hypoattenuating area deforms kidney contour) versus perirenal hematoma (does not deform kidney)
    c. Segmental infarct (sharply demarcated, wedge-shaped areas of decreased contrast enhancement)

d. Active arterial extravasation (areas of high attenuating contrast within lower attenuation hematoma)
e. Extravasation of urine (contrast extravasation on delayed images)
f. Thrombosis of renal artery (absence of perinephric hematoma, abrupt termination of renal artery just beyond its origin, or global renal infarction with or without cortical rim sign)
g. Renal artery avulsion (extensive perirenal hematoma associated with kidney infarction)
h. Renal vein thrombosis (intraluminal thrombus in distended renal vein and renal changes secondary to acute venous hypertension)
i. Ureteropelvic junction (UPJ) transection (medial perinephric urine extravasation with circumferential urinoma)

C. Urologic trauma series—trauma resuscitation/area emergency department

1. Perform the following studies:
   a. CT scan of the abdomen and pelvis with nonionic IV contrast (2 mL/kg)
   b. CT cystogram: 300 mL of dilute contrast (Cystocon) by Foley catheter and then clamping the catheter
   c. Drainage CT: Unclamp the Foley catheter and then perform another CT scan of the pelvis with the bladder drained.
   d. CT scan of the abdomen and pelvis with delayed cuts through the ureters

D. Urologic trauma series—intraoperative

1. **Perform the following studies:**
   a. Scout KUB
   b. Static cystogram
   c. "One shot" IVP performed 10 minutes after injection of 1 mL/kg IV nonionic contrast medium
2. It is recommended that a cystogram be done during the 10-minute period while waiting to shoot the IVP.
3. The primary role of IVP is to show a functioning kidney on the uninjured side and to exclude the need for renal exploration if findings are completely normal.
4. **General considerations**
   a. Hypotensive or azotemic patients will have inferior quality pyelograms.
   b. Look for prompt bilateral renal function, extravasation from the bladder (extraperitoneal, confined to the pelvis; or intraperitoneal, diffuse extravasation into peritoneum), renal or ureteral extravasation, devitalized (nonexcreting) segments of kidney, and abnormal ureteral deviations.
   c. Causes of nonvisualization of the kidney on IVP include renal absence, which may be congenital or surgical; renal ectopia; shock; renovascular spasm due to severe contusion; renal artery thrombosis; avulsion of the renal pedicle; and high-grade obstruction.

E. Ultrasound

1. Has limited use in the management of upper tract urogenital trauma

2. In blunt scrotal trauma, ultrasound can be used to distinguish testis rupture from hematocele, hydrocele, torsion, or epididymitis.

F. Selective arteriography and venography
1. Has largely been replaced by the CT scanning
2. Indicated if one is suspicious of a renovascular injury
3. Arteriography can provide more detailed information regarding anatomic area of vascular injury.
4. Arteriography with transcatheter embolization is becoming the standard of care in the treatment of patients with renal injury associated with hemorrhage and in the evaluation of vascular complications of injury (e.g., areteriovenous fistula and pseudoaneurysm).
5. Venography is performed to evaluate the renal vein or for inferior vena cava injury.

G. Retrograde pyelogram
1. Useful when ureteral, UPJ, or pelvic injury is suspected but delayed images not obtained or inadequate to exclude injury on CT or IVP

H. MRI with gadolinium
1. Used to assess renal injury in stable patient with strong contraindication to iodinated contrast

I. Renal scan
1. Used to document presence of functional kidney in patients with contraindication to iodinated contrast

J. Retrograde urethrogram
1. **Indications**
   a. History of straddle injury
   b. History of major deceleration
   c. Blood at the meatus in an injured patient
   d. High-riding prostate on rectal examination
   e. Perineal butterfly hematoma
   f. Scrotal OK or perineal crepitus suggestive of urine extravasation
   g. Inability to pass Foley catheter
2. **Technique**
   a. Position the patient obliquely at a 30- to 45-degree angle, to adequately visualize the length of the entire urethra. Hold penis on stretch and take x-ray while instilling contrast.
   b. If patient has a large urethral meatus, instill, in a retrograde fashion, 30 mL of Conray contrast into the meatus using a 60-mL catheter tip syringe.
   c. In children or patients with a small urethral meatus, insert a Foley catheter into the meatus and inflate the Foley balloon with 1 or 2 mL of water to decrease back-leak. Instill 30 to 60 mL of contrast through the Foley catheter and shoot the film.
3. **Significant positive findings**
   a. Disruption of the prostatomembranous urethra as evidenced by extravasation of contrast into the perineum

b. Extravasation of contrast from other parts of the urethra secondary to injury

III. SUGGESTED READING

Micallef M, Ahmad I, Ramesh N, et al: Ultrasound features of blunt testicular injury. Injury 32:23-26, 2001.

Genital and Perineal Trauma

Meredith Miller, MD

I. PENILE TRAUMA

A. Penile fracture (Traumatic rupture of the corpus cavernosum)
1. Rare injury, accounting for 1 in 175,000 hospital admissions
2. Almost exclusively occurs in an erect penis, usually during coitus but occasionally with other blunt trauma
3. There is usually a history of vigorous intercourse with bending of the penis accompanied by a popping sound and immediate pain, swelling, and rapid loss of erection. Often there is a delay in presentation due to patient embarrassment.
   a. Involves disruption of the tunica albuginea of the corpus cavernosa; usually only one corpus is affected but more severe trauma may injure both. Tear in tunica albuginea is usually transversely oriented and fairly proximal. Significant bleeding fills all fascial compartments between the skin and the tunica albuginea.
   b. Concomitant urethral injury is present in 20% to 38% of cases. Patients with urethral injury usually present with blood at the urethral meatus, inability to void, and/or some degree of hematuria. **These signs are absolute indications for a retrograde urethrogram**. However, absence of these signs does not exclude the possibility of urethral injury.
4. Physical examination includes deviation of the penis away from the injured side and marked swelling and ecchymosis (called "eggplant sign"). If Buck's fascia is damaged, blood and urine extravasate around Colle's fascia, producing "butterfly ecchymosis" in the perineum and a "sleeve hematoma" along the penis.
5. Diagnosis is clinical and usually obvious. Sonography and cavernosography may be helpful but are less sensitive and rarely needed. Retrograde urethrogram (RUG) should be done to evaluate the urethra.
6. Treatment is immediate surgical exploration with evacuation of the hematoma, debridement, and repair of the injury to the tunica albuginea via distal circumferential incision, with degloving of penile skin proximal to the area of injury. A Foley catheter should be placed at the beginning of the operation to guide the exploration, to help identify existing urethral injuries, and to prevent intraoperative injuries from occurring. As urethral injury is usually minor, primary repair over the catheter should be attempted.
7. Postoperatively, the patient is given benzodiazepam to minimize erectile activity while the tissues are healing.
8. Long-term prognosis is usually good with immediate intervention. Nonoperative management or delayed exploration (> 72 hours after injury) carries a 10% risk of penile deformity, curvature, and/or erectile dysfunction.

B. Penile amputation

1. This is a rare injury, usually due to self-emasculation in a psychotic patient or in an assault. Very rarely it may occur with neonatal circumcision.
2. The severed penile segment should be immediately wrapped in saline-soaked gauze, placed in a sterile plastic bag, and cooled in ice slush.
3. Control bleeding with compression, *not* tourniquet as this may compromise the viability of remaining penile tissue.
4. Reconstruction should be attempted early, preferably within 6 hours of injury, but up to 16- to 24-hour delays have also had successful results.
   a. Macroscopic anastomosis of corporal bodies and urethra followed by microscopic reconstruction of dorsal nerves and vessels is recommended whenever possible. However, some report success with macroscopic reapproximation alone, but this should be done only when microvascular repair is not available.
   b. Urethral and suprapubic catheters should be maintained until fully healed.
   c. Distal amputation should be debrided and the corpora closed. The urethra can be spatulated and imbricated to a button-holed dorsal skin flap to achieve a highly functional phallus.
5. If reanastamoses is not successful, the remaining penile stump may be elongated using several techniques or a new phallus may be constructed using various grafts augmented with a penile prosthesis
6. Psychotic patients often repeat attempts at penile amputation even after successful reattachments. Self-amputation mandates an inpatient psychiatric consult.

C. Degloving of penile or scrotal skin

1. Avulsion of penile skin may be complete or partial and frequently is accompanied by scrotal avulsion (see Scrotal Avulsion, below)
2. Mechanism of injury usually involves farm or industrial equipment in which the patient's clothes become caught or the injury may be secondary to motorcycle deceleration trauma when the rider is thrown over the handlebars.
3. Reconstruction should be delayed 12 to 24 hours and local care with moist soaks applied to the penis before debridement. A thick split-thickness skin graft is later used for coverage. Partial avulsions with remaining distal penile skin should be converted to complete avulsions by debridement to prevent distal penile edema
4. Long-term prognosis is good.

D. Penile strangulation

1. Usually due to constricting bands or metal rings
2. Strangulating material should be removed immediately and may require operative anesthesia and metal-cutting equipment.
3. Even though the distal penis may appear initially nonviable, satisfactory outcomes are usually obtained with conservative therapy.

E. Penetrating penile trauma

1. Usually gunshot wounds or stab wounds

2. Requires retrograde urethrogram especially in injuries with proximity to urethra and/or meatal blood
3. Exploration required, with corporal and urethral repair as needed

F. Human bite, zipper injury, or preputial frenula tear
1. Respond well to local care. Often wounds must heal by secondary intention due to infections from oral flora.
2. Antibiotic prophylaxis is necessary due to a high incidence of post-traumatic cellulitis.
3. Frenulum injury is usually related to coitus and must be differentiated from meatal bleeding in uncircumcised patients. The foreskin must be retracted to differentiate as these patients are almost always uncircumcised.

II. SCROTAL AND TESTICULAR TRAUMA

A. Blunt trauma
1. 85% of testicular injuries are the result of blunt trauma.
2. Despite patient's history of trauma and complaint of pain, one must rule out testicular malignancy and then consider trauma-induced torsion, epididymitis, or testicular rupture.
3. Physical examination may be difficult because of swelling and pain.
4. Ultrasound is a useful diagnostic tool. Urinalysis may demonstrate pyuria with epididymitis. Testicular radionuclide scanning may be necessary to exclude torsion.
5. **Testicular rupture**
    a. Examination may demonstrate scrotal ecchymosis, loss of palpable testicular contour, and marked pain and tenderness.
    b. Sonography with a 7.5-MHz transducer will demonstrate acute hematocele, which requires exploration. Frequently laceration of the tunica albuginea testis or loss of normal contour with extrusion of parenchymal tissue may be demonstrated, but a normal ultrasound does not rule out a testicular disruption. The overall accuracy of sonography in the detection of traumatic testis rupture is as follows: specificity, 75%; sensitivity, 64%; positive predicitive value, 78%; and negative predicitive value, 60%. If clinical suspicion is high, exploration is mandated.
    c. Requires prompt surgical exploration since the probability of testicular salvage after blunt trauma decreases from 80% to 90% to 32% to 45% if exploration is delayed more than 3 days
    d. At exploration, the affected testis must be copiously irrigated, extruded seminiferous tubules debrided, and the tunica albuginea reapproximated with placement of Penrose drains in the scrotum. The spermatic cord and epididymis should be examined and any obvious bleeding controlled prior to scrotal closure.
    e. If massive injury is sustained and little viable testicular tissue is left, then proceed with orchiectomy.

f. Follow-up sonography may be used to document healing and serum testosterone and leuteinizing hormone levels monitored if parenchymal loss has been significant. Follow-up studies show no detrimental effects on fertility following testicular salvage.
6. Hematoceles warrant prompt surgical draianage to prevent infectious complications, prolonged pain, or testicular ischemia from compression.
7. Stable scrotal hematomas and hydroceles can be managed conservatively with ice, bed rest, and elevation.

B. Penetrating injuries
1. **Scrotal lacerations**
    a. Simple skin lacerations may be debrided and closed primarily.
    b. If Dartos fascia is violated, scrotal exploration is required to rule out testicular injury or penetration of the tunica vaginalis. Fascia should be closed separately to prevent hematoma formation.
    c. Sonography may be helpful preoperatively, particularly with regard to diagnosis of testicular trauma in questionable cases.
2. **Scrotal avulsion**
    a. Usually results from rapid deceleration injury
    b. Minor avulsions can be managed as simple lacerations, with copious irrigation of the wound and immediate closure in two layers.
    c. Complex avulsions require initial judicious debridement, close observation, and either primary reapproximation or delayed reconstruction and skin grafting.
    d. Due to the elasticity and vascularity of scrotal skin, wounds can often be closed primarily even after a loss of up to 60% of skin surface area.
    e. With complete avulsion of the scrotum, the testes should be kept moist and then implanted into thigh pouches. The thigh pouches can then be mobilized as cutaneous flaps and used for later reconstruction.
3. **Testicular laceration**
    a. In face of penetrating trauma, usually a gunshot wound or stab wound, exploration is indicated.
    b. Testicular laceration is treated in the same manner as a testicular rupture (see above, Testicular Rupture, Blunt Trauma).

III. PERINEAL TRAUMA AND LACERATION

A. Mechanism of injury is generally impalement after a fall, motor vehicle or pedestrian accident, or avulsion of perineal skin due to power take-off injury.
B. Frequently associated with pelvic fracture and concurrent genitourinary and/or rectal injuries
C. May require temporary diverting colostomy and/or urinary diversion with a suprapubic tube so as to prevent contamination prior to closure. Gracilis or thigh flap may be required for definitive coverage.

IV. CHEMICAL, ELECTRICAL, AND THERMAL INJURY TO THE GENITALIA AND PERINEUM

A. Thermal burns are treated similarly to other skin burns.
1. When burns are superficial, use local topical therapy of 1% silver sulfadiazene.
2. Third-degree burns usually require excision and definitive reconstruction.
3. Burns of the glans penis tend to heal best by secondary intention; aggressive debridement can cause inferior functional and esthetic outcomes.

B. Chemical burns are usually superficial and are treated by flushing the area copiously, then treating it as a thermal burn.

C. Electrical burns can have a misleading innocent appearence. Despite minimal skin injury, the electric current is dissipated through the vessels, causing extensive destruction of deep structures. After 24 hours of conservative management, determine the limits of destruction and then debride the tissue.

V. SUGGESTED READINGS

Morey AF, et al: Consensus on genitourinary trauma: External genitalia. Br J Urol Int 94:507-515, 2004.

Peters PC, Sagalowsky AI: Genitourinary trauma. In Walsh PC, Retik AB, Vaughn ED, Wein AJ (eds): Campbell's Urology, 7th ed. Philadelphia: WB Saunders, 1998, pp 3116-3117.

Rosenstein D, McAninch JW: Urologic emergencies. Med Clin North Am 88:495-518, 2004.

Extremity Vascular Trauma

Damon S. Pierce, MD

I. EPIDEMIOLOGY

A. Typically affects young males between the ages of 20 and 40 years
B. Upper extremities are involved in approximately 15% to 25% of civilian injuries and 30% of military injuries.
C. Lower extremities are involved in approximately 20% of civilian injuries and up to 60% of military injuries.
D. Up to 80% of patients with arterial injury have other associated injuries.
E. Motor vehicle collisions are the most common cause of blunt vascular injury.

II. MECHANISM OF INJURY

A. Approximately 80% of peripheral vascular trauma occurs as a result of gunshot wounds, shotgun wounds, and stab wounds.
B. Blunt injuries are most common following dislocations, especially of the knee, shoulder, and elbow, as well as fractures.
C. Iatrogenic injuries are well documented and arise mostly from catheterizations, angiography, and surgical procedures.

III. PATHOPHYSIOLOGY

A. Local and regional effects are determined by the site and mechanism of injury.
B. High-velocity gunshot wounds can produce massive soft tissue damage and disrupt collateral circulation.
C. Blunt trauma can contuse the vessel wall or disrupt the intima, which may lead to thrombosis.

IV. EVALUATION

A. History
1. Amount of blood at the scene of injury
2. Type of bleeding—pulsatile (arterial) versus steady flow (venous)
3. Neurologic deficits
4. Associated injuries
5. Mechanism of injuries

B. Physical Examination
1. The physical examination must be meticulous and include pulse character, caliber, ankle-brachial indices (ABIs), arterial pressure index (API), and a complete neurologic evaluation of the injured extremity.

TABLE 33-1
SIGNS OF ARTERIAL INJURY

Hard Signs	Soft Signs
Circulatory deficit	Small, stable hematoma
Ischemia	Adjacent nerve injury
Pulse deficit	Shock (otherwise unexplained)
Bruit	Proximity to major vascular structures, <1 cm from anatomic position of vessel
Expanding or pulsatile hematoma	Difference in ankle-brachial indices >0.15 injured extremity
Arterial bleeding	

2. API is determined by dividing the systolic pressure in the injured limb by the systolic pressure in the uninjured limb. (normal=1.0).
3. Bone and joint integrity, temperature, capillary refill time, and venous insufficiency must be evaluated (Table 33-1).
4. Pulse changes in relation to orthopaedic maneuvers must be noted.
5. Local evaluation of the area of injury must include the direction and size of the wound, auscultation for the presence of a bruit, and palpation of a thrill, as well as assessment of any hematoma. Proximity to known major vascular structures must be noted.
6. The six Ps—pulselessness, pallor, pain, paresthesia, paralysis, and poikilothermia—are key clinical features to assess when evaluating a patient for possible arterial injury.

C. Ultrasonic flow detection
1. All patients with extremity trauma and no clinical evidence of arterial injury should be screened with Doppler arterial pressure measurements. The determination of phasic Doppler signal can provide qualitative evidence regarding collateral flow. Triphasic signal indicates no significant obstruction, whereas low-pitched monophasic signal strongly supports an obstruction.
2. Patients with normal studies (API >0.9) may be followed by serial noninvasive examinations. Arteriography or operative intervention is reserved for those patients with abnormal Doppler studies (API <0.9).
3. Limitations of Doppler examination include its inaccuracy for venous injuries, for damage to nonaxial vessels (e.g., profunda femoris artery), and for nonocclusive arterial injuries, such as pseudoaneurysms.
4. Proximal injuries (axillosubclavian and iliac arteries) continue to require arteriography as a primary screening examination.

D. Arteriography
1. Arteriograms are usually obtained for the following reasons:
   a. To plan the operative management of complex injuries
   b. To rule out a vascular injury associated with a joint dislocation
   c. To rule out vascular injuries in patients with soft signs of vascular injury
   d. To assess injury in stable patients with hard signs of vascular injury

e. To exclude the need for surgical exploration in patients who have no other indication for operation but there is suggestion of vascular injury
2. Arteriography is frequently obtained in patients who sustain shotgun wounds unless immediate exploration is indicated because of exsanguinating hemorrhage or threatened viability of the extremity.
3. Positive signs on angiography include:
   a. Obstruction
   b. Extravasation
   c. Early venous filling or arteriovenous fistula (AVF)
   d. Wall irregularity
   e. Filling defect or intimal flap
   f. Pseudoaneurysm
4. Angiographic embolization in acute trauma may be considered for distal false aneurysms or AVFs in unstable patients or in those who have no other injury if the vessel is a small muscular branch.
5. Arteriography has a complication rate of 2% to 4%.

V. MANAGEMENT

A. Preoperative preparation
1. Intravenous antibiotics should be given, primarily to cover gram-positive cocci. Broad-spectrum antibiotics should be considered depending on the degree of contamination.
2. The prepped area should include:
   a. The entire injured extremity
   b. The entire chest for proximal upper extremity injuries
   c. An uninjured lower extremity as a source of donor site for autologous vein graft

B. Operative technique for arterial injuries
1. A generous incision is used to allow proximal and distal control to be obtained prior to direct exploration of the suspected injury.
2. Following proximal and distal control of the vessel with vessel loops, the artery is carefully dissected, taking care to preserve all collateral branches if possible.
   a. Proximal and distal embolectomy is routinely performed with Fogarty catheters.
   b. Vessels are then flushed with 1:1000 heparinized saline solution both proximally and distally and clamped with a Heifetz clip or a vascular clamp.
3. Simple lacerations are repaired by lateral arteriorrhaphy using fine monofilament suture of polypropylene; 5-0 should be used for larger arteries such as femoral or axillary arteries, and 6-0 suture should be used for smaller arteries such as popliteal or brachial arteries.
4. When debridement is required, repair is attempted by primary end-to-end anastomosis if adequate vessel length can be achieved. This generally requires 4 to 5 cm of vessel mobilization for each 1 cm of lost vessel length.

a. Major collaterals should not be interrupted to achieve sufficient length.
b. The vessels are spatulated, then anastomosed with a running monofilament suture if larger than 4 to 5 mm, or interrupted monofilament suture if smaller. Occasionally spatulation can be omitted if the vessel is large enough in caliber or if length is restricted.

5. If a tension-free anastomosis cannot be achieved because of significant loss of vessel length, then repair is performed by an interposition graft.
    a. The primary choice of graft conduit is autologous vein if it is available and of adequate caliber.
    b. Foot or ankle saphenous vein is used for forearm and infrapopliteal vessels, while saphenous vein from the groin is preferred for axillary, brachial, femoral, and popliteal repair.
    c. If no satisfactory autologous tissue is available, a prosthetic interposition graft may be used.
6. Prior to completing the anastomosis, the clamps are briefly removed from the proximal and distal ends of the repair in order to flush out any clots.
7. Completion arteriography is performed in the operating room to ensure no additional injuries and to identify any residual thrombus or embolus distal to the repair.

C. Operative technique for venous injury
1. **Single injury**
    a. Repair if major vein (e.g., popliteal) in a stable patient.
    b. Ligate if a minor vein.
2. **Concomitant with an arterial injury**
    a. The arterial injury is shunted and the vein repaired first (only if a major vein).
    b. Popliteal vein injury should be repaired unless venous duplication is present.
3. Attempt to remove clots from the system by gentle use of the Fogarty catheter and flushing of the vessel.
4. Consider completion venogram to ensure no clots exist in the system that may serve as a nidus for embolization.
5. Interposition prostheses are rarely indicated.
6. Veins that can be repaired are shunted if it is necessary to harvest conduit or an orthopaedic procedure is performed prior to vascular repair.

D. Concomitant fracture. The management of concomitant fractures is dependent on both the distal perfusion status and the degree of orthopaedic instability.
1. For unstable fractures without distal perfusion, vascular exploration with placement of an arterial and, if necessary, a venous shunt is performed initially, followed by orthopaedic stabilization. This allows for definitive vascular repair to be completed without anastomotic disruption secondary to fracture motion during reduction and fixation.
2. When distal perfusion is preserved as documented by Doppler examination, fractures may be addressed prior to exploration and repair. This can also be accomplished if fracture reduction can be done expeditiously.

3. Distal pulse status is frequently assessed during all orthopaedic manipulation and stabilization procedures.

E. Neurologic injury. Associated neurologic injury is managed according to the discretion of the neurosurgical, orthopaedic, or plastic surgery consulting physician.

1. Contused nerves generally are managed conservatively.
2. Sharply transected nerves are repaired under magnification by group fascicular approximation with fine monofilament suture.
3. Nerves transected by gunshot wounds or avulsion are tagged with permanent suture and repaired electively at a later time.

F. Fasciotomy. Fasciotomy is performed prior to any repair where ischemia has been present, or will be present, for a significant period of time.

G. Closure. Exposed vascular repairs are covered with myocutaneous flaps or heterografts at the initial procedure regardless of the amount of debridement required or if subsequent debridement will be required.

VI. POSTOPERATIVE CARE

A. Pulses and/or Doppler signal must be checked frequently.
B. Compression devices are not used on any extremity with a vascular repair.
C. Ambulation is begun as soon as feasible.
D. Anticoagulants are used infrequently.
E. Antibiotics are not used for the vascular repair, but they may be indicated for concomitant orthopaedic injuries.
F. Continual observation and vigilance for the development of compartment syndrome are vital.

VII. SUGGESTED READINGS

Mullenix PS, Steele SR, Andersen CA, et al: Limb salvage and outcomes among patients with traumatic popliteal vascular injury: An analysis of the National Trauma Data Bank. J Vasc Surg 44(1):94-100, 2006.

Subramanian A, Vercruysse G, Dente C, et al: A decade's experience with temporary intravascular shunts at a civilian Level I trauma center. J Trauma Inj Infec 65(2):316-326, 2008.

Woodward EB, Clouse WD, Eliason JL, et al: Penetrating femoropopliteal injury during modern warfare: Experience of the Balad Vascular Registry. J Vasc Surg 47(6):1259-1265, 2008.

Abdominal Vascular Injury

Stephen Smith, MD

I. INTRODUCTION

A. General facts
1. Blunt trauma—5% to 10% will have an abdominal vascular injury.
2. Penetrating trauma—15% to 20% will have an abdominal vascular injury.
3. Abdominal vascular trauma accounts for 20% to 30% of all reported vascular trauma—18% of all arterial injuries and 48% of all venous injuries.
4. More than 75% of all penetrating vascular injury patients will present in shock.

B. Mechanism of injury
1. **Causes of blunt trauma**
   a. Avulsion injuries of small branches of major vessels
   b. Intimal tears with secondary thrombosis (e.g., renal artery/seat belt)
   c. The majority of hepatic vein injuries and one-third of renal artery injuries
2. **Causes of penetrating trauma**
   a. Blast effect, intimal flaps, and secondary thrombosis
   b. Lateral wall defects
   c. Complete transection with either free bleeding or thrombosis
   d. Arteriovenous fistulas
   e. Bullet embolization, which is rare

II. EVALUATION

A. Initial evaluation
1. ATLS protocol: primary survey (ABCDE)/secondary survey
2. Vascular examination: pulses/thrill/bruit/ankle-brachial index
3. Keep the patient warm; change out cold IV fluids to warm solutions.
4. At Parkland Memorial Hospital our goal is to be in the operating room within 5 minutes of arrival for an unstable penetrating torso injury.
5. Resuscitation is titrated to mentation or normal blood pressure, whichever comes first.
6. **Blunt abdominal injuries**
   a. Diagnostic modalities include focused abdominal sonography for trauma (FAST), diagnostic peritoneal lavage (DPL), and CT (if patient's condition is stable).
   b. Gross hematuria requires CT of the abdomen with CT cystourethrogram.
   c. Arteriogram of the iliac arteries is performed if there is a significant pelvic fracture (greater than type LC I (lateral compression type I)) and hypotension without other cause.

III. INITIAL MANAGEMENT

A. Exploratory celiotomy
1. Ensure availability of blood for transfusion, vascular set, sponge sticks, and vascular suture.
2. Prep the patient awake. Prep from chin to knees. If there is high suspicion of an iliac injury or there are abnormal pulses in an extremity, prep the entire leg.
3. Keep the patient warm using an upper extremity warming blanket, warm humidified oxygen, and warm fluids.
4. Broad-spectrum antibiotics
5. Midline incision from xiphoid to pubis
6. Evacuate clot.
7. Pack bleeding. If the patient has persistent hemorrhage despite packing, attempt direct aortic compression manually or with sponge stick until the bleeding vessel can be cross-clamped. Venous bleeding can usually be controlled with a sponge stick.
8. When bleeding is controlled, other intra-abdominal injuries can be addressed.

B. Retroperitoneal and peritoneal hematomas
1. **Retroperitoneal zones**
   a. **Zone I**—central hematoma. Area extending from the diaphragm down to the level of the bifurcation of the common iliac arteries with its lateral boundaries encompassing bilateral renal pedicles; includes aorta and inferior vena cava along with their associated branches
   b. **Zone II**—lateral hematoma. Encompasses area to the left and right of zone I, with its inferior border being the bifurcation of the common iliac arteries
   c. **Zone III**—pelvic hematoma. Superior boundary is at the level of the bifurcation of the common iliac arteries with its inferior boundary being the pelvic cul de sac.
2. **General rules**
   a. All hematomas secondary to penetrating injuries are explored.
   b. All zone I hematomas are explored.
   c. Blunt zone II and zone III injuries are not explored unless they are expanding or if previous urologic work-up showed nonvisualization of kidney or possible genitourinary injury.

IV. EXPOSURE AND MANAGEMENT OF INJURIES

A. Abdominal vascular injuries generally occur in one of five locations:
1. Midline supramesocolic
2. Midline inframesocolic
3. Upper lateral retroperitoneum
4. Pelvic retroperitoneum

5. Periportal
B. Zone I: midline supramesocolic area
1. **Supraceliac aortic control**
   a. In the setting of active hemorrhage, proximal subdiaphragmatic aortic control can be obtained using manual compression (aortic compressor, Richardson retractor). An alternative approach is to divide the lesser omentum, retract the stomach and esophagus to the left, split the left crus of the diaphragm, and clamp the aorta.
2. **Exposure**
   a. If active hemorrhage is not present, this area is best exposed with **left medial visceral rotation (Mattox maneuver)**. The left colon, kidney, spleen, tail of the pancreas, and fundus of the stomach are reflected medially. The majority of the time the left kidney is left in place by dividing the splenic-renal ligaments.
   b. Additional exposure is obtained by dividing the left crus at the 2 o'clock position. Left medial visceral rotation allows complete exposure of the aorta. The disadvantage is the time required and the possibility of iatrogenic injury to the spleen or pancreas.
3. **Management of specific injuries**
   a. **Aorta**: A small tear in the aorta can be repaired primarily with 3-0 or 4-0 polypropylene suture. If primary closure would cause narrowing of the aorta, a prosthetic patch can be used. Resection and end-to-end anastomosis are rarely performed due to immobility of the aorta from lumbar branches. Aortic injury requiring replacement with a prosthetic graft often occurs in combination with gastrointestinal injuries and contamination. There are data supporting the use of prosthetic grafts in these situations rather than an extra-anatomic bypass. After the vascular repair has been performed, the abdomen is irrigated and the retroperitoneum is used to provide coverage and exclude it from the abdomen.
   b. **Celiac artery**: Repair of branches of the celiac artery is often difficult because of their small size and the dense neural tissue of the celiac plexus.
      i. The left gastric and splenic artery can be ligated without consequences.
      ii. The common hepatic artery proximal to the gastroduodenal artery can be ligated because of the extensive collateral blood supply through the superior mesenteric artery.
      iii. Injuries distal to the gastroduodenal artery should be repaired when feasible.
      iv. However, if the patient is unstable and a concomitant portal vein injury has not occurred, the hepatic artery can be ligated. In this situation there will be an increased incidence of gallbladder necrosis and a cholecystectomy must also be done.
      v. If the entire celiac axis is injured, it is best to ligate all three vessels.
      vi. Ligation of the splenic artery does not necessitate splenectomy due to potential collateral blood supply. Ligation of the splenic vein,

however, usually requires splenectomy to prevent congestive splenomegaly with thrombocytopenia.

c. **Superior mesenteric artery (SMA)**. Injuries may occur at several levels. Given the small size of this vessel, repair usually requires autologous bypass.

Fullen classification of SMA injuries:
  i. Zone I—injury to the SMA beneath the pancreas. Ligation here would jeopardize the small bowel, ascending colon, two-thirds of the transverse colon, and the pancreas. Transection of the pancreas at the neck may be required for repair.
  ii. Zone II—injury to the SMA at the base of the pancreas between the pancreaticoduodenal and middle colic arteries. Ligation is often not tolerated because of vasoconstriction of the distal SMA due to massive blood loss. In a damage control situation a temporary shunt can be used until the repair can be performed in a more stable situation. A saphenous vein bypass can then be performed to the infrarenal aorta.
  iii. Zone III—injury beyond the middle colic artery
  iv. Zone IV—injury to vasa recta and distal arcades. Repair the vessel if it is large enough or perform segmental resection of the bowel.
  v. Bowel viability must be assessed by examination, Doppler, and occasionally by giving 1 g of fluoroscein and observing with a Wood's lamp.
  vi. If bowel viability is questionable, a second-look operation is required at 24 to 48 hours. This decision is made in the operating room at the time of the first operation.

d. **Superior mesenteric vein (SMV)**: Aggressive attempts to repair the SMV should be made. Division of the neck of the pancreas on rare occasions is necessary to visualize perforations of the retropancreatic SMV. The survival rate associated with ligation of the SMV varies greatly among series from 50% to 80%. In this situation aggressive resuscitation is needed to overcome the fluid sequestration in the bowel and resultant peripheral hypovolemia.

C. **Zone I: midline inframesocolic area** (includes the infrarenal aorta and the inferior vena cava [IVC])

1. **Exposure**
   a. Similar to exposure of an infrarenal abdominal aortic aneurysm. Retract the transverse mesocolon cephalad, eviscerate the small bowel toward the patient's right side, and open the midline peritoneum.
   b. Divide the ligament of Treitz and identify the left renal vein. Proximal control can be obtained just below the left renal vein. Distal exposure can be obtained by opening the midline peritoneum inferiorly, staying to the right near the origin of the inferior mesenteric artery (IMA).
   c. If the bleeding appears to be more to the right and an IVC injury is suspected, better exposure can usually be obtained by mobilizing the

right colon and duodenum (right medial visceral rotation). Once the loose retroperitoneal tissue is stripped off of the IVC, the injury can be identified.

2. **Management of specific injuries**
   a. **Infrarenal abdominal aorta**
      i. Injuries to this portion of the aorta are repaired in a similar fashion to that described for the suprarenal aorta.
      ii. This includes primary repair, patch angioplasty, and replacement with a prosthetic graft.
   b. **Inferior vena cava**
      i. **Initial control**. Extensive injuries to the IVC can usually be controlled with sponge stick compression. Back bleeding from large lumbar veins can usually be controlled with large DeBakey aortic clamps.
      ii. **Anterior injuries**. After exposure, anterior injuries can be isolated with a partially occluding vascular clamp such as a Satinsky. Anterior perforations are best repaired in a transverse fashion to avoid narrowing the lumen. In the stable patient narrowing can be avoided with a patch angioplasty.
      iii. **Injuries near the renal veins**. Perforations at the level of the renal veins can be controlled with sponge sticks temporarily. Control of the infrahepatic IVC, renal veins, and infrarenal vena cava can then be obtained with umbilical tape. Control of hemorrhage from the IVC may also be obtained with the use of a 30-mL balloon catheter by placing the catheter either proximally or distally through the injury site. Injuries to the suprarenal vena cava should be repaired or bypassed to prevent postoperative renal failure. If autogenous tissue is not available, GoreTex PTFE (polytetrafluoroethylene) may be considered.
      iv. **Posterior injuries**. Medial mobilization of the right kidney is helpful for exposure of posterior perforations of the suprarenal vena cava. Posterior perforations can also be visualized and repaired inside the vena cava by opening the anterior surface.
      v. **Distal IVC injury**. Injury at the confluence of the common iliac veins may be exposed by dividing the right common iliac artery and reflecting the aorta to the left. Repair of the right common iliac artery is accomplished after the venous repair.
      vi. **Retrohepatic caval injuries** are discussed in Chapter 27.
      vii. **IVC ligation**. If the patient is exsanguinating and extensive repair is necessary, ligation is performed. Ligation should be performed as close to the inferior edge of the renal veins as possible to avoid a cul de sac that could promote embolism. Once ligation has been performed, bilateral four-compartment fasciotomy must be considered. Most young trauma patients will tolerate this as long as circulating volume is aggressively maintained in the postoperative period. Elastic compression wraps are applied to both lower extremities for 5 to 7 days. At the time of discharge, full-length custom support hose are recommended for the patient.

D. Zone II: upper lateral retroperitoneum
1. **Exposure**
   a. Perform left or right medial visceral rotation. The standard protocol for penetrating injuries to zone II is operative exploration.
   b. If the patient is stable and there is no active hemorrhage, vascular control at the renal hilum is usually performed. Otherwise, Gerota's fascia is opened and the kidney is mobilized up into the field, where the hilum can then be clamped.
   c. A zone II hematoma from blunt trauma is not usually opened unless it is pulsatile or expanding.
2. **Management of specific injuries**
   a. **Renal artery injury**
      i. The renal artery is small and difficult to repair primarily.
      ii. Options for repair include mobilization with limited resection and end-to-end anastomosis, interposition grafting, or replacement with the right hepatic or splenic artery.
      iii. Another option to consider is explantation, cold perfusion, and autotransplantation. However, nephrectomy is often a better choice in the hypotensive patient with significant renovascular injury.
      iv. When considering revascularization versus nephrectomy, the following must be assessed:
         (a) Hemodynamic stability and magnitude of associated injuries
         (b) Extent of vascular, ureteral, and renal parenchymal damage
         (c) Intravenous pyelogram indicates a functioning contralateral kidney.
         (d) Duration of ischemia
   b. **Renal vein injury**
      i. Renal vein lacerations should be repaired primarily by venorrhaphy.
      ii. Right renal vein ligation that is necessary to control hemorrhage in a hypotensive patient should prompt a nephrectomy.
      iii. The proximal left renal vein can usually by ligated safely if there is an intact gonadal vein.

E. Zone III: pelvic retroperitoneum
1. **General notes**
   a. Penetrating iliac artery/vein injuries comprise 10% of all vascular injuries.
   b. One-third of patients die with in 24 hours. An additional 10% die of late septic complications. As many as 95% have associated visceral injuries. About 80% will be hypotensive on arrival.
   c. **Clinical triad**
      i. Hypotension
      ii. Peritoneal signs
      iii. Entrance wound below umbilicus (75% of time)
   d. A normal peripheral vascular examination does not exclude injury.

e. Mortality is usually secondary to hemorrhage, coagulopathy, or irreversible shock. Combined arterial and venous injuries have a mortality of 47%. In several large series, all deaths occurred in those who arrived hypotensive (BP<90).
f. Mortality is affected by the absence of retroperitoneal tamponade (i.e., 46% die if freely bleeding intra-abdominally), difficult exposure in the pelvis, and a high incidence of associated injuries; individuals who respond clinically to resuscitation have a good prognosis (92% survive).

2. **Exposure**
   a. Retract the small bowel to the right and open the retroperitoneum in the midline. The common iliac artery and vein can be encircled distal to the bifurcation of the aorta/IVC.
   b. On the right, the cecum may need to be mobilized cephalad to expose the iliac bifurcation.
   c. On the left, the bifurcation of the left iliac artery is covered by the mesentery of the sigmoid colon. Reflect the sigmoid colon and distal descending colon medially.
   d. The ureter crosses over the iliac bifurcation and as a result one must be conscious of associated urologic injuries in this region.
   e. In a patient with bilateral iliac injuries, total pelvic vascular isolation is performed by clamping the distal aorta and IVC at their bifurcation and bilateral iliac vessels proximal to the inguinal ligament.

3. Management of specific injuries:
   a. **Iliac arteries**
      i. Options include primary repair (be careful to avoid narrowing), patch angioplasty, and bypass.
      ii. In the setting of gross fecal contamination, the iliac artery can be ligated and a fem-fem crossover is performed after closure of the abdomen if the patient is stable.
      iii. The internal iliac can be ligated unilaterally without consequence.
      iv. Bilateral internal iliac ligation can be performed but has an increased percentage of buttock claudication and impotence.
      v. In combined arterial/venous injuries, the venous injury is dealt with first. With combined injuries, the fasciotomy should be considered.
   b. **Iliac veins**
      i. Venous injury to the right common iliac/ bifurcation of the IVC may require division of the right common iliac artery to gain exposure.
      ii. After venous repair the artery is repaired primarily.
      iii. Iliac vein injuries may require division of the internal iliac artery for exposure. This artery does not need to be repaired. Primary repair of the venous injury (i.e., lateral venorrhaphy) is preferable.
      iv. If the patient is unstable with multiple associated injuries or has multiple venous injuries, the vein is ligated.

v. If ligation of the vein is performed, the patient must have compressive wraps and the legs must be elevated postoperatively. Transient extremity edema occurs in one-third of patients, with most edema resolving at 12 weeks.
vi. A low threshold for fasciotomy (four compartment) is used in the setting of iliac ligation. Pulmonary embolus following ligation is rare. The reported incidence is <2%, with no statistical difference between repair and ligation.

F. Portal area
1. **Exposure**
   a. When a hematoma involves the portal triad in the right upper quadrant the proximal hepatoduodenal ligament should be looped with an umbilical tape or noncrushing vascular clamp (Pringle maneuver) before the hematoma is entered.
   b. Distal control should be attempted but may be difficult in those with a short portal vein.
2. **Management of specific injuries**
   a. **Portal vein**
      i. The portal vein can be repaired primarily, with end-to-end anastomosis or interposition grafting. Lateral venorrhaphy with 4-0 or 5-0 polypropylene suture is preferred. Care should be taken to completely identify the injury prior to placing sutures owing to the proximity of the bile duct.
      ii. Ligation of the portal vein in the absence of hepatic artery injury is compatible with survival (20% mortality). This may be associated with postoperative portal hypertension and encephalopathy.
      iii. If ligation is performed (e.g., in a setting of extensive injury, hypothermia, or acidosis), aggressive resuscitation must be undertaken to compensate for splanchnic hypervolemia.
   b. **Hepatic artery**
      i. The hepatic artery is small in this area and may require ligation versus autogenous bypass or patch.
      ii. Ligation is well tolerated in young patients in the absence of concomitant portal vein injuries.
      iii. Selective ligation of the right hepatic artery alone requires cholecystectomy. Selective ligation of hepatic artery and portal vein branches to one lobe of the liver will lead to necrosis of the lobe and thus mandates hepatectomy.

V. MORBIDITY/MORTALITY OF ABDOMINAL VASCULAR INJURIES

A. Morbidity
1. Infection
2. Aortoenteric fistulas
3. Thrombosis

4. False aneurysm
5. Coagulopathy—usually the result of hypothermia, multiple transfusions, acidosis

B. Mortality is affected by a number of different parameters:
1. Location of the injury
   a. Suprarenal aorta—70%
   b. IVC—50% to 70%
   c. SMA—40% to 50%
   d. SMV—30% to 40%
   e. Iliac artery/vein—30%
   f. Portal vein—20%
2. Presentation of patient: hypotensive versus normotensive
3. Number of associated visceral injuries
4. Number of associated vascular injuries (IVC is the most common associated vascular injury)
5. The presence of coagulopathy, hypothermia, and metabolic acidosis accounts for 80% of deaths.

VI. SUGGESTED READINGS

Asensio JA, Petrone P, Garcia-Nunez L, et al: Superior mesenteric venous injuries: To ligate or to repair remains the question. J Trauma 62(3):668-675, 2007.

Goaley TJ, Dente CJ, Feliciano DV: Torso vascular trauma at an urban level I trauma center. Perspect Vasc Surg Endovasc Ther 18(2):102-112, 2006.

Gunn M, Campbell M, Hoffer EK: Traumatic abdominal aortic injury treated by endovascular stent placement. Emerg Radiol 13(6):329-331, 2007.

Seamon MJ, Pathak AS, Bradley KM, et al: Emergency department thoracotomy still useful after abdominal exsanguination? J Trauma 64(1):1-7, 2008.

Thermal, Chemical, and Cold Injuries

Robert Garza, MD

I. BURN INJURY OVERVIEW

A. Approximately 50,000 patients per year require hospitalization for thermal injuries in the United States, with a 6% overall mortality.
B. Severe burns require triage to regional burn centers (Table 35-1).
C. Morbidity and mortality are a function of burn depth, size, and location; the presence of inhalation injury; and the patient's age and comorbidities.
D. The terminology of first-, second-, and third-degree burns has mostly been replaced with the terms *superficial, partial-thickness*, and *full-thickness* burns.
1. Partial-thickness burns generally heal within 10 to 21 days with mild to moderate scar formation and may or may not require skin grafting. Deep partial-thickness burns may take longer to heal and will heal with greater scarring and decreased function depending on location.
2. Full-thickness burns destroy deep dermal structures, heal poorly with severe scarring, and generally require skin grafting (Table 35-2).

II. EVALUATION OF BURNS

A. Prehospital
1. The goal is to prevent additional injury and limit microbial contamination.
2. Clean bed sheets or large absorbent dressings are used to protect the burn wound.
3. The application of cool water on partial-thickness burns in the first minutes after injury may reduce residual heat in the wound, preventing extension of tissue damage. However, hypothermia may follow excessive cooling of the patient.
4. Airway protection and initiation of fluid resuscitation are considered for all patients, depending on anticipated time of transport and the condition of the patient.

B. Emergency department
1. Standard ATLS protocol is used to evaluate burn patients with a history or mechanism of injury suggesting trauma, given the incidence of concomitant trauma (approximately 7%). A Foley catheter and nasogastric tube are placed in all major burn patients.
2. Patients with facial or neck burns and those suspected of having inhalational injuries (burns in an enclosed space, carbonaceous sputum, respiratory distress, hypoxia, singed nasal hair and/or eyebrows) are evaluated for airway compromise.

TABLE 35-1
BURN UNIT REFERRAL CRITERIA

1. Partial-thickness burns of more than 10% of total body surface area
2. Burns involving the face, hands, feet, perineum, or major joints
3. Full-thickness burns in any age group
4. Electrical burns, including lightning injury
5. Chemical burns
6. Inhalation injury
7. Burn injury in patients with significant comorbidities
8. Patients with concomitant major trauma
9. Burned children in hospitals without resources or equipment for pediatric care
10. Burn injury in patients who will require social, emotional, or long-term rehabilitative intervention

From Guidelines for the Operation of Burn Units, Resources for Optimal Care of the Injured Patient: Committee on Trauma, Chicago, American College of Surgeons, 2006, pp 79-86.

3. Intubation is frequently performed for patients with large burns prior to airway compromise associated with a large fluid resuscitation.
4. Patients who require intubation are sedated, without paralysis, to the point where nasotracheal or orotracheal intubation is tolerated. Incremental doses of morphine (0.1 mg/kg) and diazepam (0.1 mg/kg) are used with bag-valve-mask assistance until intubation is tolerated. Pharmacologic paralysis is rarely used since apnea and airway collapse can turn an elective procedure into an emergent surgical airway.
5. After an adequate airway is ensured, either with spontaneous breathing or mechanical ventilation, 100% oxygen is delivered for the presumptive treatment of carbon monoxide poisoning.

TABLE 35-2
CHARACTERISTICS OF SUPERFICIAL, PARTIAL-THICKNESS, AND FULL-THICKNESS BURNS

	Superficial	Partial-thickness	Full-thickness
Mechanism	Sunburn, minor flash or flame burn, minor scald	Scald, flash burn, some flame burns, some chemical agents	Prolonged exposure to flame or chemical agents, electrical burn
Color	Light pink or red	Pink or mottled red	Pearly white and gray, translucent, charred; deep red in infants
Texture	Dry, or small blisters	Blisters or moist, weeping surface	Dry, thrombosis of superficial vessels; spongy necrosis with alkali burn
Sensation	Painful	Painful	Insensate
Healing	3-6 days	10-21 days (may be longer for deep dermal)	Requires grafting

Adapted from Mozingo DW, et al: Acute resuscitation and transfer management of burned and electrically injured patients. Trauma Quarterly 11(2):96, 1994.

6. Two large-bore intravenous catheters are inserted for fluid resuscitation, preferably through unburned skin. This includes 14- to16-gauge peripheral intravenous lines and/or saphenous vein cutdowns. Central venous lines are not used for initial resuscitation unless no alternative exists. Catheters may be placed through burned skin without significant morbidity.
7. The patient's response to resuscitation can be assessed by obtaining frequent vital signs and monitoring urine output.
8. The secondary survey is completed to identify associated injuries and other life-threatening issues that may need to be addressed in the emergency department.
9. The extent of the burn is roughly assessed using the rule of nine's. The Berkow formula is used after the patient is stabilized to specifically quantify the surface area burned (Figure 35-1).

III. RESUSCITATION OF BURNS

A. The Parkland formula. This formula is used for resuscitation of burns >10% total body surface area (TBSA) in children and the elderly, and for burns >20% TBSA in adults.
1. The Parkland formula consists of 4 mL/kg per %TBSA burn of lactated Ringer's (LR) for the first 24 hours. Colloid and $D_5\frac{1}{2}NS$ maintenance fluid are given beginning at 24 hours post-burn as described below:
   a. 2 mL/kg per %TBSA given over first 8 hours post-burn
   b. 1 mL/kg per %TBSA given over second 8 hours post-burn
   c. 1 mL/kg per %TBSA given over third 8 hours post-burn
   d. 0.1 mL/kg per %TBSA of 25% albumin given over the first 4 hours of the second day
   e. 1 mL/kg per %TBSA $D_5\frac{1}{2}NS$ given per day of maintenance fluid
2. The Parkland formula is used only as a guide for resuscitation. The patient is continually reassessed with frequent vital signs. A Foley catheter is mandatory, as urine output is the single best indicator of adequacy of resuscitation. The resuscitation is adjusted to keep a urine output between 0.5 and 1 mL/kg per hour (30 to 50 mL/hour in adults).
3. Peripheral intravenous access is preferable and adequate during the resuscitation of the majority of burn patients. Catheters are sutured in place.
4. Central venous pressure monitoring and pulmonary artery catheterization are not routinely used and are reserved for patients who do not appropriately respond to resuscitation or who have known compromised cardiac function.
5. Salt-poor albumin solution (25% solution) is administered beginning 24 hours post-burn (after the burn-induced capillary leak has resolved).
6. Maintenance fluids are replaced with $D_5\frac{1}{2}NS$.
7. Packed red blood cells are transfused only in anemic patients.

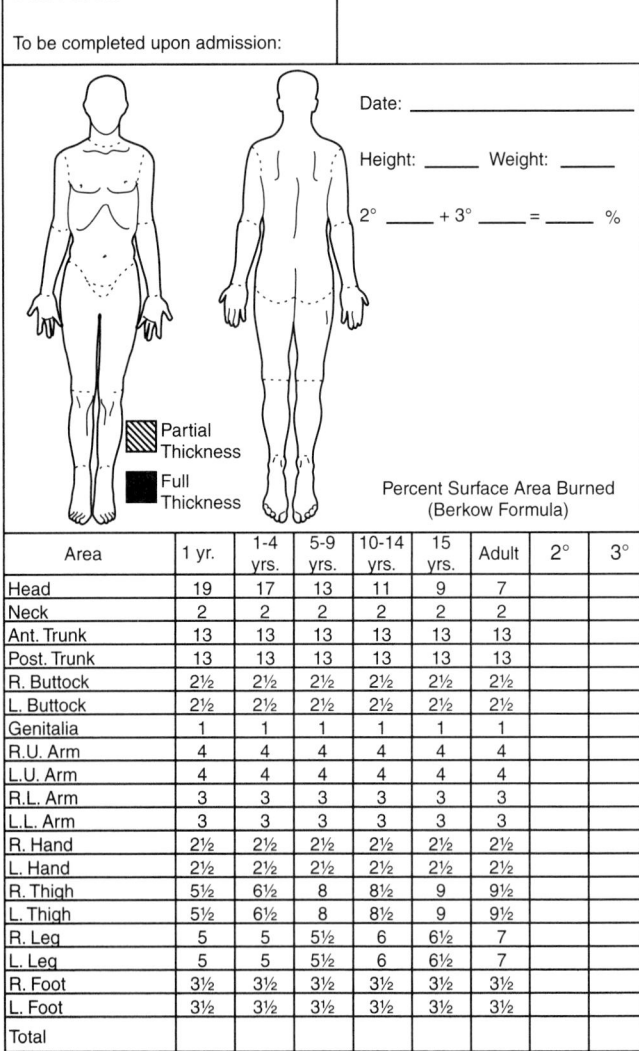

FIGURE 35-1

Berkow formula. (Courtesy of Dallas County Hospital District, Dallas, Texas.)

8. The patient is given both active and passive tetanus prophylaxis in the contralateral deltoid muscles while in the emergency department. The dose of tetanus immune globulin (Hypertet) is 4 units/kg and is the only medication that should be administered intramuscularly to the burn patient as these patients have poor skin and muscle perfusion acutely.
9. A nasogastric tube is inserted to prevent gastric dilation, vomiting, and aspiration with burns >25% TBSA because burn patients have a tendency to develop an ileus. It is also used for early initiation of enteral feeding.
10. H2 blockers are used intravenously to prevent gastric stress ulceration.
11. Prophylactic antibiotics are not administered unless there is an indication from a concomitant injury such as an open fracture or a preexisting comorbidity such as a mechanical valve replacement.
12. All adults receive subcutaneous heparin for deep venous thrombosis prophylaxis.

B. Escharotomy (Figure 35-2)
1. Escharotomy is performed for circumferential burns of the extremities only when there is evidence of vascular compromise. This is assessed with bedside Doppler evaluation of the radial and ulnar arteries as well as the palmar arch. In the lower extremities, the dorsalis pedis and posterior tibial arteries are assessed.
2. Restriction of chest wall motion by edema to the point where ventilation is compromised (elevated peak airway pressures) is an indication for chest wall escharotomy.
3. Electrocautery is used to incise the eschar on a circumferentially burned limb. Incisions are made along the midlateral and midmedial line extending the entire length of the burned area. The incisions are carried deep to the eschar and superficial fascia to a depth sufficient to allow the cut edges of the eschar to separate.
4. Escharotomies are performed in the intensive care unit. Intubation and sedation/analgesia are required.
5. Indications for fasciotomy in high-voltage electrical injury are the same as for long bone trauma, extensive soft tissue trauma, or vascular injury. Fasciotomies are performed in the operating room under general anesthetic.
6. Escharotomies should rarely be performed prior to arrival at a burn unit and can wait until arrival at a burn unit if transport time is less than 6 hours.

IV. BURN WOUND CARE

A. Initial care on arrival. All burn wounds are treated as follows:
1. Cleansed with a mild chlorhexadine-based solution
2. Debridement of nonviable skin
3. Hair shaved from the burned areas

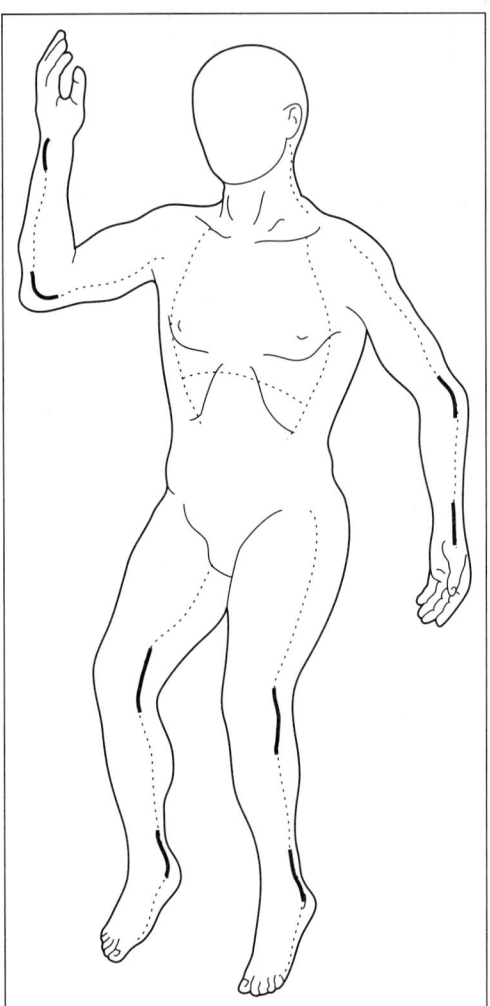

FIGURE 35-2

Escharotomy technique. (Adapted from Schwartz SI, et al: Principles of Surgery, 7th ed. New York, McGraw-Hill, *p 228*.

4. Topical antimicrobial agent applied
5. The wound is bandaged with fine mesh gauze.
6. Wound care as outlined above, is continued daily as well as frequent reassessment of burn depth and monitoring for invasive infection, is continued daily

B. Management

1. Partial-thickness burns are managed with a topical antimicrobial agent and gauze dressings.
2. Bacitracin ointment is used without a dressing for partial-thickness facial burns.
3. Silver sulfadiazine is used with gauze dressing for most partial-thickness burns other than facial burns. It is bacteriostatic and has intermediate penetration through intact eschar. Silver sulfadiazine does not cause pain, is easy to apply, and has a broad antibacterial spectrum.
4. Mafenide acetate (Sulfamylon) has excellent tissue and eschar penetration. It is primarily effective against gram-negative organisms but is associated with significant pain on application (with partial-thickness burns). It can cause carbonic anhydrase inhibition, resulting in metabolic acidosis. It is indicated for burn wounds with invasive infection, electrical burns, heavy *Pseudomonas* growth, and ear burns because of its penetration into cartilage.

V. OPERATIVE MANAGEMENT

A. Excision

1. Full-thickness burns require excision and coverage with autograft or skin substitute (see below).
2. Excision of full-thickness burns is considered when the patient's condition has stabilized from resuscitation.
3. Early excision of full-thickness burns reduces the length of stay in the intensive care unit and hospital and decreases the stress response.
4. Burn wounds are excised by either tangential excision (sequential shaving of nonviable tissue leaving a viable wound bed) or full-thickness fascial excision.
5. Extent of each burn excision is generally limited to < 20% TBSA, particularly because of the large blood loss associated with tangential excision.
6. Intraoperative blood loss can be decreased by subcutaneous infiltration (clysis) of both the burn and the graft donor site with neosynephrine and/or extremity tourniquets. The neosynephrine clysis solution is made by adding 30 mg (3 vials of 10 mg/mL 1% neosynephrine solution) to 1 liter of Ringer's lactate.
7. Excision of the burn wound to the level of fascia with electrocautery minimizes blood loss but leaves a poor cosmetic result.

B. Dressings

1. Freshly excised and grafted areas are dressed with topical antimicrobial ointment and fine mesh gauze.
2. Autograft is preferred for wound coverage. Skin substitutes are used as temporary or permanent coverage when autograft is not available. Temporary biologic dressings include homograft, xenograft (porcine),

Biobrane, and Transcyte. More permanent skin substitutes include Alloderm, Integra, and cultured epithelial autografts.
3. Operative dressings are removed on postoperative day 3. The fine mesh gauze immediately adjacent to the grafted area is left in place until postoperative day 4. The wound should continue to be dressed with fine mesh gauze impregnated with topical antimicrobial ointment until epithelialization is completed.
4. Vacuum-assisted wound devices are not routinely required. However, these can be employed as a postoperative wound dressing for difficult wounds. It should be removed on postoperative day 3, 4 or 5, and normal burn graft care should continue as outlined above.

C. Physical therapy
1. Grafted joints are exercised on postoperative day 5.
2. Ambulation is restricted in those patients who have wounds that are grafted above the knee until postoperative day 2, 3, or 4 (after operative dressings are removed). In patients with grafts below the knee, ambulation is restricted until postoperative day 3 to 10, depending on clinical status.
3. Patients with grafts above the waistline ambulate on postoperative day 1.

VI. NUTRITION

A. Metabolism
1. The metabolic rate rises in proportion to the extent of the injury and may reach levels twice those of normal individuals.
2. Post-burn hypermetabolism is manifested by increased oxygen consumption, elevated cardiac output and minute ventilation, increased core body temperature, wasting of body mass, and increased urinary nitrogen excretion.

B. Requirements
1. Protein requirements are calculated at 1.5 g/kg of protein per day.
2. The required ratio for nonprotein calories to grams of nitrogen is 150:1.
3. Nutrition requirements can be calculated by using the Harris-Benedict equation to calculate basal energy expenditure (BEE). Recommended nutritional needs are derived by multiplying the BEE by 2.
4. Nutritional support is begun immediately after resuscitation. This may be given in the form of oral diet or nasogastric/nasojejunal tube feeds. Enteral feeding is used in all patients with a functional gastrointestinal tract.

C. Pharmacology
1. The addition of oxandrolone (0.1 mg/kg orally twice daily) has an anabolic effect in burn patients and has been shown to decrease length of stay in adult burns > 20% TBSA.
2. Propanolol (0.33 mg/kg orally every 4 hours) in children with burns > 40% TBSA has been shown to reduce catabolic muscle wasting.

VII. COMPLICATIONS OF BURN INJURY

A. Pneumonia
1. Pneumonia is the most common infection in the burn patient. It is most commonly seen 3 to 5 days after an inhalation injury.
2. Diagnosis is made on the basis of a new infiltrate on chest radiograph, leukocytosis, and increased tracheal secretions.
3. Bronchoalveolar lavage specimens identify organisms and help direct antimicrobial therapy.
4. Treatment consists of ventilatory support when indicated, pulmonary toilet, and broad-spectrum antibiotics that are narrowed based on the identification and sensitivities of the organism.

B. Burn wound infection
1. Bacterial wound infections have dramatically decreased in severity and incidence over the past decade. They can cause a broad spectrum of complications, however, such as conversion to a full-thickness burn, discoloration of the wound, or hemorrhage/slough of eschar.
2. Most burn wounds become colonized. Some become locally infected, causing cellulitis, and a few cause systemic infection and overt sepsis.
3. The use of topical antimicrobial agents and early excision reduce the complications of bacterial invasion.
4. Quantitative wound cultures differentiate between colonization and infection.
5. Cultures yielding more than 1×10^5 organisms per gram of tissue indicate burn wound sepsis.
6. Treatment includes wound excision, change in topical antimicrobials, and systemic broad-spectrum antibiotics.

C. Gastrointestinal ulceration
1. Curling's ulcers are acute ulcerations of the upper gastrointestinal tract.
2. On endoscopy, they can present as either diffuse gastritis or as punctate, well-demarcated lesions in either the gastric or duodenal mucosa.
3. Its incidence is directly related to burn size and the presence of septic complications.
4. Appropriate prophylaxis with antacids or H_2 blockers have made stress ulcers virtually nonexistent.

D. Ileus
1. Patients with large burns frequently develop intestinal dysmotility.
2. Other causes include sepsis, pancreatitis, colonic pseudo-obstruction, diabetes, mesenteric ischemia, intra-abdominal sepsis, and electrolyte abnormalities.
3. Ileus is managed expectantly by decompression with a nasogastric tube and use of prokinetic agents.

E. Wound complications
1. Hyperpigmentation and hypopigmentation are common following burn injury.

2. Hyperpigmentation can be reduced by avoiding exposure to sunlight during the first year following the burn.
3. Hypertrophic scars benefit from compression garments, and keloids may benefit from steroid injection.
4. Prolonged treatment of scars is accomplished in consultation with a plastic surgeon and rehabilitation specialist.
5. Joint contractures are common where scars cross the joint surface. These are initially managed nonoperatively by aggressive physical therapy, including active and passive motion exercises. Casting can also help to prevent contractures.
6. When this fails, operative tissue contracture releases, with or without skin grafting, improve outcome.
7. Chronic burn wounds that take several years to heal may rarely develop squamous cell cancer (Marjolin's ulcer). Nonhealing ulcers should undergo biopsy.

VIII. ELECTRICAL BURNS

A. Characterization
1. Electrical burns are characterized by both cutaneous burns and deep muscle damage.
2. Mortality is dependent on burn size, associated trauma, and degree of muscle tissue damage.
3. Contact wounds may appear deceptively small even when extensive deep tissue damage may be present.
4. Approximately 14% of patients with electrical injuries have associated traumatic injuries requiring treatment.

B. High voltage/low voltage
1. Electrical injuries cause 1,000 deaths per year in the United States, and 50% of these are caused by low-voltage injuries.
2. High-voltage trauma (>1,000 V, usually from outside power lines) causes sudden, violent muscle contraction.
3. Low-voltage trauma (< 1,000 V, often caused by household current) can cause tetany, which can prolong exposure to the current.
4. Lightning strikes often have minimal cutaneous injury and secondary arc burns from metal objects on the patient at the time of injury.

C. Cardiac abnormalities
1. These are usually evident during evaluation in the emergency department.
2. Most arrhythmias are transient, and therapy is unnecessary in the absence of hemodynamic instability.
3. Observation in a telemetry or intensive care unit is mandatory for patients with loss of consciousness, arrhythmia, or electrocardiographic abnormality other than sinus bradycardia or sinus tachycardia, arrest in the field, or in a patient with a large enough cutaneous burn that would require monitoring.

D. Fluid resuscitation
1. Additional fluid resuscitation is anticipated in electrical injuries because of the underlying damage to muscle tissue.
2. The minimum fluid requirement for electrical injury is based on the size of the cutaneous injury (4 mL/kg/% TBSA burn).

E. Urine output
1. Urine output must be maintained between 0.5 and 1.0 mL/kg/hour.
2. If visible pigment (myoglobin or hemoglobin) is present, underlying muscle damage should be suspected. Urine output is maintained between 100 and 150 mL per hour until the urine is clear.
3. Prompt diuresis can be initiated by giving intravenous mannitol if gross pigment is present. The dose of intravenous mannitol is 0.25 to 0.5g/kg as a single intravenous bolus.
4. Two ampules of sodium bicarbonate may be given to alkalinize the urine if pigment is present.

F. Antimicrobial agents
1. Sulfamylon is the topical antimicrobial of choice for the deep contact point burns as a result of its broad antimicrobial spectrum and penetration of eschar.
2. Intravenous antibiotics effective against anaerobes and aerobes are given to patients with underlying devitalized muscle and are discontinued when debridement is completed.

G. Early excision
1. Early excision and surgical debridement are performed to decrease the incidence of infectious complications associated with retained nonviable muscle tissue.

H. Neurologic damage
1. Acute and chronic neurologic sequelae are often associated with high-voltage electrical injuries.
2. Repeat neurologic examinations should be performed to detect early or late neuropathology.
3. Early spinal cord deficits may be transient. However, those that appear late in the postinjury course are generally permanent.

I. Eyes
1. Early and late changes in the lenses (cataracts) may occur with electrical injury. Repeated bedside evaluations are used to evaluate visual changes. Fundoscopic and slit-lamp examination may also reveal changes.

J. Lightning injuries
1. Cutaneous thermal injuries caused by lightning may have unique serpiginous or arborizing patterns caused by the spread of the current in the skin.
2. Following a lightning strike, death may be caused by either cardiac arrhythmia or apnea.
3. Cardiopulmonary resuscitation and basic life support are initiated immediately.
4. Further care of lightning burn injuries is accomplished in the same manner as for a thermal injury.

5. Lightning injuries can cause significant extremity vasospasm, and the extremity may appear cyanotic, cold, and pulseless. However, this usually resolves spontaneously and completely within several hours.
6. Deep tissue injury or significant burn is rarely present.
7. Perforated ear drums may result from lightning injury.

IX. CHEMICAL BURNS

A. Tissue damage
1. A major problem with chemical burns is the failure to recognize and treat ongoing destruction of tissue.
2. The most important factor in the initial management of a chemical burn is dilution with copious amounts of water.
3. Neutralization of the chemical itself is not indicated as the exothermic chemical reaction can cause further tissue loss.

B. Treatment
1. Treatment includes removal of all clothing and bedding and immediate copious water lavage for at least 15 minutes, which is continued in the emergency department for a total of 2 hours using mild soap and running tap water.
2. Hydrofluoric acid (HF) is a unique chemical that causes severe burns and underlying tissue damage.
   a. HF binds to calcium in the tissues.
   b. HF is neutralized with calcium gluconate used topically, infused locally, and/or given as an intravenous or intra-arterial solution depending on the extent of the burn. Calcium carbonate or calcium chloride may also be used.
3. Universal precautions are used to protect medical personnel from chemical exposure.

X. COLD INJURY

A. Characterization
1. Freezing injuries (frostbite)
2. Nonfreezing cold injuries (immersion foot, trench foot)
3. Generalized hypothermia

B. Frostbite/cold injuries
1. Mechanisms that rapidly cause frostbite, such as contact with cold metal, cause direct cell freezing with resultant cellular destruction. Slower mechanisms of frostbite cause freezing of extracellular water with resultant cellular dehydration. Both injuries are treated in the same manner.
2. First-degree frostbite causes pallor, followed by hyperemia and edema of the skin without necrosis.
3. Second-degree frostbite causes hyperemia and vesicle formation with partial-thickness necrosis of the skin.

4. Third-degree frostbite results in full-thickness necrosis of the skin and extends to a variable degree to the underlying subcutaneous tissue.
5. Fourth-degree frostbite causes full-thickness skin necrosis and necrosis of underlying structures.
6. Accurate assessment of tissue loss may not be possible for weeks to months following cold injury.

C. Treatment of cold injuries
1. Treatment of frostbite should begin as soon as possible, including general warming of the patient.
2. Rapid rewarming of the frozen area is the single most important maneuver for preserving potentially viable tissue. The frozen area is placed in water at 40°C with frequent addition of warm water to maintain a constant temperature.
3. Narcotics are required for pain control.
4. Injured extremities are elevated, blisters are protected, and wounds are exposed to air.
5. Since the assessment of tissue viability is difficult, surgical intervention is delayed until clear demarcation of nonviable tissue has occurred.
6. Treatment of immersion foot and trench foot, which occur at temperatures above freezing, is the same as above.

XI. PEDIATRIC BURNS

A. Incidence
1. Approximately one-third of burn unit admissions are children under the age of 15 years.
2. About 10% of pediatric burn injuries are a result of deliberate abuse by adults and another 10% to 20% are the result of negligence.

B. Skin.
Children have larger surface areas relative to body mass, and have larger heads and smaller legs than adults.

C. Maintenance fluids
1. In young children (< 2 years of age), nonburned maintenance fluids are 5 to 10 times those of an adult (per kg of body mass). Nonburned maintenance fluid volume must be added to these resuscitations.
2. The standard resuscitation fluid is Ringer's lactate. Calculated maintenance fluid volume is added as 5% dextrose in lactated Ringer's solution (D_5LR).
3. Stored glucose in the liver is depleted rapidly in children. Management requires frequent monitoring of serum glucose and appropriate use of dextrose-containing intravenous fluids.
4. After the first day, children are also sensitive to changes in sodium concentration, especially hyponatremia. Seizure activity may occur at sodium levels of 130 mEq/dL.
5. The best maintenance fluid is $D_5\frac{1}{4}NS$ (1 mL/kg/% TBSA plus nonburn maintenance).
6. Hypotonic oral intake is closely monitored and appropriate restrictions applied.

7. Burn depth and size estimations must be formally reviewed and updated on the second post-burn day.
8. If abuse is suspected, skull radiographs and long-bone series ("baby-gram") are obtained on arrival in the emergency department.
9. All infants and children with burns >20% TBSA must have body temperature carefully monitored and maintained.
10. When indicated, nasotracheal intubation is the method of choice.
    a. Pediatric endotracheal and tracheostomy tubes do not have a cuff until the internal diameter reaches 5 mm.
    b. The general rule is that the size of the tube should be the same as the size of the tip of the patient's fifth finger. The following formula may also be used for endotracheal tube size: $(16 + age)/4$.
    c. The small internal diameter of the endotracheal tubes increases the risk of obstruction by secretions (mucus plugging).
11. All children receive Nystatin drops orally since they are at risk for immunosuppression and resultant thrush.

XII. SUGGESTED READINGS

Greenbaum AR, Horton JB, Williams CJ, et al: Burn injuries inflicted on children or the elderly: A framework for clinical and forensic assessment. Plast Reconstr Surg 118(2):46e-58e, 2006.

Salinas J, Drew G, Gallagher J, et al: Closed-loop and decision-assist resuscitation of burn patients. J Trauma 64(4 Suppl):S321-332, 2008.

Traber DL, Maybauer MO, Maybauer DM, et al: Inhalational and acute lung injury. Shock 24(1): 82-87, 2005.

White CE, Renz EM: Advances in surgical care: Management of severe burn injury. Crit Care Med 36(7):S318-24, 2008.

Principles of Fractures and Dislocations

Richard M. Gillespie, MD, and Joshua L. Gary, MD

I. INITIAL MANAGEMENT OF FRACTURES

A. **Examination of the patient** for orthopaedic injury is most appropriately performed during the secondary survey. Elements include a thorough musculoskeletal examination as well as evaluation of the neurovascular system in all extremities. Fractures of the small bones, including those in the hands and feet, are most commonly missed in the acute setting. Signs and symptoms that should alert the clinician to the possibility of fracture or dislocation include the following:
1. Pain
2. Deformity, angulation, shortening, rotation
3. Swelling
4. Diminished range of motion or pain and crepitus on motion
5. Abnormal vascular or neurologic examination
6. Lacerations or other soft tissue injury

Any positive findings should be pursued further with radiologic studies.

B. **Radiographic examination of fractures and dislocations**
1. Orthogonal views of the injured site should be obtained, which usually consist of at least an anteroposterior and a lateral film. These views should also include the joints above and below the site of concern.
2. Certain fractures require additional radiographs as well as other radiologic studies to better define the pattern of fracture and to assist in preoperative planning.
   a. Oblique views help define injuries at joints (e.g., Judet views of the acetabulum, inlet/outlet views of the pelvic ring, Y view of the scapula, and axillary lateral view to evaluate for shoulder dislocation).
   b. Computerized tomography (CT) scans have become the standard of care at Parkland Memorial Hospital for examining fractures at articular surfaces or areas difficult to evaluate with plain radiographs. Examples include the acetabulum, tibial plateau, scapula, pelvic ring, and especially the spine.
   c. "Dynamic" or "stress "studies can be helpful in identifying ligamentous injury by showing abnormal bony translation, but they are rarely used in the acute setting.
   d. Magnetic resonance imaging (MRI) offers views of the soft tissues and aids in the diagnosis of ligament or tendon rupture, but in the acute trauma setting MRI is most appropriate for evaluation of the spinal cord injury.

C. **Intervention in the emergency department**
1. **Open fracture wounds should be cleared of gross contaminants.** However, no bony fragments should ever be removed. Definitive washout is done in the operating room concurrently with fixation. Cover the wound with a sterile dressing and administer cefazolin for all open fractures with

the addition of gentamicin for grade III fractures or heavily contaminated wounds. Make sure the patient is protected against tetanus.
2. **Acute reduction of the fracture** should be performed in the emergency department. This reduces the risk of skin necrosis and diminishes pressure on nerves and vessels. Always obtain postreduction radiographs and document a neurovascular examination after manipulation of any injured extremity. Traction splints are used for lower extremity fractures.
3. **Splinting of the extremity** prevents further soft tissue injury and alleviates pain. Splinting also allows for transportation of the patient.

II. DEFINITIVE MANAGEMENT OF FRACTURES AND DISLOCATIONS

A. The goal of treatment of fractures and dislocations should be the rapid return of normal function, with minimal morbidity. Early definitive management (within 24 hours) of orthopaedic injuries has been shown to decrease morbidity and mortality in the patient with multiple traumatic injuries.
B. Reduction is the restoration of normal alignment of bone and joint and can be accomplished by *closed* or *open* methods, with the goal being anatomic alignment.
1. Closed reduction is manipulation of a bone or joint to restore normal alignment without opening the skin.
2. Open reduction is manipulation of a bone or joint through an incision to restore normal alignment.
C. Immobilization maintains reduction and allows healing. There are many ways to immobilize fractures.
1. **Traction and/or bedrest** is probably the oldest form of fracture treatment. Traction can be applied through Steinmann pins placed directly into bone ("skeletal traction") or through devices applied to the skin ("skin traction"), such as Buck's traction of the heel. Advantages of traction include its ease of application and the lack of need for a surgical procedure. Disadvantages include the inability to maintain reduction, as well as rotational, length, or angular deformities. Most importantly, lengthy bedrest can lead to morbidities such as deconditioning, bedsores, and contractures and increases the risk of deep venous thrombosis and pulmonary complications. Traction is most often used at Parkland Memorial Hospital in the period between presentation and definitive management to prevent shortening of the affected limb in acetabular and femur fractures.
2. **Splints ("half-casts")**. These maintain reduction while allowing for swelling around the fracture to subside and help prevent a compartment syndrome. Splints are normally used as a temporary form of immobilization, until soft tissue swelling has subsided and a cast can be placed.

3. **Casts**. Circumferential casts are made of plaster or fiberglass. They are a reliable way to maintain reduction in many fractures. Potential complications include loss of reduction and pressure sores. At Parkland Memorial Hospital, casts are usually applied after a period of splinting, usually after 1 to 2 weeks, often in an outpatient setting. Proper casting is difficult and should be performed by experienced persons.
4. **Cast braces**. These are "hinged casts" that allow for motion at a joint while maintaining reduction. They are commonly used in conjunction with limited internal fixation of articular fractures.
5. **External fixation**. Pins are placed into the bone proximal and distal to the fracture site and attached to external bars to maintain reduction. External fixations are advantageous because they can be rapidly applied and can be placed without disturbing the fracture site. They can be both temporary and definitive treatment of an acute fracture or dislocation. They can stabilize fractures where internal fixation is precluded because of soft tissue loss or in the patient who is too unstable to undergo longer operations. Disadvantages include the potential for pin tract infections, osteomyelitis at the pin sites, and loss of reduction due to instability of the external fixation.
6. **Internal fixation**. Any implanted device used to maintain reduction is a form of internal fixation. These include pins, screws, plates, rods, and bioabsorbable implants. The advantages of internal fixation include its stable and precise restoration of normal anatomy, often under direct visualization. This is especially important in articular fractures where greater than 1 mm of step-off significantly increases the risk of post-traumatic arthritis. It also allows early mobilization and limits the need for external immobilization. Disadvantages include the risk of infection, the risk of implant failure, patient discomfort, and damage to the surrounding soft tissues caused by the surgical dissection. Extensive periosteal stripping during internal fixation decreases blood supply to the bone and can delay fracture healing and increase the risk of avascular necrosis. Hardware infection, when it occurs, is a serious complication that often requires long-term antibiotics and further surgical interventions.

III. SUGGESTED READINGS

Bosse MJ, MacKenzie EJ, Kellam JF, et al: A prospective evaluation of the clinical utility lower-extremity injury-severity scores. J Bone Joint Surg (Am) 83-A(1):3-14, 2001.

Petrisor BA, Poolman R, Koval K, et al: Evidence-Based Orthopaedic Trauma Working Group: Management of displaced ankle fractures. J Orthop Trauma 20(7):515-518, 2006.

Scalea TM, Boswell SA, Scott JD, et al: External fixation as a bridge to intramedullary nailing for patients with multiple injuries and with femur fractures: Damage control orthopedics. J Trauma 48(4):613-621, 2000.

Complications of Musculoskeletal Trauma

Lee Ann Lau, MD

I. THROMBOEMBOLIC DISEASE

A. Thromboembolic disease is a common complication in trauma patients, occurring in up to 80% if no prophylaxis is used. This is because trauma patients often have all components of Virchow's triad (stasis, venous injury, and hypercoaguable state). The risk of pulmonary embolus (PE) after development of deep vein thrombosis is approximately 1%.

B. Risk factors for thromboembolic disease
1. Trauma patients are at high risk for deep vein thrombosis (DVT), especially with multiple injuries, long bone fractures, or pelvic fractures
2. Age > 40 years
3. Head and spine injuries
4. Obesity
5. Immobilization
6. Prior thromboembolic disease or malignancy
7. Blood transfusion
8. Additional iatrogenic risks such as mechanical ventilation, immobility, femoral venous catheters, and medication administration (especially sedatives and paralytics)

C. Prevention of deep venous thrombosis
1. **All** trauma patients receive some form of prophylaxis.
2. Pneumatic compression devices (calf length or foot pumps) are used. Pneumatic devices can be used on injured extremities, and foot pumps should be placed prior to casting/splinting when possible. Calf-length pumps are the device of choice at Parkland Memorial Hospital.
3. Prophylactic low–molecular weight heparin (LMVH) is used in most trauma patients. The current regimen is 30 mg subcutaneously twice a day.
4. Active mobilization is begun as soon as possible.

D. Diagnosis of DVT
1. Clinical signs are notoriously unreliable and up to 80% of DVTs are asymptomatic. Clinical symptoms may include calf pain, swelling, tachycardia, and low-grade fever. The classic Homan's sign (calf pain with passive stretch) is neither sensitive nor specific.
2. Ultrasound is useful in detecting thigh vein thrombosis and has about a 90% accuracy rate. Patients hospitalized in the intensive care unit for prolonged periods (greater than 1 week) undergo weekly ultrasound DVT screening.
3. Venography is the gold standard of DVT detection. It is highly accurate but carries the risk of allergic reaction to the contrast agent or

thrombosis at the injection site. It also requires a radiologist to perform the test and is not commonly used at Parkland Memorial Hospital.
4. Magnetic resonance venography, impedance plethysmography, and radioactive iodine-labeled fibrinogen are not used at Parkland Memorial Hospital to screen for DVT.

E. Diagnosis of pulmonary embolus (PE)

1. Clinical symptoms can be nonspecific and/or absent. Sudden death can be the presenting sign. The classic description of hemoptysis is only seen in 10% to 15% of patients. Dyspnea, shortness of breath, chest pain, or chest "tightness" is often seen. Hypotension and tachycardia are often present. Mild hypoxia, diminished Pao_2, and an Aa gradient can be present. Electrocardiogram findings can include right axis deviation but are often nonspecific ($S_1Q_3T_3$ is described). Chest radiograph may show Westermark sign (hyperlucency due to arterial occlusion) but most commonly only shows atelectasis.
2. Ventilation/perfusion (VQ) scans can be useful in some patients. However, a scan that is read as "intermediate or low probability for PE" still leaves the question unanswered with a 15% to 85% chance of PE. VQ scans are confounded by cardiopulmonary disease and must be interpreted with a pre-test index of suspicion.
3. The helical CTA scan is used almost exclusively at Parkland Memorial Hospital and is 70% sensitive and 90% specific. It will generally detect most clinically significant pulmonary emboli.
4. Pulmonary arteriogram is the gold standard but is associated with higher costs and risks than other tests.

F. Treatment of thromboembolic disease

1. **Deep venous thrombosis**. Once diagnosed, treatment is anticoagulation with a weight-based heparin infusion protocol. This is followed with oral coumadin treatment with a therapeutic INR goal of 1.5 to 2 times normal for 3 to 6 months. For patients requiring surgery, the heparin drip can be stopped 6 hours prior to surgery.
2. **Pulmonary embolus**. Once diagnosed, it should be treated with anticoagulation in the same fashion as DVT. Care in the intensive care unit is generally indicated, and ventilatory and hemodynamic support may be required. There are isolated reports of surgical removal of massive emboli; however, this is rarely done at Parkland Memorial Hospital.
3. **IVC filters**
   a. Indications
      i. Contraindication to anticoagulation in patients with pulmonary embolus or DVT (i.e., head injury, gastrointestinal bleeding, nonoperative management of solid organ injuries)
      ii. Recurrent pulmonary embolus despite anticoagulation
      iii. Free-floating thrombus in the iliac or inferior vena cava
      iv. Patients requiring multiple surgeries

b. Complications
   i. Venous insufficiency (30%)
   ii. Venous ulcers (10%)
   iii. Filter migration (30% to 50%)
   iv. Inferior vena cava (IVC) obstruction (5%)
   v. Mortality (0.12%)
c. Due to the long-term complications associated with IVC filters, retrievable filters are now being used in trauma patients. Data regarding the time to retrieval is still evolving but is currently as long as 1.5 years for certain brands.

II. COMPARTMENT SYNDROME

A. Definition. Compartment syndrome is a condition that arises when the pressure within a closed compartment becomes high enough to compromise capillary flow. Necrosis of nerves, muscles, vessels, and all other tissues will ensue if the pressure is not alleviated.

B. Causes of compartment syndrome
1. Fractures (tibia most common in adults, supracondylar humerus in children)
2. Arterial injury
3. Crush injury to soft tissues
4. Circumferential burns
5. Prolonged compression of a limb (even without obvious crush injury, as may occur when a patient is found down from drug or alcohol overdose)
6. Combined arterial and venous injuries
7. Delay between injury and repair
8. Reperfusion

C. Diagnosis of compartment syndrome
1. Clinical findings are the best guide.
   a. Tight compartment
   b. Pain is the earliest and most reliable symptom. Pain on passive stretch of muscles and pain out of proportion to the injury are hallmarks.
   c. Paresthesia is sometimes present early but later progresses to complete lack of sensation with nerve necrosis.
   d. Paralysis is a late finding.
   e. Pallor is a late finding.
   f. Pulselessness is a late finding as systolic arterial pressure is usually much higher than compartment pressures.
2. Compartment pressure monitors can be used in patients who have altered mental status or to assist with the diagnosis (Figure 37-1). If the compartment pressure is greater than 30 mm Hg or within 20 to 30 mm Hg of the diastolic blood pressure, treatment is warranted (see below).

D. Treatment of compartment syndrome
1. Compartment syndrome is a limb-threatening emergency and if present, fasciotomy should be performed immediately. The tissue viability should

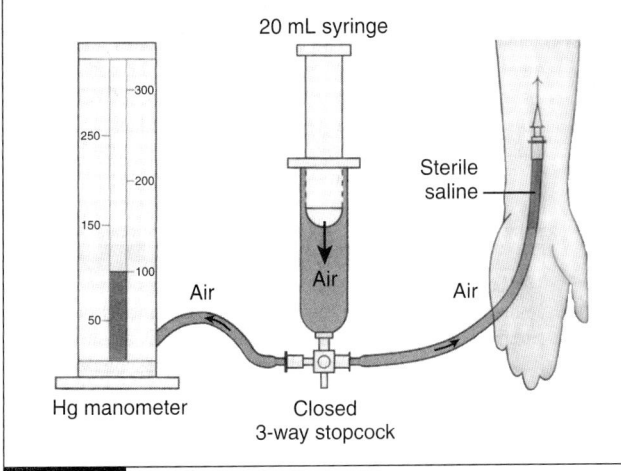

FIGURE 37-1

Whitesides' method of measuring tissue pressures. The three-way stopcock is open to the 20-mL syringe and to both extension tubes. The pressure within the closed compartment is overcome by injecting a minute quantity of saline, and the pressure required to do this is read on the mercury manometer.

be assessed at fasciotomy and any necrotic tissue should be debrided. The wounds are packed with moist gauze and can be closed in a delayed fashion as the edema resolves (usually in 3 to 5 days). Skin grafting is occasionally necessary to cover fasciotomy wounds.

2. **Technique: lower leg (two incision technique)** (Figure 37-2)
   a. The anterior and lateral compartments are released through a generous lateral incision midway between the tibia crest and fibula (Figure 37-3A). The septum between the anterior and lateral compartments is identified, and the fasciae comprising the two compartments are incised from the knee to the ankle using Metzenbaum scissors. The superficial peroneal nerve crosses through the lateral compartment's fascia at the junction of the middle and distal third of the leg and should be protected. The anterior skin flap is undermined to release the anterior compartment.
   b. The deep and superficial posterior compartments are approached through a generous medial incision about 3 cm posterior to the tibial posteromedial edge (Figure 37-3B). The saphenous nerve and vein are protected by anterior retraction while the superficial compartment's fascia is incised from the knee to the ankle. The deep posterior compartment is decompressed by taking the soleus off its origin on the proximal third of the tibia.

II. Compartment Syndrome

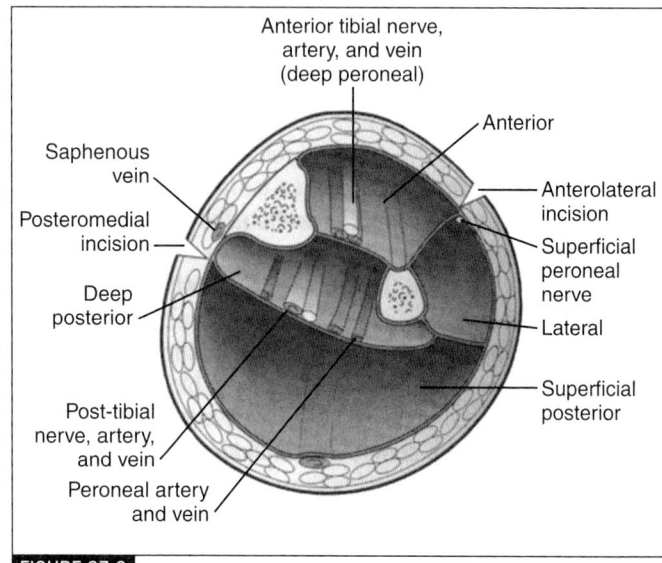

FIGURE 37-2

Fascial compartments of the leg.

3. **Technique: forearm**
   a. There are four compartments in the forearm: superficial and deep volar, dorsal, and mobile wad (Figure 37-4). A volar incision is made to decompress the volar and mobile wad compartments. It begins 2 cm proximal to the medial epicondyle and courses obliquely across the antecubital fossa to the radial side of the forearm. The incision is carried distally, and the fascia of the flexor compartment is incised longitudinally using scissors. The wrist should be crossed obliquely, and a flap of skin should be left to cover the median nerve after carpal tunnel release (Figure 37-5).
   b. A dorsal incision is made straight down the middle of the dorsal compartment of the forearm, and the underlying fascia is incised in line with the skin incision (Figures 37-6 and 37-7).
4. **Technique: thigh**
   a. The anterior and posterior compartments are decompressed first via a lateral incision from the intertrochanteric line to the lateral epicondyle. The incision is carried through the iliotibial band. The vastus lateralis is reflected off the lateral intermuscular septum. The lateral intermuscular septum is then incised for the length of the incision.
   b. The adductor compartment pressures are then checked medially; decompression of this compartment is often not necessary after the

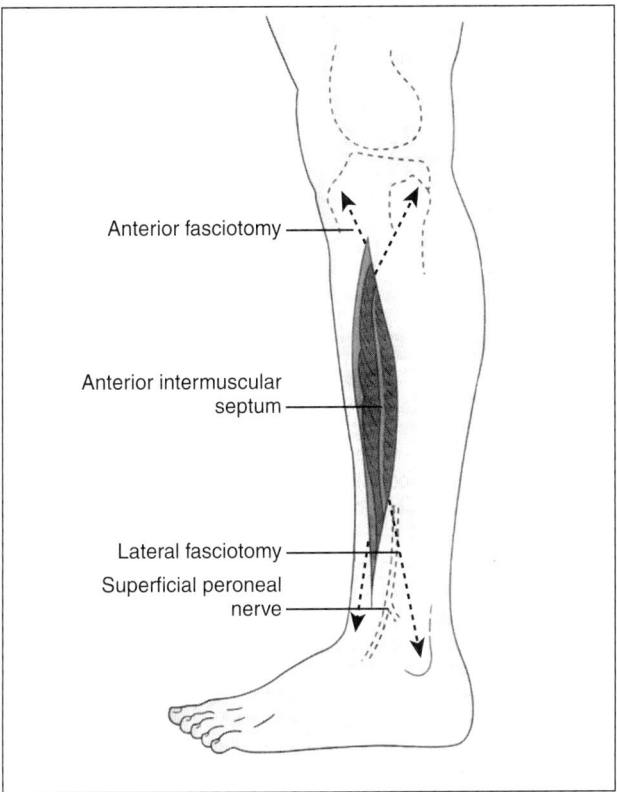

FIGURE 37-3A

An anterolateral skin incision is used to approach the anterior or lateral compartments. The incision is made halfway between the fibular shaft and the tibial crest. This is approximately over the anterior intermuscular septum, dividing the anterior and lateral compartments, and allows easy access to both. The length of the skin incision should extend the length of the compartments of the leg, unless intracompartmental pressures are monitored intraoperatively, in which case a small skin incision can be used.

anterior and posterior compartments are decompressed. Should pressures remain elevated, a medial incision is made over the adductor.

III. FAT EMBOLISM SYNDROME

A. Definition. Fat embolism is a deposition of fatty elements from the marrow of an injured bone into the blood stream. This may also occur with intravasation of fat from abdominal trauma. Fat embolism

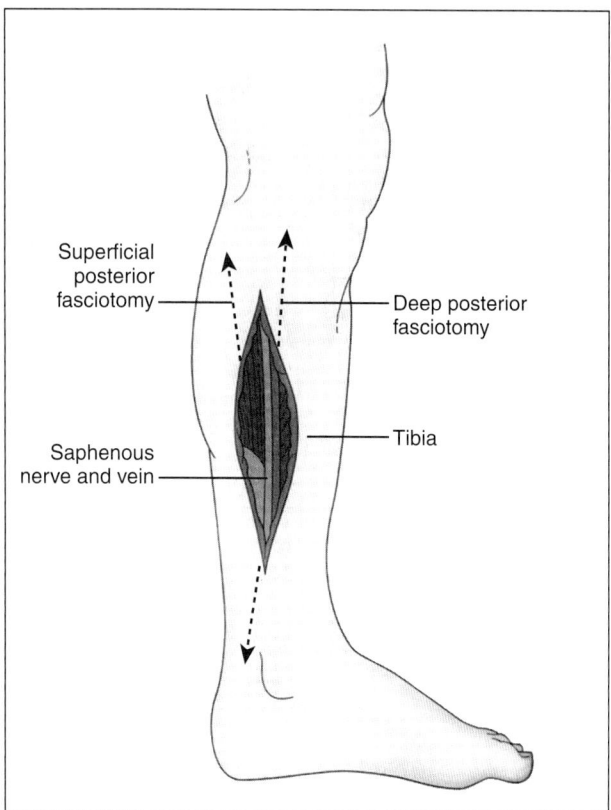

FIGURE 37-3B

A posteromedial incision is used for an approach to the superficial or deep posterior compartments. The incision is slightly distal to the previous incision and 2 cm posterior to the posterior tibial margin. By making the incision at this location, injury to the saphenous nerve and vein, which run along the posterior margin of the tibia in this area, is avoided.

syndrome is a triad of pulmonary distress, mental status changes, and a rash. It occurs when fat embolizes to lung capillaries, leading to ischemia and inflammation with increased pulmonary capillary permeability and respiratory compromise. Fat embolism is not isolated to trauma patients. The pathogenesis of the disorder is still poorly understood, but it usually occurs 24 to 48 hours after injury and is associated with 10% to 20% mortality.

- **B. Diagnosis.** Fat embolism syndrome is a diagnosis of exclusion. Other causes of respiratory compromise must first be ruled out. The symptoms are often nonspecific.
1. Shortness of breath with arterial hypoxemia (75%)
2. Restlessness/irritability
3. Confusion, disorientation, and occasionally frank coma
4. Fever to 39°C
5. Tachycardia, tachypnea
6. Nonblanching petechia on the chest, axilla, neck, and conjunctivae, which usually fades rapidly (50%)
7. Chest radiographs show "snowstorm" pulmonary infiltrates, which worsen with the patient's condition and can progress to acute respiratory distress syndrome.
- **C. Treatment.** Since the pathophysiology of fat embolism syndrome is poorly understood, the treatments described in the literature are often nonspecific and supportive in nature.
1. Oxygen should be administered immediately.
2. Intravenous fluids are given as needed.
3. Intubation and mechanical ventilation may be necessary (10%).
4. Ethanol, heparin, hypertonic glucose, and corticosteroids have all been described in the treatment of fat embolism syndrome; however, they are not used at Parkland Memorial Hospital.
- **D. Prevention.** It has consistently been shown that early (< 24 hours) stabilization of long bone fractures in multiply injured patients prevents pulmonary complications, including fat embolism syndrome. Prevention through early stabilization remains the primary method of combating fat embolism at Parkland.

IV. RHABDOMYOLYSIS

- **A. Definition.** Rhabdomyolysis is the release of myoglobin into the circulation after muscle breakdown occurs. Trauma, especially crush injuries, compartment syndrome, arterial occlusion, and electrical burns, can cause rhabdomyolysis. Other causes include sepsis (due to decreased perfusion), seizures, prolonged immobilization, inherited metabolic abnormalities, drugs (both prescribed and illicit), and heat stroke. The myoglobin and its breakdown products cause acute renal failure via acute tubular necrosis.
- **B. Diagnosis.** High clinical suspicion is necessary.
1. Muscle pain and weakness (50% of patients)
2. Dark-colored urine (75% of patients)
3. Hypocalcemia and hyperkalemia
4. Elevated creatine kinase levels (most commonly used), elevated serum and urine myoglobin (not tested frequently)
5. Acute renal failure (occurs in ~30% of patients)

298 IV. Rhabdomyolysis

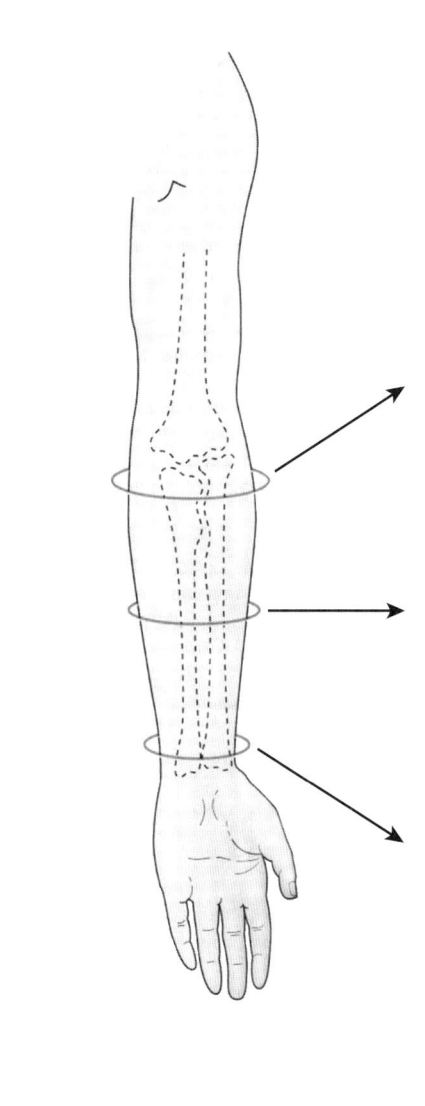

FIGURE 37-4

Forearm compartments: transverse sections through the left forearm at various levels.

Extensor carpi ulnaris muscle
Radius
Supinator muscle
Extensor digitorum muscle
Extensor carpi radialis brevis muscle
Ulna
Brachial vein
Flexor carpi radialis, palmaris longus, and flexor digitorum superficialis muscle bundle
Radial nerve (profundus)
Extensor carpi radialis longus muscle
Radial nerve (superficialis)
Radial vein
Median nerve
Medial cubital vein
Ulnar artery, vein, nerve
Posterior interosseous artery, vein, nerve
Extensor carpi ulnaris muscle
Extensor digitorum muscle
Extensor digitorum (comm) muscle
Flexor digitorum profundus muscle
Extensor carpi radialis brevis and longus muscle
Ulnar artery, vein, nerve
Pronator teres muscle
Flexor carpi ulnaris muscle
Brachioradialis muscle
Palmaris longus muscle
Radial artery, vein, nerve
Median artery, vein, nerve
Brachiocephalic vein
Flexor carpi radialis muscle
Flexor pollicis longus muscle
Extensor carpi radialis longus and brevis muscle
Extensor carpi ulnaris muscle
Antebrachial cephalic vein
Pronator quadratus muscle
Flexor carpi ulnaris muscle
Radial artery, vein, nerve
Flexor carpi radialis muscle
Ulnar nerve
Ulnar artery
Median nerve

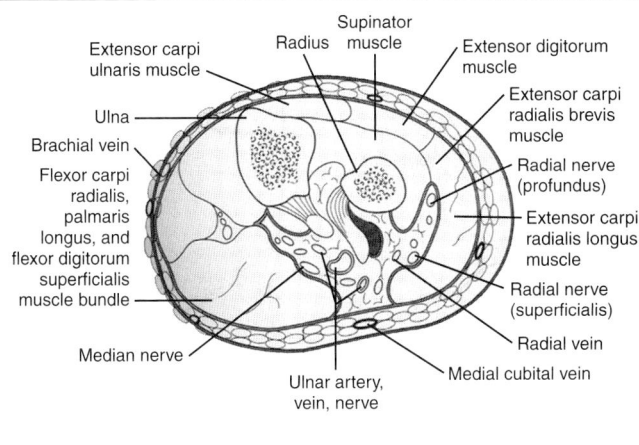

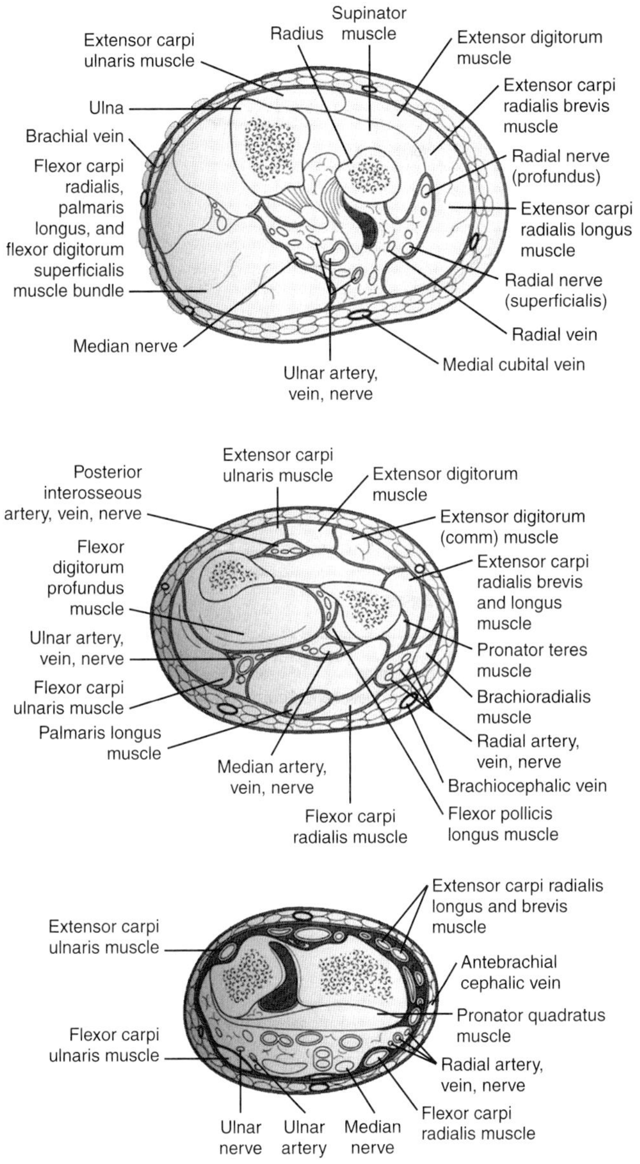

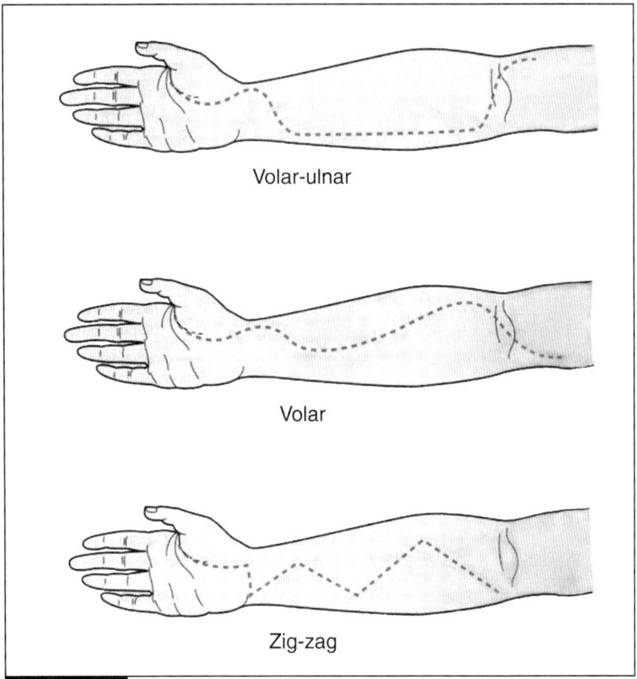

FIGURE 37-5
Various skin incisions used for performing a volar forearm fasciotomy.

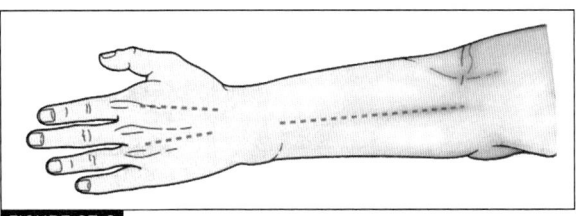

FIGURE 37-6
To decompress the dorsal and mobile wad compartments, straight incisions are done because fewer veins will be damaged.

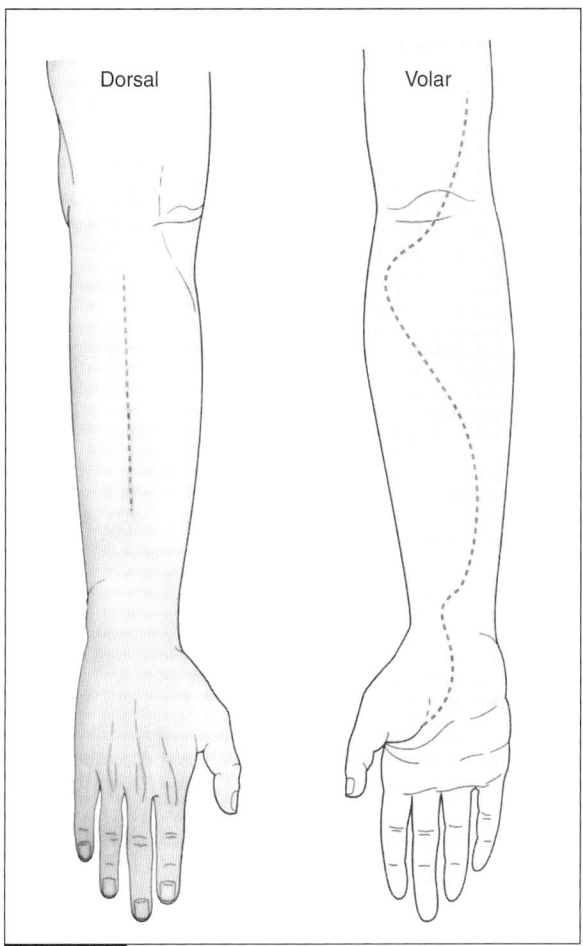

FIGURE 37-7

The dorsal and curvilinear volar incisions used for forearm decompression. The curvilinear volar incision is preferred because of the exposure afforded to major nerves, brachial artery, and mobile wad.

6. Urine dip positive for blood but without red blood cells (50% of patients)
7. Fever, tachycardia, and malaise can also be seen.

C. Treatment

1. Reversal of the underlying cause of muscle death if possible (i.e., restore perfusion, relieve compartment syndrome, etc)

2. Aggressive debridement of any necrotic tissue
3. Aggressive intravenous fluid administration with a goal urine output of 100 mL/hour or greater (may require many liters of intravenous fluid)
4. Treatment of hyperkalemia and renal failure often requires dialysis.
5. Alkalinization of the urine and treatment with mannitol/diuretics are commonly described in the literature, but this treatment has not conclusively been shown to improve morbidity or mortality. They are used at Parkland Memorial Hospital.
6. Renal failure usually resolves with time, even when hemodialysis is needed.

D. Other considerations with rhabdomyolysis
1. It is important to watch for side effects of electrolyte abnormalities with rhabdomyolysis, especially cardiac arrhythmias.
2. During fluid resuscitation, watch for compartment syndrome in injured and uninjured limbs; fasciotomies may be necessary.

V. SUGGESTED READINGS

Craig S: Rhabdomyolysis. eMed J, December, 2004.

Geerts WH, Code KI, Jay RM, et al: A prospective study of venous thromboembolism after major trauma. N Engl J Med 331:1601-1606, 1994.

Parisi DM, Koval K, Egol K: Fat embolism syndrome: A review paper. Am J Orthop Sept:507-512, 2002.

Rahimtool A, Bergin JD: Acute pulmonary embolism: An update on diagnosis and management. Curr Probl Cardiol Feb:61-114, 2005.

Wallace SB, Smith DG: Compartment syndrome, lower extremity. eMed J 4(12), December, 2003.

Wallace SB, Smith DG: Compartment syndrome, upper extremity. eMed J 4(6), June, 2003.

Fractures of the Pelvis and Acetabulum

Arsalla Islam, MD, and Jarrod King, MD

I. FRACTURES OF THE PELVIS

A. Anatomy

1. **Musculoskeletal anatomy**. The pelvis is a ring, composed of the two innominate bones and the sacrum. Anteriorly, the symphysis pubis holds the two hemipelves together. The symphysis is composed of superior and inferior ligaments, with a disk-like fibrocartilage center. Posteriorly, the sacroiliac (SI) ligaments support the sacroiliac joints. The posterior SI ligaments are up to 1 inch thick and very strong, while the anterior SI ligaments are less strong. The strong sacrotuberous and sacrospinous ligaments prevent rotation of the innominate bone away from the sacrum.

2. **Soft tissue anatomy**
   a. **Vascular structures**. The internal iliac artery bifurcates at the pelvic brim into anterior and posterior branches. The anterior division gives off the obturator and internal pudendal arteries, and the posterior division gives off the superior and inferior gluteal arteries. Due to their positions, these arteries and the veins that run with them are at risk if the SI joint is disrupted. These vessels can be the source of significant bleeding in pelvic fractures.
   b. **Neurologic structures**. The lumbosacral plexus lies anterior to the SI joint. Its components, particularly the dorsal sacral nerve roots that make up the peroneal portion of the sciatic nerve, can be injured if the SI joint is disrupted.
   c. **Urologic structures**. The urethra and bladder are occasionally injured in pelvic fracture patients.

B. Evaluation

1. **Physical examination**. Forceful stressing of the pelvis to assess stability should be avoided. Pain at the symphseal region and at the sacrum should be noted. Blood at the urethral meatus or a high-riding prostate are indicators of urologic trauma. Rectal tears or perineal lacerations are indicators of an open pelvic fracture. Neurologic deficits in the legs must be ruled out. Most importantly, the ongoing hemodynamic status of the patient must be evaluated.

2. **Radiologic studies**
   a. **X-rays**. An anteroposterior (AP) view of the pelvis is included in the initial evaluation of all trauma patients. Hemorrhage from a pelvic fracture *can* be a source of hemodynamic instability. If pelvic films are not obtained, the source of bleeding may be missed. If the AP film shows any abnormality, *inlet* and *outlet* films are obtained. The *inlet* view shows the ring of the true pelvis and reveals the presence of injury

to the SI joints. The inlet view also reveals posterior displacement of the hemipelvis. The *outlet* view reveals cephalad displacement of the hemipelvis, and offers a good look at the sacral foramina.
   b. **Computed tomography** (CT). CT scans are obtained in all pelvic fracture patients. The CT confirms fractures seen on plain films and gives better information about the posterior pelvic ring. Sacral foraminal and SI joint injuries as well as iliac wing fractures (subtle on plain films) are seen well on CT.
 3. **Urologic studies** such as urethrograms or cystograms are performed as indicated (e.g., when there is gross hematuria, urinary obstruction, high-riding prostate gland, blood at the meatus, or perineal or scrotal hematomas).
C. **Classification**. The Young and Burgess classification (Figure 38-1) is used at Parkland Memorial Hospital. This system is useful because it aids in treating the pelvic fracture and in identifying associated injuries (Tables 38-1 and 38-2)
 1. **Lateral compression injuries**. These injuries result in internal rotation of the affected hemipelvis. The are associated with injuries to the head, thorax, and abdomen and typically are not associated with the ongoing hemorrhage, as the SI joints or iliac wing are *compressed*, not blown open. However, LC III (lateral compression type III), the "windswept" pelvis (contralateral hemipelvis undergoes external rotation as the force continues from ipsilateral hemipelvis and across the midline to affect the contralateral hemipelvis) *does* have an open SI joint component and can result in massive blood loss.
 2. **Anteroposterior compression injuries**. These injuries cause widening of the symphysis pubis with or without disruption of the SI joint. They are associated with injury to the lumbosacral plexus and the pelvic vessels due to disruption of the SI joint. These patients can have *high transfusion requirements*. APC III (anterior-posterior compression type III) is the *most morbid type* because of disrupted posterior SI ligaments with resultant vertical and rotational instability. A pelvic binder is essential.
 3. **Vertical shear injuries**. The affected hemipelvis is displaced in a cranial direction. These injuries are associated with vessel and nerve injury due to disruption of the SI joint. Patients can have high transfusion requirements.(same associated injuries as seen with type III APC injuries). These patients need a pelvic binder and traction.
 4. **Combined mechanical injuries**. These patients show elements of more than one injury pattern.
D. **Treatment**. The methods of stabilizing pelvic fractures currently in use at Parkland Memorial Hospital are as follows:
 1. **Pelvic binder**. In stabilization of pelvic fractures, a strap belt is used to provide external compression of the pelvic ring and to prevent large hematomas by producing an indirect tamponade. The application of the device is easy, quick, and straightforward and requires minimal training. It should not be removed during angiography (for pelvic or abdominal hemorrhage) or celiotomy for associated injuries. It is not indicated for

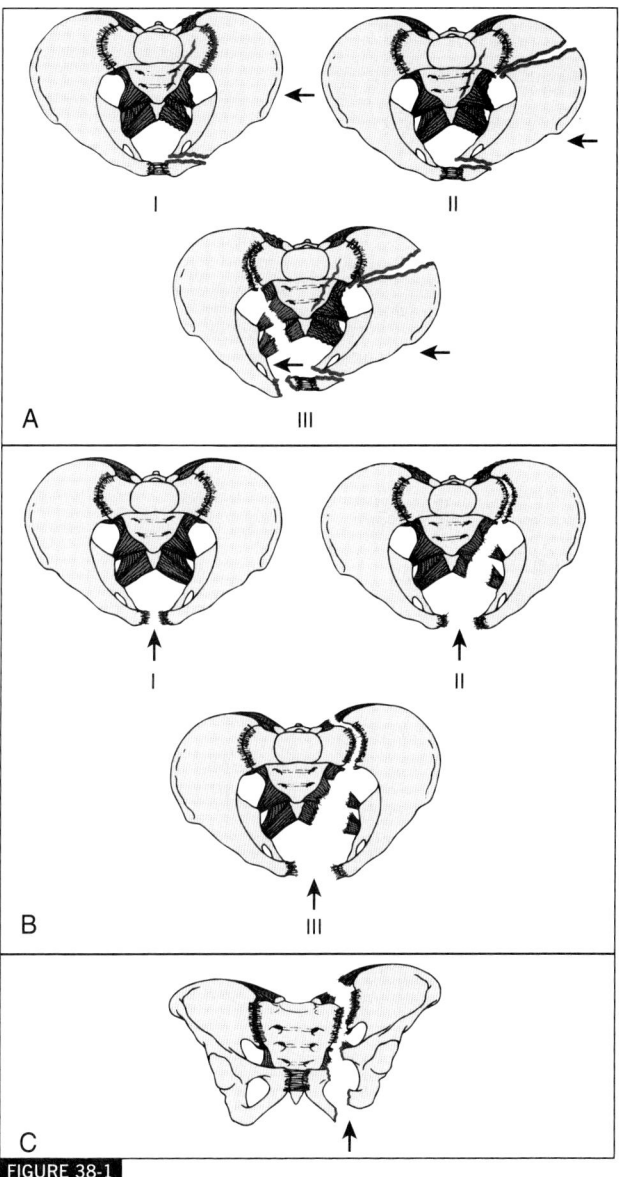

FIGURE 38-1

Young and Burgess classification. A, Lateral compression force. B, Anteroposterior compression. C, Vertical shear.

TABLE 38-1
INJURY CLASSIFICATION KEYS ACCORDING TO THE YOUNG SYSTEM

Category	Distinguishing Characteristics
LC	Transverse fracture of pubic rami, ipsilateral or contralateral to posterior injury I: Sacral compression on side of impact II: Crescent (iliac wing) fracture on side of impact III: LC-I or LC-II injury on side of impact; contralateral open-book (APC) injury
APC	Symphyseal diastasis or longitudinal rami fractures I: Slight widening of pubic symphysis or anterior SI joint; stretched but intact anterior SI, sacrotuberous, and sacrospinous ligaments; intact posterior SI ligaments II: Widened anterior SI joint; disrupted anterior SI, sacrotuberous, and sacrospinous ligaments; intact posterior SI ligaments III: Complete SI joint disruption with lateral displacement, disrupted anterior SI, sacrotuberous, and sacrospinous ligaments; disrupted posterior SI ligaments
VS	Symphyseal diastasis or vertical displacement anteriorly and posteriorly, usually through the SI joint, occasionally through the iliac wing or sacrum
CM	Combination of other injury patterns, LC/VS being the most common

TABLE 38-2
YOUNG-BURGESS CLASSIFICATION SYSTEM

Mechanism and Type	Characteristics	Hemipelvis Displacement	Stability
AP compression, type I	Pubic diastasis < 2.5 cm	External rotation	Stable
AP compression, type II	Pubic diastasis >2.5 cm, anterior SI joint disruption	External rotation	Rotationally unstable, vertically stable
AP compression, type III	Type II plus posterior SI joint disruption	External rotation	Rotationally unstable, vertically unstable
Lateral compression, type I	Ipsilateral sacral buckle fracture, ipsilateral horizontal pubic rami fractures (or disruption of symphysis with overlapping pubic bones)	Internal rotation	Stable
Lateral compression, type II	Type I plus ipsilateral iliac wing fracture or posterior SI joint disruption	Internal rotation	Rotationally unstable, vertically stable
Vertical shear	Vertical pubic rami fractures, SI joint disruption +/- adjacent fractures	Vertical (cranial)	Rotationally unstable, vertically unstable

isolated acetabular fractures. It is especially useful in hemodynamically unstable patients. The pelvic binder should be applied in all patients suspected of unstable fractures (LC II and III, APC II and III, and VS [vertical shear]) as well as all elderly patients (>65 years of age) on arrival in the emergency department.

2. **External fixation**. An anterior frame rapidly applied to the pelvis can be used to "close the book" of the pelvis in *hemodynamically unstable* patients. This reduces pelvic volume and can tamponade bleeding from pelvic vessels. Stabilizing the anterior ring and reducing pelvic volume are often all that is necessary to restore hemodynamic stability. Exploratory celiotomy can be performed with an external fixator in place. The external fixator pins can be used to aid in reduction of SI joint injuries during later placement of iliosacral screws.

3. **Iliosacral screws**. Large (6.5 mm or 7.3 mm) cannulated screws are placed percutaneously to stabilize SI joint disruptions or sacral fractures after reduction has been obtained. Safe placement of these screws requires expertise, both by the surgeon and by the fluoroscopy technician. For this reason, iliosacral screws are usually placed electively, so that all members of the surgical team are available. At Parkland Memorial Hospital, two screws are usually placed in the bodies of S1 and S2

4. **Symphyseal plating**. This is used to stabilize symphysis pubis disruptions. Open dissection can disturb a fracture hematoma and result in massive bleeding. For this reason, symphysis plating is usually delayed for 3 days after injury. If anterior stabilization is required to stop bleeding, an emergency external fixator is used. However, if emergent celiotomy is to be done, the plate can be placed through the celiotomy incision.

5. **Percutaneous screws**. These are used frequently at Parkland. These large fragment, cannulated screws can stabilize iliac wing fractures, pubic ramus fractures, and anterior and posterior column fractures of the acetabulum. Percutaneous placement limits blood loss and soft tissue stripping. As with iliosacral screws, safe placement requires expertise.

6. **Open plating**. Open plating can stabilize iliac wing fractures, ramus fractures, and fractures of the sacrum or SI joint. Open dissection permits direct anatomic reduction of these injuries but must be balanced against the *risk of bleeding from a pelvic hematoma* and the possibility of infection. As with symphyseal plating, this is normally delayed for several days after injury.

7. **Skeletal traction**. Traction can be used preoperatively to prevent proximal migration of an unstable hemipelvis. At Parkland Memorial Hospital, it is used only temporarily. Every effort is made to stabilize pelvic fractures and mobilize the patient to prevent the complications of bedrest and immobility.

E. Trauma team management of pelvic fracture patients

These patients will often have other injuries that must be addressed before the pelvic fracture is treated. The orthopaedist should make the trauma team aware of the pelvic fracture *type* to help them in their assessment. LC types are associated with intra-abdominal injuries. APC types are associated with ongoing bleeding and can be a source of hemodynamic instability. APC injuries that are hemodynamically unstable are treated with a pelvic binder placed in the emergency department and then an anterior pelvic external fixator is applied prior to or in conjunction with celiotomy. These fractures can often be plated at the time of celiotomy. Also, oral CT contrast should be avoided if possible in pelvic fracture patients, as it can make later fluoroscopic imaging of the fractures difficult. All open fractures are covered with a sterile dressing.

F. Management of specific fracture types

1. **LC types**
    a. LC I: these injuries are stable and usually require no treatment other than limited weight bearing on the affected side for pain relief.
    b. LC II: if hemodynamically stable, these can be treated with bedrest, followed by delayed open reduction-internal fixation or percutaneous fixation in elective fashion. If hemodynamically unstable, a pelvic binder is placed and later managed with an anterior pelvic external fixator, followed by surgery on the posterior ring injury.
    c. LC III: these are often hemodynamically unstable and the pelvic binder can be left on for days. These injuries are later managed with an anterior external fixator frame. If the patient is to undergo emergent celiotomy for other injuries, either an anterior external fixator or open plating of the symphysis or rami can be performed. Later, the SI joint injury can be addressed with iliosacral screws and the iliac fracture can be treated with percutaneous screws or open plating.

2. **APC types**
    a. APC I: these injuries are *rare*, with <2-cm widening of the symphysis pubis and simple stretch of the anterior SI ligaments. They are stable and require no surgical treatment. Hemodynamic instability is *rare*.
    b. APC II: there is more than 2 cm of symphyseal diastasis. Always place a pelvic binder when in doubt. If the patient is hemodynamically unstable, place a pelvic binder first and then an anterior external fixator frame. A hemodynamically stable patient can be treated with anterior symphysis plating 3 to 5 days after injury. At Parkland Memorial Hospital, the partial disruption of the SI joint is usually treated with percutaneous iliosacral screws, often on the day after injury or at the time of symphyseal plating.
    c. APC III: these patients are often hemodynamically unstable. Use a pelvic binder and apply an emergent anterior external fixator frame. A hemodynamically stable patient can be kept at bedrest for 3 to 5 days followed by symphyseal plating. The SI joint disruption should be stabilized using iliosacral screws.

3. **Vertical shear** fractures are treated much like the APC III fractures. Often the combination of skeletal traction to the lower extremity of the hemipelvis that is elevated and application of a pelvic binder can stabilize the patient until definitive operative fixation with percutaneous screw fixation or ORIF. Reduction often requires placement of Schanz pins into the ilium to aid in reduction.

4. **Combined mechanical types** must be treated according to the particular injury pattern found.

G. **Special situations**

1. **Hemorrhage**. Hemorrhage in pelvic fractures can arise from the fractured ends of bone, small torn arteries or veins, or from large, named arteries. *Significant* bleeding is most likely to occur with APC, LC III, or VS type injuries. Initial treatment to control this hemorrhage should be some form of closure of the "open pelvic book" to tamponade the bleeding. The pelvic binder is easy to use and should be placed at the scene or during transport. The definitive way to close the pelvic book in hemodynamically unstable patients is with an external fixator frame. If the patient's hemodynamic status does not improve after external fixation, arteriography and embolization of bleeding arteries can sometimes be of benefit. Direct exploration and ligation of bleeding arteries are fraught with complications and are not performed at Parkland Memorial Hospital. Disturbance of the pelvic hematoma should be avoided during a celiotomy, and the pelvic binder should be left in place.

2. **Urologic injury**. About 16% of pelvic fracture patients will have some form of urologic injury. Bladder ruptures and urethral tears are not uncommon. The urologists will manage most of these injuries with an indwelling Foley catheter and/or a suprapubic tube. Urethral ruptures (which are more common in males) are repaired about 6 months after the injury. From an orthopaedic standpoint, a suprapubic tube increases the risk of infection from the hardware placed on the anterior pelvic ring (i.e., symphyseal plates).

3. **Open pelvic fractures**. These have an increased risk of hemorrhage, infection, wound complications, and mortality. The *mortality with open pelvic fractures is about 25%*. They are divided into anterior and posterior types according to the position of the open wound.
   a. Anterior open pelvic fractures have lacerations on the thigh or flank and do not communicate with the perineum, scrotum, vagina, or rectum. These usually involve only lacerations of muscle tissue. They should be considered *high energy injuries* and be debrided aggressively. All such wounds should be left open and should undergo serial debridement.
   b. Posterior open pelvic fractures involve lacerations of the rectum or anus and can involve the distal urologic structures. Injuries of this sort are aggressively debrided and treated with *early fecal diversion* with a colostomy. The wounds should be left open and should undergo serial debridement. Hardware has to be used judiciously in these patients, due to the markedly increased risk of infection.

II. ACETABULAR FRACTURES

A. **Anatomy**. The acetabulum is made up of contributions from the *ischium, ilium, and pubis*. The arrangement of these three bones forming the acetabular cup is best seen in the immature skeleton, prior to closure of the triradiate cartilage. In the adult, the acetabulum is best thought of as an inverted Y, with anterior and posterior "columns." There are also anterior and posterior "walls," which form the boundaries defining the acetabular cup. The involvement of these four structures—anterior and posterior columns, anterior and posterior walls—determines the classification of each particular acetabular fracture. By convention, the 90-degree arc at the top of the acetabular dome is termed the *weight-bearing dome*.

B. Evaluation. Each acetabular fracture is evaluated using an anteroposterior x-ray of the pelvis, coupled with *iliac oblique* and *obturator oblique* views. (These oblique views are termed "Judet" views in honor of Robert Judet, who pioneered their use). Also, a CT bony pelvis protocol is obtained, with 5-mm sections through the iliac wings and 2-mm sections through the acetabulum itself. The CT is invaluable in demonstrating the extent of *marginal impaction* of fractures, especially at the posterior wall. It also reveals minimally displaced fractures and intra-articular bone fragments. Reformatting CT sections to produce three-dimensional images has not provided more information in our experience.

C. Classification. Emile Letournel's classification system is used at Parkland Memorial Hospital. It is comprised of five *elementary* fracture types and five *associated* fracture types. The associated types are complex and include *combinations* of the elementary types.

D. Treatment. Most patients will need to have skeletal traction. Judet's views and the CT bony pelvis protocol help to plan treatment. The principles of acetabular fracture treatment are the same as with other articular fractures: *restore anatomic alignment and stability to prevent post-traumatic arthritis, and mobilize early to prevent stiffness*. Any articular incongruity greater than 2 mm in the weight-bearing dome of the acetabulum should be treated with open reduction and internal fixation. (Ill elderly patients are *not* good candidates for acetabular fracture surgery, which can often be lengthy with significant blood loss.)

E. Perioperative management. Surgery should be delayed 3 to 5 days after injury to avoid causing excessive bleeding. Skeletal traction should be used to maintain reduction if the hip was dislocated. Traction will also prevent impaction and scuffing of the femoral head on the fracture. In selected patients, preoperative thigh sonograms and pelvic magnetic resonance venograms are used to screen for deep venous thrombosis (DVT). If a DVT is found, anticoagulation with intravenous heparin is begun. An inferior vena cava filter is placed preoperatively on the day of surgery. Patients are mobilized on the first day after surgery using a walker. They are restricted to foot flat weight-bearing for 3 months. Postoperative thigh sonograms are used to screen for DVT. *All patients who had an extensile approach undergo a single dose of 600 rad of radiation to prevent heterotopic ossification*. Indomethacin is used as prophylaxis in patients who refuse radiation treatment. We do not believe that indomethacin is as effective as radiation in the treatment of heterotopic ossification.

F. Complications

1. **Post-traumatic arthritis** is usually caused by residual articular incongruity and can be seen after *any* acetabular fracture surgery, but is most common in nonsurgical patients. Some arthritis may arise from damage to the articular cartilage itself.
2. **Heterotopic ossification** (HO) after surgery through a posterior or extensile approach. HO can severely limit hip motion. Prophylaxis at Parkland Memorial Hospital is accomplished with a single dose of 600 rad of radiation. Alternate treatments include indomethacin orally.
3. **Sciatic nerve palsy** is most common after posterior approaches. This risk can be limited by flexing the knee and limiting hip flexion during the surgery.

III. SUGGESTED READINGS

Burgess A, et al: Pelvic ring disruptions: Effective classification system and treatment protocols. J Trauma (7):848-856, 1990.

Dalal SA, Burgess AR, Siegel JH, et al: Pelvic fracture in multiple trauma: Classification by mechanism is key to pattern of organ injury, resuscitative requirements, and outcome. J Trauma 29:981-1002, 1989.

Reinert CM, Bosse MJ, Poka A, et al.: A modified extensile exposure for the treatment of complex or malunited acetabular fractures. J Bone Joint Surg (Am) 70:329-336, 1988.

Rockwood CA, Green DP, Bucholz RW, Heckman JD (eds): Fractures of the pelvic Ring. In Rockwood & Green's Fractures in Adults, 4th ed. Philadelphia, Lippincott-Raven Publishers, 2005.

Routt MLC, Kregor PJ, Simonian PT, et al: Early results of percutaneous iliosacral screws placed with the patient in the supine position. J Orthop Trauma 9:207-214, 1995.

Surgery.mc.duke.edu, Management of Pelvic Fractures, revised 11/04.

Tile M: Pelvic ring fractures: Should they be fixed? J Bone Joint Surg (Br) 70:1-12, 1988.

Vermulin B, et al: Prehospital stabilization of pelvic dislocations. Swiss Surge 5(2):43-46, 1999.

Fractures and Dislocations of the Lower Extremity

Krishna Venkatesh, MD

I. HIP DISLOCATIONS

A. Occurrence
1. **Hip dislocations usually occur** after motor vehicle collisions or falls.
2. They can be missed in multiply injured patients who have more dramatic injuries.
3. **A single anteroposterior (AP) view** of the pelvis is recommended in all trauma patients.

B. Evaluation
1. **Sciatic nerve injuries** can occur in 8% to 19% of posterior dislocations.
    a. The risk is higher with fracture dislocations.
    b. The peroneal portion of the nerve is usually affected
    c. The nerve injury is usually a neuropraxia that will improve with time after the hip is reduced.
2. **Femoral nerve and vessel injuries** have been reported after anterior dislocations, but they are more rare.
3. Search for open wounds and concomitant knee injuries.
4. Anteroposterior and oblique (Judet) views of the pelvis should be obtained.
    a. Fractures of the acetabulum and femoral head should be looked for.
    b. These views should be repeated after reduction to assess congruency.
    c. A post-reduction CT scan should be obtained to ensure that there are no intra-articular bone fragments. These loose bodies can damage the joint and cause arthritis if left in place. If closed reduction is not possible, a CT scan should be obtained to assess the femoral head and for the presence of intra-articular bone fragments and to rule out associated femoral head and acetabular fractures.

C. Classification
1. **Anterior dislocations**
    a. The femoral head lies anterior to the coronal plane of the acetabulum.
    b. These are classified into two categories:
        i. Type I – superior, including pubic or subspinous dislocations
        ii. Type II – inferior, including obturator or perineal dislocations
        iii. The injuries are further subclassified as A, no associated fracture; B, associated fracture of the femoral head or neck; and C, associated acetabular fracture.
2. **Posterior dislocations**
    a. The femoral head lies posterior to the coronal plane of the acetabulum.
    b. These are subclassified into five categories:
        i Type I – with or without a minor posterior wall acetabular fracture

ii. Type II – with a single-fragment posterior wall fracture
iii. Type III – with a comminution of the posterior wall
iv. Type IV – with fracture of the acetabular floor
v. Type V – with fracture of the femoral head
c. The type V fractures can be further subclassified according to the location of the femoral head or neck fracture.

D. Treatment
1. **Hip dislocations are an orthopaedic emergency**. Results will be worse if reduction is delayed for >12 hours.
2. **Reduction**
   a. Closed reduction is attempted first. Ideally this should be done under a general anesthetic or adequate IV sedation.
   b. No more than three attempts should be made.
   c. Repeated, forceful attempts can damage the articular cartilage, leading to poor results.
   d. If closed reduction fails, open methods must be used. In irreducible anterior dislocations, an anterior iliofemoral approach is employed.
   e. In irreducible posterior dislocations, a Kocher-Langenbeck approach is used. These approaches are used to try to preserve the remaining blood supply to the femoral head.
3. **Indications for open reduction**
   a. Dislocation irreducible by closed means
   b. Nonconcentric reduction
   c. Fracture of the acetabulum or femoral head that requires either excision or open reduction and internal fixation
   d. Ipsilateral femoral neck fracture
4. **Assessment and traction**
   a. Reduction of posterior dislocations is assessed by flexing the hip to 90 degrees. If the hip redislocates, it is deemed unstable and further diagnostic studies and surgical exploration and traction may be needed.
   b. Instability usually results from an associated posterior wall acetabular fracture.
   c. Unstable hip dislocations must be treated with open reduction and internal fixation (ORIF). (Unstable anterior dislocations are rare, so no assessment is done.)
   d. After reduction, anteroposterior and Judet radiographs of the hip are obtained to ensure no intra-articular fragments are present.
   e. A pelvic CT scan is also obtained.
   f. Any intra-articular fragments require surgical removal.
   g. If the reduction is stable, the patient is treated with 5 to 7 days of bed rest and traction. This is followed by limited weight bearing for 6 weeks.

E. Complications
1. Recurrent dislocation
   a. Rare after anterior dislocations

b. Inadequate length of immobilization is the usual cause.
   c. Recurrence is also rare after posterior dislocations (about 1% prevalence), but hip capsule laxity or bony deficiency is usually to blame with these patients.
   d. Surgery is often required for recurrent posterior instability.
2. Avascular necrosis (AVN)
   a. AVN of the femoral head may appear 2 to 5 years after the dislocation.
   b. Delay in reduction and repeated attempts at reduction have been blamed for this complication, although increased severity of the initial injury is the most likely culprit.
   c. AVN is rare after anterior dislocations (8% prevalence). The rate is higher with posterior dislocations (6% to 40%).
3. Post-traumatic arthritis
   a. The most frequent long-term complication
   b. Usually arises because of associated femoral head or acetabular fractures
   c. It can also result if AVN leads to joint incongruity. As many as one-third of anterior dislocations go on to show arthritic changes.
   d. Arthritis has been reported in 17% to 30% of posterior dislocation patients.
   e. The best treatment for this complication is prevention through congruent, stable reduction of the hip.

II. HIP FRACTURES

1. Fractures of the femoral neck and intertrochanteric region are, primarily, injuries of the elderly.
2. They frequently occur after minor trauma and are usually isolated injuries.
3. While the fractures are often fairly simple, management of these patients can be difficult.
4. Hip fracture patients often suffer from dementia, and associated medical conditions are usually present.
5. Mortality rates during hospitalization for hip fracture treatment can be as high as 10%.
6. Complications such as decubitus ulcers, urinary tract infections, and deep vein thromboses are common.
7. The reported 1-year mortality ranges from 18% to 30%.
8. In patients with more than three concurrent medical illnesses, preoperative medical treatment to optimize the patient's condition has been shown to lessen mortality.
9. In patients with fewer medical problems, immediate fracture care appears to improve results.
10. Improvements in orthopaedic implants have made stabilizing of the fracture easier.

III. FEMORAL NECK FRACTURES

A. Evaluation. Anteroposterior radiographs of the pelvis and a lateral view of the hip will generally demonstrate the fracture. If plain films are negative and there is a high index of suspicion, a magnetic resonance imaging scan may be obtained in the first 24 hours.

B. Classification. Garden classification is most commonly used (Figure 39-1).
1. Garden I – valgus impacted neck fracture; may be incomplete, sparing the inferior femoral neck
2. Garden II – complete, nondisplaced fracture on anteroposterior and lateral views
3. Garden III – complete, partially displaced fracture
4. Garden IV – compete, fully displaced fracture

C. Treatment. The choices for treatment are as follows:
1. Internal fixation
   a. Reduction is obtained with the patient on a fracture table.

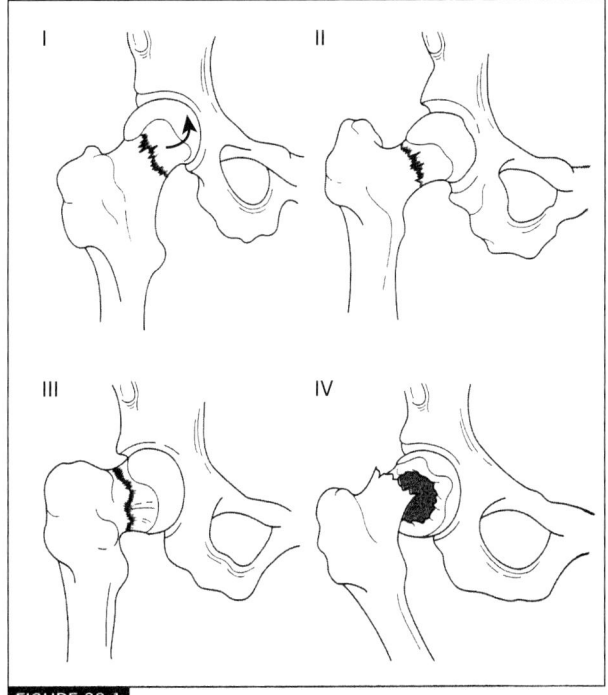

FIGURE 39-1

Garden classification of femoral neck fractures.

    b. Fluoroscopy is used to judge reduction and aid guidewire placement for cannulated screws.
    c. Three or four large fragment, cannulated screws are placed into the femoral neck and head.
    d. Percutaneous technique limits dissection and blood loss.
    e. Postoperatively, the patients are made toe-touch weight bearing with crutches or a walker.
  2. Prosthetic replacement
    a. Endoprosthetic use is indicated in patients with:
      i. Severe medical problems
      ii. Physiologic age >75 years (life expectancy < 5 years)
      iii. Pathologic hip fractures
      iv. Parkinsonism or other neuromuscular disease
      v. Recently failed internal fixation of a femoral neck fracture
    b. The above criteria are relative indications. Each patient must be considered individually.
  3. Primary total hip arthroplasty is indicated in patients with a femoral neck fracture in a hip with preexisting arthritis, such as rheumatoid arthritis.
D. Nonoperative treatment
  1. Traction has a poor track record in the treatment of hip fractures.
  2. Only severely ill patients who are not likely to survive surgery are treated with traction.
E. Complications
  1. Lack of blood supply
    a. Fracture and displacement of the femoral neck interrupts all blood flow except that through the ligamentum teres.
    b. The intracapsular position of the femoral head means that no callus will form outside the fracture to aid in union.
    c. Synovial fluid will lyse any blood clot that forms, which means the femoral neck fracture is dependent on endosteal union alone.
    d. After stabilization, revascularization of the avascular head occurs by a process of "creeping substitution."
    e. As dead segments of bone are reached by the new blood supply, they are resorbed and replaced with new trabeculae.
    f. Understanding this process is the key to understanding the two major complications after femoral neck fracture.
  2. Nonunion
    a. This occurs in about 20% to 30% of displaced femoral neck fractures after reduction and stabilization.
    b. It is rare after stabilization of nondisplaced fractures (5%).
    c. Predisposing factors include:
      i. Increased patient age
      ii. Poor reduction
      iii. Inadequate fixation
      iv. Comminution
  3. Avascular necrosis

a. Prevalence of AVN after a femoral neck fracture varies from 11% to 84%.
b. Prevalence of late segmental collapse ranges from 7% to 35%.
c. Segmental collapse of the infarcted bone results in joint incongruity and post-traumatic arthritis.
d. This segmental collapse can occur as late as 2 to 5 years after the fracture.

4. Thromboembolic phenomenon
   a. Occurs in 30% to 50% of patients but only 7% to 12% are symptomatic.
   b. All patients awaiting surgery should have deep vein thrombosis prophylaxis.

IV. INTERTROCHANTERIC HIP FRACTURES

A. Evaluation. Anteroposterior pelvis and lateral hip radiographs will generally demonstrate the fracture.

B. Classification
1. Intertrochanteric fractures are simply classified as stable or unstable at Parkland Memorial Hospital.
2. Unstable fractures involve the posteromedial cortex of the proximal femur, around the lesser trochanter and calcar femoral. They have lost the posteromedial "buttress." Stable patterns have not.
3. Unstable patterns are more likely to undergo significant bony collapse after stabilization, as the bone settles into a more stable position.

C. Treatment
1. Surgical stabilization of the fracture using a dynamic hip screw is the treatment of choice for these injuries.
2. Nonsurgical treatment is reserved for severly ill patients.

D. Complications
1. Nonunion is rare after these injuries (1% to 2%), owing to the rich cancellous blood supply.
2. AVN is also rare (< 1%).
3. Nail cutout. This hardware complication is often due to an unstable reduction or as a result of misplacement of the screw inside the femoral head. Studies have stressed the importance of placing the screw close to the subchondral bone (within 1 cm). This will provide secure fixation and central position.
4. Varus displacement and bony collapse of the neck are sometimes seen with hardware failure in an unstable fracture pattern.

V. SUBTROCHANTERIC FEMUR FRACTURES

A. Occurrence
1. Subtrochanteric femur fractures can occur after high-energy crashes in young patients, or after minimal trauma in the elderly. Ten percent of high-energy subtrochanteric fractures are due to gunshot injuries.

2. The subtrochanteric region of the femur is subjected to high compressive and tensile loads. Because of this, implant failure can occur after fixation of these fractures.

B. Evaluation. Anteroposterior and lateral radiographs of the pelvis, hip, and femur should be obtained.

C. Classification. Seinsheimer classification is most commonly used.
1. Type I – nondisplaced
2. Type II – two-part fracture
3. Type III – three-part fracture
4. Type IV – comminuted, with four or more fragments
5. Type V – subtrochanteric fracture with an intertrochanteric extension

D. Treatment
1. Nonoperative
   a. Several authors have reported acceptable results using hip-spica casting with a hinge at the knee. However, the rates of malunion and nonunion are high using conservative methods such as casting.
   b. Owing to these problems, casts and traction are not used at Parkland Memorial Hospital unless the patient is too ill to survive surgery.
   c. Subtrochanteric fractures in multiply injured patients should be immediately stabilized to prevent pulmonary complications.
2. Operative
   a. Anatomic stabilization of the fracture to allow early mobilization is the goal of treatment. The type of implant used must be determined by the fracture pattern and includes:
      i. Intramedullary (IM) devices (first- or second-generation nails)
      ii. Blade plates
      iii. Dynamic condylar screws
      iv. Dynamic hip screws with long side-plates
   b. Restoration of medial cortical contact is important, since the compressive forces across the medial subtrochanteric region are very high (2 to 3 times body weight in stance phase of gait).
      i. This force can cause implant failure if the bone has not been aligned to share some of the load.
      ii. Some authors have recommended bone grafting of the medial cortex at the time of the initial internal fixation. Closed reduction techniques have decreased the need for bone grafting.

E. Complications
1. Nonunion (5%)
2. Comminution of the greater trochanter
3. Fracture of the femoral neck
4. Rotational malalignment (21%)

VI. FEMORAL SHAFT FRACTURES

A. Occurrence
1. Femoral shaft fractures are high-energy injuries.

2. These fractures are commonly associated with other injuries and can themselves cause life-threatening complications.

B. Evaluation
1. AP and lateral radiographs of the entire femur
2. The hip and knee should be included in these views.

C. Classification. There is no commonly accepted classification system for femoral shaft fractures

D. Treatment
1. A prospective, randomized trial at Parkland Memorial Hospital showed that, compared with traction, immediate stabilization of femur fractures in multiply injured patients lessens the risk of pneumonia, fat embolism, and acute respiratory distress syndrome.
2. Early stabilization reduces the time spent intubated and in the intensive care unit as well as shortening the hospital stay.
3. Every effort is made to stabilize femur fractures within 24 hours of injury.
4. Indications
   a. Intramedullary (IM) nailing
      i. IM nailing has become the treatment of choice for fractures of the femoral shaft. The technique restores anatomy, allows for rapid mobilization, limits the time of bed rest (out of bed in 24 hours), and lessens the pain from fracture instability, and the static locking of the nails lessens the risk of a rotational malunion without adversely affecting union rates.
      ii. Methods such as cast bracing and traction for femur fractures have shown consistently poorer results in randomized trials.
      iii. Nonoperative treatment methods are reserved for very ill, elderly patients who would not survive a general anesthetic.
   b. Retrograde femoral nailing. The relative indications for this technique include:
      i. Need for concurrent celiotomy or other surgery
      ii. Floating knee (see F, below, Special situations, below)
      iii. Ipsilateral femoral neck and shaft fractures (see F, below)
      iv. Concomitant femoral vascular injury (see F, below)
      v. Morbidly obese patients with pulmonary or spine injuries
   c. External fixation
      i. External fixators used for femur fractures are often complicated by pin tract infections, knee stiffness from tethering the quadriceps to the femur, and malunions.
      ii. Delayed union is more common with external fixation.
      iii. At Parkland Memorial Hospital, external fixators are primarily reserved for open femur fractures with gross wound contamination and for fractures that clearly require a flap procedure to cover the fracture site.
      iv. External fixators can also be used to stabilize femur fractures in patients who would not survive an IM nailing.
      v. External fixators can be rapidly applied to obtain bony stability in patients with concomitant vascular injuries who present to the hospital late.

E. Complications
1. Infections are rare (< 1%).
   a. Infections should be treated with irrigation and debridement.
   b. The IM nail can usually be left in place until the fracture unites.
2. Nonunion is rare.
   a. Exchange nailing and placement of a larger nail have proven successful at Parkland Memorial Hospital.
   b. Bone grafting can be used as necessary.
   c. Rotational malunions can be treated with nail removal and osteotomy with an IM saw. Derotation and static-locked nailing can then correct the deformity.
3. Nerve injury
   a. Uncommon because the femoral and sciatic nerves are encased in muscle throughout the length of the thigh
4. Vascular injury
   a. Compartment syndrome of the thigh occurs only with significant bleeding.
   b. Injury to the femoral artery may be due to tethering of the artery at the adductor hiatus.

F. Special situations
1. Open fractures
   a. Rapid stabilization of the femur will prevent pulmonary complications and limit time spent in the intensive care unit and on the ventilator.
   b. Most open femur fractures can be safely treated with immediate IM nailing after thorough surgical irrigation and debridement (grade I, II, IIIa open fractures).
   c. Several series of open femur fractures treated with IM nails have shown functional results comparable to those seen with closed fractures. The infection rates have been reported to be about 2% to 4%.
   d. The presence of gross contaminants in the wound (gravel, dirt, etc.) is an indication for external fixation.
   e. Fractures that require flap coverage are usually treated with an external fixator.
   f. External fixators on the femur are commonly complicated by pin tract infections.
      i. Malunion and delayed union are also much more frequent than with IM nails.
      ii. Placement of the pins through the quadriceps tethers the muscle to the bone and can cause knee stiffness. (More posterior pin placement, nearer to the insertion of the lateral intermuscular septum on the linea aspera, can limit muscle tethering.)
   g. Open femur fractures that require flap coverage have a high rate of nonunion and limb loss due to the extensive nature of these injuries.
2. Ipsilateral femoral shaft and femoral neck fractures
   a. There are several ways to treat these fractures. The "recon," or second-generation nail, is one option.

b. The "miss a nail" method (antegrade femoral nailing followed by placement of percutaneous cannulated screws around the nail) is another option.

c. The third option, now in use at Parkland Memorial Hospital, is retrograde femoral nailing followed by percutaneous screw fixation of the femoral neck fracture.

3. Ipsilateral femoral and tibial fractures—the "floating knee"
   a. This difficult injury pattern is made simpler to treat by approaching both fractures through one incision at the knee.
   b. Antegrade tibia nailing in a standard fashion will stabilize the tibia. This is necessary for control of the femur, which can then be stabilized via a retrograde approach. This method saves operating time.
   c. The clinician must be aware of the risk of compartment syndrome in floating knee injuries – reported as high as 30% in some series.

4. Femur fractures with an associated vascular injury
   a. About 2% of femur fractures have an associated vascular injury.
   b. These injuries are managed with immediate fracture stabilization.
   c. If the patient arrives at the treating hospital soon enough, standard internal fixation techniques can safely be used.
   d. The vascular repair then follows.
   e. If the ischemic threshold is approaching (i.e., 3 hours or more since the time of injury), the vascular injury must be addressed first.
      i. This can be done either with direct vascular repair or with a temporary vascular shunt.
      ii. Stabilization of the fracture then follows.
   f. Close cooperation between the trauma and orthopaedic surgeons is a necessity in the care of these patients.

5. Gunshot wounds
   a. IM nailing is a safe, effective form of treatment for femur fractures caused by gunshot wounds.
   b. The entry wound is debrided, but no attempt is made to remove the bullet unless it is superficial or has entered a joint.
   c. Shotgun wounds that produce fractures are close-range, high-energy injuries.
      i. The amount of soft tissue damage is usually extensive.
      ii. Fracture comminution and bone loss are often severe.
      iii. Wadding from the shell often enters the wound.
      iv. This plastic or paper wad (even horsehair in older shells) is not visible radiographically and can be missed at debridement.
      v. Severe chronic infections can result from these injuries.
      vi. Shotgun wounds should be treated as open fractures.
      vii. Aggressive, serial irrigation and debridement are necessary.
      viii. Antibiotic coverage is mandatory.

VII. SUPRACONDYLAR FEMUR FRACTURES

A. Supracondylar femur fractures, like subtrochanteric fractures, can either result from high-energy trauma in young patients or from low-energy trauma in the elderly.

B. Evaluation
1. AP and lateral radiographs of the knee and entire femur
2. Oblique views can occasionally be helpful in delineating the fracture pattern.
3. CT scan helps to identify fracture lines in the frontal plane and can aid in operative planning.
4. Angiography is indicated with dislocation of the knee. Forty percent of such injuries are associated with vascular disruption.

C. Classification
1. The AO classification is most commonly used:
   a. Type A – extra-articular fractures (Figure 39-2)
   b. Type B – unicondylar fractures (Figure 39-3)
   c. Type C – intercondylar fractures (Figure 39-4)
2. Each type is subcategorized as 1, 2, or 3 according to the amount of comminution present.

D. Treatment
1. Nonoperative
   a. Non-weight bearing and cast bracing are the forms of nonoperative treatment used at Parkland Memorial Hospital.
   b. Nondisplaced fractures can be safely treated conservatively.
   c. Very ill, elderly patients who would not tolerate an operation can also be managed conservatively.
   d. Osteoporotic patients
   e. Infected or severely contaminated fractures (grade IIb or IIc open injuries)
2. Operative treatment should be performed within 48 hours. If surgery is delayed by more than 8 hours, tibial traction should be used.
   a. ORIF
      i. Most displaced supracondylar femur fractures will require some form of ORIF.
      ii. Side-plates, blade plates, dynamic condylar screws, and IM devices have all been used with success.
      iii. One IM device, the supracondylar nail, has been designed specifically for this fracture type.
      iv. The implant must be chosen to match the particular fracture pattern.
      v. The goal is to achieve a stable anatomic reduction, to allow early mobility, and to prevent post-traumatic arthritis.
      vi. These fractures are often technically difficult to repair.
      vii. Comminution can make exact articular restoration difficult
   b. External fixation
      i. In patients who are multiply injured, hemodynamically unstable, and near death, there is little time on the day of injury for reconstruction of the distal femoral articular surface.

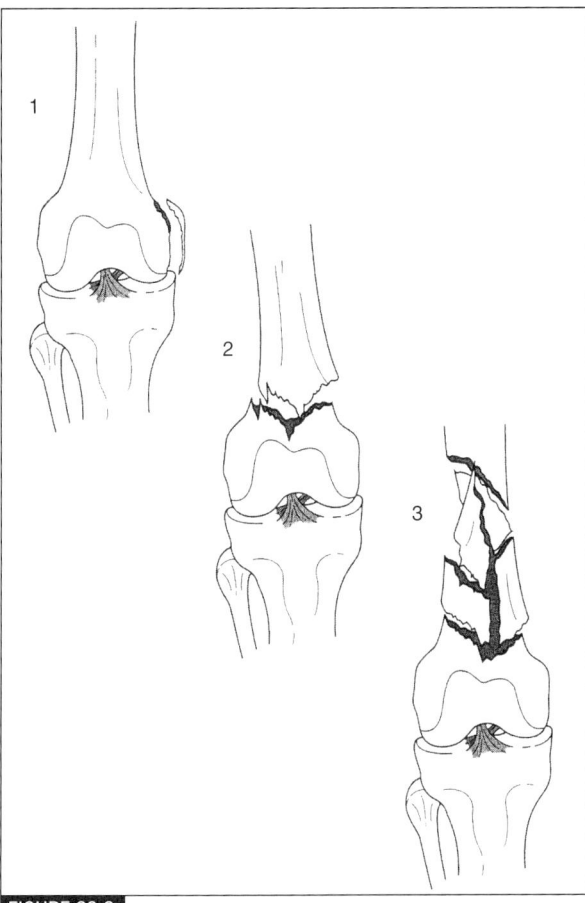

FIGURE 39-2

Type A distal femur fracture.

ii. In patients with large, open wounds with gross contamination, internal fixation is unwise due to the risk of infection.
iii. In these rare types of patients, a knee-bridging external fixator is used at Parkland Memorial Hospital.
iv. Distraction with this frame will usually give a good reduction of the major fracture fragments.
v. Fixation can be supplemented by limited internal fixation with percutaneously placed screws.

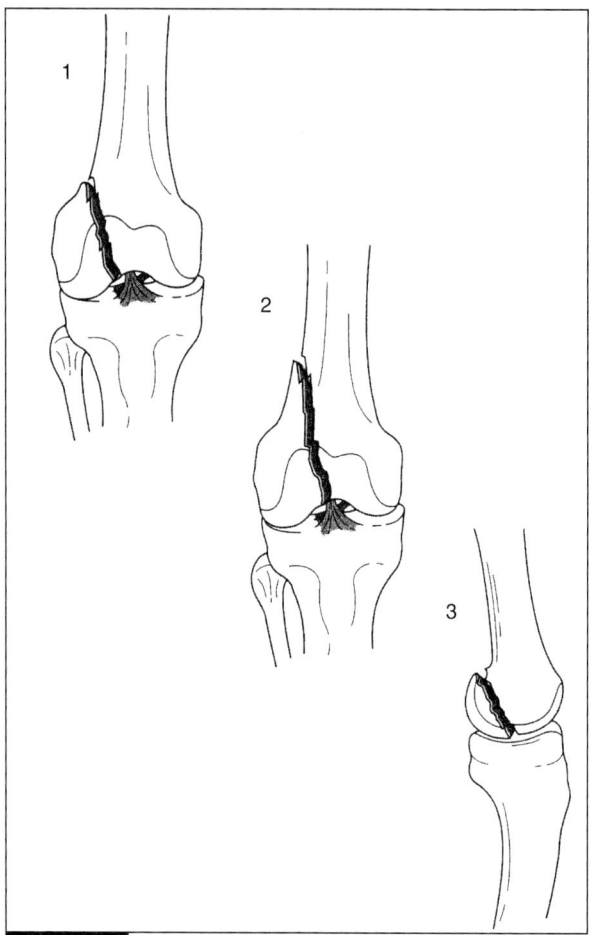

FIGURE 35-3

Type B distal femur fracture.

      vi. This type of frame can be easily applied in about 20 minutes.
     vii. Minimal blood is lost, and it achieves the goal of stabilizing the fracture.
    viii. This makes transport easier and limits further soft tissue injury.

E. Complications
1. Malunion
   a. This usually results from unstable fixation or infection.
2. Hardware failure is also fairly common and can be a sign of nonunion.
3. Nonunion

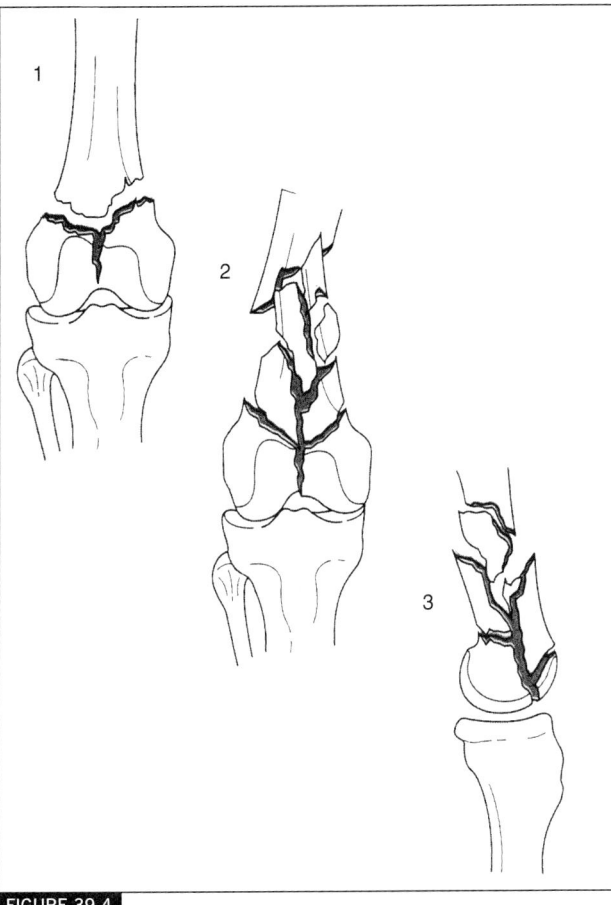

FIGURE 39-4
Type C distal femur fracture.

  a. This is infrequent due to the abundant vascular supply and predominance of cancellous bone.
  b. Occurs more commonly in the elderly
  c. Some authors have recommended primary bone grafting to improve union rates.

VIII. PATELLA FRACTURES

A. Occurrence
1. Patella fractures usually result from direct blows to the front of the knee.

2. Knee ligament injury, femoral shaft or distal femur fracture, and posterior hip dislocation can be associated with patella fractures.

B. Evaluation
1. AP and lateral views of the knee as well as bilateral axial views of patellae should be obtained.
2. The patient's ability to extend the knee must be evaluated.

C. Classification
1. Fractures are usually classified as:
   a. Transverse
   b. Vertical
   c. Upper or lower pole fractures
   d. Comminuted
   e. Stellate
2. Comminuted fractures of the lower pole are the most common.

D. Treatment
1. Nonoperative
   a. This can be used in nondisplaced or minimally displaced (maximum of 2-mm step-off) fractures, as long as the patient's extensor mechanism is intact.
   b. At Parkland Memorial Hospital these patients are placed in a cylinder cast for 6 weeks and are kept on limited weight bearing.
2. Operative
   a. This is preferable if displacement is present or if the extensor mechanism is ruptured.
   b. Surgery on the patella should be done through a longitudinal midline incision. Transverse incisions can compromise later surgery on the knee.
   c. The goal is restoration of articular anatomy with a stable construct that allows early movement.
      i. This can be accomplished with either K-wires or screws.
      ii. An anterior tension band wire is passed around the ends of the wires or screws.
      iii. Cerclage wires are not used as the sole means of stabilization.
      iv. The extensor retinaculum is usually torn transversely, and it must be repaired at surgery.
      v. Comminuted inferior pole fractures can be safely excised. The patellar tendon can then be reattached using a nonabsorbable suture woven through the tendon, and passed up through drill holes in the patella.
      vi. Postoperatively, most patients are kept in a knee immobilizer for 3 to 4 weeks and then are started on active exercises.

E. Complications
1. Post-traumatic arthritis has been reported in as many as 50% of patients in some series.
2. Nonunion is rare and has been reported in only 2% of cases.
3. Painful hardware is common, owing to the subcutaneous position of the patella. Removal of the hardware alleviates this.

IX. TIBIAL PLATEAU FRACTURES

A. Evaluation
1. AP and lateral radiographs should be obtained.
2. Oblique views are helpful.
3. CT scans are obtained to demonstrate the full extent of depression of the articular surface.
4. Ligamentous stability must be assessed, either in the operating room under anesthesia or after injection of an anesthetic in the knee.
5. Arteriography should be performed if distal pulses are decreased.

B. Classification.
The Schatzker classification is used at Parkland (Figures 39-5A and 39-5B).
1. Schatzker I – lateral plateau split

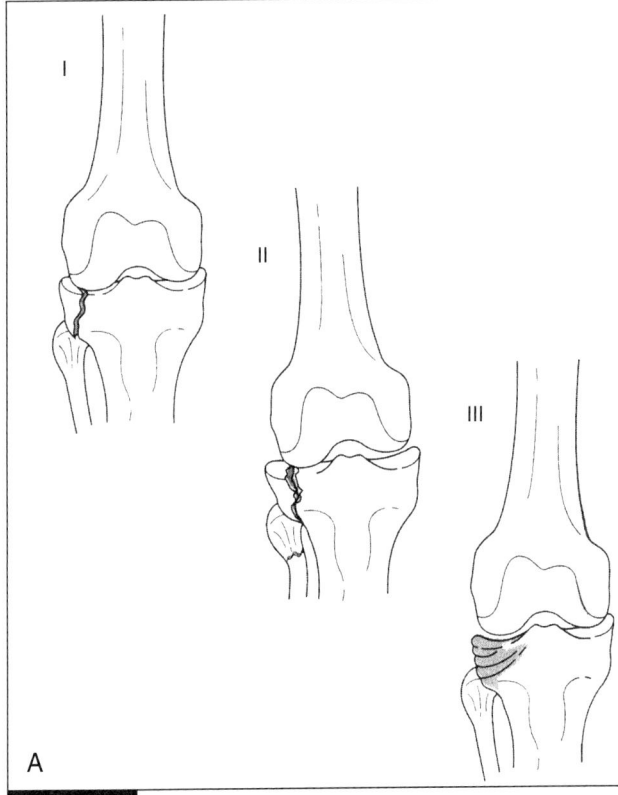

FIGURE 39-5A

Schatzker classification of tibial plateau fractures.

IX. Tibial Plateau Fractures

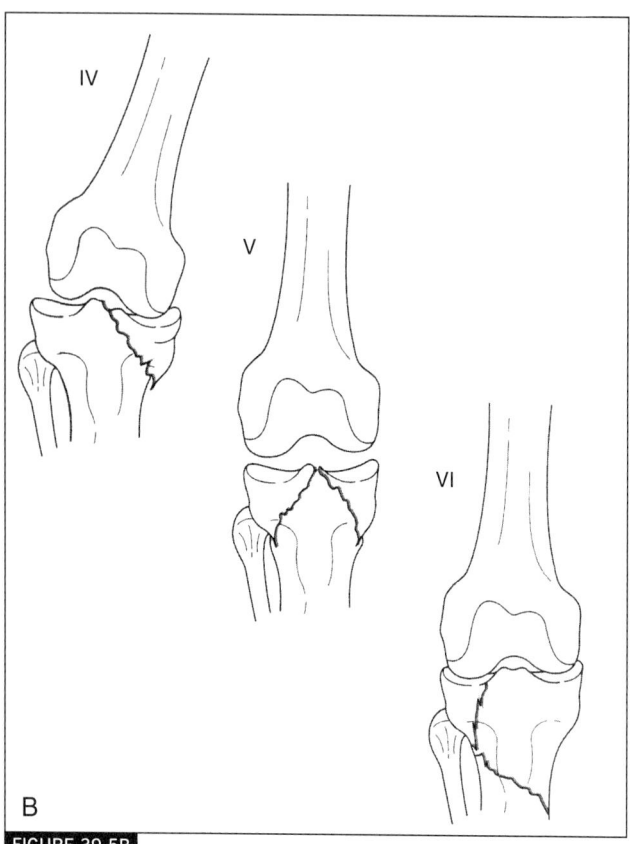

FIGURE 39-5B
Schatzker classification of tibial plateau fractures.

2. Schatzker II – lateral plateau split depression
3. Schatzker III – lateral plateau depression
4. Schatzker IV – medial plateau fracture
5. Schatzker V – bicondylar plateau fracture
6. Schatzker VI – plateau fracture, with associated fracture at the metaphyseal/diaphyseal junction

C. Treatment
1. As with other articular fractures, stable anatomic reduction, early mobilization, and prevention of post-traumatic arthritis are the goals of treatment.
2. Use of limited exposure and external fixation as an adjunct is an acceptable form of treatment.

3. Since 2 to 3 mm of displacement is commonly accepted as adequate reduction for other articular fractures, it is accepted for tibial plateau fractures as well. Greater displacement is usually an indication for operative reduction.
4. Varus or valgus instability of more than 10 degrees is also an indication for surgical stabilization.
5. Nonoperative
   a. Nondisplaced or minimally displaced tibial plateau fractures do well when treated with cast bracing.
   b. Rapid mobilization prevents stiffness, and non-weight bearing prevents further displacement.
   c. In elderly patients greater amounts of displacement can be accepted and nonoperative treatment can be successfully used.
   d. In the older population (age >60 years) post-traumatic arthritis can be treated with total knee replacement, which has good results.
   e. The best predictor of future arthritis is knee instability in the varus or valgus plane. Minor articular irregularities appear to be tolerated well as long as the knee is stable.
6. Operative
   a. Internal fixation and buttress plating
      i. ORIF allows anatomic restoration of articular surfaces.
      ii. This prevents future arthritis.
      iii. This is normally done through a lateral or medial parapatellar arthrotomy.
      iv. The meniscus is lifted off the plateau, and the plateau is reconstructed.
      v. Small fragment plates and 3.5-mm screws to limit implant size are used.
      vi. Open fractures or injuries with significant soft tissue contusion or abrasion should probably be treated with other techniques.
      vii. Patients with compromised soft tissues are at high risk for infection and wound breakdown.
   b. Limited internal fixation
      i. Depressed plateau fractures can often be elevated using a bone tamp placed through a small anterior cortical window.
      ii. Bone graft can be stuffed up into the window to buttress the articular fragment.
      iii. Reduction is judged using an image intensifier.
      iv. Stabilization is obtained with 2 to 3 percutaneously placed large fragment cannulated screws.
      v. A screw and a washer placed just below a fracture line can be used as an antiglide plate to hold up metaphyseal fragments.
      vi. After surgery, the patients are kept non-weight bearing and in a cast brace for 3 months.
   c. External fixation
      i. External fixation can be used to supplement limited internal fixation of plateau fractures.

ii. Proximal pins placed into the stable, nonfractured plateau can be used to support the fractured plateau and hold the tibia out to length.
iii. External fixation also obviates the need for cast bracing. This is a very versatile technique that is especially useful in open fractures or fractures with compromised soft tissues. Infection rates are low.
iv. As with supracondylar femur fractures, physicians at Parkland Memorial Hospital use knee-bridging external fixators in patients who have large, contaminated open wounds or who are hemodynamically unstable. The fixator can be rapidly applied and a good reduction obtained.

d. Hybrid external fixation and ring fixators
   i. Ring fixators (Ilizarov-type fixators) can be used to suspend comminuted articular fragments.
   ii. The distal rings, anchored in the stable tibial diaphysis, provide the platform for the ring holding up the plateau.
   iii. As with external fixation, ring fixators limit soft tissue stripping and are less likely to be complicated by wound breakdown and infection. They can also be supplemented with limited internal fixation using cannulated screws.
   iv. "Hybrid" fixators use standard external fixator pins in the tibial diaphysis, instead of rings. The pins are connected to the tibial plateau ring using a standard external fixation bar.

D. Complications

1. Post-traumatic arthritis is a common complication of tibial plateau fractures.
   a. The major cause of this is instability of the knee in varus or valgus stress.
   b. Articular displacement is also a cause of arthritis.
   c. Associated ligamentous injuries are repaired using standard techniques after fracture union.
2. Wound breakdown and infection are also potential complications, especially with open fractures or those with injured soft tissues.
3. Peroneal nerve injury
   a. Most common with trauma to the lateral aspect of the leg where the nerve courses in proximity to the fibular head and lateral tibial plateau

X. TIBIAL SHAFT FRACTURES

A. Occurrence

1. Tibial fracture is one of the most common long bone injuries seen in trauma centers.
2. Since much of the tibia is subcutaneous, open fractures are very common.
3. Soft tissue damage and bone loss can be extensive.
4. The severely mangled leg remains one of the most difficult injuries to treat.

B. Evaluation

1. AP and lateral views of the ankle, knee, and tibia should be obtained.

2. A thorough examination of the soft tissues and neurovascular structures must be carried out to avoid missing an injury.

C. Classification
1. No accepted classification for tibial fractures exists.
2. Most surgeons describe fractures according to site (proximal, middle, or distal third), pattern (transverse, oblique, butterfly, or comminuted), and displacement.

D. Treatment
1. Nonoperative
   a. Nonoperative treatment can give good functional results in many low-energy tibial fractures.
   b. Treatment starts with a long-leg, bent-knee cast for about 4 weeks.
   c. This is followed by a patellar tendon-bearing cast.
   d. Progressive weight bearing is allowed as fracture callus is seen on radiographs.
   e. Cast immobilization is continued until the fracture unites. Union commonly takes from 3 to 5 months in tibia fractures (longer in smokers).
   f. Maintenance of reduction can be difficult.
   g. Close monitoring and frequent radiographs are necessary.
   h. Remanipulation or cutting wedges out of the cast to move the fracture is occasionally necessary.
   i. The following indications for cast treatment are commonly quoted:
      i. <5 degrees of varus or valgus malalignment
      ii. <10 degrees of anterior or posterior angulation
      iii. <1 cm of shortening
      iv. < 5 degrees of malrotation
2. Operative
   a. Operative fixation provides excellent stabilization and maintenance of reduction.
   b. The following are commonly quoted as indications for surgical management:
      i. Ipsilateral femur fracture (floating knee)
      ii. Segmental tibia fracture
      iii. Concomitant vascular injury requiring repair
      iv. Concomitant compartment syndrome
      v. Multiply injured patient
      vi. Pathologic fractures
      vii. Inability to maintain reduction with closed methods
   c. Plating, as a means of surgical stabilization, is not used at Parkland Memorial Hospital.
   d. IM nailing is the treatment of choice at Parkland Memorial Hospital.
      i. Reamed IM nailing gives excellent stabilization of tibial fractures.
      ii. Static locking of IM nails prevents rotational deformities, and reaming deposits bone graft at the fracture site.

      iii. Reaming allows easy placement of IM nails and seems to lessen the prevalence of delayed union.
      iv. The endosteal blood supply, which reaming destroys, has been shown to return after 6 weeks.
      v. Unreamed-type nails (Delta nails) are still placed, but they are placed after reaming.
      vi. The unreamed-type nails are narrower and can be placed after fewer passes of the reamer.
      vii. IM nailing is the surgical treatment of choice for most closed tibia fractures.
   e. External fixation
      i. External fixation is useful in stabilizing open tibia fractures that cannot be managed with an IM nail.
      ii. External fixation allows further care of wounds and does not disturb the fracture site.
      iii. In fractures with no soft tissue coverage, external fixation avoids contamination of the medullary canal, which is a possible complication of nailing.

E. Complications

1. Nonunion or delayed union
   a. More common after more severe injuries
   b. Prophylactic bone grafting 6 to 8 weeks after injury is normally done in high-energy fractures, since they will predictably be very slow to unite.
   c. The posterolateral approach to the tibia is useful for bone grafting, since it avoids the original injury site.
   d. Smoking has been shown to double the time required for healing in practically all types of tibia fractures.
   e. Delayed union can be treated with dynamization of the nail or reamed-exchange nailing.
2. Malunion
   a. More common after casting
   b. Correctional osteotomies can be stabilized using plates, IM nails, or Ilizarov-ring fixators.
   c. No criteria for defining malunion exist; each case must be individually considered.
3. Infection and osteomyelitis
   a. More common after open injuries
   b. Can be prevented with aggressive surgical debridement at the first operataion
   c. Established infections should be treated aggressively with removal of all infected tissues
4. Soft tissue loss
   a. Common after high-energy injuries
   b. Should be addressed after the soft tissue envelope has healed
   c. Treatment ranges from simple iliac crest-bone grafting to bone transport using Ilizarov-ring fixators.

5. Compartment syndrome
   a. Common after tibia fractures, especially open fractures
   b. Up to 10% of open tibia fractures develop compartment syndrome.
   c. Require four-compartment fasciotomy

XI. SPECIAL SITUATIONS

A. The following guideline for open fracutres uses the Gustilo and Andersen classification system. It must be remembered that this classifications system has poor interobserver reliability.
B. Each open fracture must be treated according to the fracture's "personality."
C. Grade I or II. These injuries can usually be treated with reamed IM nailing.
D. Grade IIIA. The usual treatment is with an IM nail.
1. If soft tissue coverage of the bone is available quickly, IM nailing is usually safe and effective.
2. If any question about the viability of the soft tissue exists, external fixation is a safe, reliable alternative.
E. Grade IIIB. This classification is usually best managed with an external fixator.
1. External fixation allows good access to the wound and can easily be modified if needed.
2. Flap coverage is not much more difficult with an external fixator in place.
F. Grade IIIC. These injuries should be managed according to the size of the soft tissue defect.
1. Vascular repair distal to the popliteal fossa is difficult and can make later flap coverage harder.
2. Patients with high-energy injuries require extensive surgical care. Despite aggressive care these patients can still develop an insensate, ischemic limb.
3. These are the most difficult patients to manage, and early amputation must be considered as an option.

XII. SUGGESTED READINGS

Rozycki GS, Tremblay LN, Feliciano DV, et al: Blunt vascular trauma in the extremity: Diagnosis, management, and outcome. J Trauma 55(5):814–824, 2003.

Rudloff U, Gonzalez V, Fernandez E, et al: Chirurgica taurina: A 10-year experience of bullfight injuries. J Trauma 61(4):970–974, 2006.

Knee Ligament Injuries

Krishna Venkatesh, MD

I. EVALUATION

A. History
1. Solicit mechanism of injury (Table 40-1).
2. Inquire as to sensations—audible pop, location of pain, feeling of instability, chronology, and quality of effusion.
3. History of previous injuries or operations on the knee can be helpful.
4. History of knee problems since the time of injury is valuable information in assisting with the diagnosis.

B. Physical examination
1. Always examine the good knee first for comparison.
2. Inspection: observe gait, if possible, and look for ecchymosis, edema, effusion, and abrasions.
3. Palpation: check for ballottement of the patella as well as tenderness and crepitus along the joint line, epicondyles, apophyses, and so on.
4. Observe the limits of both active and passive range of motion.
5. Stability testing (see Section III)
6. Be systematic, yet practical. For example, performing a pivot-shift test prior to other painful stimuli may help gain a diagnosis.

C. Diagnostic tests
1. **Radiography**
   a. Routine – anteroposterior (AP), lateral, and sunrise patella views
   b. Optional – condylar tunnel and oblique views
   c. Children – comparison and stress views
2. **Joint aspiration**
   a. Approximately 70% of patients who have acute hemarthroses following an injury have an anterior cruciate ligament injury.
   b. Aspiration followed by an injection of lidocaine into the knee joint may relieve the pain and allow a more thorough examination to be obtained.
3. **Magnetic resonance imaging (MRI)**
   a. Expensive, very sensitive and specific (>95%)
   b. Often unnecessary
   c. This test should not be ordered if an objective finding is not going to be treated surgically.
4. Arteriograms are useful in excluding vascular injury following a knee dislocation.
5. **Arthrometry**. Multiple-instrumented testing devices are available for reliable assessment of AP laxity.

II. CLASSIFICATION OF KNEE LIGAMENT INJURIES

A. Grade I: usually minor tearing or stretching of the ligament with <5 mm of laxity detected

TABLE 40-1
COMMON MECHANISMS OF KNEE INJURY

Mechanism of Injury (Knee Position[*])	Ligament Injury
Valgus	
Straight medial opening	Tibial collateral plus capsular ligaments[†]
External rotation	Medial structures, medial meniscus, anterior cruciate – 'terrible triad'
Varus	
Straight lateral opening	Fibular collateral plus capsular ligaments[†]
Internal rotation	Lateral ligaments plus anterior cruciate
External rotation	Lateral ligaments plus posterior cruciate
Hyperextension	Posterior capsule and posterior cruciate[‡]
Direct blow driving tibia backward	Posterior cruciate
Direct blow driving tibia forward	Anterior cruciate

[*] Tibia moving with femur fixed.
[†] Severe opening implies injury to either one or both cruciates.
[‡] Severe hyperextension may also injure the anterior cruciate ligament.

B. Grade II: partial tearing of the ligament (50% to 75%) with 5 to 10 mm of laxity detected
C. Grade III: associated with a complete tear, >10mm laxity, and no endpoint on examination
D. Isolated laxities: involving one plane
E. Combined laxities: involving >1 plane and is usually a rotational instability (i.e., anterolateral rotatory, posterolateral rotatory, anteromedial rotatory, and posteromedial rotatory instabilities)
F. Knee dislocation: classification according to the displacement of the tibia in relation to the femur

III. STABILITY TESTING

A. Isolated laxities
1. **Anterior cruciate ligament (ACL) insufficiency**
   a. The Lachman test at 30 degrees of flexion is the most sensitive test (Figure 40-1). The quality of the endpoint (firm or soft) should be noted and compared with the contralateral side.
   b. The pivot shift phenomenon describes the anterior subluxation of the tibial plateau in extension pivoting into reduction with knee flexion.
   c. The anterior drawer test is less sensitive than the Lachman test. (Figure 40-2)
   d. Before determining anterior laxity, ensure that the tibia begins in the neutral position for all testing. If the tibia is posteriorly subluxated secondary to a posterior cruciate ligament injury, one may be fooled by anterior-posterior translation.
2. **Posterior cruciate ligament (PCL) insufficiency**
   a. Posterior drawer test

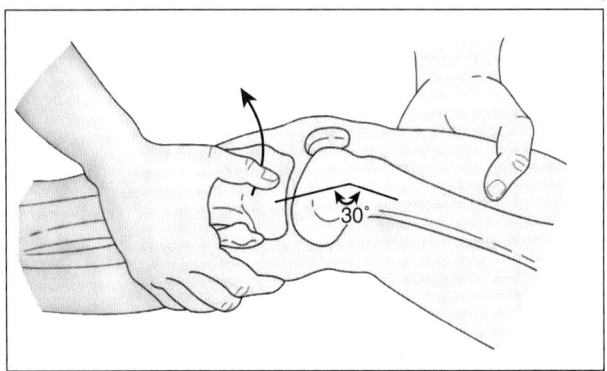

FIGURE 40-1

Lachman test for anterior cruciate instability is at 30 degrees of flexion. The extremity does not have to be lifted or the foot stabilized.

  i. The posterior drawer test is the most accurate method of detecting a PCL injury.
  ii. The test is similar to the anterior drawer test except that a posteriorly directed force is applied to the tibia, starting from the neutral position.
  iii. The latter point is important because, with a PCL-deficient knee, there is normally a posterior sag of the tibia when flexed to a 90-degree angle.
  b. Quadriceps active test
  i. The knee is flexed 90 degrees with the foot stabilized as the patient is asked to contract the quadriceps muscle.
  ii. The tibia will translate forward from the posterior subluxed position when a PCL deficiency is present.
3. **Medial collateral ligament (MCL) insufficiency with valgus or medial laxity**
  a. Valgus stress test (Figures 40-3)
  i. The primary restraint to valgus stress is the MCL with additional support afforded by the secondary stabilizers (i.e., cruciate ligments, posterior oblique ligament, and the posteromedial capsule).
  ii. The MCL should be stressed to 0 degrees and 30 degrees of flexion.
  iii. With 30 degrees of flexion, the secondary stabilizers are relaxed and the superficial and deep MCL fibers are stressed.
  iv. With full extension, medial laxity implies injury to the MCL and secondary stabilizers, giving anteromedial or posteromedial rotatory instability.
4. **Lateral collateral ligament (LCL) insufficiency with varus or lateral laxity**

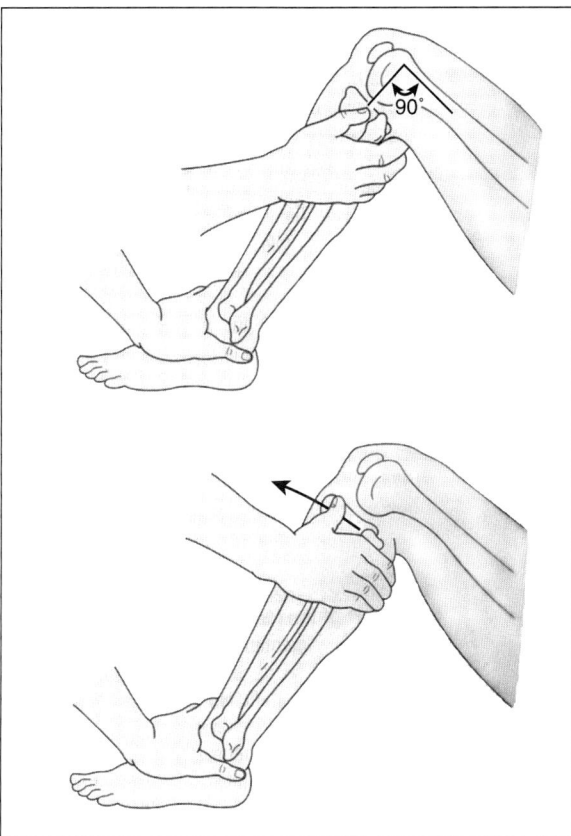

FIGURE 40-2

Anterior drawer test determines anterior cruciate instability. Flex the knee to 90 degrees and stabilize the foot. Note forward shift of the tibia.

  a. The varus stress test (i.e., varus or adduction stress testing) should be performed in the same manner as above in full extension and at 30 degrees of flexion.
  b. Isolated sectioning of the lateral posterolateral ligaments has demonstrated only a small change (1 to 4 degrees) in varus rotation at all angles of flexion with an LCL complete tear.
  c. Further increase in varus laxity or a side-to-side difference in external rotation >10 degrees indicates a posterolateral complex injury usually involving the LCL, popliteus, arcuate ligament complex, lateral head of the gastrocnemius, or posterolateral capsule.

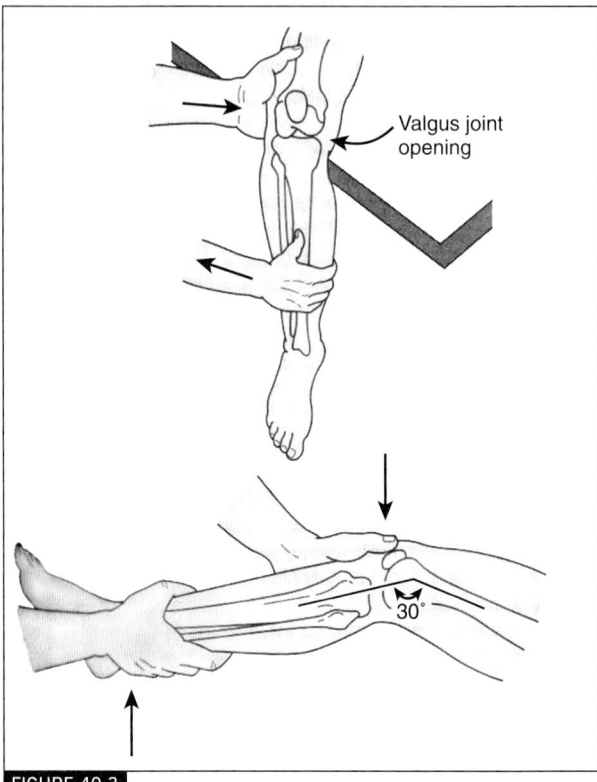

FIGURE 40-3
Valgus test in 30 degrees of flexion.

B. Combined laxities
1. Posterolateral complex with ACL deficiency is evaluated with the external rotation recurvatum test:
   a. Performed with the patient in the supine position
   b. The big toe is grasped and lifted, lifting the entire leg from the table.
   c. If the tibia externally rotates and the knee falls into varus hyperextension, a combined ACL posterolateral complex injury is present.
   d. Further side-to-side differences in external rotation and Lachman's test at 30 degrees corroborate this diagnosis.
2. **Posterolateral complex with PCL deficiency**
   a. Prone (or supine) external rotation test
      i. Performed at 30 degrees and 90 degrees of flexion

ii. Increases in varus and external rotation at 30 degrees and 90 degrees of knee flexion, compared with the opposite side, indicate an injury to the PCL and posterolateral structures.
 b. Posterolateral drawer test
  i. A posterior drawer test is applied with the knee flexed 80 degrees and externally rotated 15 degrees.
  ii. Laxity indicates a combined injury to the PCL and posterolateral complex.

IV. TREATMENT OF KNEE LIGAMENT INJURIES

A. General principles
1. Rest, ice, compression, and elevation (RICE) along with symptomatic treatment are sufficient until the inflammatory phase is completed in several weeks.
2. Gentle, passive and active range-of-motion exercises are performed as tolerated to prevent stiffness and atrophy.
3. Crutches and bracing can be helpful.

B. Collateral ligament injuries
1. Grades I and IIa
   a. Treat in a hinged brace with full range of motion until completely nontender and clinically stable.
   b. Rehabilitation should concentrate on quadriceps, hamstrings, and adductor strengthening.
2. Grade III
   a. Same as above, allowing for more time to heal
   b. MCL tears associated with cruciate ligament injuries may or may not be repaired. This is a controversial subject and should be left to the individual surgeon.
   c. Posterolateral complex tears should be repaired acutely or reconstructed in chronic situations.

C. ACL injury
1. Nonoperative treatment
   a. Treat in a hinged brace and encourage full range-of-motion exercises until the acute inflammation has resolved.
   b. Rehabilitation concentrating on hamstring and quadriceps strengthening as well as obtaining a full range of motion
   c. Use a functional brace for patients involved in athletics or work requiring pivotiong or climbing.
   d. Nonoperative treatment may involve arthroscopic surgery for meniscal tears or debridement of the ACL stump to allow a full range of motion.
2. Operative treatment
   a. Arthroscopic or open repair should be performed if the ligament has avulsed bone from the tibia or femur (more commonly the former) and is unstable. Primary repairs have a poor success rate and should be considered in only the immature person with open growth plates.

b. Reconstruction of the ACL using patellar bone-tendon-bone, hamstring, or allograft tendon is usually recommended in a young, active patient who wishes to continue an active lifestyle or those who have failed nonoperative treatment and have instability with daily activities.
c. This decision should be individualized for each patient with the understanding that the rehabilitation process is lengthy and just as important as the surgery.

D. PCL injury
1. Isolated PCL injuries are usually treated nonoperatively with a hinged knee brace and full range of motion, while emphasizing quadriceps strengthening. However, if the injury is associated with disability or combined injuries, surgical reconstruction is advocated.
2. Arthroscopic or open repair should be performed if bony avulsion has taken place.

V. KNEE DISLOCATIONS

A. Classification. This is made according to the displacement of the tibia in relation to the femur.
1. Anterior
2. Posterior
3. Medial
4. Lateral
5. Rotatory

B. Occurrence. Anterior dislocations secondary to a hyperextension force are the most common.

C. Vascular injury
1. Incidence is about 20% to 30%. Arteriograms should be performed emergently on all knee dislocations because of risk.
2. Absence of pedal pulses; tenderness, swelling, and ecchymosis in the popliteal fossa; or a cold cyanotic lower extremity are all signs of a vascular injury.
3. Warm ischemia time should not exceed 6 to 8 hours.
   a. Attempts at arterial repair after 8 hours frequently require later amputation secondary to nonviable tissues distal to the knee joint.
4. Compartment syndromes may accompany these injuries. Treat appropriately with fasciotomies.

D. Nerve injury
1. The incidence of peroneal nerve injury varies between 16% and 43%. It is more common following a posterolateral knee dislocation.
2. Prognosis for return of function should be guarded.

E. Ligament injury
1. Usually both cruciates and one or more collaterals are torn.
2. Avulsion fractures at the insertion of the PCL and ACL are common, making repair a possibility.

3. If the primary repair is tenuous, the augmentation with the semitendinosus and gracilis, or a reconstruction, should be performed.

F. Treatment

1. Physical examination documenting pulses and a neurologic examination are paramount.
2. Reduce the dislocation emergently and splint in slight flexion. Most dislocations can be reduced by closed means.
3. Re-examine the patient after reduction for vascular injury and then evaluate the popliteal artery with an arteriogram.
4. Open dislocations should undergo:
   a. Immediate irrigation and debridement
   b. Vascular exploration and possible repair
   c. Stabilization with an external fixator, splint, or orthosis
5. Ligamentous repair or reconstruction should be performed within 7 to 10 days for best results. When this is not possible, nonsurgical management in a hinged brace or cast can yield satisfactory results.
6. Rehabilitation should concentrate on range-of-motion therapy and quadriceps and hamstring strengthening.
   a. Current data suggest that stiffness and knee pain are much more common than ligamentous insufficiency following knee dislocations.
   b. Therefore, rehabilitation is of utmost importance.
7. Operative methods yield better outcomes than nonoperative methods.

VI. SUGGESTED READINGS

Abou-Sayed H, et al: Blunt lower-extremity trauma and popliteal artery injuries: Revisiting the case for selective arteriography. Arch Surg 137(5): 585-589, 2002.

Inaba K, et al: Multi-slice CT angiography for arterial evaluation in the injured lower extremity. J Trauma 60(3):502-507, 2006.

Koval JK, Zuckerman JD: Handbook of Fractures, 2nd ed. Philadelphia, Lippincott Williams & Wilkins, 2002, pp163-235.

Foot and Ankle Injuries

Taylor Smith, MD, and Henry Ellis, MD

I. INTRODUCTION

When evaluating an injured foot or ankle, the location, mechanism, and timing of the injury; the overall condition of the patient and any underlying functional disability should be determined and documented. A complete neurovascular examination must always accompany the physical examination.

II. ANKLE AND FOOT EVALUATION

A. Physical examination
1. **Circumferential visual inspection** for any skin defect that may indicate an open fracture or open joint which will require surgical debridement
2. **Inspect and document** areas of deformity/displacement.
3. **Palpate** both proximally and distally to area of deformity to evaluate for possible hidden injury prior to radiographs. Palpation of the proximal fibula may reveal a Maisonneuve fracture (a **fracture** of the medial malleolus of the ankle with disruption of the tibiofibular syndesmosis).
4. **Range of motion** of the ankle, subtalar, midtalar, and metatarsophalangeal joints should be evaluated.
5. **Vascular examination**, including bilateral comparison of posterior tibial and dorsalis pedis pulses. You can also assess capillary refill and document the color of the foot and ankle.
6. **Neurologic examination** including
   a. **Sensory** – dorsum of the foot (superficial peroneal), web space (deep peroneal), lateral border of the foot (sural), and bottom of the foot (posterior tibial); can use light touch and sharp/dull discrimination
   b. **Motor** – dorsiflexion and plantar flexion of the toes is usually acceptable.

B. Radiographic studies
1. **Initial x-rays**
   a. Ankle—anteroposterior (AP), lateral, and mortise views
   b. Foot—AP, lateral, and oblique views
2. **Computed tomography** is used in assessing calcaneal fractures and some pilon and midfoot fractures.

III. INITIAL MANAGEMENT PRINCIPLES

A. All patients with foot and ankle injuries should have their injured extremity elevated above their heart as expeditiously as possible to prevent edema.

B. Foot compression devices are useful in the management of soft tissue swelling.

C. Reduction attempts should be made, especially with a loss of pulses or severe deformity. This can dramatically improve subsequent care by reducing the risk of skin necrosis and tension on neurovascular structures.

D. Open fractures should be managed with:
1. Tetanus prophylaxis
2. Immediate IV antibiotic therapy
3. Emergent surgical irrigation and debridement

IV. ANKLE SPRAINS

A. Most likely anterior talofibular ligament
B. Use the "squeeze test" (increased pain with calf squeeze) to determine syndesmotic injury.
C. Use Ottawa ankle rules to determine if radiographs are needed to rule out fractures.
1. Distal tibia or fibula tenderness
2. Tenderness at base of fifth metatarsal or navicular bone
3. Inability to bear weight
D. An alternate general rule is that patients who are able to ambulate do not require radiographs.
E. Best treated with **r**est, **i**ce, **c**ompression and **e**levation (**RICE**)
F. Severe sprains may require a walking boot or surgical treatment

IV. ANKLE DISLOCATIONS

A. Ankle dislocations should be reduced and splinted immediately to prevent pressure or impaction injury (before radiographs if clinically evident).
B. Associated fractures and ligamentous injuries almost always accompany a dislocation.
C. Can be associated with neurovascular compromise and will necessitate immediate closed reduction
D. Require an immediate orthopaedic consultation

V. ANKLE FRACTURES

A. Open abrasions and wounds should be cleaned and dressed in a sterile fashion. Fracture blisters should be left intact and dressed with a well-padded dressing.
B. Pilon fractures are a subset of ankle fractures in which the tibial pilon has one or more fractures. They may require CT scan with both axial and coronal images.
C. Treatment options include cast immobilization, limited open reduction with internal fixation, or external fixation.

D. **Open fractures** should be reduced and splinted with sterile wet gauze over the wound. Open fractures are taken to the operating room within 8 hours of injury to decrease the incidence of infection. Do not attempt to clean, debride, or remove foreign bodies in the emergency department.
E. **Nonoperative treatment**
1. Nondisplaced stable fractures without syndesmotic injury
2. Displaced fracture with stable anatomic reduction
3. If operative treatment for patient is contraindicated due to his/her status

VI. FOOT FRACTURES

A. **Talus fractures**
1. Usually result from high-energy trauma
2. **Most important bone** in the foot to stabilize due to the large number of joints
3. **A CT may be required** to characterize fracture or assess articular involvement.
4. **Prone to avascular necrosis** depending on type and severity of fracture. This is due to the blood supply running from distal to proximal.
5. **Usually requires operative fixation** with no weight bearing for 3 months
B. **Calcaneus fractures**
1. Usually caused by **motor vehicle collision or falls** from heights of more than 6 feet
2. **May be accompanied by vertebral** fractures due to axial load and therefore mandate radiographic evaluation of the lumbar spine
3. **Most patients requires a CT scan** to define anatomy of injury and to enable planning of operative intervention.
4. **Nonoperative versus operative fixation**. There is no benefit to early surgery as long as patient is non-weight bearing. In rare cases patient may require primary fusion.
C. **Other hindfoot and midfoot fractures**
1. **Assessment** similar to other foot and ankle fractures
2. **Most common hindfoot dislocation is a subtalar dislocation**, of which medial dislocation is most common. As previously mentioned, reduction needs to be performed expeditiously.
3. **Fractures** near the midtarsal joints include talonavicular and calcaneocuboid.
4. Fracture pattern and mechanism will determine:
   a. Need for additional radiographs beyond plain films
   b. Operative vs. nonoperative treatment
D. Metatarsal fractures
1. **Most common fracture of the foot**
2. **Most are treated nonoperatively**, with early weight bearing in a hard-sole shoe or walking cast if fracture is nondisplaced.

3. **Simple avulsion fractures** of the base of the fifth metatarsal are best managed with weight bearing in a 3-dimensional boot.
4. **Jones (proximal fifth metatarsal fracture) and diaphyseal fractures** of the fifth metatarsal require cast immobilization and non-weight bearing.
5. **Displaced or open fractures will require operative reduction and fixation**.
E. **Tarsometatarsal dislocations (Lisfranc injury)**
1. **Disruption of the articulation** between the metatarsals and the cuneiform bones
2. Injury is usually the result of motor vehicle collision or industrial accident.
3. Seen on standard AP and lateral radiographs; however, may require a CT
4. **Almost all require open reduction with internal fixation** followed by cast immobilization and non-weight bearing.

VII. ACHILLES RUPTURE

A. Typical patient is middle-aged weekend athlete.
B. **Mechanism** involves eccentric loading on a dorsiflexed foot with the knee in flexion causing a maximum stretch of the gastrocnemius and soleus muscles.
C. **Thompson test** – plantar flexion produced by squeezing the calf of a kneeling patient. The injured Achilles will demonstrate less plantar flexion.
D. **Treatment**
1. Nonoperative – reserved for older patient or younger patient not expected to return to athletic sports for 1 year
2. Operative – offers reduced re-rupture rate and increased plantar flexion strength

VIII. TENDON LACERATIONS

A. **Simple lacerations** of the lesser flexors or extensors without concomitant traumatic arthrotomy or open fracture can usually be left alone with the only potential long-term problem being deformity.
B. **Repair of the flexor hallucis longus** does not change long-term outcome.
C. **Primary repair** of all other tendon lacerations is done to restore muscle balance.

XI. COMPARTMENT SYNDROME

A. An orthopaedic emergency
B. Should be expected in all crush injuries, Lisfranc injury, or midtarsal fracture dislocations
C. Unlike other areas, the foot **has no consistent signs** (e.g., pain with passive flexion), and it is therefore incumbent upon the examiner to have a high level of suspicion.
D. **Emergent surgical release is indicated**.

X. LAWN MOWER INJURIES

A. Often involve multiple toes or large areas of tissue with multiple fractures or traumatic amputations
B. All patients require **triple antibiotic coverage**.
1. Cefazolin
2. Gentamicin
3. Metronidazole or clindamycin
C. Tetanus prophylaxis
D. Immediate surgical irrigation and debridement

XI. SUGGESTED READINGS

Canale ST, et al: Campbell's Operative Orthopaedics, 11th ed. Philadelphia, Mosby, 2008.

Koval KJ, Zuckerman JD: Handbook of Fractures, 2nd ed.. Philadelphia, Lippincott Williams & Wilkins, 2002, pp 242-290.

Leddy JJ, Smolinski RJ, Lawrence J, et al: Prospective Evaluation of the Ottawa Ankle Rules in a University Sports Medicine Center. Am J Sports Med 26(2):158-165, 1998.

Rockwood CA, Green DP, Bucholz RW, et al: Fractures in Adults, 6th ed. Lippincott Williams & Wilkins, 2006, pp 2147-2235.

Stiell IG, et al: A Study to develop clinical decision rules for the use of radiography in acute ankle injuries. Ann Emerg Med 21:384-390, 1992.

Thompson JC: Netter's Concise Atlas of Orthopaedic Anatomy. Yardley, PA, Icon Learning Systems, 2002, pp 243-280.

Upper Extremity Fractures and Dislocations

Taylor Smith, MD, and Henry Ellis, MD

When evaluating any fracture or upper extremity injury, a thorough history and physical examination, including detailed neurovascular examination, should be performed. History should include age, sex, occupation, dominant hand, and how the extremity is used in daily life. Details of the mechanism of injury may give insight into the fracture pattern and help determine the best method of treatment.

I. STERNOCLAVICULAR DISLOCATIONS

- **A. Mechanism of Injury** is usually from a direct force; however, indirect forces from anterolateral or posterolateral can also cause this injury.
- **B. Physical examination** must include complete neurovascular assessment plus evaluation of the trachea and esophagus. With a posterior dislocation, one must evaluate the integrity of the pulmonary system.
- **C. Plain films** may be obtained with or without a Hobbs view (axial radiograph of the sternoclavicular joint) or serendipity view (supine, 40-degree cephalad tilt of the x-ray). However, computed tomography will be able to assess a medial clavicle fracture versus dislocation
- **D. Anterior type**
  1. Patient may complain of pain with abduction and external rotation.
  2. Treatment goals are cosmetic and symptomatic.
     a. Closed treatment if patient is unstable
     b. Reduction should be attempted under general anesthesia with immobilization for 6 weeks.
  3. If closed treatment fails, acceptance of the resulting deformity, resection of the medial clavicle head, or surgical fixation with open reduction and fixation are all viable options.
- **E. Posterior type**
  1. Mediastinal structures must be carefully examined to rule out injury. The patient may show symptoms similar to thoracic outlet syndrome.
  2. Closed reductions are usually stable.
  3. Closed reduction involves traction with the extremity in abduction and extension.

II. CLAVICLE FRACTURES

- **A.** Up to **3% may be associated with pneumothorax**. Auscultation of the chest as well as palpating for crepitus is necessary.
- **B. Anteroposterior (AP) as well as oblique (45-degree caudal tilt) radiographs** may be necessary to evaluate the acromioclavicular and

sternoclavicular joints and determine the degree of angulation, displacement, and pattern.
C. **Classification is based on fracture location and displacement**: proximal, middle, or distal thirds, with minimal to severe displacement.
D. **Closed treatment is usually successful**. Sling or figure-of-eight bandage is usually sufficient for immobilization when used for 4 to 6 weeks.
E. **Open reduction-internal fixation is indicated** in open fractures, association with neurovascular compromise, cosmetics, severely displaced distal third fractures (controversial), or when the skin is tented or its integrity threatened.

III. SCAPULOTHORACIC DISLOCATIONS

A. **Very uncommon**
B. **Usually associated with neurovascular compromise and a high mortality rate (10% to 25%)**
C. **Intrathoracic** – inferior scapula is traumatically inserted between 2 ribs.
D. **Lateral** – can be thought of as a closed, partial amputation
1. Diagnosed as lateral displacement of the scapula on standard chest film
2. Marker for devastating neurovascular injury with immediate arteriogram and vascular repair indicated
E. **Treatments** include open reduction, internal fixation, amputation, arthrodesis, forearm-hand transfers, and prosthetic fitting.

IV. ACROMIOCLAVICULAR SEPARATION

A. **Common sports-related injury**
B. **A standard shoulder physical examination**: noting palpation of acromioclavicular (AC) joint, neurovascular status, and range of motion
C. **Standard 3 views of the shoulder**
   a. AP view in plane of scapula
   b. Lateral view in plane of scapula
   c. Axillary view
D. **Classification system**
   a. Type I – sprain of AC ligament with no radiographic abnormalities
   b. Type II – AC ligament tear with coroacoclavicular ligament sprain. Radiographs reveal slight elevation of distal clavicle and AC joint widening.
   c. Type III – AC and coracoclavicular ligaments torn with widening of coracoclavicular on radiographs.
   d. Type IV – type III with posterior displacement of distal clavicle
   e. Type V – type III with clavicle severely displaced
   f. Type VI – AC dislocated with inferior displacement of the clavicle.
E. **Treatment**
   a. **Types I to III**

    i. Conservative treatment with rest, ice, and sling for comfort
    ii. For heavy laborers or athletes, surgical treatment may be indicated.
  b. **Type IV to VI**
    i. Open reduction and fixation
    ii. Repair of coracoclavicular ligaments

V. SCAPULAR FRACTURES

- **A. Most common fracture** occurs through the body.
- **B.** Commonly associated with polytrauma
- **C.** Most often found incidentally during a trauma work-up
  1. Serve as a marker for high-energy thoracic trauma with many associated injuries
  2. Most commonly associated with pulmonary injury including contusion and pneumothorax
  3. Can also see traumatic brain injuries and cervical spine and skull fractures
- **D. Radiographic evaluation** include three views of the shoulder with scapular Y view. Computed tomography is also useful to further evaluate the fracture.
- **E. Compartment syndrome** is uncommon but needs to be ruled out due to overlying supraspinatus and infraspinatus.
- **F. Symptomatic treatment** is often all that is required for a scapular body fracture, including shoulder sling and early range of motion.
- **G. Complex fractures** involving the glenoid, neck, or spine of the scapula may require internal fixation.

VI. GLENOHUMERAL DISLOCATIONS

- **A.** Anterior dislocation – most common
  1. Extremity will be slightly externally rotated and adducted
  2. A careful neurovascular examination is necessary, including evaluation of **axillary nerve** function. Deltoid muscle is not easily tested, but tactile sensation over lateral shoulder will suffice.
  3. Humeral head will be anterior, medial, and inferior with a posterior sulcus on plain films. **Three views of the shoulder are required**.
  4. Usually the result of a fall or athletic trauma
  5. **Associated injuries**
    a. Greater tuberosity or glenoid fractures
    b. Brachial plexus or axillary nerve injury
    c. Vascular injury
      i. Usually seen in association with advanced atherosclerotic disease
      ii. May lead to amputation if not recognized early
  6. **Treatment** – usually closed reduction
    a. **Hippocratic technique** – physician's foot is placed in the patient's axilla and traction is applied to the extremity.

b. **Traction-countertraction** – with one sheet wrapped around the patient's chest and another around the flexed forearm of the affected side, the physician applies traction with an assistant providing countertraction.
c. **Operative treatment** may be necessary with chronic dislocation or associated injuries.
d. **Immobilization for 2 to 5 weeks**; however, use caution with patients >40 years old due to stiffness. Early range of motion may be indicated in some cases. Young patients with recurrent dislocation may require sling with immobilization for longer periods of time.
7. **Post reduction neurovascular examination and radiographs are necessary**.
B. **Posterior dislocations**
1. Relatively rare; account for less than 10% of shoulder dislocations
2. Usually due to strong muscle contractions during a **seizure or electrical injury**
3. Physical examination and radiographic evaluation are the same as for anterior dislocation.
4. **Prompt closed reduction** with care not to externally rotate the shoulder since this may lead to a fracture of the humeral head. Open reduction may need to be done if the dislocation is fixed or due to associated injuries.
C. **Inferior/superior dislocations**
1. **Very rare**
2. Usually associated with neurovascular compromise that will resolve with reduction

VII. PROXIMAL HUMERUS FRACTURES

A. Make up 4% to 5% of all fractures and are most common in older age groups in correlation with an increased incidence of **osteoporosis**
B. **A careful neurovascular examination** needs to be done and, like for a shoulder dislocation, special attention should be placed on axillary nerve function.
C. **Radiographic evaluation** should include 3 views of the shoulder and computed tomography if there is a need to evaluate relation to articular surface.
D. **Neer classification** (Figure 42-1) is most commonly used.
1. Described as two-, three-, or four-part fractures
2. One-part fractures are nondisplaced, nonangulated regardless of the number of fracture lines.
E. **Treatment**
1. **One-part fractures** – sling and early range of motion
2. **Two-part fractures** may require open reduction and internal fixation if closed reduction fails or required due to fracture pattern.
3. **Three-part fractures** – open reduction and internal fixation

VII. Proximal Humerus Fractures

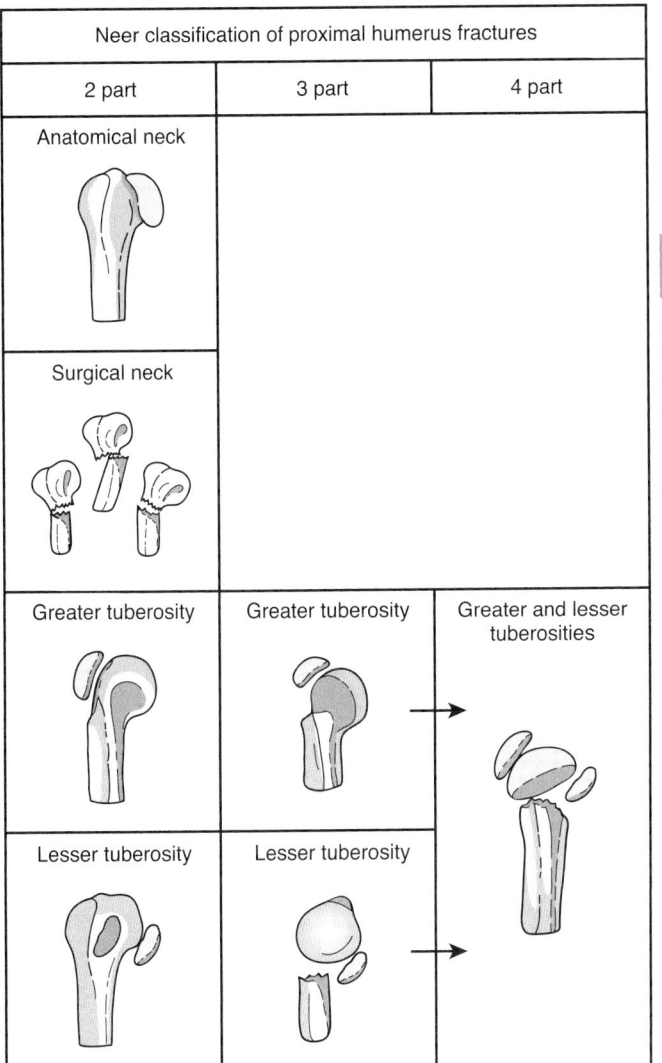

FIGURE 42-1
Neer classification for proximal humerus fractures.

4. **Four-part fractures** may require joint replacement due to the risk of avascular necrosis of the fragments.

VIII. DIAPHYSEAL HUMERUS FRACTURES

A. Site of fracture in relation to the muscular insertions on the humeral shaft will determine direction and degree of displacement.

B. Diagnosis
1. Cardinal signs of fracture: pain, swelling, deformity, crepitus. Limb shortening may be present.
2. Neurovascular examination of the entire arm must be documented. Special attention should be placed on radial nerve function.
3. Radiographs should include two views at 90 degrees to one another and include the shoulder and elbow.

C. Treatment
1. More than 90% are treated with closed reduction with immobilization in a hanging splint.
2. Operative Indications include
    a. Open fractures
    b. Polytraumatized patients
    c. Neurovascular injury
    d. Failed closed treatment
    e. Pathologic fractures
    f. Bilateral fractures
    g. Segmental fractures
    h. Floating elbow
    i. Nonunion
    j. Progressive radial nerve palsy
    k. Intra-articular extension

D. Complications
1. Radial nerve injury due to proximity to humeral shaft
2. Function should be documented before and after every intervention.

IX. DISTAL HUMERUS FRACTURE

A. Anatomy is best described as two divergent columns (condyles) supporting the articular surface.

B. Most common fracture pattern is the intercondylar fracture.

C. Physical examination and radiographs should include careful neurovascular examination, and two views of the elbow and possibly arm should be obtained. Look for the posterior "fat pad" sign.

D. Supracondylar fractures
1. **Extension type** – extra-articular, treated with posterior long arm splint in 90 degrees of flexion. Operative indication when open, displaced fracture or vascular injuries are present.

2. **Flexion type** – uncommon, but when present is associated with open fractures
E. **Transcondylar fractures**
1. Occurs in elderly with osteoporotic bone
2. Nonoperative vs. operative treatment depending on displacement and stability of fracture
F. **Intercondylar fractures**
1. **Most common**, mostly with comminution
2. **Mechanism** is usually force on posterior aspect of elbow, as if ulna is being compressed into the trochlea.
3. **Treatment** options depend on type of fracture and quality of bone.
   a. Cast immobilization
   b. Traction
   c. Gravity traction
   d. Open reduction internal fixation
   e. Total elbow arthroplasty
G. **Condylar fractures** (single-column fractures)
1. **Rare (3% to 4%)** with lateral column fractures being more common than medial
2. **Includes** capitellum, lateral epicondyle, epicondyle, and trochlea fractures
3. **Treatment with open reduction and internal** fixation is usually reserved for unstable or displaced fractures.
4. **Complications** are usually cubitus varus/valgus, arthritis, and/or ulnar nerve symptoms.

X. ELBOW DISLOCATION

A. **Occurs most commonly in younger age groups**; 5 to 25 years old is the peak age and accounts for 11% to 28% of elbow injuries.
B. **A careful neurovascular examination** should be done and documented immediately on presentation, after reduction, and then serially in cases with massive antecubital swelling.
C. **Classification** is based on relationship of the radius and ulna (Figure 42-2).
1. 80% are posterior or posterolateral.
2. May also be anterior or medial
3. Divergent dislocations or dislocation of the radius or ulna individually is very rare.
D. **Associated injuries**
1. **Vascular injury**
2. **Neurologic injury** – most commonly stretch injury to either median or ulnar nerves
3. **Supracondylar humerus** fracture must be considered.
4. **Compartment syndrome** (Volkmann contracture)
E. **Treatment**
1. **Posterior reduction** can be accomplished with forearm traction and arm countertraction

X. Elbow Dislocation

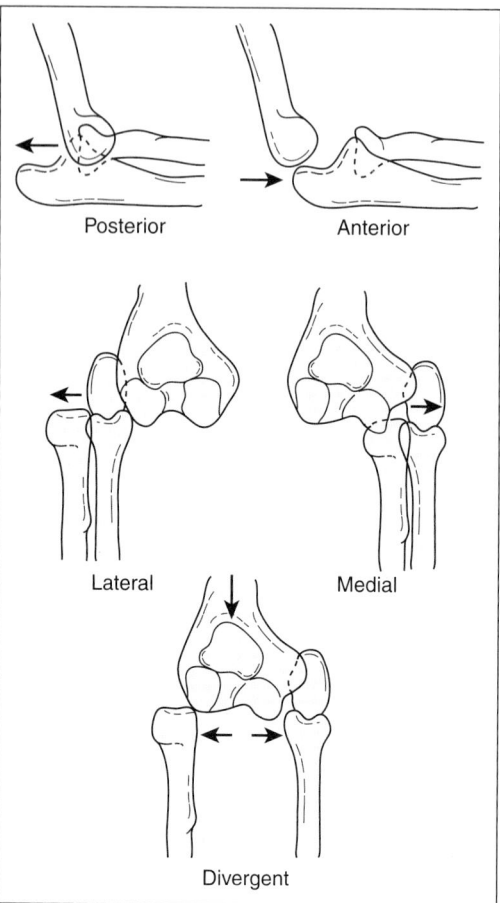

FIGURE 42-2
Elbow dislocations.

2. **Medial and lateral dislocations** may require sustained traction.
3. May require operative treatment
F. Post reduction
1. Confirm reduction with radiographs and physical examination, documenting range of motion and any residual instability.
2. Splint elbow at 90 degrees loosely to accommodate large amounts of swelling.

XI. OLECRANON FRACTURES

A. Represents the proximal articulation of the ulna
B. Presents with swelling, pain, and joint effusion due to intra-articular injury
C. **Diagnosis** using a true lateral radiograph
D. Treatment
1. **Nondisplaced** – long arm splint at 45 to 90 degrees of flexion with range of motion beginning on day 5 to 7
2. **Displaced** (greater then 2 mm) or transverse will require operative fixation.
E. Complications
1. Decreased range of motion
2. Arthritis
3. Nonunion/malunion
4. Ulnar neuropathy
5. Decreased extension power

XII. RADIAL HEAD FRACTURES

A. Found in 20% of all elbow trauma
B. Up to 30% also have associated injuries, including carpal fractures, distal radius ulnar disruption, Monteggia injuries, or capitellar fractures.
C. Mason classification
1. **Type I**: nondisplaced fractures
2. **Type II**: marginal fractures with displacement
3. **Type III**: communited fractures involving the entire head
4. **Type IV**: assocaited with dislocation of the elbow
D. Diagnosis
1. **Tenderness/swelling** over the lateral elbow or limitation of active or passive range of motion
2. **AP and lateral radiographs** – may see "sail sign" caused by intra-articular hemarthrosis elevating the anterior fat pad. If posterior fat pad is seen, additional studies to find a fracture are needed.
3. **Radiocapetellar view** –lateral film with the tube angled 45 degrees toward the shoulder
E. Treatment
1. **Type I** – splint or sling with early range of motion 24 to 48 hours after injury
2. **Type II** – operative fixation is controversial.
3. **Type III/IV** – radial head excision; the medial collateral ligament must be addressed for loss of integrity.
F. Complications
1. Decreased range of motion or contracture
2. Wrist pain
3. Arthritis
4. Loss of grip strength
5. Reflex sympathetic dystrophy

XIII. FOREARM FRACTURES

A. Examination should also include wrist and elbow to evaluate for any associated injuries. Also keep an eye out for a compartment syndrome.
B. "Nightstick" fracture – isolated ulnar shaft fracture from direct blow
1. Nondisplaced fractures may be treated with splinting.
2. Fractures with > 50% displacement or >10 degrees angulation should be treated with open reduction and internal fixation.
C. Galeazzi fracture – distal third radius fracture in association with subluxation or dislocation of the distal radioulnar joint (DRUJ)
1. Diagnosed with standard AP and lateral radiographs
2. Treatment – typically open reduction and internal fixation, but minimally displaced fractures may be managed in a long arm cast.
D. Monteggia fracture – proximal third ulnar shaft fracture associated with dislocation of the radial head
1. Categorized based on the direction of the radial head dislocation. See Figure 42-3, Bado's classification.
2. **Treatment**
   a. Closed reduction in pediatrics
   b. ORIF in adults

XIV. DISTAL RADIUS FRACTURES

A. Bimodal age distribution, 6 to10 years old or 60 to 69 years old
B. Among the most common fractures of the upper extremity
C. Colles fracture
1. >90% of distal radius fractures present as a Colles fracture.
2. Mechanism of injury is a fall on outstretched extremity.
3. Dorsal angulation, dorsal displacement, radial shift, and radial shortening
4. Reverse Colles fracture is a Smith's fracture.
D. Frykman classification widely accepted (see Table 42-1 and Figure 42-4)
E. Treatment
1. **Stable Fracture** – closed reduction and below elbow splint followed by cast and frequent follow-up films
2. **Unstable** – percutaneous pinning or open reduction internal fixation
F. Complications
1. Median nerve injury
   a. Mild sensory impairment may be observed.
   b. Progressive sensory loss must raise suspicion for compartment syndrome.
2. Ulnar nerve injury
3. Malunion/nonunion
4. Arthritis
5. Reflux sympathetic dystrophy
6. Tendon rupture
7. Midcarpal instability

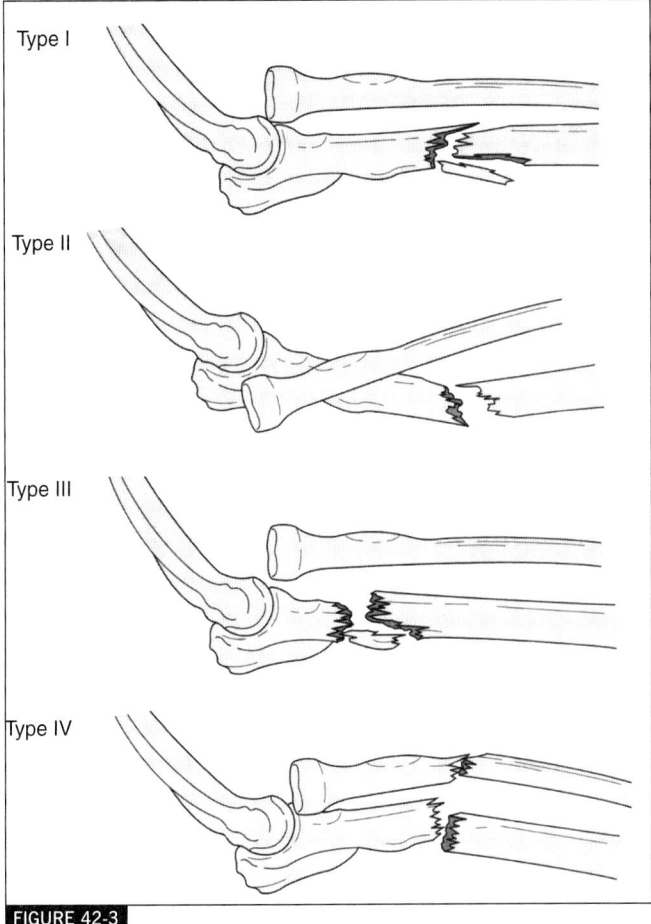

FIGURE 42-3

Types of Monteggia's fracture of the proximal third of the ulna with dislocation of the radial head.

358 XIV. Distal Radius Fractures

TABLE 42-1
FRYKMAN CLASSIFICATION OF FRACTURES TO DISTAL RADIUS

Fracture	Distal Ulna Fracture Absent	Distal Ulna Fracture Present
Extra-articular	I	II
Intra-articular involving radiocarpal joint	III	IV
Intra-articular involving radioulnar joint	V	VI
Intra-articular involving both radiocarpal and radioulnar joints	VII	VIII

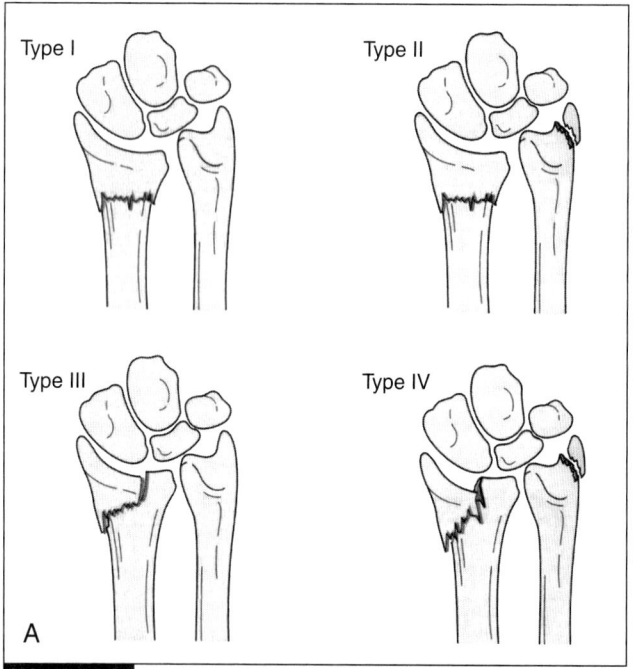

FIGURE 42-4A
Distal radius fractures types I to IV.

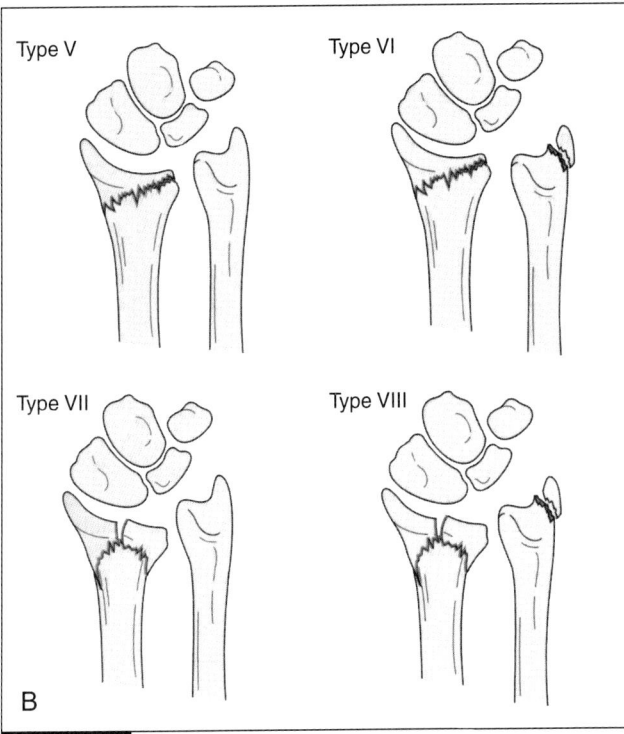

FIGURE 42-4B
Distal radius fractures types V to VIII.

XV. SUGGESTED READINGS

Canale ST et al: Campbell's Operative Orthopaedics, 11th ed. Philadelphia, Mosby 2008.

Koval KJ, Zuckerman JD: Handbook of Fractures, 2nd ed. Philadelphia, Lippincott Williams & Wilkins. 2002.

Thompson JC: Netter's Concise Atlas of Orthopaedic Anatomy. Yardley, PA, Icon Learning Systems, 2002.

Hand Injuries and Infections

Rohit K. Khosla, MD, and Tif Siragusa, MD

I. HISTORY AND MECHANISM OF INJURY

A. Timing and age of injury
B. Mechanism of injury (i.e., crush, avulsion, laceration, etc.)
C. Position of hand when injured
D. Hand dominance
E. Patient's occupation
F. Previous hand injuries
G. Age of patient
H. Medical/surgical history

II. PHYSICAL EXAMINATION

A. Inspection
1. Observe resting position of the hand and fingers. Tendon lacerations may cause asymmetry of digits in resting position.
2. Inspect soft tissue for discoloration, abrasions, lacerations, puncture wounds, erythema, edema, drainage, and extent of contamination.

B. Palpation
1. Palpate for crepitus and joint laxity.

C. Range of motion
1. **Active and passive motion of wrist and all digits**
   a. Flexor digitorum profundus (FDP) assessment (Figure 43-1)
   b. Flexor digitorum superficialis (FDS) assessment (Figure 43-2)
   c. **Scissoring effect**: when digits overlap on flexion. This indicates a significant metacarpal or phanlangeal fracture (Figure 43-3).
   d. **Tenodesis effect**: passively extend and flex the wrist. Extension produces normal flexion of digits by stretch of flexors. Flexion results in normal extension of digits by stretch of extensors. Abnormal findings here indicate tendon laceration. This test is useful when examining children and patients unable to comply with the examination (e.g., intubated, sedated, altered patients).

D. Vascular examination
assess radial and ulnar pulses or Doppler signal, Doppler signal in palmar arch, capillary refill (normal <2 seconds), and Doppler signal in both digital arteries of each digit.
1. Doppler Allen's test evaluates flow through the radial and ulnar arteries at wrist.
   a. Occlude both arteries at the wrist.
   b. The examiner releases pressure on one artery at a time to assess the flow in released artery.
   c. Should detect immediate Doppler signal in palmar arch if artery is patent. Allen's test is positive when there is no flow into the hand after release of an artery. This indicates an injury to the artery.

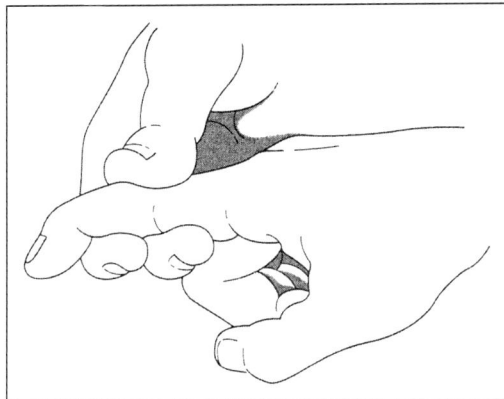

FIGURE 43-1
Actively flexing the distal interphalangeal joint while the proximal interphalangeal joint is stabilized tests integrity of flexor digitorum profundus (FDP) tendon.

   d. Perform similar technique with digital arteries when evaluating patency of digital vessels.
E. Sensory examination
1. Assess two-point discrimination of all digits. Normal discrimination is 2 to 5 mm. The open end of a paper clip can be used with ends 2 to 5 m apart.

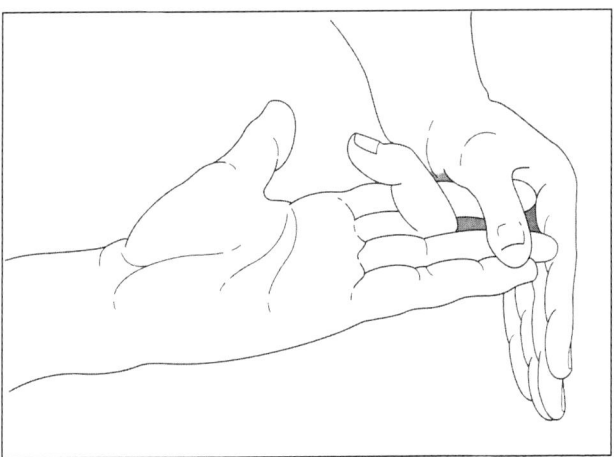

FIGURE 43-2
Actively flexing the proximal interphalangeal joint while adjacent fingers are held completely extended tests the integrity of the flexor digitorum superficialis (FDS) tendon.

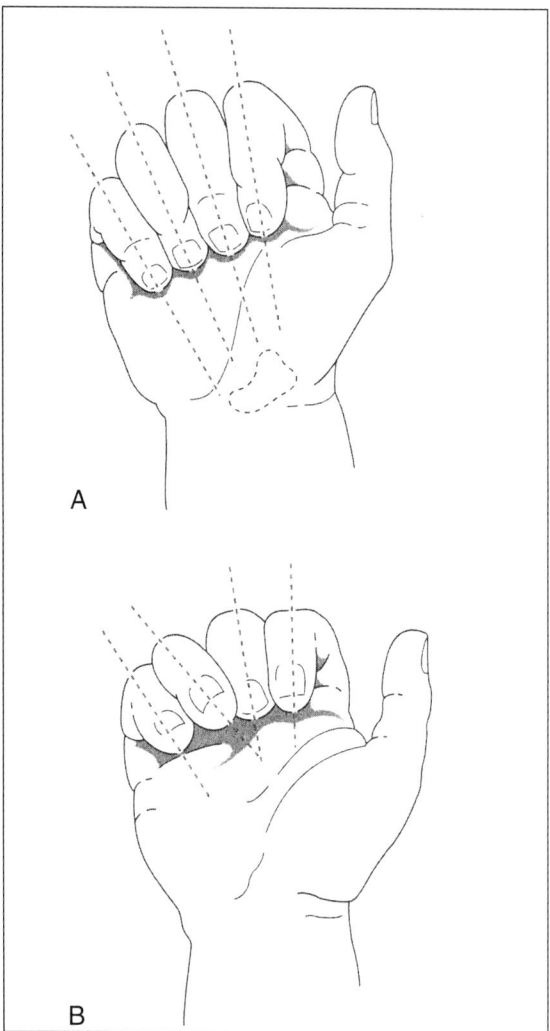

FIGURE 43-3
Scissoring effect indicates malrotation of metacarpal or phalangeal fractures
A, Normally all fingers point toward region of scaphoid when a fist is made.
B, Malrotation at fracture causes affected finger to deviate.

2. Assess sweat on palms. Normally there is a fine film of moisture on the palmar surface. Dry skin may indicate nerve injury.
3. **Prune test**: immerse the hand in water for 5 to 10 minutes. Glabrous skin that is normally innervated will wrinkle when submersed. A nerve injury will manifest as a finger without wrinkles. This test is useful when examining children and patients unable to comply with the examination (e.g., intubated, sedated, altered patients).

III. RADIOLOGIC EXAMINATION

A. **Standard views**: anteroposterior (AP), lateral, and oblique
B. **Stress views**: this is the best test if a ligament injury is suspected but requires local anesthetic.
C. **Comparison views** of the contralateral limb are essential for children and may be helpful in evaluating adult patients if the anatomy is confusing.
D. **Computed tomography scan**: this is useful for bone (e.g., carpal bone fractures) and joint evaluation. It is not routinely obtained.
E. **Magnetic resonance imaging** is useful for soft tissue evaluation. It is not routinely obtained.

IV. OTHER DIAGNOSTIC TESTS

A. **Arteriogram**: evaluate for vascular injury in the upper extremity. Risks include allergic reaction, bleeding, arterial injury, and renal failure.
B. **Electromyography**: useful >3 weeks after injury to demonstrate nerve conduction deficit in an injured peripheral nerve

V. ANESTHETIC TECHNIQUES

A. Use lidocaine 1% or 2% without epinephrine.
B. **Wrist blocks**: inject 5 to 7 mL at each location with a 25-gauge needle.
1. **Median nerve block** (Figure 43-4)
   a. Insert needle at a 45-degree angle into the carpal tunnel between the palmaris longus and flexor carpi radialis tendons at the level of the proximal wrist crease.
   b. If paresthesia is encountered, pull the needle back slightly to avoid injection directly into the nerve.
2. **Ulnar nerve block** (Figure 43-5)
   a. Insert needle at a 45-degree angle just radial to the flexor carpi radialis tendon at the proximal wrist crease.
3. **Superficial branch of radial nerve**
   a. Raise a subcutaneous weal over the radial styloid and infiltrate across the dorsal aspect of the wrist to the midline.
C. **Digital blocks**. Inject 3 to 5 mL at each location with a 25-gauge needle. Avoid circumferential injections of the digits because this can cause necrosis.

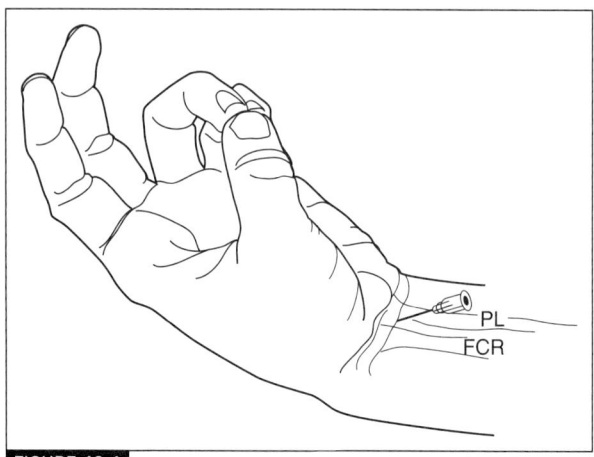

FIGURE 43-4

Median nerve block. Injection is into the carpal tunnel at a 45-degree angle between the palmaris longus and flexor carpi radialis tendon.

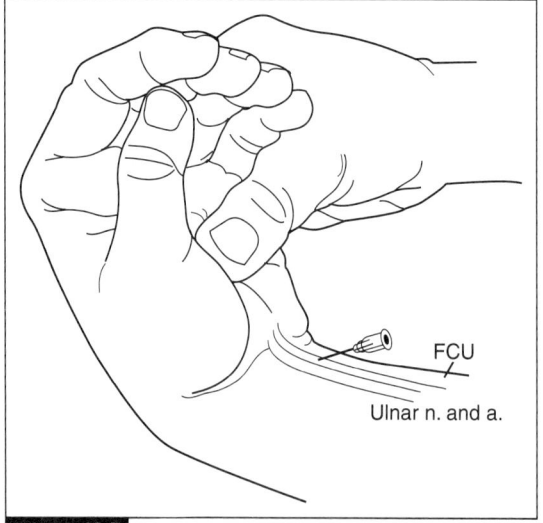

FIGURE 43-5

Ulnar nerve block. The nerve lies between the ulnar artery and the flexor carpi ulnaris tendon.

V. Anesthetic Techniques

1. **Volar approaches**
   a. **Metacarpal head approach**. Insert the needle on the volar metacarpal head until the flexor tendon sheath in reached. This will feel rubbery. Back off sheath slightly and inject 2 to 3 mL on either side of the flexor sheath. This will anesthetize both digital nerves at the bifurcation with a single stick.
   b. **Web space approach** (Figure 43-6). Insert the needle in the web space on each side of the digit. The web space is less sensate than the palm.

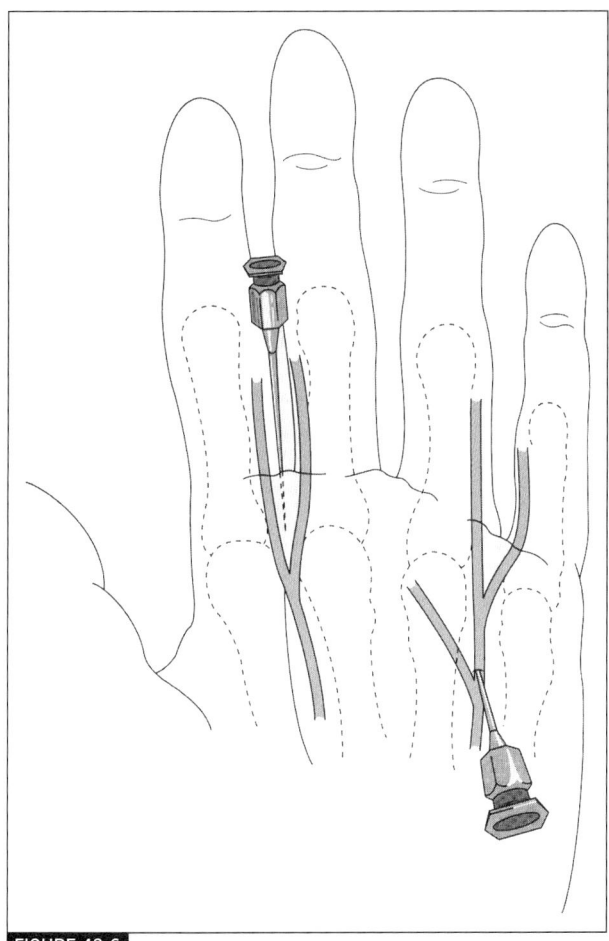

FIGURE 43-6

Web space and volar approach for digital nerve blocks.

c. **Intermetacarpal approach** (Figure 43-6). Insert the needle in the intermetacarpal space on each side of the target digit.
2. **Dorsal approach** (Figure 43-7). Inject in a volar direction on one side of the digit. Then redirect across the dorsal aspect. A second injection is made on the opposite side of the digit in a volar direction.

VI. ANATOMY

A. Flexor tendons (Figure 43-8)
1. Each digit has an FDP and an FDS tendon with an intricate pulley system.
2. The pulley system anchors the tendons, improves power, and prevents bowstringing.

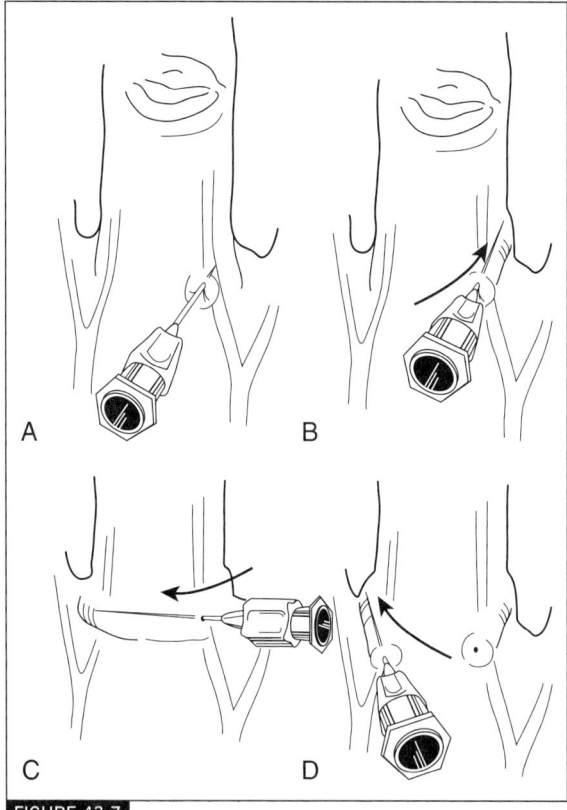

FIGURE 43-7

Dorsal approach for digital nerve block.

VII. Tendon Injury

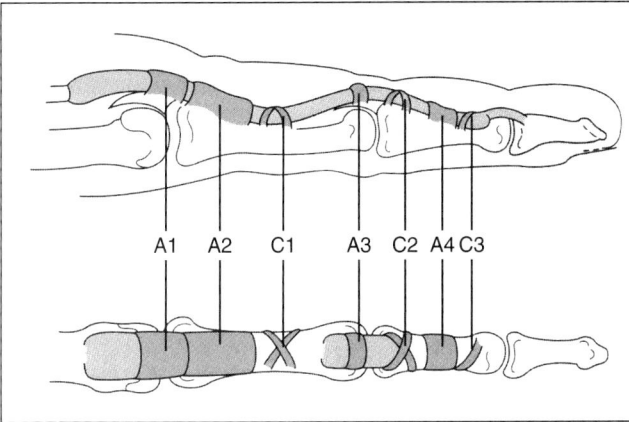

FIGURE 43-8

The components of the flexor tendon sheath and pulley system.

3. Do not disrupt A2 and A4 pulleys, as they are the most important.
4. There are five flexor tendon zones (Figure 43-9).
B. The are nine extensor tendon zones (Figure 43-10).
C. Nomenclature for classification of injuries
1. Right versus left
2. Digit: thumb, index finger, middle finger, ring finger, small finger
3. Zone of injury

VII. TENDON INJURY

A. Flexor tendon
1. **Closed injury**: commonly avulsion from insertion of tendon onto a bone
   a. Treat with open repair in the operating room.
2. **Open laceration**
   a. Level of injury may be at different level than skin laceration depending on the position of the hand at the time of injury (e.g., if fist was clenched the tendon laceration will be distal to the skin laceration).
   b. Requires operative repair. Place in dorsal extension blocking splint with metacarpophalangeal (MCP) joints at 45 to 70 degrees of flexion. Immobilize in splint for 4 weeks.
   c. If repair is to be delayed, clean and close lacerations and splint hand with digits and wrist in slight flexion.
   d. Zone II injuries are problematic secondary to poor gliding of tendons through the scar.

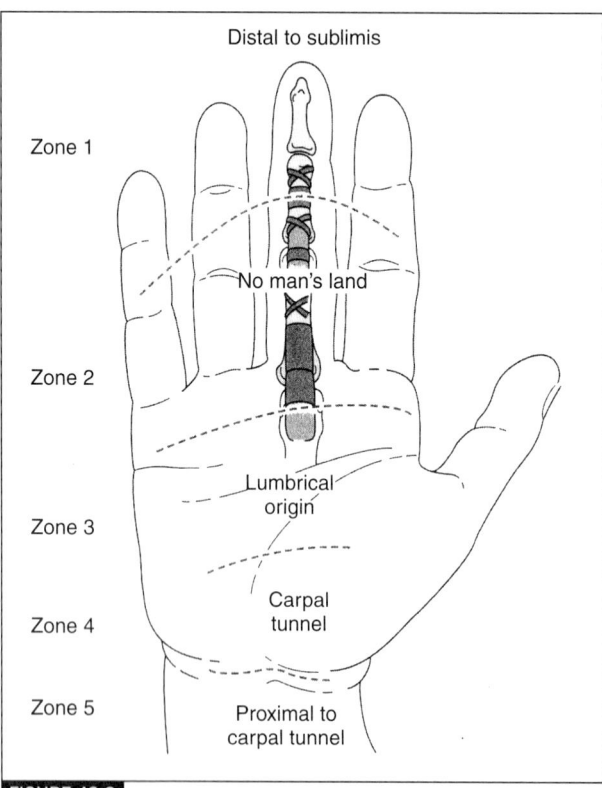

FIGURE 43-9

The five flexor zones of the hand.

   e. Rehabilitation is as important as actual repair.
B. Extensor tendon
1. **Closed injury**: commonly avulsed from dorsum of distal phalanx after hyperextension. This can lead to mallet deformity.
   a. **Treatment**: closed reduction with a stack splint for 6 weeks leaving the proximal interphalangeal (PIP) joint free
2. **Open laceration**
   a. Best repaired in the operating room
   b. If repair is to be delayed, clean and close the wound. Place in a volar splint with 45 degrees of wrist extension and with the MCP joints flexed at 30 degrees.

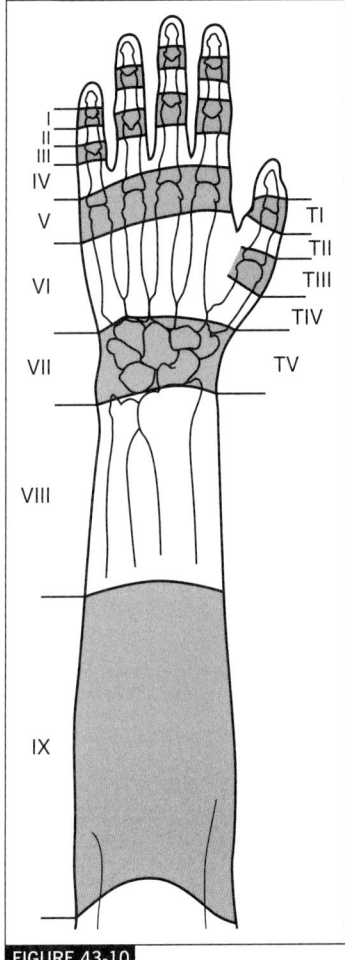

FIGURE 43-10

The nine extensor zones of the hand.

3. **Boutonniere deformity**: disruption of extensor tendon central slip at PIP joint with volar migration of lateral bands leading to flexion of the PIP joint and hyperextension of the distal interphalangeal (DIP) joint.
   a. **Open injury**: treat with debridement followed by tendon repair.
   b. **Closed injury**: splint the PIP in full extension or pin the PIP with K-wire and leave the DIP joint free for 6 weeks.

VIII. NERVE INJURY

A. At Parkland Memorial Hospital, all upper extremity nerve injuries are repaired as soon as possible.
B. Motor nerves can be repaired within 6 months of injury.
C. Sensory nerves should be repaired and can be repaired within 12 months of injury.
D. Digital nerves
1. We attempt to repair all digital nerve injuries to restore protective sensation in the hand.
2. Key nerves for pinch function and protective sensation of the hand are the following:
   a. Thumb ulnar digital branch
   b. Index radial digital branch
   c. Small finger ulnar digital branch
3. Surgical repair is done in the operating room by a microsurgeon to preserve pinch function and protective sensation.

E. Peripheral nerves
1. Microsurgical repair is mandatory for median, ulnar, and radial nerves.
2. If repair is to be delayed, clean and close the wound. Splint the hand in neutral position.
3. Nerve injury is often associated with tendon injuries.
4. If isolated nerve injury is suspected, reexamine in a few days to assess for return of sensation as neuropraxia can occur.

IX. BLOOD VESSEL INJURY

A. Microsurgical repair is necessary for any digit with complete loss of blood flow.
B. Isolated digital artery injuries do not need to be repaired if the finger is perfused and has normal capillary refill. However, sensory regeneration of an associated digital nerve repair is improved with digital vessel repair on that side of the digit.
C. Avoid blind clamping when operating on the upper extremity as nerves run very close to arteries.

X. LIGAMENT INJURY

A. The basic treatment regimen for joint dislocation is to attempt closed reduction under digital block and to stress the joint to test stability after reduction.
1. If the joint is stable, immobilize.
2. If the joint is unstable or irreducible, consider operative intervention.

B. DIP joint and thumb IP joint
1. Usually dorsally or laterally dislocated
2. Closed reduction and immobilization with slight flexion for 3 weeks

C. PIP joint
1. Most common ligament injured in hand
2. May be dorsal, lateral, or volar dislocation
3. An unstable joint may indicate a fracture dislocation.
4. Most can be treated with closed reduction and splinting at 30 degrees for two weeks, followed by buddy taping and range of motion.
5. If more than 40% of the articular surface is involved, proceed to open reduction and pinning to restore articular surface.

D. MP joint
1. Usually dorsally dislocated
2. Most commonly seen in index finger
3. Must distinguish between simple (subluxation) and complex (complete) dislocation
   a. **Simple**: reduce with flexion of wrist and place pressure on the distal dorsum of proximal phalanx in a volar direction.
   b. **Complex**
      i. **Irreducible**: metacarpal head buttonholes through volar structures and prevents reduction.
      ii. **Reducible**: hyperextension of joint (60 to 80 degrees), with dislocated phalanx directly on top of metacarpal head. The joint is commonly held in extension and may be slightly angulated, with puckering of volar skin. Closed reduction is done, with dorsal extension blocking splint in neutral position. Early range of motion is started. Open reduction and immobilization in 30 degrees flexion for 2 weeks is followed by dorsal blocking splint to 0 degrees for an additional 2 weeks

E. Carpometacarpal joint
1. Majority are dorsal.
2. Fifth joint is most commonly involved.
3. Closed reduction under wrist block is usually successful if done less than 12 hours after injury.
4. Flex the wrist and apply traction on the metacarpal with dorsal pressure on displaced metacarpal base, followed by extension of the metacarpal head. If unstable, hold it in place with K-wire and a cast for 4 weeks.
5. May require open reduction

F. Thumb MCP joint
1. **Dorsal**
   a. Apply dorsal pressure to the base of the proximal phalanx with the wrist and metacarpal flexed and adducted.
   b. Immobilize in 25 degrees of flexion for 4 weeks.
2. **Lateral**
   a. Associated with ulnar collateral ligament injury (gamekeeper's or skier's thumb)
   b. Stress joint under block; if >30 degrees of laxity, complete rupture; if <30 degrees of laxity, partial rupture

c. Treat with thumb spica cast for 4 weeks for partial rupture and surgical repair for complete rupture.
d. The radial collateral ligament is less commonly injured but the treatment is as for ulnar collateral ligament.

G. Thumb carpometacarpal joint
1. Rare injury that usually involves the volar ligament, which is thought to be main capsular reinforcement
2. Stress radiography may be helpful.
3. Immobilize the joint for 4 weeks in a thumb spica cast.
4. If grossly unstable, pin with K-wire.

XI. NAILBED INJURY

A. Administer digital block anesthesia.
B. Remove nail by gently spreading a small hemostat or Freer elevator beneath the nail.
C. Explore the nailbed and debride lacerations. Repair lacerations to nailbed with 6-0 plain gut.
D. Drill a hole in the nail to allow for drainage once it is replaced.
E. Replace the nail under the eponychial fold. This will keep this space open and allow for new nail growth and prevent future nail deformity. Secure the nail in place with nylon or chromic suture at the tip.
F. Create a spacer with a piece of sterile aluminum from the suture wrapper if the nail is not available.
G. Complete new nail growth can take from 2 to 5 months

XII. AMPUTATIONS

A. Finger tip amputation
1. Most common type of finger amputation injury in the upper extremity
2. Clean and debride under digital block.
3. Resect exposed bone and repair nail bed injury if present.
4. Open wounds <1 cm^2 can heal well by secondary intention.
5. Primary closures of tip amputations yield the best results.

B. Amputation through DIP or PIP
1. Shorten the phalanx and close primarily.
2. Do not suture flexor and extensor tendons together.

C. Amputation through middle phalanx
1. If distal to insertion of FDS, shorten bone and close primarily.
2. If proximal to insertion of FDS, preserve PIP joint if possible for cosmetic reasons.
3. Consider replantation if indicated.

D. Amputation proximal to PIP joint
1. Will have gripping motion with intrinsic muscles and common extensors
2. Preserve as much length as possible.

3. Consider replantation if indicated.
4. Perform ray amputation if close to the MP joint, as the short stump will be functionally limiting (especially in the middle and ring fingers).

E. Thumb amputation
1. Thumb amputation distal to IP joint will leave the thumb quite functional.
   a. Shortening bone and primary closure
2. Replantation is an option if the amputation is proximal to the IP joint and meets criteria.

XIII. REPLANTATION

A. The goal of replantation is to restore function of the digit.

B. Indications for replantation
1. Multiple fingers
2. Thumb
3. Amputation across palm or wrist
4. Amputation in a child

C. Contraindications for replantation
1. Severe crush or avulsion mechanism
2. Multiple level injuries
3. Extreme contamination
4. Concomitant life-threatening injuries
5. Warm ischemia time >6 hours
6. Cold ischemia time >12 hours
7. Self-mutilation cases or psychotic patients
8. Patient who cannot endure extensive postoperative rehabilitation

D. Transportation of amputated part
1. Wrap the part in moist gauze, place in a bag, and place bag on ice.

XIV. FRACTURES

A. Metacarpal head (intra-articular)
1. **Simple two-part fracture**: open reduction; internal fixation with screws
2. **Comminuted fracture**
   a. **Closed**: immobilization for 2 weeks, followed by aggressive range of motion
   b. **Open**: Incise and irrigate initially, followed by external fixation. Arthrodesis of joint is considered a salvage procedure.

B. Metacarpal neck (boxer's fracture)
1. Acceptable angulation of neck
   a. Index and middle finger (15 degrees)
   b. Ring finger (30 to 40 degrees)
   c. Small finger (50 to 60 degrees)
2. Typically managed nonoperatively in splint for 2 to 4 weeks with range of motion thereafter

3. Reduction indicated when angulation greater than above or metacarpal shortening >3 mm; utilize K-wire or plate and screw fixation if cannot hold in reduction.

C. Metacarpal shaft
1. **Types**
   a. Tranverse
   b. Oblique
   c. Spiral
   d. Comminuted
2. Most treated with closed reduction and splint immobilization
3. Percutaneous pinning or open reduction and internal fixation if reduction is unstable
4. **Indication for open reduction**
   a. Open fractures
   b. Multiple fractures
   c. Unstable fractures
   d. Rotational or angulation malalignment
5. **Fixation options**
   a. K-wires (most commonly used)
   b. Plate and screws
   c. Intramedullary pins
   d. Wiring
   e. External fixation (useful when there is significant bone loss)

D. Proximal and middle phalanx
1. **Stable, nondisplaced fractures**
   a. Place in volar splint in the position of function with 45 degrees of wrist extension, 70 degrees of MCP flexion, and IP joint extension. Immobilize for 3 to 4 weeks.
   b. Then buddy tape to adjacent finger and start gradual range of motion for 4 to 6 weeks.
2. Closed reduction of displaced fractures under digital block and splint as above.

E. Distal phalanx
1. Most common fracture of the hand.
2. Place in stack splint for protection and pain control for 3 to 4 weeks.
3. Often associated with nailbed injuries that would require evaluation and repair
4. Decompress associated subungual hematoma with 18-gauge needle placed through the nail.

F. Thumb fractures
1. Metacarpal base fracture (intra-articular)
   a. **Bennet's fracture: fracture** involving the base of the thumb metacarpal. The pull by the adductor pollicis and the pull by the abductor pollicis longus muscles on the metacarpal cause separation along the fracture line.
      i. If the fragment is <20% of the articular surface, closed reduction and fixate with K-wires.

ii. If the fragment is >20% of the articular surface, open reduction and fixate with pins or screws.
  b. Rolando's fracture: Comminuted intra-articular fracture of the base of the thumb metacarpal; requires open reduction and internal fixation with pins.
2. **Metacarpal shaft fracture**
  a. Angulation <30% is well tolerated.
  b. If angulation is greater, closed reduction and percutaneous pinning.
3. **Phalanx shaft**
  a. Splint in thumb spica for 4 weeks if nondisplaced.
  b. Percutaneously pin shaft fracture if displaced.
  c. Start early range of motion.
4. **Phalanx head**
  a. Reduce the articular surface as anatomic as possible by open reduction and internal fixation.
  b. Immobilize for 2 weeks and begin early range of motion for comminuted fractures.

XV. WRIST INJURIES

A. Sprain
1. If normal radiographs and no tenderness in anatomic snuffbox, treat with normal range of motion and anti-inflammatory drugs as needed.
2. If tender in the snuffbox with normal radiographs, place in thumb spica cast and follow up with repeat plain films to include scaphoid series in 7 to 10 days to evaluate for scaphoid fracture.

B. Dislocations
1. **Radiocarpal**
  a. Pure dislocation of the distal radius without an associated fracture is extremely rare. Perform careful neurovascular examination of the hand. Treat with closed reduction.
2. **Radiocarpal and intracarpal**
  a. This combination requires open reduction with internal fixation.
3. **Intracarpal**
  a. Seen in high-energy injury with significant soft tissue damage
  b. Perform a careful neurovascular examination as median nerve injuries are commonly seen in association with this type of injury.
  c. **Common carpal dislocations**
     i. Lunate dislocation: volar dislocation of the lunate
     ii. Perilunate dislocation: dorsal dislocation of the capitate
        (a) Closed reduction often successful. Place in longitudinal traction with finger traps for 5 to 10 minutes prior to attempted reduction. Then reduce with longitudinal traction of hand while stabilizing the lunate with the opposite thumb. Slowly flex at the wrist to allow the capitate to slip

back into the concavity of the lunate. May require pinning to hold the reduction.
- (b) Open reduction required in the operating room if unable to achieve a closed reduction
- (c) Splint in 30 degrees of wrist flexion with dorsal thumb spica splint.

C. Carpal fractures

1. **Scaphoid**
   a. Usually caused by a fall on dorsiflexed wrist. Examine for pain in the anatomic snuffbox.
   b. Need to obtain scaphoid views if suspicious for fracture. This includes films with radial and ulnar deviation of the hand.
   c. If clinically tender and radiographs are negative, treat in thumb spica cast with repeat plain films in 7 to 10 days.
   d. Place in thumb spica cast for 8 to 12 weeks if fracture is nondisplaced.
   e. Treat with open reduction and internal fixation with pins or screw if there is presence of flexion, angulation, or >1 mm displacement of fracture.
   f. High risk of avascular necrosis or non-union requiring future bone grafting if symptomatic

2. **Lunate**
   a. Fracture of the volar pole is most common. Treat with open reduction and internal fixation for fractures with displaced volar pole.
   b. High risk of avascular necrosis of the bone (Keinbock's disease)

3. **Triquetrum**
   a. Seen with impaction mechanism and associated with other carpal fractures
   b. Treat with cast immobilization for 6 weeks.

4. **Pisiform**
   a. Occurs with direct force to bone; often need supination oblique or carpal tunnel views to make the diagnosis
   b. Treat with cast immobilization for 4 to 6 weeks.

5. **Trapezium**
   a. Associated with fractures of the first metacarpal and radius
   b. Treat nondisplaced fractures in thumb spica for 4 to 6 weeks.
   c. Treat displaced or intra-articular fractures with open reduction and internal fixation with pins or screws.

6. **Trapezoid**
   a. Splint if nondisplaced.
   b. Open reduction and internal fixation if displaced

7. **Capitate**
   a. Most often are nondisplaced
   b. Non-unions are common and will require future midcarpal arthrodesis, bone grafting, or excision arthroplasty.

8. **Hamate**
   a. Most often involves the hook; seen in athletes who play racquet sports; best seen with carpal tunnel view
   b. Cast immobilization if acute
   c. Splint for 4 to 6 weeks for a nondisplaced body fracture.

XVI. COMPARTMENT SYNDROME

A. Early findings
1. Tense forearm and/or hand compartments
2. Pain with passive extension and flexion of digits is the most reliable finding. The pain tends to be out of proportion to the injury.
3. Paresthesias

B. Late findings
1. Paralysis
2. Pallor
3. Pulselessness

C. Clinical suspicion is of paramount importance. Compartment pressure >30 mm Hg is an absolute indication for fasciotomy.

D. Forearm and hand fasciotomies
1. Avoid longitudinal incisions across the wrist and elbow crease in order to prevent flexor contractures.
2. Must open the carpal tunnel. Loosely approximate the skin over the carpal tunnel to cover the median nerve and tendons at this level.
3. Extend incision up proximal to the elbow and also release the lacertus fibrosus (this is the ulnar fascial extension of the biceps aponeurosis that inserts on the ulna and covers the neurovascular structures).
4. The dorsal longitudinal forearm incision allows release of the dorsal and mobile wad compartments.
5. Dorsal incisions over the second and fourth metacarpals allow entrance into the dorsal and volar interosseous compartments as well as the adductor compartment of the thumb.

XVII. INFECTIONS

A. Human bites
1. Perform aggressive irrigation and debridement in the operating room and leave the wound open.
2. May have injury to MCP or PIP joints if mouth struck with a closed fist.
3. Extended-spectrum IV penicillins are antibiotics of choice.
4. Oral agent of choice is amoxicillin-clavulanate.
5. Common organisms are gram-positive cocci and anaerobes (e.g., *Eikanella corrodans*).

B. Animal bites

1. Common organisms in dog and cat bites are gram-positive cocci and *Pasteurella multocida*.
2. Antibiotic of choice is amoxicillin-clavulanate.

C. Herpetic whitlow
1. Common in medical and dental personnel caring for orotracheal area (e.g., respiratory therapists)
2. Herpes simplex infection: patches of clear fluid-filled vesicles often with a rim of erythema
3. Viral incubation period of 2 to14 days. Infection is self-limiting.
4. Do not incise and drain. Treat with splinting and elevation.
5. Antiviral medication such as acyclovir may be considered.

D. Flexor tenosynovitis
1. **Kanavel's four cardinal signs**
    a. Fusiform swelling of the entire digit
    b. Semiflexed finger at rest
    c. Tenderness along the flexor sheath tracking into the proximal hand
    d. Marked pain with passive extension of the digit, mostly at the proximal end
2. Requires tendon sheath irrigation in the operating room

E. High pressure injection injuries
1. Benign-appearing pinpoint wound that is very painful
2. Must be treated aggressively with surgical debridement as the injected material often enters tendon sheath and travels proximally in hand or forearm
3. Oil-based material may be especially difficult to remove completely and rarely leads to good long-term outcome.
4. Amputation rate approaches 60% to 70%.

XVIII. SUGGESTED READINGS

Canale ST, Beaty JH (eds): Campbell's Operative Orthopaedics, 11th ed. Philadelphia, Mosby; 2008.

Green DP, Hotchkiss RN, Pederson WC (eds): Green's Operative Hand Surgery, 5th ed. Philadelphia, Churchill Livingstone; 2004.

Gutowski KA: Hand II: Peripheral nerves and tendon transfers: Selected readings in plastic surgery,Vol 9, No 33. Dallas, University of Texas Southwestern Medical Center and Baylor University Medical Center; 2003.

Hill NA: Fractures and dislocations of the carpus. Orthop Clin North Am 1:275-284, 1970.

Masson JA: Hand I: Fingernails, infections, tumors and soft-tissue reconstruction. Selected readings in plastic surgery, Vol 9, No 32. Dallas, University of Texas Southwestern Medical Center and Baylor University Medical Center; 2002.

Seiler JG: Essentials of Hand Surgery. Philadelphia, Lippincott Williams & Wilkins, 2002.

Fractures in Children

Amy Brazda, MD, and Kevin Crawford, MD

I. ETIOLOGY

Etiologies are strongly age dependent.
A. Thirty-seven percent of all childhood fractures occur in the home environment

II. PATHOPHYSIOLOGY

A. The immature skeleton of a child is a more dynamic system than that of an adult.
B. Pediatric bone is more narrow and flexible.
C. A large potential for remodeling exists in the bones of children.
D. Pediatric bones may contain cartilaginous components of varying size that are radiolucent on radiographs and thus may cause difficulty in diagnosing fractures.
E. Immature bones contain a physis, or "growth plate."
F. The periosteum of the child's bone is a much more significant structure when compared to that of the adult bone.

III. FRACTURE PATTERNS

A. Incomplete patterns
1. Torus (buckle fracture)
   a. An impaction fracture primarily involving the metaphysis
   b. This is a stable injury that presents as pain without deformity.
2. Greenstick
   a. Commonly seen in the ulna and fibula, in which the cortex is incompletely fractured, with plastic deformation of the remaining intact cortex and periosteum
   b. This fracture often results in angular deformity, which may require conversion to a complete fracture to correct the deformity.
3. Longitudinal
   a. These fractures occur along the axis of the bone.
   b. They may be associated with other fracture patterns.

B. Complete patterns
1. Transverse
2. Oblique
3. Spiral
4. Comminuted

C. Epiphyseal and apophyseal injuries
1. Avulsion fractures (e.g., tibial spine, ulnar styloid, etc.)
   a. Stronger soft tissues (e.g., ligaments) avulse a portion of the bone.

2. Osteochondral fractures (e.g., capitellum, femur)
   a. Intra-articular bone and cartilage fragments may result in loose bodies within the joint.

D. Physeal injuries
1. These are most commonly categorized by the Salter-Harris scheme.
2. The more recent classification is by Peterson.
   a. Type I
      i. Transverse fractures of the metaphysic with one or more fracture lines extending to the physis
      ii. No fracture along the physis and no displacement of the epiphysis
      iii. No Salter-Harris equivalent
   b. Type II
      i. Separation of part of the physis with a portion of the metaphysis attached to the epiphysis
      ii. Salter-Harris II
   c. Type III
      i. Separation of the epiphysis from the diaphysis through any of the layers of the physis, disrupting the complete physis
      ii. Salter-Harris I
   d. Type IV
      i. Fracture of the epiphysis extending to and along the physis
      ii. More common in older children in whom part of the physis has begun to close
      iii. Salter-Harris III
   e. Type V
      i. Fracture traversing the metaphysis, physis, and epiphysis
      ii. Salter-Harris IV
   f. Type VI
      i. Fracture with missing physis
      ii. No Salter-Harris equivalent
3. Type II injury is most common (54%).
4. The need for both immediate and later surgery increases with increasing type number.

IV. PRINCIPLES OF PEDIATRIC FRACTURE MANAGEMENT

A. Ligament injuries are rare in children, whereas physeal fractures are common.

B. Stress radiographs or other imaging modalities may clearly delineate a suspected fracture through the physis.

C. Vascular injuries
1. Occur in association with fractures in children, but are rare
2. Prompt recognition and treatment are essential.
3. Most commonly seen with supracondylar fractures of the humerus

D. Compartment syndrome does occur in the pediatric population, especially with fractures of the distal humerus and tibia.

V. CHILD ABUSE

A. Approximately 2.4 million reports of child abuse are filed annually in the United States.
B. The incidence of physical abuse is roughly 4.9 children per 1000.
C. The risk of abuse is greatest for children under 3 years of age, firstborn children, premature infants, stepchildren, and disabled children.
D. Radiographic evidence for child abuse includes the following:
1. Multiple fractures in various stages of healing. This finding indicates child abuse and should be considered as such until proven otherwise.
2. Fractures of the extremities (usually humerus, femur, or tibia), skull, and ribs are most frequently seen.
3. Suspicious patterns include:
    a. Fractures in children under the age of 3 years without reasonable explanation
    b. Metaphyseal and epiphyseal fractures of the long bones
    c. Buckle fractures of the metaphyses are commonly associated with child abuse.
    d. Spiral long bone fractures
    e. Periosteal hematomas from direct trauma will be evident on radiographs at 10 to14 days after injury.
    f. Bucket-handle fractures of the metaphyses are thought to be pathognomonic of abuse. Radiographs reveal a "chip" at the edge of the metaphysis with no gross displacement of the epiphysis.

E. Any injured child should be undressed completely and examined for other signs of abuse.
F. Several states have laws requiring physicians to report any case of suspected abuse, and physicians should be aware of such laws in their areas of practice.

VI. OPEN FRACTURES IN CHILDREN

A. The majority of open fractures are the result of high-energy trauma.
B. Ten percent of open fractures are seen in multiply injured children.
C. Fifty percent will have additional injuries.
D. Classification is principally based on the Gustilo-Anderson system.
E. Treatment
1. Initial resuscitation (ABCs) and a detailed musculoskeletal examination to include neurologic and vascular examination of the extremities
2. Tetanus prophylaxis
3. Removal of gross contamination and sterile coverage of wound
4. Application of a splint with realignment of the limb to prevent further soft tissue injury
5. Intravenous antibiotics are initiated in the emergency department.
    a. Type I fractures require a first-generation cephalosporin for 48 to 72 hours.

b. Type II and III fractures require a cephalosporin and aminoglycoside for 48 to 72 hours.
c. Injuries sustained on a farm benefit from the addition of penicillin to the above regimen.
d. Regimen may be repeated at the time of delayed closure or bony reconstruction.
e. Emergency department cultures are of questionable benefit.

F. Surgical debridement
1. All open fractures should be treated in the operating room.
2. Wound edges should be excised and the open wound extended to explore the depths of the wound and to debride all necrotic tissues and contamination.
3. Fasciotomies should be performed as indicated.
4. Debridement should be aggressive since multiple modalities now exist for soft tissue and bony reconstruction.
5. The patient should be returned to the operating room as many times as needed to gain control of the wound.
6. Decisions on definitive fracture treatment can be made at this time, depending on fracture type and location and the condition of the soft tissues. Options include:
   a. Splint or cast with or without percutaneous pins (e.g. radius)
   b. External fixation (commonly used for the tibia and femur)
   c. Internal fixation
   d. Intramedullary fixation (e.g., type 1 open femur fracture)

VII. AMPUTATION

A. Every attempt should be made to salvage amputated limbs in children.
B. Even type IIIC injuries, which may suggest amputation in the adult, should be salvaged, if possible, in the child.
C. Length should be preserved, given the potential for growth in children.
D. As in adult trauma patients, multiply injured children benefit from early fracture stabilization and definitive treatment of all fractures as soon as they are stable.

VIII. FRACTURES AND DISLOCATIONS OF THE UPPER EXTREMITY

A. Hand
1. **Basic principles**
   a. The incidence of hand fractures peaks around age 13 years.
   b. Almost all hand fractures in children can be treated by closed reduction and splinting for 3 to 4 weeks.
   c. Repeated attempts at reduction of physeal fractures are not advised.
   d. Repeat radiographs should be obtained at 5 to 7 days to confirm maintenance of reduction.

e. "Buddy-taping" and short arm immobilization are acceptable for fractures of the phalanges and metacarpals, but more proximal fractures should be addressed with long arm immobilization.
f. The most common hand fractures are of the distal phalanx and Peterson type II (Salter II) of the proximal phalanx.
g. Open reduction is generally reserved for:
   i. Displaced intra-articular fractures
   ii. Displaced Peterson type IV or V fractures (Salter-Harris type III and IV)
   iii. Unstable fractures

2. **Distal phalanx**
   a. Extraphyseal injury
   b. Nail removal with careful debridement, irrigation, and nail-bed repair may be in order.
   c. If there is insufficient stability, the fracture may be pinned.
   d. Most can be treated simply by splinting the tip of the distal interphalangeal joint, leaving the proximal interphalangeal joint free.

3. **Mallet finger** (distal phalanx physeal injury)
   a. There are five types:
      i. Peterson type III or II (Salter-Harris I or II)
      ii. Peterson type IV or V (Salter-Harris III or IV)
      iii. Peterson type III or II with joint dislocation
      iv. Avulsion of extensor with Salter-Harris fracture
      v. Reverse mallet with flexor avulsion with bone
   b. Treatment depends on the type of fracture.
      i. Closed, nonoperative treatment; open injuries may require nail-bed repair, etc.
      ii. Nonoperative treatment is favored except in the presence of inadequate reduction or joint subluxation, both of which require operative treatment.
      iii. Open reduction to restore joint and extensor mechanism
      iv. Treat as Peterson type III or type II with joint dislocation.
      v. Repair under minimal tension within 1 week through volar approach.

4. **Proximal phalanx**
   a. Fracture classification:
      i. Physeal fractures
      ii. Shaft fractures
      iii. Condylar and phalangeal neck fractures
   b. Treatment for type A fractures includes closed reduction and immobilization for 3 weeks.
   c. Indications for operative reduction include:
      i. Irreducibility
      ii. Unstable reductions
      iii. More than 25% articular surface involvement
      iv. Displacement of >1.5 mm

B. Fractures of the radius and ulna

1. Distal radius fractures are the most common of childhood fractures.
2. Classification
   a. Type A–dorsally displaced
   b. Type B–volarly displaced
3. Treatment is nonoperative.
   a. Timely and gentle closed reduction is ideal.
   b. For type A fractures, a good three-point mold of the splint or cast with the wrist in neutral is essential.
   c. For type B fractures, a three-point mold with the wrist dorsiflexed 30 degrees and the forearm in full supination is desirable.
   d. Acceptable results for a child with 1 year of growth remaining are at least 50% apposition (which should remodel to almost normal) and <25% of angulation.
   e. Immobolize for 4 to 6 weeks in a short or long arm cast with follow-up radiographs at 4 to 6 months to ensure the resumption in normal growth.
4. Operative treatment may be required in patients with:
   a. Severe local soft tissue or ipsilateral proximal fractures
   b. Open fractures
   c. Median nerve compression or compartment syndrome
   d. Comminuted epiphyseal fractures
   e. Failure to obtain an adequate closed reduction

C. Fractures of the shaft of the radius and ulna

1. **Basic principles**
   a. Rotation and angular deformities must be corrected.
   b. Less than 10 degrees of deformity in all planes is desirable.
   c. Children <10 years of age have more potential for remodeling.
   d. Bayonet apposition does not limit rotation.
   e. Avoid narrowing of the interosseous membrane and use the bicipital tuberosity to aid in rotational alignment.
2. **Greenstick fractures**
   a. Necessity of "completing" the fracture is controversial.
   b. Angular components must be corrected as follows:
      i. For apex-volar angulation, a pronation force must be applied during reduction.
      ii. For apex-dorsal angulation, a supination force must be applied during reduction.
      iii. Immobilize in a well-molded, sugar-tong splint or long arm cast.
      iv. Slight overcorrection may be preferable to prevent recurrence of deformity.
      v. Repeat radiographs within the first few days, then every week for 2 to 3 weeks to ensure maintenance of reduction.
      vi. Remanipulate fracture if reduction is lost after 2 to 5 days.
3. **Complete fractures of the radius and ulna**
   a. **Closed reduction**

i. Confirm correct rotational and angular alignment by radiographic examination.
ii. Bayonet apposition is acceptable if the interossesous distance and angular and rotational alignment are acceptable.
iii. Apply a well-molded, sugar-tong splint and change to a long arm cast as swelling permits.
iv. In older children, difficulty in obtaining or maintaining the reduction may require open reduction and plate fixation.
v. Close radiographic follow-up is required to confirm maintenance of alignment.

4. **Monteggia fractures—fractures of the ulnar shaft associated with radial head dislocation**
   a. Treatment varies with the direction of the dislocation.
      i. Anterior or later dislocation require closed reduction and immobilization of the arm in a long arm splint or cast for 6 to 8 weeks.
      ii. Flexion and supination are the appropriate positions for these variants.
      iii. Posterior dislocation may require immobilization in extension to maintain stability of the reduction.
      iv. Check for alignment of the proximal radius with the capitellum on the anteroposterior (AP) and lateral radiograph.

5. **Galeazzi fractures—fracture of the radial shaft with distal radioulnar joint dislocation**
   a. Results are good with closed reduction in children, unlike the results in adults.
   b. Closed reduction of the radius and long arm immobilization in supination or pronation (depending on the deforming forces) is recommended.
   c. Operative reduction is reserved for unstable closed reduction.

D. Fractures of the elbow
1. Radiographic evaluation should include AP, lateral, and oblique views.
2. Comparison views may be helpful.
3. Stress radiographs may be helpful if ligamentous or physeal injury is suspected.
4. Documentation of neurologic and vascular examination is critical.
5. If there is suspected fracture but negative radiographs, splint the extremity and reevaluate at 10 to 14 days.

E. Supracondylar humerus fractures
1. Initial treatment includes:
   a. Complete neurologic and vascular examination
   b. Reduction of gross displacement
   c. Splint application
   d. Radiographic evaluation
2. These fractures are one of the most common causes of compartment syndrome in children and require a high index of suspicion, with careful examination and frequent monitoring.

3. Inpatient observation is recommended for at least 24 hours for the majority of supracondylar humerus fracture.
4. **Classification**
   a. Type I–nondisplaced or minimally displaced
   b. Type II–displaced with an intact posterior cortex
   c. Type III–a completely displaced fracture or one lacking intrinsic stability with the elbow flexed
5. **Treatment**
   a. Type I fractures are treated with splinting in 90 degrees of flexion, with conversion to a long arm cast (when swelling permits) for 3 to 4 weeks.
   b. Type II and III fractures are treated with closed reduction and, after assessment for stability, treated by either splint, cast, or percutaneous pin fixation if unstable.
   c. At Parkland Memorial Hospital, the majority of type III and type II fractures are stabilized with K-wires; crossed medial and later pins are used.
   d. Anatomic reduction is crucial.
   e. The reduction maneuver involves longitudinal traction to obtain length and the correction of angulation (restoring a normal carrying angle), followed by hyperflexion and then pronation.
   f. Open reduction may sometimes be necessary.
   g. Anteromedial or anterolateral exposure may be used as appropriate.
   h. Frequent, early radiographic follow-up is mandatory to ensure maintenance of the reduction.
6. **Associated injuries and vascular compromise**
   a. The incidence of associated nerve injury, previously estimated at 7%, is now felt to be somewhat higher, with the anterior interosseous nerve most commonly affected.
   b. Vascular compromise is not uncommon, especially with type III fractures.
      i. Fractures that present with diminished or absent pulses are best treated by immediate reduction followed by percutaneous pin fixation if pulses return after reduction.
      ii. There is very little role for angiography in the treatment of these patients because it may result in a significant delay in appropriate treatment.
      iii. Persistent vascular compromise after reduction mandates open vascular exploration.
      iv. Loss of reduction after closed treatment is an indication for percutaneous pin fixation.

F. Medial epicondyle fractures
1. The injury mechanism is an extension force at the wrist and valgus force at the elbow.
2. Comparison radiographs are frequently helpful for diagnosis, although children <5 years of age will not have an ossified epicondyle.

3. **Treatment**
   a. Nondisplaced fractures are treated in a long arm cast for 3 to 4 weeks.
   b. Fractures with >5 mm displacement, instability of the elbow joint, or a fragment incarcerated in the joint require open reduction and internal fixation.
   c. Carefully document ulnar nerve status prior to instituting therapy.
   d. Lateral epicondyle fractures are very rare and are treated the same as fractures of the medial epicondyle.

G. **Lateral condyle fractures**
1. Peterson type V (Salter-Harris type IV) pattern
2. The injury mechanism is commonly elbow extension with a valgus force.
3. Nondisplaced fractures are treated with a long arm cast for 3 to 4 weeks with radiographic follow-up at 3 to 4 days to ensure maintenance of reduction.
4. Anatomic reduction is mandatory for displaced fractures.
   a. Closed reduction with percutaneous pins is acceptable if reduction is anatomic.
   b. Most of these fractures require open reduction and pin fixation.

H. **Medial condyle fractures**
1. These fractures are a relatively uncommon injury in children.
2. **Classification**
   a. Milch Type I is a Peterson type V (Salter-Harris type IV) pattern.
   b. Milch Type II is a Peterson type II (Salter-Harris type II).
   c. Also classified in terms of displacement, which may assist in determination of appropriate treatment
      i. Type I–fracture line from the medial condylar metaphysis extending to the physis; generally nondisplaced
      ii. Type II–fracture line from the medial condylar metaphysis extending into the medial condylar physis
      iii. Type III–fragment is displaced and rotated.
3. **Treatment**
   a. Type I is best treated with a long arm splint or cast for 3 to 4 weeks.
   b. Types II and III are treated at Parkland Memorial Hospital by open reduction and pin fixation.

I. **Radial head and neck fractures**
1. These are often associated with other fractures or dislocations.
2. Angulation of 30 degrees requires an attempt at closed reduction.
3. Poorer results are associated with initial angulation of >30 degrees or translocation >3 to 4 mm.
4. **Treatment**
   a. For fractures with <30 degrees of angulation and no translation, long arm immobilization for 7 to 10 days followed by early motion is usually adequate.
   b. Angulation of >30 degrees requires closed manipulation followed by long arm immobilization for 1 to 2 weeks.

c. Angulation of >45 degrees requires closed manipulation or percutaneous pin reduction followed by long arm immobilization for 1 to 2 weeks.
d. Open reduction, with or without fixation, is required for fractures with residual angulation fixed at >40 degrees with translation >3mm, and <60 degrees of supination or pronation, or complete displacement of the radial head.
e. Acceptable results are <45 degrees of angulation, no translation, and supination or pronation arc of 50 to 60 degrees.

J. Olecranon fractures
1. Very uncommon and highly associated with other injuries
2. Most minimally displaced fractures and nondisplaced fractures can be treated by simple immobilization in 75 to 80 degrees of flexion.
3. Displaced fractures require open reduction and internal fixation.

K. Elbow dislocation
1. Commonly associated with other fractures and injuries
2. Closed reduction is generally the successful treatment for these injuries.
3. Confirm joint congruity on postreduction radiographs, and examine the joint for stability.
4. Beware of entrapment of the median nerve or a nonossified medial condyle, which may prevent reduction.
5. Treatment is long arm immobilization for 5 to 7 days, followed by active range of motion.

L. Subluxation of the radial head (nursemaid's elbow)
1. Commonly the result of pulling the outstrectched arm, although about one-third of presentations may be atypical
2. The child will usually present with the elbow flexed and pronated and will refuse to use the arm.
3. Radiographs may be negative.
4. The reduction maneuver involves supination and gentle traction in extension, followed by hyperflexion.
5. The child will usually begin to use the arm immediately and without pain with a successful reduction.
6. Parents should be warned against causing recurrence by pulling on the child's arm.

M. Fractures of the humerus
1. **Humeral shaft fractures**
   a. Frequently transverse or spiral fracture patterns, which can be treated in a coaptation splint, humeral cuff orthosis, or collar and cuff for 3 to 4 weeks
   b. Be wary of child abuse when spiral fractures are seen.
   c. Overgrowth of the humerus by 1 cm can be expected.
   d. Neuropraxic injury to the radial nerve can be apparent on presentation and is managed as follows:
      i. Observation only is recommended if nerve palsy is present at initial patient presentation.

ii. If neuropraxic injury occurs after manipulation, surgical exploration is warranted.
e. Rarely, soft tissue interposition may block an adequate reduction and require surgical intervention.

2. **Metaphyseal fractures**
   a. These are usually greenstick injuries and can be treated in a sling for 3 to 4 weeks.
   b. Displaced fractures require closed reduction and immobilization.
   c. The fracture may buttonhole through the deltoid and require surgical extraction to achieve reduction.

N. Injuries around the shoulder girdle

1. **Proximal humerus fractures**
   a. AP and axillary lateral radiographs are necessary for adequate evaluation.
   b. These injuries are usually Peterson type II (Salter-Harris II) patterns caused by a variety of mechanisms.
   c. The vast majority of these fractures can be treated by nonoperative means.
   d. No hard and fast rules exist for operative treatment, but possible indications include the following:
      i. Marked displacement with little growth remaining
      ii. Multiple trauma
      iii. Open fracture with significant periosteal disruption

2. **Traumatic shoulder dislocations**
   a. AP and axillary lateral or trans-scapular views are necessary to evaluate.
   b. Occurrence is more frequent in the adolescent with closed physes.
   c. Treatment is by closed reduction, sling immobilization, and early motion.
   d. Anterior dislocations far exceed posterior dislocations in frequency.
   e. The axillary nerve is the most frequently injured neurovascular structure with anterior dislocations.
   f. Open reduction may rarely be required if closed reduction is unsuccessful.

3. **Clavicle fractures**
   a. **Shaft fracture**
      i. Very common in the pediatric population and usually the midshaft is fractured
      ii. Treated in a figure-of-eight splint for 3 to 6 weeks.
      iii. Most heal in malunited position, but remodel within 1 year.
      iv. Occasionally may be implicated in brachial plexus or vascular injury
      v. Greenstick fractures with posterior bowing may also result in neurovascular compromise.
   b. **Proximal clavicle fracture**
      i. Usually represents an epiphyseal separation, which can occur up to 25 years of age
      ii. Anterior displacement is manifested by prominence of the clavicle and may be treated conservatively.

  iii. Posterior displacement may compromise the trachea or vascular structures.
  iv. Reduce to anatomic position by closed or open means.
  v. Unstable reductions may require internal fixation.
  vi. Rockwood 45-degree upshot view provides the best radiographic visualization.
4. **Distal clavicle fracture**
 a. Usually epiphyseal separation
 b. Treated in a sling for 2 to 3 weeks

O. Scapular fractures
1. Usually associated with severe trauma
2. Majority may be treated with a sling, analgesia, and early motion.
3. Avulsion of the coracoid with complete acromioclavicular separation may require open reduction and internal fixation.
4. Some glenoid fractures with joint incongruity or instability may require open reduction and internal fixation.

IX. FRACTURES OF THE PELVIS AND ACETABULUM

A. Apophyseal fractures are usually the result of sudden, violent muscle contractions.

B. Anterior superior iliac spine and ischial avulsions are most commonly seen.

C. Symptomatic treatment is sufficient unless there is marked displacement.

D. "Isolated" fractures of the pubi ramus, ischium, or ilium
1. Pubic ramus fractures are common pelvic injuries in children.
2. They are associated with high-energy trauma.
3. The superior ramus fracture is most commonly seen.
4. Treatment is symptomatic, but these patients have a high incidence of associated injuries.
5. Ischial fractures are rare and treatment is generally symptomatic.
6. Iliac wing fractures result from high-energy trauma and are highly associated with other injuries.
7. The majority are nondisplaced or minimally displaced.
8. Treatment is conservative with protected weight bearing on the affected side for 4 to 6 weeks.

E. Fractures of the sacrum and coccyx
1. These fractures may be associated with neurologic injury.
2. Most are treated conservatively.

F. Pelvic ring disruptions
1. Classification in children is the same as in adults.
2. Most are treated conservatively with protected weight bearing.
3. Pelvic ring disruptions can be associated with other significant injuries.

G. Acetabular fractures
1. These fractures are uncommon in the pediatric population.
2. Classification in children is similar to that in adults.

3. Most are treated conservatively with protected weight bearing, traction, or spica cast.
4. The goal is to maintain a congruent joint until healing has occurred.
5. Injuries to the triradiate cartilage may lead to growth arrest and acetabular insufficiency.

X. FRACTURES AND DISLOCATIONS OF THE LOWER EXTREMITIES

A. **Fractures and dislocations of the hip**
1. Hip fractures are rare injuries in the pediatric population.
   a. **Transepiphyseal fracture, with or without hip dislocation**
      i. Expect poor results.
      ii. Treatment is closed or open reduction with secure pin fixation.
      iii. In very young children, closed reduction and traction can be used.
   b. **Transcervical fracture**
      i. These account for the majority of pediatric hip fractures.
      ii. There is a 15% to 40% incidence of associated avascular necrosis.
      iii. Anatomic reduction with internal fixation is standard treatment.
   c. **Cervicotrochanteric fracture**
      i. A nondisplaced fracture is treated in an abduction hip spica cast and followed by frequent radiographs to confirm maintenance of reduction.
      ii. A displaced fracture is treated with closed or open reduction with internal fixation.
   d. **An intertrochanteric fracture** is generally treated with skin or skeletal traction followed by spica cast or internal fixation in the older child.
2. **Hip dislocations**
   a. Careful neurovascular examination is important.
   b. Obtain prereduction radiographs to identify associated fractures.
   c. Treatment is urgent, gentle reduction, usually under a mask anesthesia.
   d. If closed reduction fails or the joint is incongruent, open reduction is indicated.
   e. Beware of occult physeal injuries, which may displace during reduction.
   f. Document joint congruency with good postreduction radiographs or CT scan if necessary.
   g. After reduction, traction is followed by protected weight bearing.

B. **Fractures of the shaft of the femur**
1. Infants 0 to 2 years of age
   a. Consider the possibility of child abuse.
   b. Almost all can be treated by immediate hip spica application for 4 to 6 weeks.
   c. Acceptable reduction is <1.5 cm of shortening and 30 degrees of angulation.
2. Children 2 to 6 years of age

a. Most can be treated by closed reduction and immediate hip spica application.
b. Shortening of >2 to 3 cm or multiple injuries contraindicate immediate spica cast application.
c. Treat with skeletal or split Russell's traction for 2 to 3 weeks until fracture is stable
d. Spica cast for 4 to 6 weeks
e. Acceptable reduction is up to 2 cm of shortening and angulation of 20 to 30 degrees in the sagittal plane and 15 to 20 degrees in the coronal plane.

3. Children 6 to 16 years of age
   a. Treatment goal currently revolves around healing the fracture without deformity, low cost of care delivery, and rapid return to function.
   b. Treatment modalities are currently evolving with several options.
   c. Immediate spica cast
      i. This is still the best and arguably the least expensive form of treatment.
      ii. Tends to apply to the younger children in this age group
   d. Traction followed by spica cast; low major complication rate, and a cost comparable to surgical treatment.
   e. External fixation:
      i. May be useful for open injuries or comminuted fractures, but is associated with high major and minor complication rates (and complications are expensive, making this procedure less cost-effective)
      ii. Performs poorly on purely transverse fractures
      iii. Average time to device removal in the above series was 18 weeks and full weight bearing at 22 weeks.
   f. Flexible intramedullary nails:
      i. Excellent choice for transverse fractures, with early healing and a low complication rate
      ii. Also useful for other fracture patterns, but use is technique dependent with a learning curve
      iii. Average time to device removal is 44 weeks, and to full weight bearing 8 weeks.
      iv. This modality is currently used at Parkland Memorial Hospital for patients up to age 14 years.
   g. Plate fixation: this technique is useful in special situations.
   h. Reamed intramedullary nails:
      i. This may have a use in older children, but sporadic cases of avascular necrosis of the femoral head are being reported.
      ii. For this reason, this method is not currently used at Parkland Memorial Hospital.

4. Acceptable reduction is no more than 1.5-mm shortening, 5 to 10 degrees of varus or valgus, and 10 to 15 degrees of AP angulation, with more exacting standards applied with increasing age of the child.

5. **Hardware removal**
   a. Timing of hardware removal is controversial.
   b. At Parkland Memorial Hospital, hardware is generally removed in children under age 10 to 11 years or if parents are insistent.
C. **Supracondylar femur fractures**
1. These are often occult fractures.
2. They are often misdiagnosed as a knee sprain or ligament injury.
3. Comparison views of the unaffected leg are often helpful, as are stress views of the injured extremity.
4. These injuries are usually Peterson type II or III injuries but often result in growth arrest or deformity because of the undulating nature of the femoral physis.
5. Supracondylar metaphyseal fractures in young children may be the result of child abuse.
6. Long term follow-up is necessary to assess growth.
7. Treatment of nondisplaced fractures should be immobilization in a cast.
8. Displaced fractures need closed reduction followed by cast application for 4 to 6 weeks.
9. Unstable fractures may require smooth pin fixation or internal fixation.
10. Document neurovascular status pre- and post-reduction.
D. **Knee injuries**
1. **Knee dislocation** is uncommon in the pediatric population.
   a. Physeal injury is much more common.
   b. There is a high incidence of vascular injury with knee dislocation.
   c. Treatment is by closed reduction and casting; in some instances, ligament repair may be appropriate.
   d. External fixation is required for:
      i. Open joint injuries
      ii. Vascular injury
      iii. Gross instability
2. **Knee ligament injuries**
   a. Variable prognosis
   b. Be alert for epiphyseal fractures presenting as a ligament sprain.
3. **Patellar dislocations**
   a. These are common pediatric injuries.
   b. Diagnosis is arrived at by history and physical examination.
   c. Dislocations commonly reduce spontaneously with knee extension, and frank dislocation may not be present by the time the patient seeks out the physician.
   d. Treatment is with a long leg cast for 3 to 6 weeks.
   e. If a dislocation is present on presentation, closed reduction by knee extension, followed by cast application, is required.
   f. In the presence of an associated chondral or osteochondral fracture, this may be addressed by closed reduction and fixation or excision of the fragment.
4. **Patella fractures**

a. AP, lateral, and sunrise patella views should be obtained.
b. A nondisplaced fracture with preserved active extension is treated in a cylinder cast for 6 weeks.
c. Greater than 2 mm displacement or loss of active knee extension needs open reduction and internal fixation.

E. Tibial spine fractures
1. These injuries are usually caused by a direct blow or fall on the knee.
2. **Classification and treatment**
   a. Type I (nondisplaced)–requires casting for 6 weeks.
   b. Type II (hinged fracture of the spine)–requires closed reduction and casting in 0 to 10 degrees for 6 weeks.
   c. Type III (displaced tibial spine fracture)–may be treated by closed reduction with casting for 6 to 8 weeks, otherwise failed closed reduction requires open reduction and internal fixation.

F. Proximal tibial epiphyseal fracture
1. Assess for vascular injury.
2. Stress radiographs and comparison views may aid diagnosis.
3. Treatment for nondisplaced fractures is a long leg cast for 6 weeks.
4. Displaced fractures require anatomic closed reduction and cast for pin fixation, or open reduction and internal fixation.

G. Tibial tubercle fractures
1. Similar to avulsion of the patellar ligament
2. **Classification**
   a. Type I–fracture at the secondary ossified center
   b. Type II–fracture at the primary and secondary ossification centers
   c. Type III–fracture extending across the tibial epiphysis into the knee joint
3. Treatment is with closed reduction and immobilization if anatomic reduction is obtained and the patient is able to extend the knee.
4. Open reduction and internal fixation are necessary for any displacement in this epiphyseal fracture.

H. Proximal tibial metaphyseal fractures
1. Assess for vascular injury.
2. All valgus greenstick fractures should be reduced anatomically or over-reduced into varus.
3. Overgrowth into valgus is common.
4. Warn parents of possible valgus deformity.
5. Most valgus deformities correct spontaneously over time.

I. Tibial shaft fractures
1. **Greenstick fractures**
   a. Greenstick deformity of the fibula may prevent reduction of the tibia.
   b. Anatomic reduction should be attempted.
   c. Treatment is long leg cast for 6 weeks.
2. **Nondisplaced fractures**
   a. These injuries can be treated in a long leg cast for 6-8 weeks.
   b. Some may need hospital admission for observation.

3. **Displaced fractures**
   a. Treatment is closed reduction and a long leg cast for 6 to 8 weeks.
   b. Most warrant overnight observation to rule out compartment syndrome.
4. **Unstable fractures**
   a. Treatment is closed reduction and pin fixation with cast immobilization.
   b. Internal and external fixation may be used if above treatment is unsuccessful.

J. Intra-articular fractures of the distal tibia
1. Best results are obtained with anatomic reduction.
2. A CT scan may be necessary to evaluate fracture or reduction.
3. Closed reduction is successful if anatomic reduction is achieved, and it is followed by immediate immobilization in a long leg cast for 4 to 6 weeks.
4. If unable to achieve anatomic reduction, perform open reduction and internal fixation.

K. Fractures of the distal tibial physis
1. AP, lateral, and mortise radiographs are helpful.
2. Most of these are Peterson type II or III.
3. Beware of "triplane" fractures in older children in whom the physis has begun to close.
4. Treatment is closed reduction by reversing the mechanism of injury, followed by a long leg cast for 6 weeks.
5. Intra-articular fractures require anatomic reduction.

XI. SUGGESTED READINGS

Bhatnagar R, Nzegwe NI, Miller NH: Diagnosis and treatment of common fractures in children: Femoral shaft fractures and supracondylar humeral fractures. J Surg Orthop Advances 15(1):1-15, 2006.

Heyworth BE, Galano GJ, Vitale MA, et al: Management of closed femoral shaft fractures in children, ages 6 to 10: National practice patterns and emerging trends. J Pediatr Orthop 24(5):455-459, 2004.

Bites

Marc Labat, MD

I. INTRODUCTION

A. Approximately 4 million Americans are victims of animal and human bites each year.
B. The majority of bite wounds are minor and resolve without complications.
C. Wound infection is the most common bite-related complication.

II. DOG BITES

A. Dog bites are responsible for approximately 0.4% of all emergency department (ED) visits and for 60% to 90% of bite injuries treated in EDs in the United States.
B. The lower extremities are the most frequently bitten areas of the body in adults. However, children are more susceptible to face, neck, and scalp injuries. This may lead to skull fractures, brain lacerations, and meningitis in severe cases when the victim is less than 2 years of age.
C. Large dogs may generate jaw pressures greater than 450 psi, which result in significant avulsion or crush injury.
D. Bite wounds to the hand are at an increased risk for tenosynovitis, septic arthritis, and abscess formation.
E. The incidence of infection from dog bites is 5% to 10%, which is slightly higher than for non-bite lacerations. However, the risk of infection is higher in bites involving the hand (12% to 30%). Infections are usually polymicrobial, but common pathogens include the following:
1. Aerobic organisms such as *Staphylococcus aureus*, α-hemolytic and β-hemolytic streptococci, *Klebsiellla*, *Bacillus*, *Pseudomonas*, and Enterobacteriaceae
2. Anaerobic organisms such as *Bacteroides*, *Fusobacterium*, *Peptostreptococcus*, and *Actinomyces*
3. *Pasteurella multocida*: found in approximately 13% of dog mouths and results in intense inflammation, localized pain, and swelling, usually within 24 hours of the initial bite

III. CAT BITES

A. Cat bites are the second most common type of mammalian bites in the United States.
B. From 60% to 70% of bite injuries occur in the upper extremity with an associated infection rate of 30% to 50%. Approximately 25% of infected cat wounds require hospital admission.
C. Septic arthritis or osteomyelitis may result from penetrating bone injuries.

- **D.** Cat scratches inoculate the same microorganisms as bites and should be treated in the same manner.
- **E.** *Pasteurella multocida* is isolated in the oral cavities of 70% to 90% of healthy cats. Infection usually develops rapidly (<24 hours), and complications include abscess, tenosynovitis, and osteomyelitis. Rare complications include endocarditis and meningitis.
- **F.** Cat scratch disease is a chronic infection that is a result of a cat bite or scratch. It is caused by *Bartonella henselae* and results in painful regional lymphadenopathy that presents 1 to 2 weeks after the initial injury. Serology or biopsy of the lymph node can confirm the diagnosis. It is usually a self-limiting disease, with resolution of symptoms within 2 months. Azithromycin may reduce the duration of lymphadenopathy.

IV. HUMAN BITES

- **A.** Human bites are less common than dog or cat bites but cause more serious infection owing to the mechanism of injury and oral flora. Most complications result from bites involving the hand. Serious infection is associated with 25% to 50% of these injuries. Human bites in locations other than the hand result in a similar incidence of infection as non-bite lacerations.
- **B.** Clenched fist injuries (CFI), or fight bites, are the most serious of human bite wounds and usually occur at the third or fourth metacarpophalangeal joint of the dominant hand.
  1. The metacarpophalangeal joints are in flexion at the time of injury, facilitating tooth penetration into the joint space.
  2. Tendon or nerve laceration, or phalangeal or metacarpal fracture, may occur occasionally.
  3. Joint penetration is present in 62% of these wounds, and 58% of CFIs may have bone involvement. CFIs should be evaluated by a hand surgeon for possible joint injury, tendon involvement, or the need for exploration.
- **C.** Occlusional bites to the hand, not involving the clenched fist, have a higher risk of infection and complication than simple occlusional bites to other areas.
- **D.** Human bite infections are usually polymicrobial with a higher incidence of gram-negative rods and anaerobes.
- **E.** *Eikenella corrodens* is a facultative anaerobic gram-negative rod identified in approximately 25% to 30% of CFI infections. It results in higher morbidity in human hand bites by acting synergistically with aerobic bacteria.

V. OTHER MAMMALIAN BITES

- **A.** Rodent bites usually are associated with a low risk of local infection. However, systemic diseases, including leptospirosis, tularemia, sporotrichosis, murine typhus, rat-bite fever, and plague, may be transmitted by rodent bites or scratches.

B. Monkey and other primate bites have a high infection rate. Old World macaque monkeys may transmit herpesvirus simian (B virus), which presents with vesicles at the site of injury, followed by paresthesias, encephalopathy, and death in approximately 70% of cases. Immediate wound care and early aggressive treatment are required in this infection.

VI. INITIAL MANAGEMENT

A. In patients sustaining animal bites, determine the type of animal involved, the captivity status, and whether the attack was provoked or unprovoked. This information is useful in establishing the need for rabies prophylaxis.
B. Elicit a history of allergies to local anesthetics or other medications, as well as tetanus and rabies immune status.
C. Record important medical data, including history of splenectomy, diabetes, HIV infection, liver disease, malignancy, or immunosuppressive therapy.
D. Perform a thorough neurovascular examination with emphasis on wound type and depth, as well as tendon, ligament, bone, or joint involvement.
E. Document initial and subsequent range of motion and level of discomfort.
F. Obtain a radiograph to exclude bone or joint involvement, as well as to determine if a foreign body (e.g., tooth) is present in the wound.
G. Obtain Gram stain and culture of all infected wounds before treatment, as 90% of infected dog bite wounds yield pathogenic bacteria.
H. Irrigate under 15 lb (6.75 kg) of pressure using an 18- to 20-gauge angiocath, a 60-mL syringe, and a minimum of 150 mL of normal saline. Pressure irrigation significantly decreases the bacterial inoculum and may reduce the rate of infection by up to 20 fold.
I. Apply ice, immobilize, and elevate the wounded area.
J. Human hand bites, primate bites, or cat bite wounds should not be closed because secondary infection is common.
K. Dog bites without signs of infection or hand involvement may be sutured if less than 12 hours old.
L. Bite wounds that are contaminated, more than 12 hours old, or infected at presentation should be left open.
M. Bites to the head and face may be closed at the discretion of a plastic or oral-maxillofacial surgeon.

VII. ANTIBIOTIC TREATMENT

A. Prophylactic antibiotic therapy for 5 days is indicated for the following:
1. Dog or human bites involving the hand, deep punctures, heavy contamination, or those with tendon, joint, or bone involvement
2. Wounds more than 12 hours old
3. All cat bites

4. Diabetic, asplenic, or immunocompromised patients, including those with cirrhosis or peripheral vascular disease

B. Antibiotic choices

1. For dog bite prophylaxis, an antibiotic such as cephalexin or dicloxacillin that covers *Staphylococcus aureus* and streptococci is usually sufficient.
2. Either a second- or third-generation cephalosporin, amoxicillin-clavulanic acid, or clindamycin and a fluoroquinolone are necessary for a documented dog bite infection to cover *Pasteurella multocida*.
3. Clindamycin and trimethoprim-sulfamethoxazole is an alternative in penicillin-allergic pediatric patients who have documented dog bite infections and offers sufficient coverage against *P. multocida*.
4. All cat bites should receive antibiotic prophylaxis for 5 days, including one of the above regimens, to cover *P. multocida*. Dicloxacillin plus penicillin and macrolides such as azithromycin are additional alternatives in pediatric patients who cannot receive a fluoroquinolone. A first dose of prophylactic IV antibiotics should be given in the ED, and most documented cat bite infections should be admitted to the hospital.
5. All human hand bites should receive prophylaxis with antibiotics such as a second-generation cephalosporin or amoxicillin-clavulanate. Infected wounds should receive antibiotic coverage against gram-positive and anaerobic organisms as well as *E. corrodens*. Options include amoxicillin-sulbactam, cefoxitin, and ticarcillin-clavulanate. For penicillin-allergic patients, TMP-SMX or clindamycin plus a fluoroquinolone is indicated.
6. Antibiotic prophylaxis is usually not indicated for rodent bites
7. Management of monkey bites should follow the treatment guidelines for human bites. Immediate local wound care should be initiated to prevent herpesvirus simiae infection.

VIII. INDICATIONS FOR HOSPITAL ADMISSION

A. Systemic signs of infection
B. Head injury
C. Severe cellulitis
D. Peripheral vascular disease
E. Poorly controlled diabetes mellitus
F. Penetration of a joint, nerve, bone, tendon, or central nervous system
G. Failed outpatient therapy, or likelihood of noncompliance with outpatient treatment

IX. TETANUS IMMUNIZATION

A. Patients with an unknown tetanus immunization history or those who have received fewer than 3 doses should receive tetanus immunoglobulin 250 units IM plus the first of three doses of tetanus toxoid (0.5 mL IM). The second and third doses are given 1 month and 6 months later.

B. Tetanus toxoid 0.5 mL IM is recommended for patients who have not received a booster in 5 years

X. RABIES

A. There were 32 deaths in the United States between 1990 and 2000 as a result of rabies infection.
B. Transmission is usually accomplished through the saliva from the bite or scratch of an infected animal. Wild animals accounted for 93% of the 7369 cases of rabies reported in animals in the United States in 2000.
C. Common wildlife vectors in decreasing order include raccoons (37.7%), skunks (30.2%), bats (16.8%), and foxes (6.2%) as well as others.
D. The primary domestic animal vectors include cats (3.4%), dogs (1.6%), and cattle (1.1%). Of note, rodents are very rarely identified as the cause of rabies transmission.
E. The need for post-exposure prophylaxis is dependent on the location of the incident, the type of animal, and whether or not the exposure was provoked. All unprovoked attacks should be considered high risk, especially those involving the hand and face.
F. Post-exposure prophylaxis should be strongly considered when any high-risk contact with a wild animal has occurred. If captured, wild animals and stray or unwanted dogs or cats should be sacrificed and refrigerated. The brain should be examined for Negri bodies.
G. A healthy domestic dog or cat should be confined and observed for 10 days. If aggressive behavior occurs, the animal should be sacrificed and brain tissue should be examined for signs of rabies.
H. Once the animal is sacrificed, the first dose of the rabies vaccine should be initiated (human diploid cell vaccine [HDCV] or rabies vaccine adsorbed [RVA] 1.0 mL IM in the deltoid area) and rabies immunoglobulin should be administered around the wound (20 IU/kg). Any remaining volume should be administered IM elsewhere in a separate syringe from the vaccine.
I. Additional vaccine doses should be given on days 3, 7, 14, and 28 if the animal is rabid. The vaccine may be discontinued if the animal is not rabid. Public health officials or the Centers for Disease Control and Prevention should be contacted for specific recommendations if the animal has escaped.
J. Previously vaccinated patients do not need rabies immunoglobulin but should receive rabies vaccine on days 0 and 3.
K. Pregnancy is not a contraindication to post-exposure rabies prophylaxis when indicated.

XI. SNAKE BITES

A. It is estimated that more than 40,000 snake bites occur yearly in the United States and from 2000 to 8000 of these are caused by poisonous snakes.

- **B.** Mortality rates from poisonous snake bites are around 0.5%. About 25% of poisonous snake bites are dry bites, meaning the patient will show no signs or symptoms of envenomation.
- **C.** There are two families of venomous snakes in the United States—Crotalinae and Elapidae.
- **D.** Snakes in the Crotalinae family are copperheads, cottonmouths, and rattlesnakes.
  1. Members of the Crotalinae family are also known as pit vipers because of a heat-sensitive pit located between the eye and nostril.
  2. Pit vipers can be distinguished from nonvenomous snakes by their elliptical pupils, curved fangs, single subcaudal scale pattern, and rattles (only in rattlesnakes).
  3. Pit viper venom contains more than 15 proteolytic enzymes. These enzymes alter cell membrane permeability, disrupt hemostasis, and catalyze disseminated intravascular coagulation (DIC). In addition to proteases, Mojave rattlesnake venom contains neurotoxins, which can lead to cranial nerve weakness, respiratory failure, and altered mental status.
  4. Signs of pit viper envenomation are more caustic. Initial symptoms include severe pain and burning, followed by edema, ecchymosis, vesicle and bleb formation, nausea, vomiting, hypotension, hemolysis, and DIC. Other complaints include perioral numbness, a metallic taste in the mouth, lethargy, muscle weakness, ptosis, tremors, and seizures.
  5. Factors that must be taken into consideration include the amount and type of snake venom injected, the location of the bite, and the age, size, and health of the patient.
- **E.** Coral snakes belong to the Elapidae family.
  1. Coral snakes are small snakes with black snouts and alternating bands of yellow, red, and black. Remember the following saying when differentiating between coral snakes and similar appearing nonvenomous snakes: "Red on yellow, kill a fellow; red on black, venom lack."
  2. The effects of a coral snake bite are delayed. Initially, there is a minimal local tissue reaction. Systemic symptoms may present up to 13 hours after envenomation and include cranial nerve weakness, intense salivation, paresthesias, muscle fasciculations, generalized weakness, and respiratory failure as a result of neurotoxins.

XII. TREATMENT

- **A.** Prehospital treatment should include calming the patient, immobilizing the extremity in a dependent position, and marking the induration. Lymphatic constriction bands are a controversial option. Incision and suction, ice water immersion, arterial tourniquets, electric shock, and alcohol consumption are contraindicated methods of care.
- **B.** Initial emergency department management should include assessing for ABCs, placing 2 large-bore IV lines, early typing and cross-matching of blood, laboratory studies, and analgesia. The progression of swelling

should be monitored every 30 minutes and neurovascular checks should be repeatedly performed.
- **C.** Recommended laboratory studies include complete blood count, PT, PTT, fibrin split products, fibrinogen, bleeding time, electrolytes, CPK, and urinalysis for myoglobinuria.
- **D. Grades of crotalid envenomation:**
1. **None**: fang marks, no local or systemic side effects, or a dry bite
2. **Mild**: local pain and swelling (6 to 12 inches from fang marks) with no systemic involvement
3. **Moderate**: progressive swelling from fang marks (>12 inches) with some systemic symptoms including vomiting, diaphoresis, hemoconcentration, and mild coagulopathy
4. **Severe**: rapid and marked swelling of extremity, severe coagulopathy, hypotension, altered mental status, and pulmonary edema
- **E.** The antivenin now used, Crofab, is a mixture of sheep-derived immunoglobulin Fab fragments against the cottonmouth and various rattlesnakes found in the United States. Antivenin is indicated for moderate or severe envenomations.
- **F.** The recommended treatment is to give 4 to 6 vials of Crofab to start and repeat as needed to control progression of local swelling, systemic signs or symptoms, and coagulopathy. Each vial is diluted in 250 mL of crystalloid and infused slowly over 10 minutes (total time of infusion is approximately 1 hour). Monitor and be prepared for anaphylaxis!
- **G.** After initial control is established, maintenance dosing of 2 vials every 6 hours is recommended for 3 additional doses.
- **H.** The number of vials given to pediatric patients is the same as for adults but may be given in a smaller volume.
- **I.** If the patient is stable, the bite wound may be cleansed and debrided.
- **J.** Tetanus prophylaxis should be given as well as broad-spectrum antibiotics when indicated.
- **K.** Laboratory work should be repeated every 6 hours until abnormal parameters stabilize.
- **L.** Pit viper bite victims who present without signs or symptoms of envenomation and remain asymptomatic in the emergency department for 6 hours may be discharged.

XIII. SUGGESTED READINGS

Kerins M, Greene S, O'Connor N: A human bite to the scrotum: A case report and review of the literature. Eur J Emerg Med. 11(4):223–224, 2004.

Staiano J, Graham K: A tooth in the hand is worth a washout in the operating theater. J Trauma 62(6):1531–1532, 2007.

Woolgar JD, Cliff G, Nair R, et al: Shark attack: Review of 86 consecutive cases. J Trauma 50(5):887–891, 2001.

Trauma in the Pregnant Patient

Julie Grimes, MD, and Frances Rosenbaum, MD

I. INTRODUCTION

A. Etiology
1. Trauma is the most frequent cause of death in women younger than 35 years of age.
2. One in twelve pregnancies is associated with trauma. Most cases of significant trauma during pregnancy are caused by motor vehicle collisions, falls, and assaults.

B. Providing **prompt and proper care** to the injured obstetric patient requires not only knowledge of the specific anatomic and physiologic changes that occur in pregnancy, but also the cooperation of a complete trauma team, including the trauma surgeon, the obstetrician, the emergency department physician, and the pediatrician.
1. Treatment goals should be directed toward evaluation and stabilization of maternal injuries.
2. Attention to fetal assessment during the acute evaluation may divert attention from life-threatening maternal injuries.

II. ANATOMIC AND PHYSIOLOGIC CHANGES OF PREGNANCY

Unique anatomic and physiologic changes occur during pregnancy and have a direct bearing on the care and evaluation of the injured pregnant patient. These changes include the following::

A. Cardiovascular changes
1. Maternal blood volume begins to increase in the first trimester and near term averages 40% to 50% above nonpregnant values.
   a. Increased blood volume is the result of an increase in plasma volume and an increase in red blood cell volume.
   b. A dilutional anemia results from a disproportionate plasma volume increase without normal expansion of maternal hemoglobin mass.
   c. With proper iron supplementation throughout pregnancy, normal hematocrit levels in the pregnant woman in the second and third trimesters should be between 30% and 36%.
2. Cardiac output increases by 30% to 50% by 28 to 32 weeks (6.2 +/− 1.0 L/minute).
3. Resting heart rate increases by 10 to 20 beats per minute (83 +/− 10 bpm).
4. Blood pressure (BP) decreases in the first trimester (mean BP 105/60) and reaches a nadir in the second trimester (mean BP 100/54).

a. BP then begins to return to the prepregnant baseline in the latter part of the third trimester (mean BP 110/70).

B. Pulmonary changes
1. Minute ventilation increases by 50%, tidal volume increases by 40%, and minute oxygen consumption increases.
2. There is a decrease in functional residual capacity (FRC) and residual volume (RV) as a result of the elevated diaphragm during pregnancy.
3. Hormonal changes cause hyperventilation and a sensation of dyspnea, although the respiratory rate does not change in pregnancy.
   a. Hyperventilation produces an increase in the partial pressure of oxygen (Po_2 100 to 105 mm Hg), as well as a respiratory alkalosis (Pco_2 30 mm Hg). This is compensated for by a reduction in plasma bicarbonate level.

C. Hematopoietic changes
1. Several coagulation factors (fibrinogen, VII, VIII, IX, X) as well as the white blood cell count are increased in normal pregnancy.
2. Fibrinogen levels average 450 mg/dL in late pregnancy, so if a trauma patient presents in the latter half of pregnancy with a normal or low fibrinogen level as well as with elevated fibrin degradation products, consider a consumptive coagulopathy.
   a. This is commonly noted with placental abruption.

D. Gastrointestinal changes
1. Due to hormonal factors in pregnancy, there is an increased risk of gastroesophageal reflux and aspiration.
   a. This is from a decreased lower esophageal sphincter pressure, in addition to delayed gastric emptying and intestinal transit time.
2. There is displacement of abdominal viscera cephalad in the latter part of pregnancy, which increases the risk of complex bowel injuries with penetrating trauma to the upper abdomen.
3. Abdominal tenderness and peritoneal signs are less obvious in later pregnancy due to stretching of abdominal musculature and peritoneum.

E. Genitourinary changes
1. Glomerular filtration rate and renal plasma flow increase about 50% in pregnancy.
   a. As a result, glucosuria may be present and is not necessarily abnormal.
   b. Proteinuria and hematuria are not normal and require evaluation.
2. There is a mild to moderate amount of hydroureter and hydronephrosis (R > L) in the second and third trimesters due to compression of the ureters by the gravid uterus.

III. INITIAL EVALUATION AND CARE: PRIMARY SURVEY

A. Treatment priorities for an injured pregnant woman are the same as for a nonpregnant patient.

1. If attention is focused on the fetus before the mother has been adequately resuscitated and stabilized, life-threatening maternal injuries may be overlooked.
   a. Assessment of fetal status is appropriate after an adequate maternal evaluation.
   b. There should be no restriction in using the usual diagnostic, pharmacologic, or resuscitative procedures or maneuvers.

B. Airway/breathing
1. Maintaining a patent airway is of primary importance.
2. Supplemental oxygen should be given because small increases in maternal oxygen concentration will improve the blood oxygen concentration and reserve for the fetus.
3. Maternal SaO_2 should be maintained above 92%.

C. Circulation
1. Due to the hypervolemia of pregnancy, the patient's blood loss may be substantial before she manifests signs of shock.
   a. Minor volume depletion may shunt blood from the placenta and compromise fetal blood supply.
   b. Two large-bore peripheral intravenous lines should be placed and crystalloid infused generously.
   c. It may be necessary to administer large quantities of fluid and blood to adequately resuscitate the pregnant patient because of her expanded blood volume.
2. If the patient is more than 20 weeks pregnant and her spine has been stabilized, she should be placed in the left lateral decubitus position to avoid the supine hypotension syndrome.
   a. Supine hypotension syndrome consists of hypotension, dizziness, pallor, tachycardia, sweating, and nausea.
   b. In late pregnancy, the gravid uterus will impede blood return to the heart and therefore decrease cardiac output in the supine position.
   c. The uterus may also compress the aorta and reduce blood flow to the fetus.
3. If the patient is strapped to a backboard, a wedge can be placed beneath her right side to deflect the uterus.
4. A Foley catheter should be inserted to decompress the bladder, to monitor urine output, and to detect hematuria or hemoglobinuria.

IV. SECONDARY SURVEY

A. Once resuscitation is complete, a complete history and physical examination are performed.
B. Obstetricians should be summoned immediately to help with determination of fetal gestational age as well as fetal condition, management of the fetus, and any obstetric emergencies.

1. Fetal heart rate auscultation, fundal height measurement, cervical examination, assessment of the presence and frequency of contractions using electronic monitoring, and sonographic evaluation of the placenta and fetus are all important in determining fetal age and status and the need for obstetric intervention.
2. A fetus with an estimated gestational age greater than 25 weeks is considered viable.

C. Adjunctive studies

1. It may be necessary to further evaluate the pregnant patient using diagnostic peritoneal lavage or radiographic studies.
2. Radiologic evaluation, including computed tomography and angiography, should be performed when indicated regardless of fetal age. However, the uterus should be shielded when possible.
3. Unnecessary and duplicate films should be avoided to minimize fetal doses of radiation.

D. Special consideration should be given to the presence of splenic injury and retroperitoneal hemorrhage following blunt trauma, as these are thought to occur more frequently in the pregnant patient when compared to the nonpregnant patient.

V. OPERATIVE MANAGEMENT

A. Indications for exploratory celiotomy are unchanged by pregnancy.
B. Before celiotomy, the fetus should be examined for gestational age and condition using sonography, electronic monitoring, and possibly amniocentesis, if time permits.
C. All gunshot wounds should be explored, but some advocate close observation for selected stab wounds.
D. If the patient has been adequately resuscitated, the fetus will usually tolerate the stress of surgery and anesthesia.
E. During the exploration, the uterus may be retracted out of the operative field provided that blood flow to the uterus is not compromised.
F. During the exploration, the uterus must be carefully examined for evidence of penetrating injury.

1. If the uterus has been injured and there is evidence of fetal jeopardy in a viable fetus, cesarean delivery should be considered.
2. If the fetus appears to be in good condition or is not yet viable, repair of the uterus and expectant management may be indicated.
3. If the fetus is dead, either cesarean delivery or induction of labor for a vaginal delivery may be indicated, depending on the location and extent of the uterine injury.

G. Celiotomy itself is not an indication for cesarean section.

1. Consideration is given to fetal age and condition, extent of uterine injury, and whether treatment or evaluation of the mother's injuries at the time of celiotomy is hindered by the gravid uterus.

2. Cesarean section prolongs the operative procedure and increases blood loss by approximately 1 liter, but should be performed when indicated.

VI. OBSTETRIC EMERGENCIES IN THE TRAUMA PATIENT

The following is a brief list of complications unique to the pregnant trauma patient that should be considered at the time of the secondary survey. The help of obstetricians is required in the diagnosis and management of each.

A. Traumatic placental abruption

1. Abruptio placentae, or premature separation of the normally implanted placenta, complicates 1% to 6% of minor injuries and up to 50% of major injuries.
   a. This should be high on the list of differential diagnoses when the injured gravid patient presents with shock, disseminated intravascular coagulation, uterine tenderness, vaginal bleeding, ruptured fetal membranes, fetal jeopardy, or fetal death.
2. In some cases of abruption, there may be no vaginal bleeding or other physical findings and the abruption may be confused with labor.
3. Fetal electronic monitoring is the most sensitive method for detecting abruption and subtle signs of fetal jeopardy.
   a. Monitoring should begin as soon as possible after maternal stabilization in women whose fetuses are 20 to 22 weeks estimated gestational age (EGA).
   b. Women are typically monitored for a minimum of 4 hours.
   c. Contractions or nonreassuring fetal heart rate tracings warrant an extended monitoring period of at least 24 hours.
4. Blood for laboratory tests (CBC, PT/PTT, d-dimers, Kleihauer-Betke stain, fibrinogen, group and screen, and a thrombin clot tube) should be drawn while the patient is in the trauma bay.
5. Placental abruption is one of the most common causes of obstetric consumptive coagulopathy.
   a. Blood loss accompanied by hypofibrinogenemia may be substantial.
6. In the setting of placental abruption with a live fetus of viable gestational age, the decision to deliver the fetus and the mode of delivery must be made by experienced obstetricians after stabilization of the mother.
7. In Rh-negative women with evidence of fetomaternal hemorrhage, anti-D immunoglobulin (Rhogam) must be given to prevent Rh isoimmunization.

B. Uterine rupture

1. This uncommon event occurs in fewer than 1% of blunt trauma patients.
   a. This must be considered if the patient has suffered direct and intense force to the abdomen/uterus.
2. When uterine rupture occurs, rapid deterioration of the mother and the fetus is likely.

3. The diagnosis of uterine rupture may be suspected by history, physical examination, or radiologic studies, but often the diagnosis is not confirmed until celiotomy.
4. Repair of the uterus is possible, but emergency hysterectomy is often required.

C. Fetal injury/fetal jeopardy
1. The risk of fetal injury is high when factors such as hypoxia, head injury, pelvic fracture, placental injury, and shock are present in the mother.
2. Direct fetal injury occurs two thirds of the time when the uterus sustains penetrating trauma.
    a. Fetal skull and brain injuries are especially common with pelvic fractures in gravid women when the fetal head is presenting and engaged in the pelvis.
3. Fetal jeopardy in a viable fetus can be diagnosed with electronic monitoring and an experienced obstetrician.
    a. If the mother has been adequately stabilized, emergency cesarean section may be considered

D. Umbilical cord prolapse
1. Spontaneous rupture of fetal membranes has been seen both with and without contractions after blunt trauma.
2. If the presenting fetal part is not well engaged in the maternal pelvis, the fetal umbilical cord may prolapse into the vagina.
3. Cord prolapse requires emergent cesarean delivery in a viable fetus, as fetal hypoxia and death will quickly ensue.

E. Impending maternal death
1. In the case of a dead or moribund pregnant patient, the decision to perform emergency cesarean delivery must be made quickly, as fetal survival is unlikely if more than 20 minutes have elapsed since the death of the mother.
2. There is an inverse correlation between neurologically intact neonatal survival and the cardiac-arrest-to-delivery interval in women delivered by perimortem cesarean.
3. During cardiopulmonary resuscitation, left lateral uterine displacement is essential for adequate cardiac output in a gravid female.
4. Consideration is given to fetal age and fetal condition (presence and rate of fetal heart tones).
5. The senior pediatrician, his or her resuscitation team, and, if possible, the neonatologist should be present at delivery.

VII. SUGGESTED READINGS

Alger L, Crenshaw M Jr: Management of the obstetric patient after trauma. In Siegel JH (ed): Trauma—Emergency Surgery and Critical Care. New York, Churchill Livingston, 1978, pp 1075–1098.

American College of Obstetricians and Gynecologists: Trauma during pregnancy. ACOG Technical Bulletin No. 161, November 1991.

Chames MC, Pearlman MD: Trauma during pregnancy: Outcomes and clinical management. Clin Obstet Gynecol 51(2):398–408, 2008.

Cokkinides VE, Coker Al, Sanderson M, et al: Physical violence during pregnancy: Maternal complications and birth outcomes. Obstet Gynecol 93(5 Pt 1):661–666, 1999.

Patteson SK, Snider CC, Meyer DS, et al: The consequences of high-risk behaviors: Trauma during pregnancy. J Trauma. 62(4):1015–1020, 2007.

Pediatric Trauma

Ian Mitchell, MD, and Kshama Jaiswal, MD

I. ANATOMIC DIFFERENCES AND THEIR SEQUELAE

A. **Relatively larger head**—increased frequency of head injury and changes in the most common cervical spine injury patterns from C5-C7 in adults to C1-C2 in children
B. **Lax ligaments and incomplete ossification**—yield more ligamentous injuries not identifiable by plain film or computed tomography
C. **Larger tongue and anterior larynx**—different intubation technique
D. **Increased body surface area**—increased heat and fluid loss
E. **Compliant chest and abdomen**—may have significant internal injury without evidence of external trauma/bony injury
F. **Widely transmitted breath sounds**—may obscure significant pneumothorax

II. PHYSIOLOGIC DIFFERENCES

A. **Stroke volume relatively fixed**; thus increased heart rate required for increased cardiac output
B. **Hypotension** is a late manifestation of blood loss.
C. **Hypothermia** is common, especially with increased body surface area.
D. **Low total blood volume**—a small amount of bleeding may be significant in infants/younger children.
E. **More prone to gastric dilatation after injury** due to redistribution from splanchnic bed and tachypnea

III. OCCULT INJURIES

A. **Spine dislocation or cord tear** from torn ligaments in the absence of a fracture
B. **Myocardial and pulmonary contusion** without rib or sternal fracture
C. **Vascular injury**—intimal disruption with delayed occlusion
D. **Nondisplaced fractures** in the unconscious child
E. **Intestinal injuries** from lap belt use. Associated with lumbar spine fractures

IV. PRIMARY SURVEY

A. Airway
1. **Airway obstruction or compromise** may be caused by decreased mental status allowing relatively large tongue to fall back in pharynx and is manifest by wheezing, stridor, retractions, or nasal flaring.
   a. **Initial management is similar to the adult**:
      i. Chin lift/ jaw thrust
      ii. Placement of an orotracheal airway

IV. Primary Survey

      iii. Suctioning
      iv. Supplemental oxygen administration
2. **Indications for intubation** include:
    a. Apnea
    b. Traumatic brain injury with Glasgow Coma Scale (GCS) score <9
    c. Facial injury
    d. Severe hypotension
3. **Intubation is accomplished without neck extension** using a noncuffed endotracheal tube.
    a. Tube size should approximate the size of the child's fifth finger or nare.
    b. Tube size can also be calculated with the equation: $(Age + 16)/4$.
4. **A tracheostomy** may be performed in children under the age of 7 years.
5. **Children over the age of 7 years** may safely have a cricothyroidotomy performed.
6. **Surgical airways are rarely necessary**.
7. **Nasogastric or orogastric tube placement** as soon as feasible

B. Breathing
1. **Oxygen is indicated** whether or not the patient is intubated.
2. **Tidal volumes** of 10 to 15 mL/kg with respiratory rate varying by age (see Table 47-1)

C. Circulation
1. **Normal heart rate and good capillary refill** are signs of adequate volume status.
2. **Do not rely on blood pressure alone**.
3. **Total blood volume is 75 to 80 mL/kg**.
4. **Preferred vascular access**:
    a. Two upper extremity IV lines
    b. Intraosseous (IO) lines are indicated if unable to gain expeditious IV access for children under 7 years of age. Older children may have a central line.
    c. To perform an IO line:
        i. Prep and drape the anterior tibial surface.
        ii. Insert IO needle 2 cm below tibial tuberosity.
        iii. Avoid placement near fracture sites and avoid multiple passes as this may lead to fluid leakage and iatrogenic compartment syndrome.
5. **Fluid administration** is 20 mL/kg of Ringer's lactate as a bolus.
    a. Bolus may be repeated 1 to 2 times.
    b. If the patient remains unstable, transfuse with 10 mL/kg of packed red blood cells.

TABLE 47-1
NORMAL PEDIATRIC VITAL SIGNS BY AGE

Age	Heart Rate	Blood Pressure	Respirations
0–1	120	80/40	40
1–5	100	100/60	30
5–10	80	120/80	20

TABLE 47-2
GLASGOW COMA SCORE ADAPTED FOR CHILDREN

Verbalization:

Appropriate for age, fixes and follows, social smile	5
Cries but consolable	4
Persistently irritable	3
Restless, lethargic	2
None	1
Motor:	
Spontaneous movements	6

All other motor and all eye-opening scores are the same as for an adult.

6. **Cardiopulmonary resuscitation** in accordance with the Pediatric Advanced Cardiac Life Support guidelines is indicated for the patient in cardiac arrest.
D. **Disability**
1. **Establish the patient's GCS score** (Table 47-2)
2. **Rapid assessment** of pupillary function as well as extremity, motor, and sensory function
E. **Exposure**
1. **Remove all clothing and roll the patient**, removing the backboard as quickly as possible, while maintaining cervical spine immobilization
2. **Be wary of iatrogenic hypothermia**; all blankets should be warmed.
F. **Perform secondary survey and obtain indicated adjunctive studies.**

V. SPECIFIC INJURIES

A. Brain injury
1. **Brain injury is the primary cause of death** and disability in children
2. **Most injuries are traumatic brain injuries** with intraparenchymal hematoma and/or diffuse axonal injuries.
3. **After neurologic assessment is complete**, the indications for CT scan include:
   a. Loss of consciousness
   b. Neurologic deficit
   c. GCS <15
   d. Large cephalohematoma
4. With a persistent GCS less than 8 **despite adequate resuscitation**, an intracranial pressure monitor should be placed with the goal of cerebral perfusion pressure (CPP) of 60 mm Hg. (CPP = mean arterial pressure − intracranial pressure).
5. **Bulging fontanelles** can be an indication of intracranial swelling or bleeding in the very young child.
B. Spine

1. **Plain radiographs are negative** in 25% of pediatric patients with spinal cord injury. Cervical spine tenderness and careful neurologic examination must remain the mainstay of diagnosis.
2. **Children with altered** consciousness, or those under 8 years of age, should be maintained with the neck in neutral position until cervical spine films are obtained regardless of the presence or absence of tenderness.
3. **Tenderness or neurologic** deficit requires evaluation for fracture or dislocation with plain films or CT and assesment of ligaments.
4. **The neutral position of the spine in children** under age 5 is accomplished by having the shoulders elevated 2.0 to 2.5 cm on a foam pad or blanket.
5. **Pain without neurologic deficit and normal imaging** warrants evaluation of intraspinous ligaments with flexion/extension or magnetic resonance imaging (MRI).
6. **Persistent neurologic deficit or unreliable examination** and normal imaging mandate MRI for evaluation of possible ligamentous injury.
7. **Lumbar spine injury** (Chance fracture) must be ruled out in children with lap belt injuries.

C. Chest

1. **Pulmonary contusion, pneumothorax, and hemothorax** may be present in the absence of rib fractures. If such fractures are present, maintain a high index of suspicion for the above as well as for cardiac contusion, aortic injury, and abdominal solid organ injury.
2. **Of all penetrating chest injuries** only 2% of pneumothoraces and 10% of hemothoraces treated with tube drainage require thoracotomy
3. **If tube thoracostomy is required** the tube size should be equivalent to the size of the patient's intercostal space.
4. **Immediate thoracotomy** is indicated if hemothorax greater than 20 mL/kg is present or if bleeding persists after tube placement.

D. Abdomen

1. **CT of the abdomen** remains the standard for evaluation of children with blunt abdominal trauma.
2. **Diagnostic peritoneal lavage** (DPL) is occasionally performed in patients with lap-belt imprints and suspected bowel injury.
    a. **Warmed Ringer's lactate** should be infused into the peritoneal cavity:
        i. 500 mL in a child
        ii. 250 mL in an infant
    b. **DPL** is considered positive if:
        i. Frank blood is aspirated.
        ii. The red cell count is >100,000/mm^3 (adjusted for volume infused).
        iii. The white cell count is >500/mm^3 (adjusted for volume infused).
        iv. There is bile, amylase, or particles in the lavage fluid.
3. **A positive focused abdominal sonography for trauma** (FAST), in conjuction with hemodynamic instability refractive to resuscitation, is an indication for immediate operative intervention.

4. **The majority of solid organ injuries** are managed nonoperatively with close monitoring of hemodynamic status and hematocrit.
5. **Most clinicians** will accept hemoglobin as low as 7 g/dL with stable vital signs before transfusion. An ongoing transfusion requirement greater than 40 mL/kg is a relative indication for operation.
6. **A contrast blush on CT in the liver or spleen** is a sign of active bleeding and is a relative indication for operation or embolization.
7. **Most deaths from abdominal trauma** result from injuries to the liver, which involve either the portal or hepatic veins.
8. Successful nonoperative management of solid organ injury depends on:
   a. Hemodynamic stability
   b. No other need for intra-abdominal procedure
   c. Transfusion requirement less than 40 mL/kg
9. Hollow viscus injuries may be missed initially by CT, and if the clinical examination fails to improve after an observation period, DPL, laparoscopy, or laparotomy may be warranted.
10. **Pancreatic contusions** may be treated conservatively with nasogastric decompression and hyperalimentation; however, a transection left of the superior mesenteric vessels warrants distal pancreatectomy with attempted splenic salvage.
11. **Renal injuries** are most often managed by observation.
    a. Nonfunctioning of a kidney by CT requires angiographic evaluation.
    b. A shattered kidney, continued haemorrhage, and renal pedicle injury are operative indications. One-shot intravenous pyelogram should be obtained either prior to or during operation to ensure the function of the contralateral kidney.
    c. Operative intervention should proceed within 4 to 6 hours to salvage renal function.
12. **Hyperflexion mechanisms**, secondary to lap belts plus deceleration, are associated with injuries to the:
    a. Small bowel
    b. Duodenum
    c. Pancreas
    d. Lumbar spine
    e. Liver and spleen

E. Musculoskeletal trauma

1. **Radiologic examination** of the contralateral extremity is helpful in making an accurate diagnosis.
2. **Supracondylar fractures of the humerus** and fracture dislocations of the knee and ankle have a high likelihood of vascular injury.
3. **Concern for child abuse should be raised** any time there is variation in the history or the history is not consistent with the injuries present.
4. **Abuse should be suspected** if a young child has had multiple previous injuries or old fractures are seen radiographically.
5. **When abuse is suspected** the appropriate authorities must be notified.

6. **Patients with physical abuse** should be worked up completely for injuries as would any patient suffering an assault.

VI. SUGGESTED READINGS

Acierno SP, Jurkovich GJ, Nathens AB: Is pediatric trauma still a surgical disease? Patterns of emergent operative intervention in the injured child. J Trauma 56(5):960–964; discussion 965–966, 2004.

Grisoni E, Stallion A, Nance ML, et al: The New Injury Severity Score and the evaluation of pediatric trauma. J Trauma 50(6):1106–1110, 2001.

Geriatric Trauma

Severn Barloco, MD

I. DEMOGRAPHICS

A. According to the US Census, data from the year 2000 indicate that people age 65 or older make up approximately 12% of the country's population; this number is expected to grow to greater than 20% by the year 2030.
B. Age is an independent risk factor for trauma-related mortality. Elderly trauma patients have a six-fold higher mortality rate than younger trauma patients, even after controlling for injury severity.
C. Patients 65 years of age or older make up an estimated 23% of all trauma admissions, and they account for approximately 28% of all trauma-related hospital costs.

II. PHYSIOLOGIC CHANGES WITH INCREASING AGE

A. Chronologic age versus physiologic age
1. Significant preexisting conditions are predictors of increased mortality in trauma patients, independent of age; however, chronologic age for patients 65 years of age or older is the predominant predictor of mortality, and generally the presence or absence of preexisting conditions does not significantly affect the already increased risk of mortality.
2. The "normal" effects of aging may profoundly limit an elderly patient's physiologic reserve in response to traumatic injury.

B. Cardiovascular changes
1. Independent of the presence of significant atherosclerotic coronary artery or peripheral vascular disease, there is a steady decline in cardiac output (estimated 50% reduction from age 20 to age 80) related to a decrease in myocardial compliance.
2. There is a decrease in the number of β-adrenergic receptors, resulting in decreased responsiveness to catecholamines.
3. Medications, especially those for the treatment of hypertension or coronary artery disease, may severely affect a patient's cardiovascular function.
4. Normal vital signs may mask severe physiologic derangements.

C. Renal changes
1. There is a decrease in glomerular filtration rate and concentrating ability of the kidneys; this can limit the usefulness of the urinary output as an end point for resuscitation.
2. The loss of lean muscle mass must be considered when following the serum creatinine. A normal serum creatinine may not translate into normal kidney function.

D. Central nervous system changes
1. Traumatic brain injury is considered a predictor of poor outcome in geriatric trauma patients.

2. An initial Glasgow Coma Scale (GCS) score of <8 is associated with an approximately 80% mortality in elderly trauma patients; if there is not significant improvement in the GCS score within 72 hours after admission, the limitation of further aggressive interventions must be considered.

III. TREATMENT

A. Triage
1. There is sufficient evidence to suggest that there should be a low threshold for triaging elderly patients with traumatic injuries directly to a trauma center.
2. At Parkland Memorial Hospital, the trauma team evaluates all patients age 70 years or older with any traumatic mechanism of injury other than patients who have fallen from standing without any signs of injury.

B. Initial treatment
1. Although initial resuscitation of an elderly patient is no different than for other patients (ABCs), these patients require close monitoring and consideration of their physiologic reserve; subtle signs of decompensation must be recognized early.
2. Because geriatric patients tend to have limited physiologic reserve in response to traumatic injury, nonoperative management of significant blunt solid organ injury is generally not recommended.
3. Post-injury complications are significantly less well tolerated in geriatric trauma patients and have been associated with adverse outcomes; priority should be given to preventing such complications.

C. Monitoring
1. Early invasive monitoring in the intensive care unit with pulmonary artery catheterization may improve survival in geriatric blunt trauma patients.
2. Patients who appear hemodynamically stable may be found to have dangerously low cardiac outputs after placement of pulmonary artery catheters; perfusion/oxygen delivery is optimized with the administration of intravenous fluid, blood, or inotropes as indicated.

D. Prevention
1. Given the trend toward poorer outcomes in geriatric patients who sustain traumatic injury, greater efforts should be made toward injury prevention.

E. Withdrawal of care
1. There is some evidence that geriatric trauma patients with severe chest and/or abdominal trauma with moderate shock and mild to moderate head injury have a dismal prognosis, and early withdrawal of care may be a consideration in these circumstances; however, there is no evidence to support limitation or denial of care by any criteria on initial presentation.
2. At Parkland Memorial Hospital, an initial course of aggressive therapy is pursued in all geriatric trauma patients.

IV. SUGGESTED READINGS

Godley CD, et al: Nonoperative management of blunt splenic injury in adults: Age over 55 years as a powerful indicator for failure. J Am Coll Surg 183(2):133–139, 1996.

Hannan EL, et al: Elderly trauma inpatients in New York state: 1994-1998. J Trauma 56:1297–1304, 2004.

Jacobs DG: Special considerations in geriatric injury. Curr Opin Crit Care 9(6):535–539, 2003.

Jacobs DG, Plaisier BR, et al: Practice management guidelines for geriatric trauma: The EAST Practice Management Guidelines Work Group. J Trauma 54(2):391–416, 2003.

Kauder DR, Schwab CW, Shapiro MB: Geriatric trauma: Patterns, care, and outcomes. In Moore EE, Feliciano DV, Mattox KL (eds): Trauma, 5th ed. New York, McGraw-Hill, 2003, pp 1041–1058.

Longo WE, et al: Nonoperative management of adult blunt splenic trauma. Criteria for successful outcome. Ann Surg 210(5):626–629, 1989.

McKevitt EC, et al: Geriatric trauma: Resource use and patient outcomes. Can J Surg 46(3):211–215, 2003.

Nirula R, Gentilello LM: Futility of resuscitation criteria for the "young" old and the "old" old trauma patient: A National Trauma Data Bank analysis. J Trauma 57:37–41, 2004.

Scalea TM, et al: Geriatric blunt multiple trauma: Improved survival with early invasive monitoring. J Trauma 30(2):129–136, 1990.

Anesthesia in Trauma

Nabil N. Dagher, MD

I. PREOPERATIVE PREPARATION

A. Initial patient assessment:
Physical examination and evaluation of the patient's airway by the trauma team are essential. Prior medical history (if obtainable from the patient or family) is important, concentrating especially on cardiac and pulmonary problems. All severely injured patients should be considered at risk for aspiration, cervical spine and traumatic brain injuries, hypovolemia, alcohol abuse, and the possibility of a difficult intubation.

B. Designated operating room: a well-equipped operating room must be available at all times.

1. **Standard anesthesia equipment** for this trauma room includes the following:
   a. Anesthesia machine checked and operational, suction apparatus, and monitors
   b. Airway equipment: several sizes of endotracheal tubes
   c. Laryngoscope and blades (wide variety of sizes)
   d. Other emergency airway equipment (tube exchanger, fiberoptic scope)
   e. Laryngeal mask airways (rescue and intubating)
   f. Cricothyroidotomy and/or tracheostomy instruments
   g. High-flow IV fluid infusion devices, blood warmers (e.g., Level I), and automatic transfusers (e.g., cell saver)
   h. Vasoactive medications and anesthetic agents (drawn up and clearly labeled)
   i. Warming devices for the patient as well as a warm ambient temperature in the room
   j. Adequate personnel

C. Anesthetic drugs

1. **Induction/sedation agents**
   a. Etomidate (0.2 mg/kg)
   b. Ketamine (1 to 2 mg/kg)
   c. Other induction agents may be used if the patient is hemodynamically normal and shows no signs of hypovolemia (e.g., sodium thiopental, propofol).

2. **Neuromuscular blockade agents**
   a. Succinylcholine (1 to 2 mg/kg)
      i. May cause bradycardia with repeated doses, especially in the pediatric population
      ii. May cause hyperkalemia and cardiovascular collapse in patients with severe burns, spinal cord injury, upper motor-neuron injury, or muscular dystrophy

        iii. Is contraindicated in patients with genetic disorders of plasma pseudocholinesterases, a family history of malignant hyperthermia, and penetrating eye injuries
    b. Rocuronium (1 mg/kg)
        i. Rapid onset—within 60 seconds
        ii. Useful for rapid sequence induction when succinylcholine is contraindicated
3. **Maintenance agents**
    a. Rocuronium (0.06 to 0.6 mg/kg)
    b. Vecuronium (0.01 to 0.05 mg/kg)
    c. Pancuronium (0.01 to 0.05 mg/kg)
4. **Inhalational anesthetic agents**
    a. Carefully titrated
    b. Avoid nitrous oxide to prevent expansion of possible pneumothorax, bowel distention.
5. **Benzodiazepines** (use intra-operatively to prevent recall)
    a. Midazolam (1 to 4 mg IV q 1-2 hours)
    b. Lorazepam (1 to 4 mg IV q 6-12 hours)
6. Analgesics/narcotics
    a. Carefully titrated
    b. Avoid histamine-releasing agents such as morphine during the initial resuscitation.
7. **Vasopressors/resuscitation adjuncts**
    a. Epinephrine 10 to 100 µg (1.0 mg IV every 3 to 5 minutes for cardiac arrest)
    b. Sodium bicarbonate (1 mL/kg)
    c. Atropine (0.5 to 1.0 mg IV)
    d. Calcium chloride (500 to 1000 mg IV)
    e. Lidocaine (0.5 to 1.0 mg IV)
    f. Ephedrine (5 to 10 mg IV)
    g. Phenylephrine (50 to 100 µg IV)

II. INTRAOPERATIVE TECHNIQUES AND PEARLS

A. Anesthetic technique
1. General anesthesia is required for most trauma patients, especially those with multiple injuries.
2. Regional techniques may be appropriate for isolated injury to the limbs and if the patient is hemodynamically normal, though these are infrequently used at Parkland Memorial Hospital.

B. Airway
1. Hypotensive patients often arrive in the operating room already intubated.
2. Endotracheal intubation (ETI) must be confirmed with bilateral breath sounds and evidence of end tidal CO_2 on capnography.

3. All trauma patients should be considered to have a full stomach; therefore, a nasogastric tube should be inserted, preferably in the emergency department.
4. Awake intubation or rapid sequence induction should always be performed with cricoid pressure to compress the esophagus and prevent reflux.
5. Cervical spine stabilization must be held during intubation if the cervical spine has not been cleared.
6. Airway management can be particularly complex and requires careful planning in facial, head, and neck trauma.
7. Consider awake tracheostomy under local anesthesia if there is uncertainty about the airway.
8. In emergency situations, the best sequence for intubation is as follows:
    a. Give Bicitra 30 mL orally and preoxygenate with 100% oxygen for 5 minutes.
    b. Remove anterior portion of cervical collar and have assistant hold manual stabilization of cervical spine.
    c. Have another assistant hold cricoid pressure starting with induction and continued until endotracheal intubation is confirmed.
    d. Perform direct laryngoscopy and insert the endotracheal tube with minimal head movement.
    e. Confirm endotracheal intubation and replace cervical collar.
    f. If attempts at endotracheal intubation fail in the presence of hemodynamic instability and/or hypoxia, proceed directly to emergent cricothyroidotomy.

C. Maintenance of anesthesia

1. Arterial catheters are placed prior to or during induction and are useful for continuous blood pressure monitoring and serial arterial blood gas/hematocrit determinations.
2. Central venous catheters are avoided if possible but are used in critically ill patients.
3. Oxygen, muscle relaxants, and lorazepam may be the sole anesthetic agents until hypotension/hypovolemia resolve.
4. Communication between all members of the surgical team is essential.
5. Aggressive prevention of hypothermia is crucial to combat the "vicious triad of trauma": hypothermia, acidosis, and coagulopathy. Measures employed at Parkland Memorial Hospital to avoid hypothermia include:
    a. Warm operating suite prior to patient arrival.
    b. Monitor patient core temperature (esophageal probe).
    c. Warm all IV fluids and blood products.
    d. Use a heated humidifier to warm inhaled gases.
    e. Use a warming blanket on the operating room table, and BAIR hugger anywhere on the patient outside the operative sterile field.
    f. If the above attempts at rewarming fail, consider continuous arteriovenous rewarming (CAVR).

D. Fluid resuscitation and blood replacement

1. Patients in mild to moderate hemorrhagic shock (class I and II) respond well to crystalloid fluid replacement (Ringer's lactate or Plasmalyte) without need for immediate blood transfusion.
2. Patients in severe shock (class III and IV) have sustained massive blood loss (>30% of blood volume) and require blood transfusion to restore intravascular volume and improve oxygen delivery.
3. If blood transfusion is required prior to a formal typing and cross-matching, type O Rh-negative blood should be used.

E. Massive transfusion

1. Massive transfusion is defined as a complete replacement of a patient's blood volume (approximately 10 units of packed red blood cells in an adult) in a 24-hour period.
2. During intraoperative massive transfusion, laboratory values are reassessed every 30 to 60 minutes: hemoglobin, hematocrit, platelet count, PT, PTT, fibrinogen, and electrolytes.
3. Note: Due to the large citrate load, calcium chloride is administered after each patient blood volume in packed red blood cells has been transfused.
4. Table 49-1 lists the Parkland Memorial Hospital Massive Transfusion Protocol.
   a. Once patients meet criteria for massive transfusion, this protocol is immediately activated (often in the operating room).
   b. Product delivery is automatic according to protocol (see Table 49-1).
   c. Preplanned product delivery removes the need to order blood products individually and allows the blood bank to stay ahead of the operative/anesthesia team.
5. Thrombocytopenia is the most likely contributor to clotting abnormalities in these patients. Keep platelet counts >20,000/µL in nonbleeding patients and >100,000/µL if there is evidence of ongoing bleeding.
6. Should shipment 10 be reached and the patient requires further resuscitation with blood products, the protocol cycles back to shipment 1.

TABLE 49-1
MASSIVE TRANSFUSION PROTOCOL

Shipment	RBC	TP	PLT	CR	rVIIa
1a	5(O-Neg)	2(AB)			
1b	5	2			
2	5	2	1		2.4 mg
3	5	2		10	
4	5	2	1		2.4 mg
5	5	2			
6	5	2	1	10	2.4 mg
7	5	2			
8	5	2	1		
9	5	2		10	
10	5	2	1		

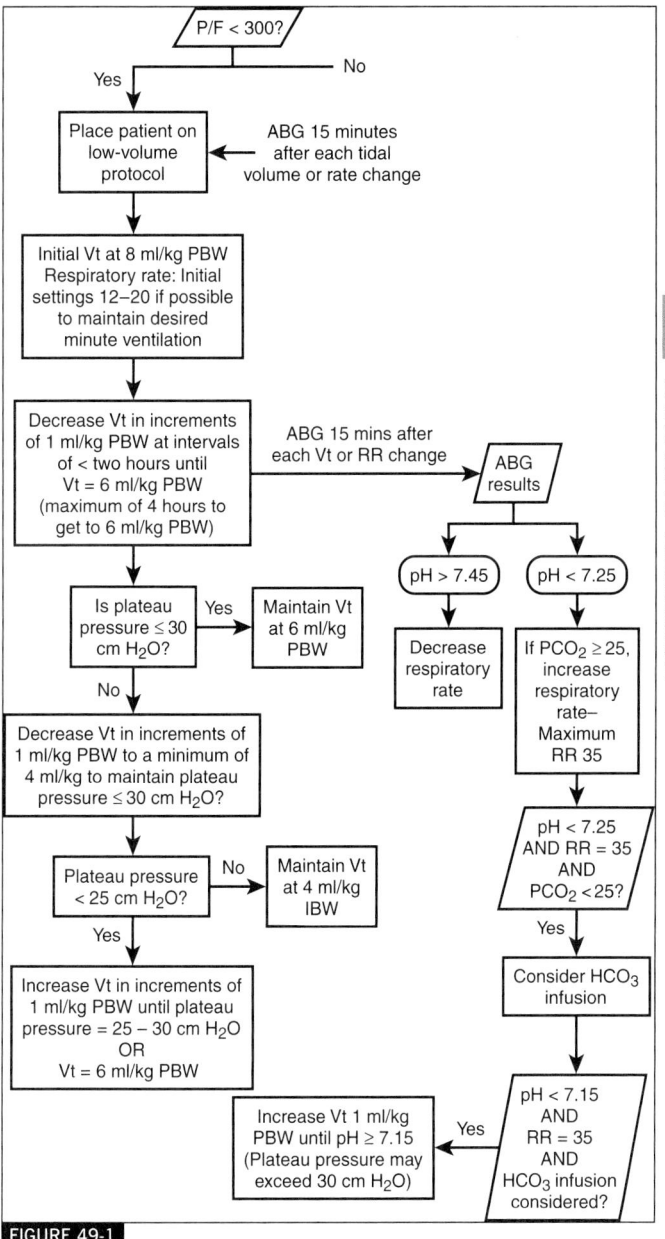

FIGURE 49-1

Low-volume protocol for patients with ALI/ARDS at Parkland Memorial Hospital. (Courtesy of the Respiratory Care Department at Parkland Memorial Hospital, Dallas, Texas.)

7. Constant communication between surgeon and anesthesiologist as to the degree of blood loss and presence of ongoing hemorrhage is critical.

III. ANESTHESIA MANAGEMENT IN SPECIFIC PATIENT GROUPS

A. The pregnant trauma patient
1. Though often not possible, surgery should be delayed until the second trimester.
2. Use pentothal for induction and narcotics and inhalational agents for maintenance; a decreased minimum alveolar concentration for inhalational agents is needed in pregnant patients.
3. Place a wedge under the patient's right hip for left uterine displacement to relieve the weight of the uterus on the aorta and inferior vena cava.
4. Avoid nitric oxide.
5. Treat hypotension aggressively to maintain uteroplacental blood flow. Keep in mind that pregnancy is a vasodilated state and there may be natural alterations in vital signs.
6. Monitor fetal heart rate/intraoperative uterine activity if gestational age is > 24 weeks.

B. The patient with acute lung injury (ALI)
1. Recent data have shown that in patients with ALI and acute respiratory distress syndrome (ARDS), mechanical ventilation with lower tidal volumes (Vt) than traditionally used (6 mL/kg vs. 12 mL/kg) reduces mortality and decreases the number of days of ventilator use.
2. In patients who have a Po_2/Fio_2 ratio < 300, a low-volume (low-stretch) protocol is instituted intraoperatively (Figure 49-1).
3. Goals include maintaining a plateau pressure of <30 mm Hg and tidal volume of 6 mL/kg.
4. If plateau pressures continue to be ≤ 30 mm Hg, Vt can be decreased further to 4 mL/kg.
5. Fio_2 and PEEP are adjusted to a ratio of ≤ 5, to maintain Pao_2 at 55 to 80 mm Hg or Spo_2 at 88% to 95%.

IV. SUGGESTED READINGS

The Acute Respiratory Syndrome Network, Ventilation with lower tidal volumes as compared with traditional tidal volumes for acute lung injury and the acute respiratory distress syndrome. N Engl J Med. 342(18):1301–1308, 2000.

Moore EE, Feliciano D, Mattox KL (eds): Trauma, 5th ed. New York, McGraw-Hill, 2004, Chapters 13 and 17.

Cardiovascular Support and Management in the Intensive Care Unit

Sean Dineen, MD, and Paul Schumacher, MD

I. SHOCK AND ITS ETIOLOGIES

Shock occurs when tissue metabolic demands are inadequately supplied by the delivery of oxygen and nutrients. Though reversible in its early phase, untreated shock progresses to cellular injury, multiorgan dysfunction, and ultimately death.

A. Hypovolemic shock (Table 50-1)

1. Hypovolemia is the most common etiology of shock and the most common cause of early mortality in trauma. It occurs from hemorrhage, extravascular fluid sequestration ("third-space fluid losses"), or from losses from the gastrointestinal tract.
2. Physiologic compensatory mechanisms maintain cerebral and coronary perfusion by increasing sympathetic activity, releasing stress hormones, and expanding the effective circulatory volume through fluid conservation by the kidneys and mobilization of intracellular and interstitial fluid.
3. The clinical signs of hypovolemia that suggest inadequate resuscitation or persistent hemorrhage include hypotension, oliguria, metabolic acidosis, sinus tachycardia, and narrow pulse pressure.
4. Invasive monitoring with an arterial catheter and a central venous or pulmonary artery catheter is recommended for patients with persistent hypotension.
5. Treatment involves restoration of intravascular volume and correction of ongoing bleeding or fluid losses.

B. Cardiogenic shock

1. Cardiogenic shock is inadequate tissue perfusion from inability of the heart, as a result of pump impairment, to deliver sufficient substrate to the peripheral tissues.
2. *Intrinsic* mechanisms of cardiogenic shock include myocardial ischemia, blunt cardiac injury, cardiomyopathy, valvular heart disease, and acute dysrhythmias.
3. The development of cardiogenic shock reflects a complex interaction between the heart, peripheral circulation, and maladaptive compensatory mechanisms.
4. The clinical presentation of cardiogenic shock is a consequence of peripheral hypoperfusion, increased adrenergic tone, and inability of the heart to accommodate pulmonary or systemic venous return.
5. *Compressive* (or obstructive) cardiogenic shock results from extrinsic compression of the heart that impedes diastolic filling, reducing preload

TABLE 50-1
PHYSICAL FINDINGS IN HEMORRHAGIC SHOCK

	Class I	Class II	Class III	Class IV
Blood loss (mL)	<750	750–1500	1500–2000	>2000
Blood loss	Up to 15%	15%–30%	30%–40%	>40%
Pulse rate	<100	>100	>120	>140
Blood pressure	Normal	Normal	Decreased	Decreased
Pulse pressure (mm Hg)	Normal	Decreased	Decreased	Decreased
Respiratory rate	14–20	20–30	30–40	>35
Urine output (mL/hr)	>30	20–30	5–15	Negligible
CNS/mental status	Slightly anxious	Mildly anxious	Anxious, confused	Confused, lethargic

From Nathens AB, Maier RV: Shock and resuscitation. In Norton JA, et al (eds): Surgery: Basic Science and Clinical Evidence. New York, Springer-Verlag, 2001.

and thus stroke volume and cardiac output. Pericardial tamponade and causes of increased intrathoracic pressure, such as tension pneumothorax, mediastinal hematoma, and occasionally excessive positive pressure ventilation, may precipitate compressive cardiogenic shock. Typical clinical findings of pericardial tamponade include jugular venous distention, muffled heart tones, and hypotension (Beck's triad). Pulsus paradoxus and a narrow pulse pressure may also be observed.

6. If hypervolemia is the etiology of cardiogenic shock, diuretic administration will reduce ventricular end-diastolic volume and improve cardiac contractility as well as peripheral perfusion.
7. Management principles include establishing adequate oxygenation and ventilation, correction of electrolyte abnormalities, and restoration of sinus rhythm, including electrical cardioversion. If shock persists despite adequate intravascular volume, inotropic or vasopressor therapy should be instituted.
8. Dobutamine is a preferred agent because of its ability to reduce afterload and augment cardiac contractility. In moderate hypotension, dopamine is preferred, whereas in profound shock norepinephrine is often utilized. Afterload reduction may be beneficial in cardiogenic shock but may worsen or precipitate hypotension. Nitroprusside and nitroglycerin are recommended agents for afterload reduction. Of note, patients with right ventricular dysfunction related to ischemia or infarction are volume sensitive. Restoration of left ventricular filling pressure, despite significantly elevated central venous pressure, is paramount.

C. Distributive shock
1. **Distributive shock** refers to septic shock and neurogenic shock.
2. **Septic shock** presents within days to weeks of injury and is the most common cause of late mortality in the intensive care unit at Parkland Memorial Hospital (PMH).
   a. Septic shock is frequently caused by invasive bacterial infections originating most commonly from the lungs, abdomen, or urinary tract.
   b. Local and systemic responses to bacteria and their structural and metabolic products mediate septic shock and the release of

endothelial and macrophage-derived proinflammatory cytokines, especially TNF-α and IL-1.
   c. Cardiac dysfunction, decreased vasomotor tone, arteriovenous shunting, and increased endothelial permeability characterize the pathophysiology of septic shock and explain the clinical manifestations of the disorder, namely fever, tachycardia, hypotension, oliguria, and altered mental status.
   d. The collaborators of the Surviving Sepsis Campaign have developed recent evidence-based guidelines for the treatment of sepsis. These guidelines, followed strictly in the surgical intensive care unit at PMH, include:
      i. Early goal-directed therapy
      ii. Prompt fluid resuscitation and appropriate introduction of vasopressor and inotropic support
      iii. Rapid diagnosis of sepsis and institution of effective empiric antimicrobial therapy
      iv. Septic source control
      v. Judicious blood product administration
      vi. Institution of adjunctive measures, namely corticosteroid replacement therapy in states of relative adrenal insufficiency administration of recombinant human activated protein C (drotrecogin alfa) in severe sepsis, and strict glycemic control
3. **Neurogenic shock**, a constellation of features that occur following acute cervical or high thoracic spinal cord injury, results from disruption of sympathetic tone and unopposed vagal tone.
   a. Neurogenic shock is manifest by hypotension, bradycardia, dry skin, adequate urine output, and a neurologic deficit. Brief hemodynamic support with vasopressors may be required.
   b. Spinal cord injuries above L-1 are at risk of developing neurogenic shock.
   c. The cardiovascular abnormalities are only transient and typically resolve in 2 to 6 weeks.

See Table 50-2 for the differential diagnoses for the various types of shock.

TABLE 50-2
DIFFERENTIAL DIAGNOSIS OF SHOCK STATES BASED ON HEMODYNAMIC PARAMETERS

Type of Shock	CVP or PCWP	Cardiac Output	Systemic Vascular Resistance	Mixed Venous O_2 Saturation
Hypovolemic	↓	↓	↑	↓
Cardiogenic	↑	↓	↑	↓
Septic	↓↑	↑	↓	↑
Neurogenic	↓	↓	↓	↓

Adapted from Nathens AB, Maier RV: Shock and resuscitation. In Norton JA, et al (eds): Surgery: Basic Science and Clinical Evidence. New York, Springer-Verlag, 2001.

II. MEASUREMENT AND ESTIMATE OF CARDIAC FUNCTION AND PERIPHERAL PERFUSION

A. During resuscitation from shock, especially septic shock, specific, early, goal-directed therapy has improved survival. Early resuscitation in sepsis requires prompt correction of tissue hypoperfusion by attaining specific hemodyamic goals:
1. A central venous pressure (CVP) of 8 to 12 mm Hg
2. A mean arterial pressure (MAP) of ≥ 65 mm Hg
3. A urine output of ≥ 0.5 mL/kg/hour
4. A mixed venous oxygen saturation (Svo_2) or central venous oxygen saturation ($Scvo_2$) ≥ 70%
5. Normalization of serum lactate and base deficit

B. The introduction of the flow-directed, rapid-thermistor pulmonary artery catheter has permitted the measurement of important hemodynamic variables. Pulmonary artery catheters conveniently measure the following:
1. Pulmonary artery wedge pressure (PAWP)
   a. Balloon occlusion of the proximal pulmonary artery estimates left atrial pressure and closely approximates left ventricular end-diastolic pressure (LVEDP).
   b. Increases in the PAWP in response to a fluid challenge are a more useful indicator of volume status than an absolute measurement.
   c. Measurements of the PAWP are influenced by ventricular compliance, pulmonary hypertension, elevations in positive end-expiratory pressure (PEEP), and the position of the catheter tip in relationship to the lung zones of West.
   d. Normal PAWP is 6 to 12 mm Hg.
2. Right ventricular end-diastolic volume (RVEDV)
   a. The RVEDV is derived from the measurements of stroke volume and right ventricular ejection fraction (RVEF) and is an estimate of preload.
   b. The RVEDV is more predictive of recruitable increases in cardiac output in response to volume administration than PAWP, especially in the setting of elevated PEEP.
   c. The RVEDV is an accurate estimate of left ventricular function in patients with normal ventricular compliance.
   d. Normal RVEDV is 113 to 225 mL or 88 mL/m^2.
3. Cardiac output (CO)
   a. Cardiac output is measured as the area under a thermodilution curve.
   b. Cardiac output is the most useful indicator of cardiac function and is used to differentiate the various etioloiges of shock.
   c. Pulmonary artery catheters monitor CO continuously through a thermal filament device.
   d. The normal range of CO is 4 to 6 L/min.
   e. Cardiac output can be indexed to body surface area with a normal range of 2.5 to 3.5 L/min/m^2.

4. Mixed venous oxygen saturation (Svo_2)
   a. Pulmonary artery catheters equipped with an oximeter at the catheter tip can continuously measure the saturation of mixed venous blood in the pulmonary artery.
   b. The central venous oxygen saturation ($Scvo_2$) is a convenient surrogate measure of tissue oxygenation in patients without a pulmonary artery catheter.
   c. The mixed venous oxygen saturation is a function of cardiac output, blood oxygen saturation, hemoglobin concentration, and oxygen consumption.
   d. A decreased Svo_2 may indicate hemorrhage, hypoxemia, decreased cardiac output, or increased oxygen utilization by peripheral tissues.
   e. An elevated Svo_2 may indicate reduced peripheral oxygen utilization, such as occurs in sepsis or cyanide poisoning.
   f. Normal Svo_2 is 70% to 75%.
5. Systemic vascular resistance (SVR)
   a. Systemic vascular resistance is a measure of afterload and is derived from the equation (MAP–CVP) ÷ CO.
   b. The SVR is used to determine the need for vasodilator therapy in states of depressed cardiac output.
   c. Normal SVR is 800 to 1400 dynes sec cm^{-5}.
   d. The SVR can be indexed to body surface area (SVRI) with normal values of 1500 to 2400 dynes sec cm^{-5} m^{-2}.
6. Oxygen delivery (Do_2)
   a. The amount of oxygen delivered to peripheral tissues (DO_2) depends on the cardiac output (CO) and the oxygen content of blood (Cao_2):

   $$Do_2 = CO \times Cao_2 = CO \times Hgb \times Sao_2 \times 1.34$$

   b. Increasing the determinants of the above equation, namely cardiac output, hemoglobin concentration, and blood oxygen saturation, may augment oxygen delivery.
   c. No survival advantage has been realized by achieving supranormal values of oxygen delivery, however.
   d. Normal oxygen delivery is 400 to 660 mL/min/m^2.
7. Oxygen consumption (Vo_2)
   a. Oxygen consumption is the difference between the content of oxygen delivered by the heart (Cao_2) and the content returned to the heart (Cvo_2):

   $$Vo_2 = CO \times (Cao_2 \times Cvo_2)$$

   b. Decreases in oxygen consumption may indicate reduced peripheral oxygen utilization, as in sepsis.
   c. Increases in Do_2 attempt to achieve a flow-independent Vo_2 (dependent solely on metabolic rate and not oxygen delivery).
   d. Normal Vo_2 is 115 to 165 mL/min/m^2.

III. CARDIAC DYSRHYTHMIAS

A. Pathophysiology
1. All cardiac dysrhythmias occur as the result of reentry or increased automaticity.
2. Reentrant dysrhythmias occur from conduction delay related to myocardial ischemia, necrosis, or fibrosis.
3. Causes of increased automaticity include:
   a. Drugs
   b. Hypoxemia
   c. Hyperadrenergic states
   d. Cardiac dilatation or hypertrophy
   e. Electrolyte abnormalities, especially hypokalemia and hypercalcemia

B. Evaluation and management
1. During the evaluation of a patient with an acute dysrhythmia, it is less important to identify the precise rhythm disturbance than it is to rapidly recognize several clinical features that will determine initial therapy.
2. A patent, secure airway and adequate ventilation and oxygenation should be ensured. Effective chest compressions and timely defibrillation should be administered when indicated. After the identification of the electrical rhythm, preferably with a 12-lead electrocardiogram, vasoactive drugs should be promptly administered as reversible causes are investigated.
3. The reader is referred to the current ACLS Provider Manual (2008) for a more detailed and comprehensive description of dysrhythmia management. The text provides an overview of the management of common select dysrhythmias.

IV. CARDIAC SUPPORT: AN ALGORITHM

A. The principal determinants of cardiac output and tissue perfusion are:
1. Preload
2. Afterload
3. Contractility
4. Heart rate

B. These variables are related to the mean arterial pressure (MAP) by the following equation:

$$MAP = CO \times SVR$$

Thus, MAP is proportional to the heart rate and some measure of myocardial preload, afterload, and contractility (determinants of CO). Cardiac dysfunction, predominantly manifested as hypotension, occurs from decreases in any one of these variables.

1. Because of the inaccuracy of physical assessment in determining hemodynamic status, the placement of invasive hemodynamic monitors is often useful diagnostically and therapeutically.

2. Physiologic determinants in the treatment of shock (e.g., CVP or PAWP) center on the optimization of cardiac preload, contractility, afterload, and heart rate.

C. Preload management

1. Since hypovolemic and septic shock are the most common etiologies of shock in patients brought to the intensive care unit, the administration of intravenous fluid to increase preload, and thereby cardiac output, is a logical initial step.
   a. A PAWP of 12 to 16 mm Hg is optimal.
   b. An elevated PAWP (>16 mm Hg) suggests volume overload and, when it exists with pulmonary edema, warrants diuresis.
   c. A low PAWP (<12 mm Hg) suggests inadequate intravascular volume and is treated by administering intravenous crystalloid (lactated Ringer's solution).
   d. Repeated infusions of volume are administered until no further recruitable increases in cardiac output are observed by invasive measurement (Starling relationship).
2. If hypotension persists after the optimization of preload, mean arterial pressure is restored by agents that increase afterload.

D. Afterload management

1. A number of α-adrenergic agonists are employed to achieve and maintain an acceptable mean arterial pressure, approximately 65 mm Hg. Conventional vasopressors include dopamine, norepinephrine, epinephrine, and phenylephrine.
2. The SVR (or SVRI) provides an estimate of afterload and assists in differentiating the etiology of shock. A normal SVR is 800 to 1400 dynes/sec/cm^{-5}.
3. Vasopressin is a novel agent that may be beneficial in hypotension that is refractory to conventional vasopressors.

E. Inotropic support

1. Several inotropic agents are available to treat shock related to myocardial failure.
2. The preferred inotropic agents are dopamine and dobutamine.
   a. Dopamine possesses a dose-dependent action and induces tachycardia.
      i. Dopamine causes significant peripheral vasoconstriction at infusion rates above 15 µg/kg/minute.
      ii. At lower doses, dopamine enhances renal perfusion, a phenomenon that does not confer renal protection, however.
   b. Dobutamine is a potent inotropic agent that produces less tachycardia than dopamine but that causes peripheral vasodilation, especially at doses in excess of 2 µg/kg/minute.
      i. Dobutamine is a particularly useful agent if a depressed cardiac output exists concurrently with an elevated SVR.
      ii. A significant disadvantage of dobutamine is that it increases myocardial oxygen demand and is arrhythmogenic. Thus, use in patients with existing myocardial ischemia is cautioned.

TABLE 50-3
VASOACTIVE DRUGS AND RECEPTOR ACTIVITIES FOR THE TREATMENT OF SHOCK

Class and Drug	Blood Pressure	SVR	Cardiac Output	Heart Rate	Inotrope Low-Dose	Inotrope High-Dose	Renal Blood Flow	Coronary Blood Flow	SvO$_2$
Alpha only									
Phenylephrine	↑↑	↑↑↑	↓↓↓	↓↓↓	±	±	↓↓↓↓	±↑↑	↑
Alpha and beta									
Norepinephrine	↑↓	↑↑	↓↑	↓↓±	↑	↑	↓↓↓	↑↑	↑↓
Epinephrine	↑±	±↑	↑↑	↑↑	↑↑	↑↑↑	↓±	↑↑	↑↑↑
Dopamine	↑↑	↑↑	↑↑	↑	±	↑↑	↑↑↑	↑↑	↑↑
Beta only									
Isoproterenol	↑±↓	↓↓	↑↑↑↑	↑↑↑	↑↑↑	↑↑↑↑	±	↑↑↑	↑↑↑
Dobutamine	↓↓	↓↓↓	↑↑↑	↑↑	↑↑↑	↑↑↑	±	↑↑↑	↑↑↑
Beta-blocker									
Propranolol	↑↓	±↑	↓↓↓	↓↓↓↓	↓↓	↓↓↓	↓	↓↓	↓↓
Metoprolol	↓↓	→	↓↓	↓↓↓	↓↓	↓↓	±	↓↓	↓↓
Other									
Nitroglycerine	±↓	↓↓	↑↑	±↑	±	±	±↑	→→→	↓↓
Hydralazine	↓↓↓	↓↓↓	↑↑	↑↑	±	±	±↑	±	↓↓
Prazosin	↓↓↓	↓↓	↑↑	±↑	±	±	±↑	→→	↓↓
Nitroprusside	↓↓	↓↓↓	↑↑↑	±↑	±	±	±↑↑	±	↓↓

From Cobb JP: Critical care: A system-oriented approach. In Norton JA, et al (eds): Surgery: Basic Science and Clinical Evidence. New York, Springer-Verlag, 2001.

c. Other inotropes include epinephrine and norepinephrine, agents that are effective for cardiac and peripheral vascular support in patients with profound septic shock.

d. Table 50-3 lists the vasoactive drugs most commonly used in shock.

3. When pharmacologic support of the heart is unsuccessful, intra-aortic balloon counterpulsation (IABP) may be used temporarily until cardiac function improves or is corrected, or as a bridge to cardiac transplantation.

   a. IABP is not a permanent solution to poor cardiac contractility and the determination that cardiac dysfunction is correctable or reversible should be established before its use.
   b. The principles of balloon counterpulsation include maintenance of coronary perfusion and decrease in myocardial oxygen demand by afterload reduction.
   c. An IABP is placed through the femoral artery and the balloon tip is positioned distal to the origin of the left subclavian artery.
   d. Balloon inflation and deflation are synchronized with the electrocardiogram such that inflation occurs during diastole while deflation occurs at the commencement of ventricular systole.

V. SUGGESTED READINGS

American Heart Association: ACLS Provider Manual. Dallas, American Heart Association, 2005.

Cobb JP: Critical care: A system-oriented approach. In Norton JA, et al (eds) Surgery: Basic Science and Clinical Evidence. New York, Springer-Verlag, 2001.

Cooper MS, Stewart PM: Corticosteroid insufficiency in acutely ill patients. N Engl J Med 348:727–734, 2003.

Dellinger RP: Current therapy for sepsis. Infect Dis Clin North Am 13:495–509, 1999.

Durham RM, Neunaber K, Mazuki JE, et al: The use of oxygen consumption and delivery as endpoints for resuscitation in critically ill patients. J Trauma 41:32–39, 1996.

Hashmi S, Rogers SO: Current concepts in critical care. J Am Coll Surg 200:88–95, 2004.

Heyland D, Cook DJ, King D, et al: Maximizing of oxygen delivery in critically ill patients: A methodologic appraisal of the evidence. Crit Care Med 24:517–524, 1996.

Holmes CL, Walley KR: The evaluation and management of shock. Clin Chest Med 24: 775–789, 2003.

Hotchkiss RS, Karl IE: The pathophysiology and treatment of sepsis. N Engl J Med 348: 38–150, 2003.

Levi L, Wolf A, Belzberg H: Hemodynamic parameters in patients with acute cervical cord trauma: Description, intervention, and prediction of outcome. Neurosurgery 33:1007–1017, 1993.

Moscucci M, Bates ER: Cardiogenic shock. Cardiol Clin 13:391–406, 1995.

Nathens AB, Maier RV: Shock and resuscitation. In Norton JA, et al (eds): Surgery: Basic Science and Clinical Evidence. New York, Springer-Verlag, 2001.

Shoemaker WC, Appel PL, Kram HB, et al: Prospective trial of supranormal values of survivors as therapeutic goals in high-risk surgical patients. Chest 94:1176–1186, 1988.

Bedside Procedures in the Surgical Intensive Care Unit

Steven A. Vela, MD, and Kousta I. Foteh, MD

I. DECOMPRESSIVE CELIOTOMY

A. Indications: abdominal compartment syndrome (ACS) and inability to take patient to the operating room

B. ACS is a constellation of physiologic derangements associated with intra-abdominal hypertension or intra-abdominal pressure elevation.

C. Causes of ACS include:
1. Extensive abdominal trauma
2. Closure of abdominal wall under tension
3. Bowel obstruction
4. Aggressive fluid resuscitation resulting in third space fluid accumulation
5. Severe burns

D. Signs of ACS include:
1. Decreased cardiac output and stroke volume (from decreased venous return due to compression of the inferior vena cava)
2. Elevated central venous pressure and pulmonary capillary wedge pressure despite low intravascular volumes
3. Respiratory failure (i.e., high peak airway pressures, decreased tidal volumes, decreased compliance, increased pulmonary vascular resistance, and hypercarbia)
4. Decreased urine output and elevated bladder pressures unresponsive to a fluid challenge

E. Abdominal decompression should be performed with symptoms above and bladder pressures exceeding 25 mm Hg.

F. Procedure
1. After the diagnosis of ACS, a midline celiotomy incision is made from the sternum to the pubis. If a prior incision is present, it should be reopened.
2. The abdomen should be decompressed, fluid and blood evacuated, and hemostasis obtained or ensured.
3. The results of a decompressive celiotomy are sudden and dramatic with almost instantaneous improvement in gas exchange, decreased systemic vascular resistance, and increased oxygen delivery and cardiac output.
4. Once decompression is obtained, temporary abdominal closure is performed.
5. There are several approaches for temporary closure.
   a. At Parkland Memorial Hospital, the preferred method of temporary closure involves the following steps:
      i. Irrigation of the abdomen with saline
      ii. Placement of an occlusive "bowel bag" over the abdominal contents
      iii. Sterile operating room towels on top of the bowel bag
      iv. Placement of two suction Jackson-Pratt drains over the towels

v. Large occlusive/adhesive dressing (Ioban) should cover the towels, drains, and entire wound.
vi. The suction catheters should then be placed to low wall suction.
b. Commercial, more expensive devices for temporary abdominal closure are available.

G. Complications
1. Bowel injury
2. Bleeding
3. Loss of domain
4. Enterocutaneous fistula
5. Death

II. FIBEROPTIC BRONCHOSCOPY

A. Indications include the following:
1. Difficult airway for intubation
2. Atelectasis
3. Hemoptysis
4. Bronchopleural fistula
5. Foreign body aspiration
6. Diagnosis and treatment of inhalation injury
7. Acute upper airway obstruction

B. Materials
1. Yankauer suction catheter
2. ECG, blood pressure, and pulse-oximetry monitoring
3. Bronchoscope adapter for endotracheal tube
4. Laryngoscope
5. Regional anesthetic and/or sedative (i.e., propofol, morphine, versed, ativan, fentanyl, used alone or in combination)
6. Fiberoptic bronchoscope
7. Use of a video-assisted bronchoscope may be advantageous over a traditional bronchoscope because of better image resolution.

C. Procedure
1. Before bronchoscopy is performed, the surgeon must ensure that all equipment is present and functioning properly.
2. Proper anesthesia is vital to successful bronchoscopy.
   a. The goals of anesthesia are to inhibit coughing, provide amnesia, limit excessive sympathetic response, and blunt the protective reflexes of the upper airway and tracheobronchial tree.
   b. Effective anesthesia allows for a controlled examination of the bronchopulmonary tree in an unhurried fashion.
   c. This allows for greater patient safety and comfort.
3. A bronchoscope adapter is placed over the endotracheal tube.
4. A respiratory technician should be at the bedside to provide maximal ventilatory support in order to facilitate the procedure.

5. If a video-assisted system is used, the camera should be "white-balanced" prior to the start of the procedure.
6. Once proper function of the bronchoscope is verified, lubricating jelly should be placed over the tip of the bronchoscope.
7. The bronchoscope should be placed through the endotracheal adapter carefully and advanced slowly until visualization of the tracheal rings.
8. Continue to advance the bronchoscope until the bifurcation of the right and left main bronchi is visualized.
9. The bronchoscope can be used to irrigate and suction secretions and mucus or to help break up plugs.
10. A post-procedure chest x-ray should be obtained to verify the absence of a pneumothorax, improvement in atelectasis, and absence of foreign bodies.
11. Respiratory monitoring should be diligent up to 4 hours post-procedure.

D. Complications
1. Hypoxemia
2. Barotrauma
3. Hypertension
4. Aspiration
5. Infection
6. Hypercapnia
7. Hypotension
8. Hemorrhage
9. Intracranial hypertension
10. Laryngospasm
11. Cardiac arrhythmias

III. CONTINUOUS ARTERIOVENOUS REWARMING (CAVR)

A. Indications: hypothermia (core body temperature < 35°C)
B. Contraindications: systolic blood pressure < 80 mm Hg
C. Materials
1. Two hemodialysis catheters, either 8.5 or 10 French
    a. Note: At Parkland Memorial Hospital, we use a commercially available kit that contains all necessary equipment.
2. Warming device: H-500 or System 250 fluid warmer (level 1)
3. Luer-Lok connection adapters
4. Tubing
5. Intravenous solution

D. Description
1. The first step is to cannulate the femoral artery on either side, with a dialysis catheter, using an 8.5 or 10 French catheter. This procedure is done utilizing the modified Seldinger technique.
2. Next, either the contralateral femoral vein or ipsilateral subclavian or internal jugular vein is used for venous access in a similar fashion.

3. The arterial catheter is connected to the inflow side of a rewarming system using the Luer-Lok connection adapters and tubing.
4. Next, the venous side is connected to the outflow side of a rewarming system using the Luer-Lok connection adapters and tubing.
5. A side port located on the arterial hemofiltration catheter allows the operator to connect an intravenous fluid line. This completes the circuit.
6. The arterial blood and the intravenous fluid will mix in the heating chamber in the warming device (allowing for rapid rewarming of blood).
7. The warmed blood is then returned to the body through the venous access catheter, causing rapid rewarming of the body and increasing core body temperature.
8. CAVR should be stopped once core body temperature reaches 36°C.
9. When warming is complete, the catheters should be clamped and removed and firm digital pressure should be applied over the puncture site for at least 20 minutes.
10. Catheters may be left in place until the correction of any coagulopathies.
11. The site should always be inspected for oozing and hematoma formation.
12. Once hemostasis is obtained, a sterile dressing should be placed over the puncture sites.
13. Core body temperature should be monitored continuously even after rewarming.

E. Complications
1. Hematoma formation, surgical site oozing, and inability to gain arterial or venous access

IV. SUGGESTED READINGS

Gentilello LM, Cobean RA, Offner PJ, et al: Continuous arteriovenous rewarming: Rapid reversal of hypothermia in critically ill patients. J Trauma 32:316–325, 1992.

Hata JS, Schenk DA, Dellinger RP: Fiberoptic endoscopy. In Civetta, Taylor, Kirby: Critical Care Medicine. Philadelphia, Lippincott Williams & Wilkins, 1997, pp 683–702.

Ivatury RR, Latifi R, Malhotra AK: Abdominal Compartment Syndrome. In Cameron: Current Surgical Therapy. Philadelphia, Mosby; 2004.

Pulmonary Disorders

Makram Gedeon, MD

I. RESPIRATORY PHYSIOLOGY

A. Tissue oxygenation and CO_2 production

1. **Tissue oxygenation**: Factors important in the process include blood oxygen content, delivery of oxygen to tissues, and consumption of oxygen by tissues.

   a. **Oxygen content (Cao_2)** describes the concentration of oxygen in arterial blood and represents the sum of oxygen bound to hemoglobin ($1.34 \times Hb \times Sao_2$) and oxygen dissolved in plasma ($0.003 \times Pao_2$).

   $$Cao_2 = (1.34 \times Hb \times Sao_2) + (0.003 \times Pao_2)$$

   Normal value is 20 mL O_2/100 mL blood.

   Pao_2 exerts a very small influence in Cao_2 and is often excluded in calculations.

   b. **Oxygen delivery (Do_2)** represents the amount of oxygen transported to tissues and is defined as the product of cardiac output (CO) and oxygen content.

   $$Do_2 = CO \times (1.34 \times Hb \times Sao_2) \times 10$$

   Normal value is 520 to 570 mL/min/m².

   Oxygen delivery can be improved by increasing cardiac output, oxygen saturation, or hemoglobin.

   c. **Oxygen uptake (Vo_2)** represents oxygen consumption by tissues and is a function of cardiac output and the difference in oxygen content between venous and arterial blood.

   $$Vo_2 = CO \times 13.4 \times Hb \times (Sao_2 - Svo_2)$$

   Value is dependent on the total body metabolic rate.
   Normal range is 110 to 160 mL/min/m².

   d. **Oxygen extraction ratio (O_2ER)** represents the fraction of delivered oxygen used by tissues.

   $$O_2ER = Vo_2/Do_2$$

   Normal O_2ER is 0.2 to 0.3.

   In conditions of impaired oxygen delivery, Vo_2 is constant with decreasing Do_2 down to a critical Do_2 level where the oxygen extraction ratio is maximal (0.5 to 0.6). Further decrease in Do_2 will result in a proportional decrease in Vo_2, a condition where oxygen supply is not able to meet the needs of aerobic metabolism (shock). An oxygen debt ensues where a proportion of glucose metabolism is shifted to the production of lactate.

2. **Carbon dioxide transport**

   a. Carbon dioxide is one of the major byproducts of metabolism. The rate of CO_2 production is related to the rate of oxygen consumption by the respiratory quotient (RQ = V_{CO_2}/V_{O_2}). The RQ depends on the type of fuel used for metabolism. Normal RQ = 0.8; for lipids RQ = 0.7; for protein RQ = 0.8; for glucose RQ = 1.0

b. Carbon dioxide is highly soluble in plasma as it combines with water in the hydration reaction catalyzed by carbonic anhydrase, which is found in high concentrations in the red blood cell.

$$CO_2 + H_2O \leftrightarrow H_2CO_3 \leftrightarrow HCO_2^- + H^+$$

c. CO_2 enters the red blood cell by simple diffusion. The hydrogen ion generated is buffered by hemoglobin and the bicarbonate ion generated enters plasma in exchange for chloride through the red cell membrane. The CO_2 molecule is reconstituted when blood reaches the pulmonary circulation and it is eliminated in the lungs by diffusion through the capillary-alveolar interface.

d. Minute ventilation (V_E) is the quantity of air moved into and out of the lungs in a minute and dictates CO_2 elimination from alveoli. It is the product of tidal volume and respiratory rate. Normal values range from 5 to 8 L/minute. When V_E is greater than 10 to 12 L/min, spontaneous patient breathing is difficult.

B. Ventilation-perfusion balance: The ventilation-perfusion (V/Q) ratio describes the balance between pulmonary ventilation and capillary blood flow in the lungs. The normal V/Q ratio is 1. Discrepancy between ventilation and perfusion leads to V/Q mismatch and inadequate gas exchange.

1. **Dead space ventilation** describes the situation where ventilation exceeds perfusion. This results in a V/Q ratio greater than 1. The excess ventilation does not participate in gas exchange. It has two components:
   a. **Anatomic dead space** describes the volume of gas in the conducting airways (i.e., trachea and bronchi). This does not come in contact with alveolar capillaries and does not contribute to gas exchange.
   b. **Physiologic dead space** describes the volume of ventilated but nonperfused alveoli.
   c. Dead space ventilation normally accounts for 20% to 30% of the total ventilation (Vd/Vt = 0.2 to 0.3).
   d. An increase in dead space ventilation will lead to both hypoxemia and hypercapnea.
   e. An estimation of dead space ventilation can be obtained from the Bohr equation:

   $$Vd/Vt = (Pa_{CO_2} - P_E{CO_2})/Pa_{CO_2}$$

   Where $P_E{CO_2}$ represents end tidal CO_2.

2. **Intrapulmonary shunt** describes the situation where perfusion exceeds ventilation. This results in a V/Q ratio less than 1. The excess perfusion does not participate in gas exchange. It can be of two types:
   a. **True shunt** occurs when there is no contact between capillary blood and alveolar gas and is equivalent to an anatomic shunt in the heart.

b. **Venous admixture** occurs when capillary blood does not equilibrate completely with alveolar gas.
c. Shunt fraction is the proportion of cardiac output lost as intrapulmonary shunt. This is normally less than 10%.
d. An increase in intrapulmonary shunt leads to hypoxemia. When the shunt fraction exceeds 50%, arterial Po_2 will not improve by increasing Fio_2.
e. The Pco_2 is often normal or even decreased in patients with intrapulmonary shunt as a result of compensatory hyperventilation. When shunt fraction exceeds 50%, minute ventilation cannot keep up with CO_2 production and hypercapnea occurs.
f. Shunt fraction can be calculated:

$$Qs/Qt = (Cco_2 - Cao_2)/(Cco_2 - Cvo_2)$$

Where Cco_2 is the pulmonary capillary O_2 content, Cao_2 is the arterial O_2 content, and Cvo_2 the mixed venous O_2 content. Cco_2 cannot be measured directly but can be estimated by placing the patient on 100% oxygen to achieve 100% hemoglobin saturation in pulmonary capillary blood.

3. **Alveolar-arterial gradient (A-a gradient)** can be used as an indirect measure of the adequacy of the ventilation-perfusion ratio.
   a. The A-a gradient is the alveolar Po_2 (P_{AO_2}) minus the arterial Po_2 (Pao_2).

   $$\text{A-a gradient} = P_{AO_2} - Pao_2$$

   $$P_{AO_2} = Fio_2 \times (P_B - P_{H_2O}) - (Paco_2/RQ)$$

   Where Fio_2 is the fraction of inspired oxygen (0.2l in room air), P_B is the barometric pressure (760 mm Hg at sea level), P_{H_2O} is the partial pressure of water vapor (47 mm Hg at body temperature), $Paco_2$ is the arterial Pco_2, and RQ is the respiratory quotient.
   - The normal range of A-a gradient is 15 to 60 mm Hg.
   - A-a gradient increases with age.
   - A-a gradient increases with increasing Fio_2 as higher Fio_2 levels increase shunt fraction.
   - In patients on positive-pressure ventilation, the mean airway pressure should be added to the atmospheric pressure in calculating P_{AO_2}.
4. A simpler way of estimating the adequacy of the V/Q ratio at the bedside is by calculating the ratio of arterial Po_2 and fraction of inspired oxygen **(p/f ratio)**.
   a. A ratio less than 300 is consistent with acute lung injury.
   b. Improvement in the p/f ratio is correlated with improvement in the pulmonary condition.

C. Acute respiratory failure is defined as functional lung impairment resulting in hypoxemia, hypercapnea, or both.
1. **Hypoxemia**. Conditions to consider:
   a. Alveolar hypoventilation is usually secondary to a decrease in minute ventilation and is associated with hypercapnea. In this situation the

A-a gradient is normal and the P_{CO_2} is increased. Examples are drug-induced respiratory depression and neuromuscular disorders.
   b. Pulmonary disorder: the A-a gradient is increased. The P_{CO_2} can be low, normal, or increased. Examples include acute respiratory distress syndrome, pneumonia, and pulmonary embolism.
   c. Mismatch of oxygen delivery and uptake: this is accompanied by an increase in the oxygen extraction ratio, resulting in a low mixed venous O_2 (<40 mm Hg) and subsequently a low Pao_2. Examples include low cardiac output or severe anemia.
4. **Hypercapnea**. Conditions to consider:
   a. Alveolar hypoventilation secondary to a decrease in minute ventilation
   b. Dead space ventilation
   c. Hypermetabolism. Can be the result of overfeeding. Minute ventilation normally increases to compensate for the increased CO_2 production. In patients with underlying pulmonary disorders, however, CO_2 accumulates and hypercapnea ensues.
D. Indications for endotracheal intubation include but are not limited to:
- Airway protection. In the trauma setting this includes patients with decreased Glasgow Coma Scale <8.
- Impending airway compromise. Burn patients with large surface area burns expected to receive large amounts of intravenous fluids for resuscitation
- Increased work of breathing
- Acute respiratory failure as evidenced by the arterial blood gases

II. MODES OF MECHANICAL VENTILATION

Ventilators use positive pressure to inflate the lungs.
- Volume-cycled ventilation uses a set volume as an end point of inflation.
- Pressure-cycled ventilation uses a set pressure as an end point of inflation.

A. Lung mechanics
1. Proximal airway pressures can be measured by ventilators and help monitor lung mechanics:
   a. Expiratory peak pressure ("peak pressure") reflects both airway resistance and compliance of the lungs and chest wall.
   b. End inspiratory plateau pressure ("plateau pressure") measured at the end of inspiration (respiratory pause) reflects the compliance of the lungs and chest wall.
   c. The difference between the peak pressure and the plateau pressure is proportional to the resistance in the airways.
   d. Measurement of proximal airway pressures is helpful in managing ventilated patients:
      i. When peak airway pressure increases but plateau pressure is unchanged, the problem is an increase in airway resistance (bronchospasm, secretions, etc.).
      ii. When both peak and plateau pressure increase, the problem is a decrease in thoracic compliance (pneumothorax, pulmonary edema, acute respiratory distress syndrome, etc.).

e. Thoracic compliance is the compliance of both the lungs and chest wall.
      i. Calculated as the ratio of change in lung volume to change in airway pressure
      ii. Static compliance is the compliance when there is no airflow and can be measured as the ratio of tidal volume to plateau pressure (Vt/Ppl).
- The normal value for static compliance is 0.05 to 0.08. This value is lower in patients with stiff lungs (e.g., acute respiratory distress syndrome).
- The level of positive end-expiratory pressure (PEEP) should be subtracted from the plateau pressure in the compliance equation.
- The exhaled tidal volume should be used in the equation because part of the delivered volume is wasted in the ventilator tubing.

B. Modes of ventilation

1. **Assist-control ventilation**. The ventilator delivers breaths at a preselected tidal volume and rate and assists each patient-triggered breath with a full tidal volume.
   a. Volume cycled
   b. Disadvantage is in tachypneic patients as it can cause respiratory alkalosis and hyperinflation which leads to auto-PEEP.

2. **Intermittent mandatory ventilation (IMV)**. The ventilator delivers breaths at a preselected volume and rate but allows spontaneous breathing between breaths. When the ventilator breaths are made to coincide with spontaneous patient breaths, this is called synchronized IMV (SIMV)
   a. Volume cycled
   b. The work of breathing is increased in patients on SIMV as spontaneous breaths are through the high resistance of the ventilator circuit.
   c. Pressure support can be added to each patient-triggered breath to reduce the work of breathing.

3. **Pressure-controlled ventilation**. The ventilator delivers breaths at a preselected pressure and rate. The airflow delivered decreases with inspiration to keep the airway pressure at the pre-selected value.
   a. Pressure cycled
   b. Reduces the risk of barotrauma by ensuring that a maximum airway pressure is not exceeded.
   c. Inflation volume decreases as airway resistance increases or thoracic compliance decreases.

4. **Inverse-ratio ventilation**. Pressure-controlled ventilation combined with lower airflow during inspiration prolongs time spent in inspiration and reverses the inspiration:expiration (I:E) ratio from 1:2-4 to 2-1:1.
   a. Pressure cycled
   b. The prolonged inflation time helps prevent alveolar collapse.
   c. Can lead to hyperinflation and auto-PEEP, which tends to decrease cardiac output

5. **Pressure-support ventilation**. The ventilator supports each patient-triggered breath with a preselected pressure.

a. Pressure cycled
b. The level of pressure is adjusted in accordance with the patient's respiratory rate. Pressure is increased until the respiratory rate is less then 28 breaths/min.
c. Requires a spontaneously breathing patient
d. Can be added to SIMV to augment spontaneous patient breaths

C. Ventilator settings

1. **Fio_2** is the concentration of oxygen in the delivered gas, usually 40% to 100%. Values more then 60% are considered toxic.
2. **Tidal volume** is the volume of each ventilator-delivered breath—4 to 6 mL/kg body weight for protective lung strategy.
3. **Respiratory rate** is the preselected rate at which the ventilator delivers breaths, usually 8 to 16 breaths/min. It is adjusted to keep the Pco_2 in the normal range.
4. **Pressure support** is the preselected pressure that supports each spontaneous patient-initiated breath, usually 5 to 20 cm H_2O.
5. **Positive end expiratory pressure (PEEP)** is airway pressure at the end of expiration; it helps keep alveoli open and usually is 5 to 15 cm H_2O.
   a. High levels of PEEP can reduce cardiac output. This is especially pronounced when hypovolemia or cardiac dysfunction is present.
   b. High levels of PEEP can be used for short intervals of time to open atelectatic alveoli (recruitment maneuvers).
6. Inspiration to expiration ratio (I:E): this is usually maintained at 1:2-4.
   a. Can be changed to 2-1:1; called inverse ratio ventilation

D. Protective lung strategy

1. Traditionally, large inflation volumes (10 to 15 mL/kg predicted body weight) were used in volume-cycled ventilation to decrease alveolar collapse, improve oxygenation, and achieve a normal arterial Pco_2 and pH. In recent years, hyperinflation has been shown to have deleterious effects on the lungs in the form of overstretch of alveoli and airways, leading to barotrauma.
2. The Acute Respiratory Distress Syndrome network study specifically compared ventilation with lower tidal volumes to ventilation with traditional tidal volumes for patients with acute lung injury and ARDS and found a decrease in mortality and an increase in number of days without ventilation in patients who were ventilated with lower tidal volumes. At Parkland Memorial Hospital we use a lung-protective strategy for all patients with evidence of acute lung injury.
   a. The predicted body weight (kg) is calculated as follows:
      i. For males: IBW = $50 + 0.91 \times$ (height in cm $- 152.4$)
      ii. For females: IBW = $45.5 + 0.91 \times$ (height in cm $- 152.4$)
   b. The initial tidal volume is set at 6 mL/kg predicted body weight and reduced by 1 mL/kg to maintain a plateau pressure less then 30 cm H_2O or a minimum of 4 mL/kg predicted body weight.
   c. Minute ventilation is maintained by increasing the respiratory rate to compensate for lower tidal volumes.

d. Adequate oxygenation is achieved by adding PEEP and decreasing FiO_2. Generally a ratio of FiO_2 to PEEP of 5 is desired.
e. Some amount of CO_2 retention is allowed. This is called permissive hypercapnea.

III. GUIDELINES FOR WEANING FROM MECHANICAL VENTILATION

A. Patients receiving mechanical ventilation should be considered for discontinuation of ventilation if the following criteria are met (Table 52-1):
1. Evidence of reversal of the underlying cause of the respiratory failure
2. Adequate oxygenation (i.e., p/f >150 to 200, PEEP <5 to 8, FiO_2 <0.4 to 0.5) and pH > 7.25
3. Hemodynamic stability
4. Capacity to initiate an inspiratory effort
B. Weaning parameters help predict patients who will fail a ventilator discontinuation attempt and are measured at the bedside:
1. The rapid shallow breathing index (RSBI) is calculated as the ratio of tidal volume (TV) in liters to respiratory rate (RR) in breaths/minute: RSBI = TV/RR.
   a. With RSBI <105, a weaning attempt can be expected to be successful 78% of the time.
   b. With RSB >105, a weaning attempt can be expected to fails 95 % of the time.
   c. The RSBI is thus useful in predicting patients who will fail the weaning attempt.

TABLE 52-1
CRITERIA USED IN WEANING/DISCONTINUATION STUDIES

Criteria	Description
Objective measurements	Adequate oxygenation (e.g., Po_2 ≥ 60 mm Hg on FiO_2 ≤ 0.4; PEEP ≤ 5 to 10 cm H_2O; Po_2/FiO_2 ≥ 150 to 300)
	Stable cardiovascular system (e.g., HR ≤ 140; stable BP; no (or minimal) pressors)
	Afebrile (temperature < 38°C)
	No significant respiratory acidosis
	Adequate hemoglobin (e.g., Hgb ≥ 8 to 10 g/dL)
	Adequate mentation (e.g., arousable, GCS ≥ 13, no continuous sedative infusions)
	Stable metabolic status (e.g., acceptable electrolytes)
Subjective clinical assessments	Resolution of disease acute phase; physician believes discontinuation possible; adequate cough

Hgb = hemoglobin: HR = heart rate: GCS = Glasgow coma scale.

2. Negative inspiratory force (NIF) is measured by asking the patient to inhale as forcefully as possible and measuring the maximum negative pressure generated.
   a. With an NIF < 20 cm H_2O, 100% of the weaning attempts are expected to fail.
   b. With an NIF > 20 cm H_2O, 60% of the weaning attempts are expected to succeed.
   c. NIF is thus useful in predicting patients who will fail weaning.
C. A ventilator discontinuation effort should be performed during spontaneous breathing rather than while the patient is still on substantial ventilator support. This is called the "spontaneous breathing trial" (SBT).
1. Performed with low levels of CPAP (5 cm H_2O)
2. Minimal or no pressure support (0 to 10 cm H_2O)
3. The trial is considered successful if tolerated for 120 minutes.
D. Tolerance of an SBT is defined by both objective and subjective assessments:
1. **Objective assessments**
   a. Adequate gas exchange: Spo_2 >85% to 90%, Po_2 >50 to 60 mm Hg, pH >7.32, increase in Pco_2 < 10 mm Hg
   b. Hemodynamic stability: heart rate <120 to 140 or not changed by more than 20%, systolic blood pressure <180 to 200 and >90; blood pressure not changed by more then 20%, no pressors required
   c. Stable ventilatory pattern: respiratory rate <30 to 35 or not changed by more then 20%
2. **Subjective assessment**
   a. Change in mental status (e.g., somnolence, coma)
   b. Onset or worsening of dyspnea
   c. Diaphoresis
   d. Increased work of breathing (use of accessory respiratory muscles, paradoxical breathing)
   e. Patients should be considered for extubation if:
      i. They pass an SBT.
      ii. They have a patent airway, as evidenced by a cuff leak.
      iii. They are able to protect their airway, that is, they have a GCS > 8 and have an adequate cough reflex.

IV. MISCELLANEOUS DISORDERS

A. Acute respiratory distress syndrome. Acute respiratory distress syndrome (ARDS) is a condition characterized by hypoxemia refractory to supplemental oxygen and is defined by the following:
1. Acute onset
2. Bilateral infiltrates on the chest radiograph
3. Pulmonary artery wedge pressure ≤ 18 or the absence of clinical evidence of left atrial hypertension

4. $PaO_2/FiO_2 \geq 200$

Acute lung injury is considered present when the PaO_2/FiO_2 ratio is less then 300.

B. Many conditions predispose to ARDS, some of which, like pneumonia, cause a direct injury to the lungs but others, like sepsis, represent a more systemic condition. In general, ARDS is thought to represent a localized (pulmonary) manifestation of systemic disease (Table 52-2).

C. ARDS is characterized clinicopathologically by three phases:

1. **The acute or exudative phase** is manifested by the rapid onset of respiratory failure with arterial hypoxemia and the appearance of bilateral patchy infiltrates. Histologic findings include diffuse alveolar damage with disruption of the alveolar epithelium, loss of surfactant, and filling of the alveoli with protein-rich fluid, hyaline membranes, and inflammatory cells. The end result is atelectasis, loss of lung compliance, intrapulmonary shunting, and hypoxemia.

2. **The fibrosing alveolitis phase** is manifested by persistent hypoxemia and a further decrease in pulmonary compliance due to evolving fibrosis. Chest radiographs show linear opacities and sometimes bullae. Histologically there is fibrosis and partial resolution of the edema. Pulmonary hypertension may develop due to obliteration of capillary beds. Some patients do not enter the fibrosing alveolitis phase and go on to have complete resolution of their acute lung injury.

3. **The recovery phase** is manifested by the gradual resolution of hypoxemia and lung compliance. The radiographic abnormalities resolve. Pulmonary function returns to normal within 6 to 12 months, with mild residual impairment in pulmonary mechanics.

D. Treatment of ARDS focuses on a search and treatment of the underlying cause and on adequate supportive care of the patient.

TABLE 52-2
CLINICAL DISORDERS ASSOCIATED WITH THE DEVELOPMENT OF THE ACUTE RESPIRATORY DISTRESS SYNDROME

Direct Lung Injury	Indirect Lung Injury
Common causes	**Common causes**
Pneumonia	Sepsis
Aspiration of gastric contents	Severe trauma with shock and multiple transfusions
Less common causes	**Less common causes**
Pulmonary contusion	Cardiopulmonary bypass
Fat emboli	Drug overdose
Near-drowning	Acute pancreatitis
Inhalational injury	Transfusions of blood products
Reperfusion pulmonary edema after lung transplantation or pulmonary embolectomy	

1. The majority of deaths are due to multiorgan dysfunction and sepsis as a consequence of the underlying cause of ARDS rather than to ventilatory failure.
2. Adequate supportive care of the patient includes:
   a. Ventilation using a protective lung strategy with lower tidal volumes, reducing iatrogenic lung injury
   b. Avoiding oxygen toxicity with use of high PEEP levels that allow lower Fio_2 levels to be administered
   c. Restricting resuscitation fluids to a minimum needed for adequate tissue perfusion
   d. No pharmacologic agent has been proven beneficial in the treatment of ARDS to date.

E. Pulmonary thromboembolism

1. Deep venous thrombosis (DVT) and pulmonary thromboembolism (PE) constitute an important cause of morbidity and mortality in general surgical and trauma patients.
   a. Approximately 150,000 patients die annually as a result of PE.
   b. The reported three month mortality rate from PE has been estimated as 17.5%.
   c. DVT and PE should be considered part of the same pathophysiological process.
   d. 40% of patients with DVT will have evidence of PE on CT scans.
   e. 30% of patients with PE will have abnormal ultrasound examinations of the lower extremities.
   f. The outcome of a PE will depend on both the size of the embolus and the cardiopulmonary reserve of the patient.
2. **Pathophysiology.** Endothelial damage, hypercoagulability, and venous stasis (Virchow's triad) lead to thrombosis in the deep veins of the lower extremities. As thrombus propagates proximally, all or part of it can dislodge and embolize centrally to the pulmonary circulation.
   a. Serotonin released by platelets leads to pulmonary vasoconstriction. This added to the obstructing thrombus leads to an increase in pulmonary vascular resistance and results in right ventricular strain.
   b. Reflex bronchoconstriction results in an increase in airway resistance.
   c. Ventilation-perfusion mismatch occurs, resulting in hypoxia, tachypnea, and alveolar hyperventilation.
3. **Risk factors.** Risk factors for PE are the same as those for DVT and include the following:
   a. History of prior DVT
   b. Prolonged immobility
   c. Surgery requiring >30 min of anesthesia
   d. Trauma
   e. Major medical illness (e.g. stroke, recent myocardial infarction, nephrotic syndrome)
   f. Exogenous estrogens
   g. Malignancy

h. Fracture of pelvis, femur, or tibia
i. Age>40
j. Hypercoagulable states (acquired or hereditary)
k. Obesity
l. Pregnancy
m. Inflammatory bowel disease or presence of infection
n. Smoking
o. Indwelling central venous line

4. **Diagnosis.** Pulmonary embolism should be considered in any patient with risk factors for DVT having respiratory difficulty.
   a. Dyspnea is the most frequent symptom and tachypnea the most frequent sign.
   b. Right ventricular dysfunction can be evident on physical examination by finding distended neck veins and an increased pulmonic component of the second heart sound.
   c. A radiograph, electrocardiogram (ECG), and blood gases should be obtained as part of the workup
      i. The most frequent ECG abnormality is an inverted T wave in the anterior precordial leads. The S1Q3T3 pattern occurs when right ventricular strain is present.
      ii. Chest radiograph findings are often nonspecific (atelectasis, pleural effusion, elevated hemidiaphragm) but can be suggestive of the diagnosis and include focal oligemia (Westermark's sign), a peripheral wedge-shaped density above the diaphragm (Hampton's hump), or an enlarged right descending pulmonary artery (Palla's sign).
      iii. Arterial blood gases are usually notable for hypoxemia and respiratory alkalosis.
   d. The presence of DVT on ultrasound examination of the lower extremities in the setting of high clinical suspicion can be evidence for the diagnosis, but normal results do not rule out PE.
   e. Ventilation perfusion lung scanning is a useful initial test to rule out clinically significant pulmonary embolism.
      i. Can be interpreted in four ways: normal scan or high, intermediate, or low probability scan for PE
      ii. A normal scan essentially rules out PE.
      iii. A high probability scan is strongly correlated with the presence of embolism.
      iv. An intermediate or low probability scan in the presence of high clinical suspicion should prompt further diagnostic workup.
   f. Spiral CT scanning of the chest with intravenous contrast has been a major advance in the workup of pulmonary embolism in recent years and is being relied on more heavily in diagnosing PE, allowing direct visualization of emboli.
      i. The sensitivity and specificity are highest for emboli involving the proximal pulmonary arteries and decrease significantly for

emboli involving more peripheral segmental and subsegmental pulmonary vessels.
  ii. Advantages of CT scanning include providing alternative explanations of the patient's symptoms (e.g., pneumonia or pleural effusion) by allowing examination of the pulmonary parenchyma and pleural cavities.
  g. Pulmonary angiography remains the gold standard for diagnosing PE when other modalities are nondiagnostic and clinical suspicion is high.
5. **Treatment.** Goals of therapy include the prevention of recurrent thromboembolism and stabilizing the patient's cardiopulmonary status.
  a. Anticoagulation with intravenous heparin is the treatment of choice in preventing recurrent PE, the risk of which is greatest in the first 48 hours after the occurrence of PE
     i. Anticoagulation is directed at treating the associated DVT and should be started as soon as a high or moderate clinical suspicion of PE is present.
     ii. An initial intravenous bolus of 80 units/kg of unfractionated heparin is given, followed by a continuous infusion at 18 units/kg for a goal PTT of 60 to 80. Heparin normograms facilitate subsequent dose adjustments.
     iii. Adverse effects include bleeding and heparin-induced thrombocytopenia (HIT).
     iv. Low-molecular-weight heparins can be given to hemodynamically stable patients with comparable safety and efficacy.
  b. Oral warfarin should be started once a therapeutic PTT is obtained, with a goal INR of 2.0 to 3.0 and should be continued for 3 to 6 months in patients with a first episode of PE.
  c. Inferior vena cava filter placement should be considered in patients in whom anticoagulation is contraindicated, in patients who develop a complication of anticoagulation, and in patients in whom anticoagulation fails (i.e., recurrent PE despite therapeutic anticoagulation).
  d. Thrombolytic therapy should be considered in patients who show hemodynamic instability in the setting of PE.
     i. Thrombolytics improve pulmonary perfusion and right ventricular function by dissolving thrombi. They can be delivered intravenously or through catheter-directed therapy. No data to date favor one method of administration over the other.
     ii. They are most effective when given in the first 14 days following a PE.
     iii. Their usefulness is uncertain in patients who have right ventricular dysfunction but stable arterial blood pressure.
  e. In hemodynamically unstable patients with contraindication for thrombolytic therapy, options include transvenous catheter embolectomy, percutaneous thrombofragmentation, and surgical embolectomy.

6. **Prevention**
   a. **Mechanical**
      i. Early postoperative ambulation
      ii. Graduated compression stockings
      iii. Intermittent compression devices and foot pumps. These increase venous flow in the legs and stimulate the vascular endothelium, activating endogenous fibrinolysis.
   b. **Pharmacologic**
      i. Low-dose subcutaneous unfractionated heparin administered as 5000 units bid or tid
         (a) Reduces the rate of fatal PE by two thirds
         (b) First dose given 2 hours prior to surgery
         (c) Risk includes HIT
      ii. Low-molecular-weight heparins (LMWH)
         (a) Reduces the risk of HIT
         (b) Has similar efficacy to unfractionated heparin in general surgical patients; superior efficacy in trauma patients
      iii. Hirudin
         (a) Direct thrombin (IIa) inhibitor
         (b) Used as DVT prophylaxis in patients with HIT
F. **Ventilator-associated pneumonia**. Ventilator associated pneumonia (VAP) is defined as pneumonia that occurs 48 hours or more after endotracheal intubation. It occurs in 9% to 27% of intubated patients and carries a high associated mortality.
1. The incidence of VAP increases with the duration of mechanical ventilation and has been estimated as 3%/day in the first 5 days of intubation, 2%/day between days 5 and 10, and 1%/day thereafter.
2. Bacterial pneumonia constitutes the majority of patients with VAP. Viral and fungal etiologies are rare.
3. Specific bacterial pathogens to consider in VAP are aerobic gram-negative bacilli, such as *Pseudomonas aeruginosa, Klebsiella pneumoniae, Acinetobacter spp*, and gram-positive cocci such as *Staphylococcus aureus*, the majority of which are methicillin resistant (MRSA).
   a. Late onset VAP (after 5 days) is associated with higher rates of drug-resistant organisms and higher mortality rates.
   b. The process of VAP begins with aspiration of oropharyngeal organisms or leakage of secretions around endotracheal tube cuffs into the lower tracheobronchial tree. Sources of infection include health care devices, medical staff, and the environment. This is followed by colonization of the respiratory epithelium and ultimately by the overwhelming of the host defense mechanisms, resulting in infection.
4. **Diagnosis.** The diagnosis of VAP should be suspected with the clinical findings of fever, purulent secretions, leukocytosis, and a decline in oxygenation or by the appearance of new pulmonary infiltrates on the chest radiograph. In patients with ARDS, any deterioration of a patient's hemodynamic status or oxygenation should raise suspicion of VAP.

a. Blood cultures should be sent but are seldom helpful.
b. Cultures of the lower respiratory secretions in the form of bronchoalveolar lavage (BAL) should be sent if suspicion of VAP is high. At Parkland Memorial Hospital we use the clinical pulmonary infection score (CPIS) developed by Pugin and coworkers to help in the management algorithm (Table 52-3).

5. **Treatment.** Antibiotic treatment should be started as soon as VAP is considered and after appropriate cultures are taken.
   a. Empiric broad-spectrum antibiotics are started (e.g., fourth-generation penicillin with aminoglycoside) to cover for the likely organisms, including *Pseudomonas aeruginosa*.
   b. In patients who have been in the intensive care unit for more then 5 to 7 days or who have been on antibiotics, therapy should include methicillin resistant staphylococcus aureus (MRSA) coverage (e.g., vancomycin).
   c. Antibiotic coverage can then be tailored to the specific microorganism isolated from the BAL culture.

TABLE 52-3
PARKLAND MEMORIAL HOSPITAL CLINICAL PULMONARY INFECTION SCORE

CPIS: Variable	Score
1. Temperature (C)	
≥36.5 and ≤38.4	0
≥38.5 and ≤38.9	1
≥39.0 and ≤36.5	2
2. WBC Count	
≥4,000 or ≤11,000	0
<4,000 or >11,000	1
<4,000 or >11,000 & band forms ≥50%	2
3. Tracheal Secretions	
None or scant	0
Presence of nonpurulent secretions	1
Presence of purulent secretions	2
4. Oxygenation (Pao$_2$/Fio$_2$)	
>240, ARDS or Pulmonary contusion	0
≤240 and no ARDS	2
(ARDS is defined as p/f ≤200, PAWP ≤18 mm Hg and acute bilateral infiltrates.)	
5. Chest X-ray	
No infiltrate	0
Diffuse (or patchy) infiltrate	1
Localized infiltrate	2

Total score from 5 variables

CPIS Total	Action
≤6 and low suspicion for VAP	Evaluate for other potential sources of infection
≤6 and high suspicion for VAP	Evaluate as if CPIS>6
>6	Order BAL cath culture and start antibiotics

d. In general, the duration of antibiotic treatment should be 8 days except if the isolated organism is *P. aeruginosa* or *Acinetobacter spp*, in which case relapse is higher if the duration of treatment is shorter than the traditional 14-day antibiotic course.
   e. Specific antibiotic choice will depend on a particular ICU local microbiology, cost and availability, and formulary restrictions.
6. **Prevention.** Some risk factors can be modified to reduce the incidence or severity of VAP:
   a. Hand washing between patient visits reduces cross-infection with multi-drug-resistant organisms.
   b. Avoiding intubation and reintubation if possible as this increases the risk of VAP
   c. Adherence to sedation protocols in managing intubated patients has been shown to decrease length of intubation and facilitate weaning.
   d. Prevention of aspiration by keeping patients in the semirecumbent position, especially when receiving enteral feeding
   e. Stress bleeding prophylaxis with sucralfate rather then an H_2 blocker is favored, but this has to be weighed against a slightly increased risk of bleeding.
   f. Intensive insulin therapy to maintain glucose levels between 80 and 110 mg/dL
   g. Using a restricted blood transfusion trigger policy

IV. SUGGESTED READINGS

Acute Respiratory Distress Syndrome Network: Ventilation with lower tidal volumes as compared with traditional tidal volumes for acute lung injury and the respiratory distress syndrome. N Engl J Med 342(18), 2000.

American Thoracic Society Documents: Guidelines for the Management of Adults with Hospital-acquired, Ventilator-associated, and Healthcare-associated Pneumonia. Am J Respir Crit Care Med 171, 38–416, 2005.

Cameron JL: Current Surgical Therapy, 8th ed. Philadelphia, Mosby, 2004, pp 876-879; 884-889.

Evidence-based guidelines for weaning and discontinuing ventilatory support. Chest (Suppl) 120(6), 2001.

Fedullo PF, et al: The Evaluation of Suspected Pulmonary Embolism. N Engl J Med 349(13), 2003.

Goldhaber SZ: Pulmonary Embolism. N Engl J Med 339(2), 1998.

Marino PL: The ICU Book, 3rd ed. Philadelphia, Lippincott Williams & Wilkins, 2007,Chapters 2, 21, 23, 26, 27, 29.

Tobin MJ: Advances in mechanical ventilation. N Engl J Med 344(26), 2001.

Ware LB, et al: The acute respiratory distress syndrome. N Engl J Med 342(18), 2000.

Disorders of Thermoregulation in the Intensive Care Unit

Jason Hall, MD

I. TEMPERATURE HOMEOSTASIS

A. Core temperature is normally 36.7° to 37.6°C with typical variations of ±1.5°C.
B. Children and the elderly are less able to compensate for unusual ranges of temperature.
C. Continuous rectal temperature probes are used to monitor temperature in the intensive care unit (ICU) at Parkland Memorial Hospital.

II. HYPOTHERMIA

A. Etiology
1. **Primary accidental hypothermia**. These patients have normal homeostatic mechanisms and hypothermia is due to overwhelming outside exposure.
2. **Secondary accidental hypothermia**. This is more common than primary hypothermia and carries a more lethal prognosis. It occurs when patients are no longer able to regulate their body temperature in an environment in which healthy patients are unaffected and may arise from a number of causes:
    a. Long intra-abdominal operations
    b. Cardiopulmonary bypass
    c. Sepsis
    d. Multiple metabolic abnormalities can contribute or cause hypothermia, such as hypoglycemia, hypopituitarism, hypothyroidism, and hypothalamic dysfunction.
    e. Chemicals such as ethanol, barbiturates, phenothiazines, and anesthetics can also cause hypothermia.
B. Pathophysiology. Hypothermia in the surgical or trauma patient is usually in the 32°C to 35°C range. These temperatures are not associated with significant risk of problems such as ventricular fibrillation, altered pH regulation, cold-induced diuresis, respiratory depression, rewarming shock, or core afterdrop. The primary problems in this setting are alterations in oxygen supply and demand and coagulopathy.
1. **Increase in oxygen consumption**
    a. Hypothermic patients generate a vigorous sympathetic response that is designed to produce enough heat to restore body temperature to normal. This may increase oxygen consumption beyond supply, leading to a shift to anaerobic metabolism and lactic acidosis.
    b. Patient energy expenditure to overcome or to simply maintain hypothermia is detrimental. The thermoneutral temperature (28°C) is

the ambient temperature at which the basal rate of thermogenesis is sufficient to offset ongoing heat losses. Maintaining euthermia when the temperature around the body drops below the thermoneutral zone requires an increase in heat production. Because humans produce heat by combustion, extra oxygen is needed as substrate. The thermoregulatory drive is so powerful that it takes precedence over many other homeostatic functions and may deprive vital organs of needed oxygen, leading to anaerobic metabolism, acidosis, and significant cardiopulmonary stress.

2. **Coagulation**
   a. Hypothermia can prolong coagulation. Because the prothrombin time (PT) and partial thromboplastin time (PTT) are temperature-standardized tests, the extent of the hypothermia-induced coagulopathy is often underestimated.
   b. Hypothermia also **reversibly** affects platelet function. Platelets sequester in the portal circulation during hypothermia, and at temperatures less then 20°C platelets are nearly absent from the peripheral circulation. Additionally, the production of thromboxane A2 is temperature dependent, and bleeding time is significantly prolonged in hypothermia secondary to a defect in the platelets' ability to produce this prostaglandin at the bleeding site.
   c. Transfusions of fresh-frozen plasma and platelets may not correct coagulopathic bleeding if their activity is affected because the patient is cold.
   d. Blood viscosity is increased during hypothermia, and thrombotic complications are seen with severe hypothermia.

3. **Cardiovascular**
   a. Initially, the cardiovascular response is tachycardia, followed by progressive bradycardia beginning at about 34°C and resulting in a 50% heart rate decrease at 28°C.
   b. With intense vasoconstriction, blood pressure is initially maintained but begins to fall when the reduction in cardiac output becomes severe.
   c. On the electrocardiogram, the PR, then the QRS, and finally the QT interval become progressively prolonged.
   d. An Osborne wave, or J wave (hypothermic hump), is sometimes seen at the junction of the QRS and ST segments in leads II and V_6.
   e. Below ~32°C, atrial and then predominantly ventricular dysrhythmias occur, and below 25°C virtually all patients are asystolic.

4. **Respiratory**
   a. During the early stages of hypothermia, the respiratory drive is increased, but progressive respiratory depression occurs at temperatures below 33°C. This decreases minute ventilation.
   b. Noncardiogenic pulmonary edema is frequently reported after prolonged hypothermia.

5. **Central nervous system**

a. As the core temperature falls, progressive confusion, slurred speech, and incoordination occur, and at temperatures less than 32°C patients are often amnestic.
   b. Below 31°C, most patients lose consciousness; shivering and deep tendon reflexes are lost, the pupils become dilated with slow or absent light response, and the patient has a flaccid appearance.
6. **Renal**
   a. Decreases in blood pressure and cardiac output cause a concomitant decrease in the glomerular filtration rate (GFR), but urine output (UOP) is maintained because of impairment in renal tubular Na^+ reabsorption (cold diuresis).
   b. The initial vasoconstriction that occurs in response to hypothermia also causes an increase in central blood volume that prompts a diuresis.
7. **Gastrointestinal**
   a. Hypothermia causes decreased gastrointestinal motility and results in gastric dilatation, ileus, and colonic distention.
   b. Hepatic dysfunction occurs as well, secondary to a decrease in splanchnic blood flow.
   c. Gastric mucosal erosions are also common.
8. **Endocrine**
   a. Hypothermia inhibits insulin release and insulin uptake at receptor sites. Therefore, hyperglycemia is common especially at temperatures less than 30°C.

C. Diagnosis. Hypothermia is a core temperature <35°C. Hypothermia has been divided into ranges based on physiologic changes that occur at each level.

1. Mild hypothermia: 32°C to 35°C
2. Moderate hypothermia: 28°C to 32°C
3. Severe hypothermia: 20°C to 28°C
4. Profound hypothermia: 14°C to 20°C
5. Deep hypothermia: <14°C

D. Treatment

Prospective studies demonstrate that aggressive rewarming of trauma victims lowers mortality rates and decreases blood loss, fluid requirements, episodes of organ failure, and length of ICU stay.

1. **Passive external rewarming.** Usually employed for patients with temperatures >30°C who have intact homeostatic mechanisms (primary accidental hypothermia). In these patients, 100% O_2 is administered, external heat is applied, and IV fluids and inspired air are warmed. Attempts are made to achieve a temperature of 35°C by raising the body temperature by 1 to 1.5°C per hour.
2. **Active external rewarming**. Because skin temperature may be 10°C to 15°C cooler then core temperature in hypothermic patients, external rewarming techniques cannot transfer heat to the core until the temperature of the skin is raised to at least the level of the core.

During the time that skin rewarming is occurring, core temperature can continue to decrease by a phenomenon called *afterdrop*.
   a. Warm water immersion is the only external rewarming technique that transfers a significant amount of heat, but this method is associated with a high rate of cardiovascular collapse secondary to vasodilatation and is only advocated in the treatment of frostbite.
   b. Covering the head with reflective material is helpful. Scalp vessels do not undergo vasoconstriction, and 50% of radiant heat loss occurs above the neck.
3. **Active core rewarming**. Typically used for temperature <30°C or when regulatory mechanisms are impaired (secondary accidental hypothermia). This includes: airway rewarming, heated peritoneal or pleural lavage, warm IV fluids, and hyperthermic extracorporeal circulation.
   a. Airway rewarming has little effect on core temperature, but pleural or peritoneal lavage results in significant heat transfer.
   b. Effects of pleural and peritoneal cavity rewarming techniques are roughly equivalent, although fluid return may be better with pleural lavage. The pleural cavity may be preferred in a patient with arrhythmias because the heart may be rewarmed faster than with peritoneal lavage.
      i. With pleural lavage, two ipsilateral chest tubes are used to enable a continuous flow of water.
      ii. With peritoneal lavage, the liver is more likely to be warmed, thereby restoring its synthetic and metabolic properties more quickly. However, **this method is not feasible in patients who have undergone celiotomy.**
      iii. When lavaging body cavities, a temperature of 44°C is acceptable in patients who are not hemodynamically unstable. However, in the setting of cardiac arrest or severely diminished blood flow, bowel necrosis can occur with lavage fluid temperatures this high.
   c. Giving warm IV fluids is critical in preventing hypothermia. A bolus of cold IV fluids into the central circulation can increase cardiac irritability by directly affecting the conducting system.
   d. Using warm IV fluids is associated with reduction in intraoperative cardiac arrest, coagulopathy, and acidosis and better temperature preservation as compared to room temperature IV fluids.
   e. Warm IV fluids also provide the simplest means of transferring significant amounts of heat to patients requiring massive fluid resuscitation.
   f. Cardiopulmonary bypass is the most efficient warming technique and should be employed for the rewarming of fibrillating patients with primary accidental hypothermia who will require prolonged cardiopulmonary resuscitation (CPR) during rewarming.
   g. Continuous arteriovenous rewarming (CAVR) is a very effective method of rewarming that relies on the patient's blood pressure to drive an extracorporeal circuit and does not require heparinization or

membranous oxygenation. CAVR is analogous to the use of continuous arteriovenous hemofiltration.

4. **Other considerations**
   a. **Oxygen consumption**
      i. By preventing shivering, anesthetics and neuromuscular blocking agents can attenuate the increase in oxygen consumption associated with hypothermia.
      ii. During anesthesia, aggressive rewarming should be pursued so that emergence from anesthesia does not overly stress the patient from a cardiovascular standpoint.
      iii. In the absence of shivering, the catecholamine response to hypothermia causes an increase in metabolic rate, making prevention and treatment of hypothermia very important in the care of the critically ill surgical patient.
   b. **Cardiovascular**
      i. In the event that a patient does not have an organized rhythm and field conditions are such that CPR cannot be instituted, rewarming should not be undertaken until CPR can be instituted.
      ii. Vasoconstrictors should be used with extreme caution in cases of refractory hypotension because they may be arrhythmogenic, may deleteriously affect frostbitten tissues, and may decrease the effectiveness of external rewarming techniques.
      iii. Electrolytes should be monitored frequently during rewarming (more frequently during more rapid rewarming) to prevent adverse metabolic consequences.
   c. **Endocrine**
      i. Hyperglycemia at temperatures less than 30°C should not be treated because of rebound hypoglycemia that will occur during rewarming.

III. HYPERTHERMIA

A. **Malignant hyperthermia**
1. Occurs in 1/15,000 episodes of general anesthesia
2. Inherited disorder (autosomal dominant)
3. Untreated mortality ~80%
4. It is due to excessive release of calcium from the sarcoplasmic reticulum of skeletal muscle secondary to volatile anesthesia (halothane, enflurane, isoflurane, and depolarizing muscarinic relaxants such as succinyl choline).
5. Can occur up to 24 hours after induction of anesthesia
6. **Clinical signs**
   a. Increased end tidal CO_2
   b. Hyperpyrexia
   c. Depressed level of consciousness (LOC)
   d. Muscle rigidity (masseter)

e. Metabolic acidosis
f. Hypernatremia
g. Hyperkalemia
7. The syndrome will progress quickly to rhabdomyolysis, renal failure, and autonomic instability if left untreated.
8. **Treatment**
   a. Stop anesthetic agent.
   b. Hyperventilation with 100% Fio_2
   c. Give dantrolene 2.5 mg/kg IV every 15 minutes, up to 10 mg/kg
   d. Maintain urine output with IV fluids and mannitol.
   e. Check laboratory test results, including disseminated intravascular coagulation (DIC) panel and CPK.
   f. Use surface cooling for temperatures >39°C.

B. Neuroleptic malignant syndrome

1. Physiologic heat-dissipating mechanisms and hypothalamic regulation of temperature may be impaired.
2. Hypothalamic temperature set-point regulation may be affected by drug-induced dopamine receptor blockade.
3. Associated drugs: phenothiazines, butyrophenones, thiozanthenes, dibenzoxepines, dopamine-depleting drugs, and dopamine agonist withdrawal
4. Characterized by profound muscular rigidity
5. Administration of certain neuroleptic drugs may cause a reaction similar to malignant hyperthermia, although the elevation of core temperature is usually less.
6. Treatment is the same as for malignant hyperthermia

C. Heat stroke

1. 70% overall mortality if untreated
2. Exertional heat stroke typically occurs in young, healthy adults who overexert themselves at times of high ambient temperatures, high humidity, or in an environment to which they are not acclimatized.
   a. Thermoregulatory mechanisms are intact, but endogenous heat production outstrips heat-dissipating mechanisms.
   b. Usually there is little clinical warning. Body temperature climbs rapidly, and patients can quickly lapse into coma with high core temperatures.
   c. Cardiac muscle damage and infarction occur frequently and are related to the toxic effects of heat on myocytes and to coronary artery hypoperfusion in the face of hypovolemia.
3. Nonexertional heat stroke affects elderly and debilitated persons with chronic medical illnesses during times of increased ambient temperatures.
   a. Thermoregulatory mechanisms are impaired from the outset. Advancing age decreases the ability to produce sweat and impairs perception of changes in ambient or body temperatures.
   b. Drugs that may be associated with nonexertional heat stroke include alcohol, diuretics, phenothiazines, anti-parkinsonians, anticholinergics,

beta-blockers, tricyclic antidepressants, amphetamines, hallucinogens, and butyrophenones.

4. **Diagnosis**
   a. Body temperatures of 41°C or greater
   b. Irritability or irrationality
   c. Elevated creatine kinase
   d. Disseminated intravascular coagulation is rare but is a poor prognostic marker if present.
   e. Results of arterial blood gases will show the $PaCO_2$ and PaO_2 to be falsely low and the pH falsely high unless the gas is corrected for temperature

5. **Treatment**
   a. Survival is inversely related to the intensity and duration of hyperpyrexia.
   b. Effective lowering of the core temperature is usually possible with external techniques such as immersion in an ice water bath, wetting the skin with tepid water or alcohol, and using fans to help with heat dissipation and evaporation. Gastric or peritoneal lavage with iced saline is rarely needed in refractory cases or if thermogenesis is ongoing as in malignant hyperthermia.
   c. Vigorous skin massage should accompany immersion cooling to prevent dermal stasis of cooled blood in vasoconstricted skin.
   d. Once the temperature approaches 39°C, cooling efforts should be terminated.
   e. IV chlorpromazine (10 to 50 mg every 6 hours) may help to prevent shivering and associated thermogenesis.
   f. Dantrolene may decrease the time required to cool persons with heat stroke. Isoproterenol is the traditional inotropic drug of choice for heat stroke with myocardial dysfunction and inadequate cardiac output because it has very little agonist affect on peripheral alpha-receptors.

D. **Acute adrenocortical insufficiency**. This can occur in patients who are being weaned from steroids and suddenly develop increased temperature and hypotension. In elective surgical cases, acute adrenal insufficiency usually develops within the first 72 hours postoperatively. Also, the severe metabolic stress resulting from systemic sepsis or multisystem organ failure (MSOF) may produce acute adrenal insufficiency.

1. If the diagnosis is suspected, the patient should be immediately treated. Hydrocortisone (200 mg) is given IV, followed by 50 to 100 mg every 6 hours, unless there is a question of underlying sepsis or MSOF. For these patients, higher steroid doses may be necessary. Dramatic clinical improvement may be expected within minutes of steroid administration when adrenocortical insufficiency is the cause of fever and hypotension.

E. **Complications of hyperthermic illness**

1. **Heat stroke**
   a. **Cardiac:** myocardial pump failure, dysrhythmias, myocardial infarction

b. **Renal:** acute renal failure (multifactorial); more common in exertional heat stroke
   c. **Musculoskeletal:** rhabdomyolysis (exertional). Severe hypocalcemia often develops in these patients, but exogenous calcium should be avoided unless the patient develops serious ventricular ectopy secondary to hyperkalemia because calcium may worsen the rhabdomyolysis.
   d. **Central nervous system:** seizures. With hyperpyrexia, widespread cell death occurs, with the Purkinje cells of the cerebellum being the most affected. Cerebral edema and petechial hemorrhages can also occur. Marked depression of mental status is frequent. Survivors often have residual evidence of cerebellar dysfunction.
   e. **Gastrointestinal:** hepatic failure that is reversible. Cholestasis and centrolobular necrosis elevate the bilirubin and serum transaminases.
   f. **Respiratory:** acute respiratory distress syndrome
   g. **Hematologic:** disseminated intravascular coagulation (DIC). Heat enhances plasma fibrinolytic activity and directly activates platelets and may specifically trigger DIC.
2. **Malignant hyperthermia:** complications are similar to those of heat stroke but may be more severe because temperature elevations are more extreme. DIC is more common.
3. **Neuroleptic malignant syndrome:** complications are similar to those for heat stoke. There may also be at increased risk for aspiration pneumonia secondary to dystonia and impaired ability to handle secretions.

IV. FEVER

Fever is discussed in Chapter 55.

V. SUGGESTED READINGS

Civetta JM, Taylor RW, Kirby RR: Critical Care, 2nd ed. Philadelphia, JB Lippincott, 1992.

Martin RS, Kilgo PD, Miller PR, et al: Injury-associated hypothermia: An analysis of the 2004 National Trauma Data Bank. Shock 24(2):114–118, 2005.

Sugrue M, D'Amours SK, Joshipura M: Damage control surgery and the abdomen. Injury 35(7):642–648, 2004.

Wolberg AS, Meng ZH, Monroe DM 3rd, et al: A systematic evaluation of the effect of temperature on coagulation enzyme activity and platelet function. J Trauma 56(6):1221–1228, 2004.

Disorders of Acid-Base, Fluids, and Electrolytes

Sean Dineen, MD, and Paul Schumacher, MD

I. ANATOMY OF BODY FLUIDS

A. Total body water (TBW) constitutes approximately 60% (50% to 70%) of total body weight.
B. Skeletal muscle contains more water than adipose tissue, and therefore women and obese patients have less TBW.
C. Both women and men lose TBW as they age
D. Intracellular fluid (ICF)
1. Two-thirds (67%) of TBW
2. Potassium and magnesium are the major cations of ICF.
3. Phosphates and proteins are the major anions.
E. Extracellular fluid (ECF)
1. Makes up one-third (33%) of total body water
2. ECF is further divided into two compartments: interstitial fluid and plasma.
   a. Interstitial fluid is 75% of the extracellular fluid.
   b. Plasma is 25% of the extracellular fluid.
3. Sodium and calcium are the major cations of extracellular fluid.
4. Chloride and bicarbonate are the major anions.
F. "Third space" fluid is nonfunctional extracellular fluid sequestration following surgery, inflammation, burns, and infection. It does not contribute to the normal ECF or ICF.

II. DAILY FLUID AND ELECTROLYTE REQUIREMENTS AND MAINTENANCE

A. Water requirements in the hemodynamically normal patient
1. Adults require 35 mL/kg per 24 hours.
2. For children, the following formula can be used for 24-hour requirements:
   a. For the first 10 kg of body weight, multiply by 100 mL/kg.
   b. For the second 10 kg of body weight, multiply by 50 mL/kg.
   c. For each additional kg, multiply by 20 mL/kg.
3. For an hourly basis in children, this is simplified as the "4/2/1" rule.
   a. 4 mL/kg/hour for the first 10 kg of body weight
   b. 2 mL/kg/hour for the second 10 kg of body weight
   c. 1 mL/kg/hour for each additional kg
4. Sustained fever increases insensible fluid losses from the skin by approximately 250 mL/24 hours for each 1°F over 101°F.
5. Tachypnea increases insensible fluid losses as well.
B. Electrolyte requirements
1. Sodium: 1 to 2 mEq/kg per day for adults; 1 mEq/day for children

2. Chloride: 1 to 2 mEq/kg per day for adults; 1 mEq/day for children
3. Potassium: 0.5 to 1 mEq/kg per day

III. VOLUME DISORDERS

A. Hypovolemia. Most common in trauma patients. Primary concern is loss of intravascular volume. The signs and symptoms are those of volume depletion:
1. **Mild volume deficit**
   a. 4% to 6% weight loss
   b. Agitation
   c. Asymptomatic or possibly mildly increased heart rate
   d. This degree of volume depletion may be unnoticed.
2. **Moderate volume depletion**
   a. 6% to 8% weight loss
   b. Orthostatic hypotension
   c. Tachycardia
   d. Collapsed veins
   e. Apathy
   f. Anorexia
   g. Drowsiness
   h. Decreased skin turgor
   i. Oliguria (urine output less than 30 mL/hour)
   j. Increase in hematocrit
   k. Elevated BUN/Cr ratio
3. **Severe volume deficit**
   a. 8% to 10% weight loss
   b. Hypotension
   c. Stupor, coma
   d. Atonic muscles
   e. Sunken eyes
   f. Marked decrease in body temperature
   g. Anuria

B. Volume overload. The signs and symptoms include:
1. Distended jugular veins
2. Rales
3. Anasarca

C. Monitoring volume status
1. Urine output. Accurate measurement requires placement of a urinary catheter.
2. Strict intake and output
3. Daily weights
4. Measurement of central venous pressure can aid in assessing volume status.
5. In complex patients with comorbid disease, particularly congestive heart failure and renal insufficiency, placement of a pulmonary artery catheter may be necessary to assess volume status

IV. REPLACEMENT OF FLUID LOSSES

A. Deficit calculation
1. Quantify measurable losses:
   a. Urine output
   b. Nasogastric tube
   c. Drains
   d. Output from fistulas
   e. Vomiting
   f. Diarrhea
2. In postoperative patients consider that extracellular fluid losses average 750 to 800 mL/hour during celiotomy.

B. Maintenance fluid requirements
1. Insensible losses are 600 to 900 mL per day and must be replaced. The amount may increase with tachypnea or fever.
2. Replacement for urine output is about 1000 mL per day

C. Ongoing fluid losses should be replaced with a solution of similar electrolyte composition.
1. Extracellular fluid losses are replaced with a balanced salt solution, such as Ringer's lactate.
2. This includes most measurable losses, such as nasogastric output, vomitus, diarrhea, and fistula drainage, whether biliary or enteric.
3. Fluid losses due to a gastric outlet obstruction are replaced with normal saline.
4. Maintenance fluids (insensible losses and urine output) are generally given as half-normal saline but in the absence of a salt-wasting nephropathy can be supplied as D_5W.

V. HYPERNATREMIA

All forms of hypernatremia are hypertonic.

A. Signs and symptoms
1. Thirst
2. Lethargy
3. Convulsion

B. Hypovolemic hypernatremia. Burns, excessive sweating, respiratory losses, and renal failure are common causes.
1. First need to correct volume depletion with isotonic fluid (lactated Ringer's or normal saline)
2. If this does not correct hypernatremia, calculate a free water deficit and correct with hypotonic fluid. Give only hypotonic fluid (i.e., D_5W) when the patient is euvolemic.

C. Euvolemic hypernatremia
1. A patient that is euvolemic should have free water deficit calculated and corrected accordingly with hyptonic fluids.

2. Avoid correcting too quickly as this may cause brain edema.
3. Diabetes insipidus is a common cause among brain-injured patients.
   a. Characterized by large volume of dilute urine. The patient may produce as much as 1 L of urine per hour.
   b. Urine osmolarity less than 300 mEq/L in a patient with a serum sodium of >150 is consistent with diabetes insipidus.
   c. DDAVP can be given for severe cases.

D. Hypervolemic hypernatremia is caused by excess of sodium and is typically iatrogenic. It commonly occurs after IV administration of sodium bicarbonate.
1. Administer loop diuretics to reduce load of sodium.
2. D5W may be needed to restore free water.
3. Patients in renal failure who do not respond to loop diuretics will need dialysis to normalize sodium.

E. Free water deficit should be corrected slowly.

VI. HYPONATREMIA

Hyponatremia reflects an excess of total body water. In contrast to hypernatremia, hyponatremia may be hypotonic, isotonic, or hypertonic.

A. Hypotonic hyponatremia
1. Hypovolemic – replacement with hypotonic fluids
2. Euvolemic – common with renal failure, SIADH, and adrenal insufficiency
3. Hypervolemic – caused by fluid-retaining states such as in congestive heart failure, cirrhosis, nephrotic syndrome, or renal failure

B. Isotonic hyponatremia is caused by isotonic infusion of solutions such as glycine or mannitol. Pseudohyponatremia is caused by hyperlipidemia or hyperproteinemia but is less common with advances in laboratory measurements.

C. Hypertonic hypnonatremia is commonly caused by hyperglycemia and rarely by infusions of hypertonic glycine.

D. Treatment
1. Avoid correcting too fast as this may cause central pontine myelinolysis.
2. Treatment goal is to correct serum sodium to 120.
3. Correct underlying cause if possible.
4. Restrict fluids to <1500 mL/day.
5. If severe may treat with 3% NaCl
   a. Aim to correct at 1 to 2 mEq/L per hour initially.
   b. Maximum correction in one day should be 8 mEq/L unless the patient remains symptomatic.

VII. HYPERKALEMIA

A. Occurs when serum sodium exceeds 5.0 mEq/L
B. Under normal circumstances extracellular [K^+] is tightly controlled. During trauma, acidosis, or other catabolic states, the intracellular water concentration of potassium leaks into the extracellular water.

- **C.** Renal failure and rhabdomyolysis can cause rapid increases in plasma sodium.
- **D.** Hyperkalemia should be anticipated after sudden reperfusion of an ischemic limb.
- **E.** Succinylcholine may precipitate hyperkalemia.
- **F. Electrocardiographic changes**
1. Peaked T waves
2. Prolonged QRS
3. Depressed ST segments
4. Loss of T waves, heart block, and cardiac arrest are associated with increasing potassium levels.
- **G. Treatment of acute hyperkalemia**
1. Aim treatment at correcting the underlying cause
2. Stop all potassium supplementation and potassium in IV fluids.
3. Patients in renal failure need dialysis.
4. For patients with potassium levels of 5 to 6.5 and without ECG changes, loop diuretics or Kayexalate may be given.
5. For patients with ECG changes or $K^+ > 6.5$:
   a. Calcium gluconate is given for cardiac protection. Calcium antagonizes the depolarizing effect of hyperkalemia.
   b. Lasix and kayexalate are given.
   c. Insulin and glucose will drive K^+ into the cells.
   d. Bicarbonate will also force K^+ into the cells.
   e. Albuterol and other beta-agonists may also be used to shift K^+ into cells.

VIII. HYPOKALEMIA

A. Causes
1. Gastrointestinal losses. Patients with normal renal function should be able to reduce urinary excretion to less than 20 mEq/day. If daily urinary excretion is greater than this, some element of renal failure or hyperaldosteronism is present.
2. Undersupplementation particularly in the setting of diuretic use
3. Shift of potassium into cells
4. Alkalosis causes excretion of K^+ rather than H^+ in the kidney and may cause hypokalemia.

B. Signs
1. U waves on the ECG
2. Atrial tachycardia with or without a block
3. Flattening of ST segments on the ECG
4. Ileus
5. Paralysis
6. Patients on digoxin are at increased risk of toxicity.

C. Treatment
1. Oral supplementation, particularly for patients on loop diuretics

2. Intravenous supplementation should be given to correct K⁺ to greater than 4.0 in intensive care patients.
3. The dose of potassium that can be administered through a peripheral IV line should not exceed 10 mEq/L per hour (in 100 mL of normal saline). More than 10 mEq/L may be given through a central line with ICU monitoring.

IX. HYPERCALCEMIA

A. Occurs when calcium exceeds 10.5 mEq/L. Ionized calcium levels better reflect the biochemically active form of calcium. An ionized calcium greater than 1.4 mmol/L confirms hypercalcemia.
B. Uncommon in trauma
C. Causes
1. Use of thiazide diuretics
2. Thyrotoxicosis
3. Hyperparathyroidism
4. Hypophosphatemia
D. Signs and symptoms
1. Fatigue
2. Lethargy
3. Weakness
4. Polyuria due to a renal concentrating defect. This can lead to volume depletion.
5. Bradycardia, which may progress to complete heart block
E. Treatment
1. Isotonic fluid
2. Loop diuretics to shed calcium into the urine
3. Bisphosphonates
4. Intranasal or intravenous calcitonin
5. Dialysis

X. HYPOCALCEMIA

A. May be related to citrate accumulation during massive transfusion
B. Ionized calcium less than 0.8 mmol/L is diagnostic of hypocalcemia.
C. Causes
1. Rhabdomyolysis
2. Acute pancreatitis
3. Renal failure
4. Sepsis
5. Hypoparathyroidism (following thyroid surgery)
D. Signs and symptoms
1. Chvostek's sign – gently tapping along the facial nerve elicits twitching of facial muscles.

2. Trousseau's sign – inflating a blood pressure cuff above the brachial artery for 3 minutes induces carpopedal spasm.
3. Circumoral numbness and tingling
4. Paresthesias of the hands and feet
5. Prolonged QT interval
6. Decreased myocardial contractility
7. Ventricular fibrillation

E. Treatment
1. Infusion of calcium gluconate or calcium chloride
2. Calcium chloride has a greater amount of elemental calcium per volume.
3. Repleting magnesium is essential to correcting calcium.

XI. HYPERMAGNESEMIA

A. This is a rare condition.

B. Causes
1. Renal failure
2. Acidosis
3. Excessive exogenous administration (iatrogenic)

C. Signs and symptoms
1. Lethargy
2. Decreased deep tendon reflexes
3. ECG changes
   a. Prolonged PR interval
   b. Widened QRS complex
   c. Elevated T waves

D. Treatment
1. Calcium may help control symptoms.
2. Dialysis is necessary in renal failure.

XII. HYPOMAGNESEMIA

A. Causes
1. Heavy alcohol intake
2. Chronic diarrhea
3. Long-term use of diuretics

B. Signs and symptoms
1. Hyperactive deep tendon reflexes
2. Tremors
3. Chvostek's sign
4. Tetany

C. Potassium levels cannot be corrected if hypomagnesemia exists.

D. Treatment consists of replacement with 2 g of intravenous magnesium sulfate.

XIII. HYPERPHOSPHATEMIA

A. Most commonly caused by renal failure
B. Treatment
1. Stop external supplementation.
2. Oral phosphate-binding agent (Amphojel)
3. Lasix or acetazolamide
4. Dialysis in severe cases

XIV. HYPOPHOSPHATEMIA

A. Causes
1. Gastrointestinal losses
2. Renal losses
3. Starvation
4. Inadequate replacement in total parenteral nutrition
5. Use of phosphate-binding antacids

B. Signs and symptoms
1. Rhabdomyolysis
2. Weakness
3. Erythrocyte dysfunction
4. Respiratory insufficiency
5. Cardiomyopathy

C. Treatment
1. Severe deficits are corrected with sodium phosphate or potassium phosphate, depending on the electrolyte composition.
2. Less severe deficits can be corrected with oral agents (Neutrophos or Fleet's Phosphosoda).

XV. ACID-BASE DISTURBANCES

A. Regulation of a normal pH is essential for homeostasis. Most cellular processes function over a narrow pH range. These include enzyme function, coagulation pathways, oxygen delivery, and cardiovascular function.

B. Normal arterial blood gas values
1. pH 7.36 to 7.44
2. $Paco_2$ 35 to 45 mm Hg
3. Pao_2 80 to 100 mm Hg
4. Base excess –3 to 3 mEq/L

C. Buffers
1. The bicarbonate buffer system is the most important in the extracellular fluid compartment.
2. In the intracellular compartment proteins are the most important component.
3. Respiratory system regulates CO_2 and therefore H^+.

4. Renal excretion of HCO_3
D. Arterial blood gases are essential to identify the acid-base disturbances (e.g., pH), to aid in the identification of the disturbance (respiratory vs. metabolic), and to follow therapeutic interventions.
E. Shock, hemorrhage, and massive transfusion are causes of acid-base disturbances in trauma patients.
F. Respiratory disturbances
1. **Respiratory acidosis**
    a. Arises from poor ventilation, which causes retained carbon dioxide. Causes include brain injury, intoxication, oversedation, and agonal states.
    b. The pH will decrease by 0.08 for each 10 mm Hg rise in the Pa_{CO_2}.
    c. Metabolic compensation occurs
        i. In acute hypercapnia, the HCO_3 increases by 1 mmol for each 10 mm Hg in P_{CO_2} above 40.
        ii. In chronic hypercapnia, the bicarbonate will increase by 4 mmol for each 10 mm Hg increase of P_{CO_2} above 40.
    d. The degree of metabolic compensation is important to estimate so a mixed acid-base disturbance, which is common in trauma patients, is not missed.
    e. **Treatment**
        i. Correction of underlying cause
        ii. If underlying cause is not quickly reversed, mechanical ventilation is necessary.
2. **Respiratory alkalosis**
    a. Hyperventilation is the most common cause in the trauma patient.
    b. For each 10 mm Hg decrease in the Pa_{CO_2}, the pH will increase 0.08.
    c. Metabolic compensation can be estimated by:
        i. Acute hypocapnia in which the bicarbonate decreases 2 mmol/L for each 10 mm Hg decrease of Pa_{CO_2} below 40 mm Hg
        ii. Chronic hypocapnia in which the bicarbonate decreases 5 to 7 mmol/L for each decrease of Pa_{CO_2} below 40 mm Hg
    d. **Treatment**
        i. Ventilator control
        ii. Possible mechanical ventilation
G. Metabolic disturbances
1. **Metabolic acidosis**
    a. Anion gap = $Na - (Cl + HCO_3)$
    b. Normal anion gap is 8 to 14.
    c. In trauma, an anion gap acidosis is most commonly caused by under-resuscitation.
    d. Other causes of anion gap acidosis include lactic acidosis; ketoacidosis; aspirin overdose; ingestion of ethylene glycol, methylene glycol, or paraldehyde; and chronic renal insufficiency.
    e. Common causes of non-anion gap acidosis include diarrhea, fistulas, and renal tubular acidosis.

2. Hyperventilation causes respiratory compensation and inappropriate compensation may reveal a mixed disorder.
3. **Treatment**
   a. Correct underlying cause.
   b. Adequate fluid resuscitation
4. A pH <7.2 may require bicarbonate administration.
   a. Bicarbonate administration may worsen the acidosis if the patient cannot ventilate the excess CO_2.
   b. Bicarbonate may be administered using the bicarbonate deficit formula.
      i. 0.4 x body weight (kg) x (HCO_3 desired – HCO_3 measured)
      ii. One half of this amount should be administered over 8 hours, with frequent monitoring of arterial blood gases.
5. Dialysis is indicated for patients in renal failure

H. Metabolic alkalosis
1. Classified as chloride responsive or chloride resistant
2. **Chloride responsive**
   a. Urine chloride <20 mEq/L
   b. **Causes** include
      i. Large volume nasogastric output or vomiting with an obstructed pylorus
      ii. Use of diuretics
      iii. Volume contraction
   c. **Treatment**
      i. Administer chloride-containing fluids such as normal saline.
      ii. Acetazolamide 250 to 500 mg IV
3. **Chloride resistant**
   a. Urine chloride >20 mEq/L
   b. **Causes**
      i. Hyperaldosteronism
      ii. Cushing's syndrome
      iii. Hypokalemia
   c. **Treatment**
      i. Correction of underlying cause
      ii. Stop exogenous steroids

XVI. ACUTE RENAL FAILURE

A. Classification
1. **Oliguric acute renal failure**: urine output < 400 mL per 24 hours
2. **Nonoliguric acute renal failure**: urine output > 400 mL per 24 hours. Mortality of nonoliguric acute renal failure is one-half that of oliguric renal failure.

B. Etiology
1. **Prerenal**
   a. Decrease in intravascular volume is common in trauma patients after hemorrhage, third-space fluid loss, or fluid drainage.

b. Impaired cardiac function
   c. Renal vascular obstruction
2. **Renal**
   a. Prolonged pre-renal or postrenal states
   b. Parenchymal lesions of the glomerulus or tubules due to nephrotoxins such as aminoglycosides, amphotericin B, and radiologic contrast agents
      i. Acute renal failure is more likely to occur after the administration of radiologic contrast agents if the patient is diabetic or has preexisting chronic renal failure, decreased intravascular volume, hypertension, or peripheral vascular disease, or is of increased age or if other nephrotoxic drugs are being used concomitantly.
      ii. Myoglobin precipitates in the renal tubules, causing obstruction.
      iii. Nonsteroidal anti-inflammatory drugs may increase renal vasoconstriction in patients with preexisting pre-renal conditions.
3. **Postrenal: anatomic obstruction of the urinary tract**
C. **Diagnosis of acute renal failure**
1. Acute renal failure can be assessed by an accurate history and physical examination focusing **on pre-renal or postrenal etiologic factors.**
2. **Laboratory assessment**
   a. Blood urea nitrogen (BUN) and creatinine will rise with decreased renal function.
   b. Urine electrolytes should be determined before diuretics are administered.
   c. Fractional excretion of sodium (FENa) is a measure of the kidneys' concentrating ability.
      i. (Urine Na × serum creatinine)/(urine creatinine × serum Na) × 100%
      ii. FENa <1 % consistent with prerenal ARF
      iii. FENa >3% consistent with renal parenchymal injury
   d. Prerenal patients will have unremarkable urinalysis.
      i. Urine osmolality >350 mOsm
      ii. Urine Na <10 mEq/L
   e. Patients with intrinsic renal failure may have:
      i. Proteinuria
      ii. Pyuria
      iii. Casts (protein, white blood cells, or epithelial) in their urine
      iv. Urine osmolality will equal plasma osmolality.
      v. Urine Na will be >10 mEq/L.
   f. Patients with postrenal failure will have:
      i. An unremarkable urinalysis
      ii. Unremarkable urine electrolytes
      iii. Imaging studies that confirm the diagnosis
   g. Patients with rhabdomyolysis will have a positive urine dip for blood but no microscopic red blood cells.
D. **Treatment**
1. **Prerenal**
   a. Restoration of intravascular volume
   b. Correction of cardiac output

    c. Correction of renal vascular perfusion
    d. Swan-Ganz catheter may be necessary for hemodynamic monitoring.
    e. Establish urine output.
2. **Renal**
    a. Withhold nephrotoxic agents.
    b. Myoglobinuria will require vigorous fluid administration until urine is free of myoglobin.
       i. Mannitol is given for osmotic diuresis.
       ii. Urine alkalization is achieved with bicarbonate (50 mEq/50 mL).
3. **Postrenal**. Urinary obstruction should be corrected.

E. Management

1. Establish urine output (0.5 to 1.0 mL/kg per hour).
2. Optimize intravascular volume and hemodynamic status for appropriate renal perfusion.
3. Use osmotic or loop diuretics to increase urine output for fluid management.
4. Prevent hyperkalemia.
5. Dialysis for acute renal failure
    a. Acidosis
    b. Volume overload
    c. Hyperkalemia (and other electrolyte disturbances)
    d. Ingestion of toxins
    e. Signs and symptoms of uremia
6. Intermittent hemodialysis is the standard therapy for acute renal failure.
7. **Peritoneal dialysis**
    a. Inappropriate after recent celiotomy
    b. Risk of peritonitis
    c. In selected patients has advantages including no need for anticoagulation; technically easy, less associated hypotension
8. Continuous venovenous hemodialysis and arteriovenous hemodialysis have benefits over intermittent hemodialysis.
    a. **Advantages**
       i. Precise fluid and metabolic control
       ii. Less accidental hypotension
       iii. Ability to administer nutritional support
    b. **Disadvantages**
       i. Need for prolonged anticoagulation
       ii. Constant need for surveillance

XVII. SUGGESTED READINGS

Adrogue HJ, Madias NE: Hypernatremia. N Engl J Med 342:1493–1499, 2000.

Adrogue HJ, Madias NE: Hyponatremia. N Engl J Med 342:1581–1589, 2000.

Australian and New Zealand Intensive Care Society (ANZICS) Clinical Trials Group: Low dose dopamine in patients with early renal dysfunction: A placebo-controlled randomized trial. Lancet 356:2139–2143, 2000.

Kellum JA, Decker JM: Use of dopamine in acute renal failure: A meta-analysis. Crit Care Med 29:1526–1531, 2001.

Mehta RL, Pascual MT, Soroko S, Chertow GM for the PICARD Study Group: Diuretics, mortality, and nonrecovery of renal function in acute renal failure. JAMA 288:2547–2553, 2002.

Mullins RJ: Shock, electrolytes, and fluid. In Townsend CM (ed): Textbook of Surgery: The Biological Basis of Modern Practice, 17th ed. Philadelphia, Saunder, 2004, pp 67–112.

O'Brien WJ: Fluids and electrolytes. In Berry SM (ed): The Mont Reid Surgical Handbook, 4th ed. St Louis, Mosby, 1997, pp 17–31.

Singri N, Ahya SN, Levin ML: Acute renal failure. JAMA 289:747–751, 2003.

Infection in the Surgical Intensive Care Unit

Alan E. Harzman, MD

I. INTRODUCTION

A. Infection and inflammation are among the most common causes of admission and extended length of stay in the surgical intensive care unit.
B. Early recognition and institution of therapy are paramount in decreasing the morbidity and cost associated with this disease process.

II. DEFINITIONS OF INFECTION/INFLAMMATION

A. Infection
1. Microbiologic diagnosis
B. Systemic inflammatory response syndrome (SIRS)
1. The systemic inflammatory response to a variety of clinical insults
2. American College of Chest Physicians (ACCP) / Society of Critical Care Medicine (SCCM) Consensus[1]
   a. Two or more of the following criteria:
      i. Temperature >38°C or < 36°C
      ii. Heart rate > 90 beats per minute (bpm)
      iii. Respiratory rate >20 or $Paco_2$ <32 mm Hg
      iv. White blood cell count (WBC) >12,000 or < 4000 or bandemia >10%
3. Early phase characterized by elevated cardiac output and decreased systemic vascular resistance
4. Cardiac output below normal in late phases; precedes cardiac failure
C. Sepsis
1. SIRS + **infection** = sepsis
2. Hypermetabolic response associated with increased oxygen demand
3. Systemic inflammation in response to infection
D. Septic shock
1. Sepsis + (hypotension, hypoperfusion, or organ dysfunction) = septic shock
2. Associated with decreased tissue oxygen extraction and oxygen debt, increased Svo_2
3. Signs may include lactic acidosis, oliguria, or acute mental status change.
E. Multiple organ dysfunction syndrome (MODS)
1. Predisposing factors include sepsis and SIRS
2. Functional abnormality of more than one organ system; unable to maintain homeostasis without support
3. Pathophysiology related to overwhelmed host defense
4. Theories of MODS (under investigation)[2]
   a. Gut

i. Splanchnic hypoperfusion during SIRS/sepsis may cause release of cytokines, exacerbating SIRS/sepsis, and later allow translocation of bacteria during relative immunosuppression.
   b. Two-hit hypothesis
      i. Following priming of immune system by first hit, any second hit can produce an exaggerated response leading to MODS.

III. HOST DEFENSE/INFLAMMATORY RESPONSE

A. Acute inflammatory response
1. **Cellular**
   a. Tissue injury leads to polymorphonuclear chemotaxis and adhesions.
   b. Neutrophil degranulation and phagocytosis affect bacterial killing.
   c. Stimulated macrophages produce cytokines in response to bacteria, lipopolysaccharides, and complement.
2. **Cytokines**
   a. Factors released in response to injury that potentiate inflammatory response
   b. Controlled production attempts to reinstate homeostasis but overproduction is potentially deleterious.
3. **Immunologic**
   a. Humoral immunity mediated by B lymphocytes
   b. Cellular immunity mediated by T lymphocytes

IV. EVALUATION OF THE FEBRILE RESPONSE

A. Temperature
1. Normal oral temperature: 37°C (98.6°F)
2. Diurnal variation: 1.3°C (2.4°F) greatest from 4 to 6 PM
3. Core temperature is 0.5°C (0.9°F) higher than oral temperature.
4. Fever: temperature >38.0°C (100.4°F)
5. Temperatures run higher in burn patients, and at Parkland Memorial Hospital we routinely treat patients with temperatures >39.5°C as fever in burn patients.

B. Vital signs
1. Heart rate increases approximately 5 to 10 bpm/°C
2. Hypotension associated with advanced sepsis/SIRS
3. Tachypnea manifests as respiratory rate >20

C. Physical examination
1. **Neurologic**
   a. Decreased level of consciousness
   b. Focal neurologic deficit
2. **Head, eye, ear, nose, and throat (HEENT)**
   a. Facial tenderness
   b. Nuchal rigidity

c. Nasal/sinus drainage
3. **Lungs**
   a. Abnormal breath sounds
4. **Cardiac**
   a. Murmur
   b. Pericardial friction rub
   c. Sternal instability (after cardiac surgery)
5. **Abdomen**
   a. Abdominal tenderness
   b. Mass
   c. Distention
   d. Bowel sounds
6. **Rectal**
   a. Perirectal mass/tenderness
7. **Skin/soft tissue**
   a. Erythema, tenderness, swelling, heat
   b. Line sites
8. **Extremities**
   a. Take down casts/splints to inspect skin.
   b. Lower extremity edema (e.g., deep venous thrombosis)

D. Hematology (CBC)
1. WBC increased; may be decreased with overwhelming infection
2. Left shift or bandemia with infection
3. Thrombocytopenia sometimes associated with sepsis

E. Cultures (before initiation of antibiotic therapy)
1. Obtain two sets of peripheral blood cultures.
2. Obtain blood culture from each central line unless placed more than 48 hours prior.
3. Obtain cerebrospinal fluid, bronchial washings, wound cultures as indicated.

F. Urinalysis
1. Urinalysis looking for WBCs, nitrite, and leukocyte esterase
2. Urine culture

G. Chest x-ray
1. Infiltrate, with signs of infection suggestive of pneumonic process
2. Effusion (parapneumonic, sympathetic)
3. Air-fluid level suspicious for lung abscess
4. Subdiaphragmatic air is a sensitive indicator of hollow visceral perforation but a normal variant in post-celiotomy period.

H. Computed tomography (CT)
1. Suspicious for intra-abdominal process/abscess
2. Obtain 8 to 10 days postoperatively after abdominal surgery
3. Some patients will be too unstable to go to CT.

I. Bedside surgeon-performed ultrasound
1. When available, may detect presence of lower extremity deep venous thrombosis

V. ETIOLOGY OF HYPERTHERMIA

A. Infection/inflammation
1. Discussed in remainder of chapter

B. Deep venous thrombosis (DVT)/pulmonary embolus (PE)
1. Up to 11% of DVT are in the upper extremities (risk factors are central venous lines and cancer).
2. DVT precipitates local inflammatory reaction, whereas the deleterious effects of PE are associated with an acute systemic inflammatory insult.
3. Diagnosis of DVT is based on duplex evaluation of the venous system directed by physical examination.
4. Diagnosis of PE is confirmed by CT angiogram or ventilation-perfusion scan and/or pulmonary angiogram as directed on the basis of risk factors, history, and presence or absence of hemodynamic instability.
5. Treatment of both processes requires anticoagulation unless contraindicated.
6. Vena cava filter devices are optionally placed prophylactically in high-risk populations with contraindication to anticoagulation or as subsequent therapy of anticoagulation failures. We have rarely placed superior vena cava filters in patients with upper extremity DVT in whom anticoagulation was contraindicated.
7. The option of the retrievable filter allows for short-term protection until anticoagulation is no longer contraindicated.

C. Transfusion reaction[3]
1. **Minor**
    a. Reaction to foreign leukocyte antigens
    b. Treatment mainly for comfort measures
2. **Major**
    a. Usually hemolytic reactions associated with ABO or Rh incompatibility
    b. Majority related to clerical errors
    c. Precipitates systemic inflammatory reaction. Shock, renal failure, hemoglobinuria are possible.
3. Treatment requires cessation of transfusion (change IV tubing), re-crossmatch of blood, and return of remaining blood to the blood bank.
4. Hemodynamic support
5. Correction of coagulopathy

D. Drugs
1. Antibiotics (penicillins, cephalosporins, rifampin, vancomycin)
2. Antifungals (amphotericin B)
3. Antiarrythmics (procainamide, quinidine)
4. Thrombolytics (streptokinase)
5. Anticonvulsants (dilantin, carbamazepine)

E. Hypothalamic dysfunction
1. Dysfunction of preoptic nucleus of anterior hypothalamus
2. **Etiologies**
    a. Trauma

b. Malignancy
   c. Infarction (cerebrovascular accident)
   d. Hemorrhage (hypertension)
F. Endocrine/metabolic
1. **Thyroid storm**
   a. Extreme manifestation of thyrotoxicosis associated with fever, disproportionate tachycardia relative to fever, and central nervous system aberrations
   b. Inciting factors include thyroid manipulation, infection, trauma, diabetic ketoacidosis, myocardial infarction, and drugs.
   c. Diagnosis is based on thyroid function tests.
   d. Treatment is aimed at minimization of thyroid hormone and acute control of hemodynamic effects of thyroid hormone excess by beta blockade.
2. **Adrenal insufficiency**
   a. Pathophysiology related to adrenocortical dysfunction with decreased production of glucocorticoids
   b. Primary causes are adrenal in origin, including trauma, hemorrhage, infarction, and malignancy.
   c. Secondary causes are associated with suppression of hypothalamic-pituitary-adrenal axis by exogenous steroids.
   d. Signs may include hyperthermia and refractory hypotension.
   e. Diagnosis is based on an ACTH stimulation test to document cortisol production in response to exogenous hormone administration. Check serum cortisol. Give 250 µg ACTH IV and repeat cortisol in 30 to 60 minutes. Increase in cortisol of >9 µg/dL is evidence of normal adrenal function.[4]
   f. CT of the head may be useful to rule out central nervous system abnormality.
   g. Treatment is intravenous steroid and supportive measures, including possible necessity for inotropic support.
   h. If suspected, treatment should be started in patients in shock with dexamethasone. ACTH stimulation test can then be performed and treatment converted to hydrocortisone 200 to 300 mg/day divided tid or qid or in continuous infusion for 7 days. (Dexamethasone does not interfere with cortisol assay.)
   i. If ACTH stimulation test is normal, steroids are stopped immediately.
   j. Consideration must be given to weaning steroids after the 7 days.
3. **Gout**
   a. Manifest by increased serum urate in conjunction with arthritis, most common at first metatarsophalangeal joints
   b. Treatment is supportive.
G. Cardiac
1. Acute myocardial infarction
H. Drug withdrawal
1. Ethanol
   a. Sympathetic response associated with hypertension, tachycardia, and mental status changes

2. Narcotics
I. Iatrogenic
1. Warming blanket
2. Infusion devices/blood warmers
3. Ventilator circuit warming
J. Miscellaneous
1. **Malignant hyperthermia**[4]
    a. Hyperthermia usually associated with general anesthetics (e.g., halothane, enflurane, isoflurane) and depolarizing neuromuscular blockade (e.g., succinylcholine)
    b. Occurs in 1 in 50,000 general anesthetics in adults, 1 in 15,000 in children
    c. Mortality in untreated cases is 80% and in treated cases is <10%.
    d. May occur intraoperatively or within 24 hours postoperatively
    e. Etiology is excess release of Ca^{2+} by sarcoplasmic reticulum of skeletal muscle associated with sustained contraction.
    f. Symptoms include temperature >104°C, mental status changes, and muscular rigidity.
    g. Rise in end-tidal CO_2 is the first sign in ventilated patients.
    h. Laboratory findings are consistent with coagulopathy, metabolic acidosis, and progressive renal insufficiency associated with rhabdomyolysis.
    i. **Treatment**:
        i. Immediate discontinuation of anesthetic
        ii. Dantrolene 2 mg/kg bolus, subsequently followed every 10 minutes by 2 mg/kg, to a total dose of 10 mg/kg.
        iii. Aggressive cooling including gastric lavage
        iv. Correct coagulopathy.
        v. Maintain brisk urine output. May require diuretics or mannitol. Rhabdomyolysis may induce acute tubular necrosis and renal failure.
        vi. May require hemodynamic and/or ventilatory support or $NaHCO_3$ to correct acidosis
    j. Consider terminating operative procedure until malignant hyperthermia is controlled.
2. **Neuroleptic malignant syndrome**
    a. Similar presentation to maliganant hyperthermia
    b. Associated with neuroleptic therapy, most commonly haloperidol (commonly used in intensive care unit settings)
    c. Originates centrally/presynaptic
    d. Treatment same as for malignant hyperthermia

VI. ETIOLOGY OF INFECTION/INFLAMMATION

A. Intravascular catheter
1. **Peripheral**
    a. **Pathogenesis**

- i. Related to ascending infection from intravascular device
- ii. May lead to superficial or suppurative thrombophlebitis
- iii. Lines placed in emergency situations are at high risk and should be changed in less than 24 hours.

b. **Signs/symptoms**
  - i. Fever, local erythema, tenderness

c. **Diagnostic evaluation**
  - i. Physical examination
  - ii. Complete blood count (CBC)

d. **Treatment**
  - i. Catheter removal
  - ii. Anti-staphyloccal therapy (nafcillin, first-generation cephalosporin)
  - iii. Elevation/comfort measures
  - iv. Phlebectomy required for suppurative thrombophlebitis

2. **Central**
   a. **Pathogenesis**
      - i. Bacterial migration along indwelling catheters
      - ii. Hematogenous spread
      - iii. Risk factors include prolonged site utilization, catheter manipulation, and poor sterile technique on insertion.
      - iv. Antiseptic- and antimicrobial-coated catheters are now available and may reduce catheter-related bloodstream infections. However, **catheters impregnated with silver sulfadiazine are contraindicated in patients with allergies to sulfa drugs**.

   b. **Signs/symptoms**
      - i. Fever, localized pain
      - ii. Erythema, tenderness, drainage, swelling

   c. **Diagnostic evaluation**
      - i. Blood cultures: two peripheral and one through central line
      - ii. Central line culture
      - iii. CBC
      - iv. **Diagnostic criteria**
         - (a) Colonization: line with >15 colony-forming units (CFU), cultures negative
         - (b) Infection: line with >15 CFU, cultures positive with same organism

   d. **Treatment**
      - i. Antibiotics directed at gram-positive organisms (S. aureus, S. epidermidis)
      - ii. Central line removal
      - iii. Consider removal of central line prior to culture results in patients with sepsis or septic shock in whom no other obvious source is identified.

B. **Wound/soft tissue**

1. **Superficial**
   a. **Pathogenesis**

i. Cellulitis and subcutaneous abscess usually have gram-positive etiology.
   b. **Signs/symptoms**
      i. Fever, pain
      ii. Erythema, tenderness, rubor, lymphangitis
   c. **Diagnostic evaluation**
      i. Physical examination
      ii. CBC
   d. **Treatment**
      i. Antibiotics directed against most likely gram-positive pathogens (nafcillin)
      ii. Incision and drainage of superficial abscess
2. **Invasive**
   a. **Pathogenesis**
      i. Rapidly progressive invasive soft tissue infection
      ii. Pathogenesis related to host immunocompetence and aggressiveness of organism
      iii. Risk factors include immunosuppression, diabetes, advanced age, malnutrition, exogenous steroids, radiation, chemotherapy
      iv. Types of Infection
         (a) Polymicrobial
         (b) Clostridial: produces progressive myonecrosis
         (c) Streptococcal: exotoxin/lytic enzymes that cleave prefascial tissue planes associated with rapidly advancing infection
   b. **Signs/symptoms**
      i. Fever, pain, symptoms of shock
      ii. Tenderness, erythema, skin discoloration/bullae, crepitus
      iii. *Clostridium* associated with characteristic "dishwater-colored" effluent
   c. **Diagnostic evaluation**
      i. No special diagnostic studies; therapy based on clinical judgment
   d. **Treatment**
      i. Surgical emergency; hallmark of therapy is wide debridement of nonviable tissue.
      ii. Broad-spectrum antibiotic therapy instituted, including a high-dose penicillin (against clostridia and streptococci) and clindamycin

C. Pulmonary/thoracic
1. **Pneumonia**
   a. **Prevention**
      i. Hand washing between patients
      ii. Head of bed elevated ≥30 degrees
      iii. Avoid gastric overdistention.
      iv. Routine oral hygiene
   b. **Pathogenesis**
      i. Community acquired (<72 hours after admission); mostly gram-positive

ii. Common nosocomial infection, many gram-negative
iii. After one week in the hospital, methicillin-resistant *Staphylococcus aureus* (MRSA) must be considered.
iv. Predisposing conditions include endotracheal airway with loss of mucociliary clearance, nasogastric intubation, H2 blocker therapy, prolonged recumbency.

c. **Signs/symptoms**
   i. Fever, dyspnea, cough, chest pain
   ii. Abnormal breath sounds, hypoxia

d. **Diagnostic evaluation**
   i. Chest x-ray to rule out infiltrate
   ii. Sputum culture
   iii. Bronchoscopically directed bronchoalveolar lavage and culture: 10^4 organisms/mL 70% to 100% sensitivity for pneumonia

e. **Treatment**
   i. Chest physiotherapy
   ii. May require ventilatory support
   iii. Antibiotics directed by culture results. *Pseudomonas* species require double antibiotic coverage

2. **Ventilator-associated pneumonia (VAP)**[5,6]
   a. **Diagnosis**
      i. Clinical suspicion of pneumonia 72 hours after admission and intubation
      ii. Clinical Pulmonary Infection Score (CPIS) (see Table 55-1)

TABLE 55-1
CLINICAL PULMONARY INFECTION SCORE

	Points
Temperature (C)	
Between 36.5° and 38.4°	0
38.5° to 38.9°	1
<36.5 or >39.0	2
White blood cell count	
Between 4000 and 11000	0
<4000 or >11000	1
<4000 or >11000 and band >50%	2
Tracheal secretions	
None or scant	0
Nonpurulent	1
Purulent	2
Oxygentation (Pao_2/Fio_2)	
>240, ARDS or pulmonary contusion	0
<240, no ARDS	2
(ARDS defined as Pao_2/Fio_2 <200, PAWP 18 mm Hg and acute bilateral infiltrates)	
Chest x-ray	
No infiltrate	0
Diffuse (or patchy) infiltrate	1
Localized infiltrate	2

iii. CPIS <6 and low suspicion: not treated nor further evaluated
iv. CPIS >6 or high suspicion: bronchoalveolar lavage (BAL) and initiate therapy
v. BAL specimens with ≥10^4 CFU are considered positive.

b. **Treatment**
   i. Empiric therapy should be broad and include "double-coverage" for *Pseudomonas*, based on the hospital's antibiogram. If onset is 5 to 7 days after hospitalization, coverage for MRSA should be included.
   ii. Therapy is tailored to the isolated organism when culture results are obtained. They are continued until the patient is afebrile and has a normal white blood cell count, to a maximum of 10 days.
   iii. If the BAL is negative, antibiotics are stopped.

3. **Empyema**
   a. **Pathogenesis**
      i. Risk factors include penetrating thoracic trauma, retained hemothorax, tube thoracostomy, and parapneumonic effusion.
   b. **Signs/symptoms**
      i. Fever, chest pain, dyspnea
   c. **Diagnostic evaluation**
      i. Chest x-ray to evaluate for gross pathology
      ii. CT scan of chest
      iii. Thoracentesis
         (a) Exudate: pH <7.2, pleural fluid to serum protein ratio >0.5, pleural fluid to serum LDH >0.6, and LDH >200 IU
         (b) Cell counts and pleural fluid culture
   d. **Treatment**
      i. Antibiotics depend on source of contamination; endogenous (broad spectrum) or exogenous (gram positive)
      ii. Tube thoracostomy drainage
      iii. Thoracoscopy/thoracotomy with decortication reserved for conservative treatment failures

4. **Mediastinitits**
   a. **Pathogenesis**
      i. Posterior mediastinitis usually related to inflammatory esophageal pathology/perforation
      ii. Anterior mediastinitis associated with post-sternotomy procedures
   b. **Signs/symptoms**
      i. Fever, chest pain, dyspnea
      ii. May present with signs of shock, especially posterior mediastinitis
      iii. Sternal instability (anterior mediastinitis)
   c. **Diagnostic evaluation**
      i. Chest x-ray may show left basilar effusion consistent with esophageal perforation or pneumomediastinum.
      ii. Cineradiographic evaluation if esophageal perforation suspected
   d. **Treatment**

     i. Anterior mediastinitis: gram-positive coverage (vancomycin)
     ii. Surgical debridement with pectoralis major flap coverage
     iii. Posterior mediastinitis: broad-spectrum coverage
     iv. Esophageal repair or exclusion
5. **Pericarditis**
   a. **Pathogenesis**
      i. Post-sternotomy, uremia, viral
   b. **Signs/symptoms**
      i. Fever, chest pain
   c. **Diagnostic evaluation**
      i. Chest x-ray
      ii. Echocardiography if suspect significant effusion
   d. **Treatment**
      i. Supportive
      ii. Anti-inflammatory
      iii. Percutaneous or open subxiphoid drainage for suspected purulent pericarditis or tamponade

D. Urinary tract
1. **Pathogenesis**
   a. Microorganism migration along indwelling catheter.
   b. Accounts for 35% to 40% of nosocomial infections
   c. Gram-positive organisms predominate.
2. **Signs/symptoms**
   a. Fever, dysuria
   b. Flank/suprapubic tenderness
3. **Diagnostic evaluation**
   a. Urinalysis: white cell count, leukocyte esterase, nitrite
   b. Urine culture
4. **Treatment**
   a. Removal of foley catheter as soon as possible
   b. Antibiotics directed at gram-positive pathogens (combination penicillin/β-lactamase inhibitor)

E. Intra-abdominal
1. **Intra-abdominal abscess**
   a. **Pathogenesis**
      i. Perforated ulcer, diverticultits, appendicitis, gallbladder
      ii. Post-celiotomy
      iii. Missed traumatic injury
   b. **Signs/symptoms**
      i. Fever, abdominal pain, nausea, vomiting
      ii. Abdominal tenderness (local tenderness/diffuse peritonitis), mass
   c. **Diagnostic evaluation**
      i. Chest x-ray may show free air or sympathetic effusion.
      ii. KUB obtained to rule out obstruction
      iii. CT scan of the abdomen single best diagnostic test; highly sensitive and specific

d. **Treatment**
      i. Broad-spectrum antibiotics to cover especially gram-negative pathogens and anaerobes
      ii. Percutaneous CT-guided drainage
      iii. Surgical drainage
2. **Cholecystitis (acalculous)**
   a. **Pathogenesis**
      i. Predisposing factors: burns, trauma, ischemia, biliary stasis, cystic duct obstruction
   b. **Signs/symptoms**
      i. Fever, abdominal pain, nausea, vomiting
      ii. Right upper quadrant (RUQ) abdominal tenderness
   c. **Diagnostic evaluation**
      i. RUQ ultrasound for gallbladder distention/sludge, pericholecystic fluid, or wall thickening
   d. **Treatment**
      i. Gram-negative antibiotic coverage, ± anaerobe coverage
      ii. Cholecysytectomy
      iii. Unstable patients may be temporized by CT-guided percutaneous cholecystostomy.
3. **Cholangitis**
   a. **Pathogenesis**
      i. Associated with common bile duct obstruction, biliary stasis, and transendothelial migration of bacteria
   b. **Signs/symptoms**
      i. Charcot's triad: fever, jaundice, right upper quadrant (RUQ) abdominal pain
      ii. Shock
   c. **Diagnostic evaluation**
      i. RUQ ultrasound to evaluate biliary system
   d. **Treatment**
      i. Gram-negative antibiosis
      ii. Endoscopic retrograde cholangiopancreatography (ERCP) with sphincterotomy
      iii. Percutaneous or open cholecystostomy in patients who are not ERCP candidates
      iv. Percutaneous transhepatic drainage
4. **Pancreatitis**
   a. **Pathogenesis**
      i. Associated factors include ductal obstruction, ethyl alcohol, trauma, ischemia, drugs/antibiotics
   b. **Signs/symptoms**
      i. Epigastric abdominal pain, nausea, vomiting, ± fever
      ii. Epigastric abdominal tenderness, signs of shock consistent with necrotizing infection or abscess
   c. **Diagnostic evaluation**
      i. Amylase, lipase, liver function tests

ii. RUQ ultrasound to rule out common bile duct obstruction or cholelithiasis
iii. CT scan of the abdomen to evaluate for phlegmon/abscess

d. **Treatment**
  i. Broad-spectrum antibiotics
  ii. Surgical drainage/debridement for necrotizing infection or abscess
  iii. Supportive measures; may require vigorous volume support

F. Enteric
1. Pseudomembranous enterocolitis
   a. **Pathogenesis**
     i. Enteric overgrowth of *Clostridium dificile* with production of mucosal pseudomembrane and enterotoxin
     ii. Predisposing factor related to antecedent antibiotic therapy
     iii. Associated with increased risk of toxic megacolon
   b. **Signs/symptoms**
     i. Fever, abdominal pain, diarrhea
     ii. Abdominal tenderness
   c. **Diagnostic evaluation**
     i. Stool analysis: *C. dificile* toxin and fecal white blood cells
     ii. KUB to rule out colon distention (toxic megacolon)
     iii. Lower endoscopy: pseudomembrane visualization and culture/biopsy
   d. **Treatment**
     i. Parenteral or enteral metronidazole is first line of therapy. Enteral vancomycin is reserved for refractory illness.
     ii. Toxic megacolon may require surgical intervention.

G. Sinus
1. Sinusitis
   a. **Pathogenesis**
     i. Related to obstruction of the paranasal sinus ostia
     ii. Predisposing factors include paranasal sinus fracture, prolonged nasogastric or nasotracheal intubation, or nasal packing.
   b. **Signs/symptoms**
     i. Fever, headache, facial pain
     ii. Maxillary or frontal tenderness, nasal discharge
   c. **Diagnostic evaluation**
     i. Facial series x-rays
     ii. CT scans of face to paranasal sinuses
     iii. Sinus aspiration (>10^3/mL organisms indicative of infection)
   d. **Treatment**
     i. Antibiotics
     ii. Caldwell Luc approach to drainage of maxillary sinuses

H. Central nervous system
1. Meningitis
   a. **Pathogenesis**
     i. Inflammation of meninges in response to infection

ii. Associated with hematogenous spread, trauma, and post-craniospinal surgery
   b. **Signs/symptoms**
      i. Fever, headache, obtundation
      ii. Nuchal rigidity
   c. **Diagnostic evaluation**
      i. CT of head to rule out mass lesion
      ii. Lumbar puncture
   d. **Treatment**
      i. Antibiotics (must cross blood-brain barrier)
2. **Abscess**
   a. **Pathogenesis**
      i. Associated with hematogenous and continuous modes of spread
      ii. Risk factors include trauma, systemic infection, immunosuppression, etc.
   b. **Signs/symptoms**
      i. Fever, headache
      ii. Focal neurologic symptoms, depressed level of consciousness
   c. **Diagnostic evaluation**
      i. CT scan of head to rule out mass lesion
   d. **Treatment**
      i. Antibiotics
      ii. Stereotactic/surgical drainage

I. Miscellaneous
1. **Toxic shock syndrome (TSS)**
   a. **Pathogenesis**
      i. Mucocutaneous colonization/infection with exotoxin-producing *S. aureus*
      ii. Predisposing factors include retained tampons, nasal packs, etc.
   b. **Signs/symptoms**
      i. Fever, headache, diarrhea
      ii. Diffuse erythematous rash
   c. **Diagnostic evaluation**
      i. Culture of affected tissue
   d. **Treatment**
      i. Mainly supportive
      ii. ±Antibiotics (blood cultures usually sterile)
2. **Tetanus**
   a. **Signs/symptoms**
      i. Trismus
      ii. Dysphagia
      iii. Fever
   b. The interval between the first symptoms and the first severe spasms may be from 24 hours to more than 10 days.

c. In severe cases, muscular spasms are superimposed on the baseline muscular hypertonicity, leading to crush fractures of vertebrae and death from respiratory failure.
d. Any wound may be a nidus for tetanus although deep penetrating injuries with a necrotic focus create the highest risk.
e. The toxin attacks nerve synapses.
f. **Treatment**
   i. Passive immunization with human tetanus toxoid immune globulin
   ii. Active immunization with tetanus toxoid
   iii. Penicillin
   iv. Debridement and drainage of wounds
   v. Supportive care with mechanical ventilation and complete muscle paralysis may be necessary for 6 to 8 weeks.
   vi. The diagnosis is completely clinical because cultures are rarely positive.

3. **Meleney's ulcer**
   a. A rare synergistic infection usually due to a microaerophilic streptococcus and hemolytic *S. aureus*.
   b. It is a tender lesion with a central area of purple-appearing necrosis surrounded by cellulitis.
   c. It can occur around surgical drains, sutures, and stomas after 1 to 2 weeks.
   d. The lesion progressively enlarges but seldom involves underlying fascia.
   e. **Treatment**
      i. Antistaphylococcal drug
      ii. Minor debridement

VII. THERAPY OF INFECTION/INFLAMMATION

A. Volume resuscitation
1. Isotonic fluid resuscitation (lactated Ringer's, 0.9% saline) instituted to restore intravascular volume
2. Ongoing evaluation of volume status by hemodynamics and urine output
3. Patients refractory to simple methods of monitoring require invasive hemodynamic monitoring with a pulmonary artery catheter.
4. **Initial resuscitation goals** (Surviving Sepsis Study)[4]
   a. Central venous pressure ≥8 to 12 mmHg
   b. Mean arterial pressure ≥65 mm Hg
   c. Urine output ≥0.5 mL/kg/hour
   d. Svo_2 ≥70%

B. Antimicrobial
   a. See following section.

C. Invasive physiologic monitoring
1. High fluid volume support

2. High ventilatory support (PEEP >10)
3. Cardiac disease (congestive heart failure, coronary artery disease, etc.)
4. Pulmonary disease (chronic obstructive pulmonary disease, pulmonary contusion, pulmonary hypertension, etc.)
5. Age >65 years

D. Vasopressor support
1. Dependent on hemodynamic and oxygen transport/extraction variables
2. Goal to optimize oxygen consumption and delivery
3. Surviving Sepsis Study recommends dopamine or norepinephrine as first-line agent.[7]
    a. Dopamine:
        i. 2 to 5 μg/kg/min exerts renal effect via dopaminergic receptors.
        ii. 5 to 10 μg/kg/min affects mainly chronotropy via receptors.
        iii. >10 μg/kg/min is associated with vasoconstriction via alpha receptor binding.
    b. Dobutamine
        i. 2 to 5 μg/kg/min. Selective beta-receptor effect produces inotropy and decreased systemic vascular resistance and is associated with improved cardiac output. It may cause hypotension in the hypovolemic patient
    c. Phenylephrine: pure alpha-agonist; used sparingly. It produces vasoconstriction and increases afterload, which may impair cardiac output and oxygen delivery in the face of increased metabolic demand.
    d. Norepinephrine has alpha and beta effects, and it simulates the epinephrine response. It is useful for unstable patients and patients refractory to dopamine therapy. Complications include myocardial and visceral ischemia.

E. Recombinant human activated protein C[7]
1. Anticoagulant, anti-inflammatory shown to improve survival in patients with sepsis-induced organ dysfunction. Benefits must be weighed against risks related to bleeding.

F. Blood products[4]
1. In the absence of tissue hypoperfusion, significant coronary artery disease, acute hemorrhage, or lactic acidosis, red blood cell transfusion should be used only when hemoglobin is <7.0g/dL. Transfuse to a target of 7 to 9 g/dL.

G. Blood glucose control[7]
1. After initial stabilization, blood glucose is tightly maintained at 80 to 110 mg/dL with an insulin infusion protocol and close monitoring.

H. Surgical control of infection/inflammation
1. DVT prophylaxis[7]
    a. Low-dose unfractionated heparin or low-molecular weight heparin. Mechanical means (intermittent compression device or graduated compression stockings) are used in patients with contraindication to heparin.

2. Stress ulcer prophylaxis[7]
    a. H$_2$ receptor antagonists are first-line therapy.
3. Source control
4. Debridement
5. Drainage

VIII. ANTIBIOTIC THERAPY

A. General principles
1. **Bacteriostatic**
    a. Action of antibiotic inhibits bacterial cell growth and division.
    b. Bacteria subsequently cleared by host defenses
2. **Bacteriocidal**
    a. Antibiotic that exerts direct effect on organism to effect cell killing
    b. Crucial form of therapy in the immunocompromised host
3. **Synergy**
    a. Combinations of antibiotics that act by different mechanisms
4. **Resistance**
    a. Antibiotic associated; penicillins and cephalosporins especially susceptible due to bacterial mutations conferring increased β-lactamase resistance
5. **Complications**
    a. Allergy/hypersensitivity
    b. Fever
    c. Nephrotoxicity (e.g., aminoglycosides)
    d. Seizures (e.g., imipenem)
    e. Bone marrow toxicity
6. **Empiric therapy**
    a. Azole antifungal or broad-spectrum antibiotic therapy
    b. Indications
        i. Unstable/deteriorating patients with clinical sepsis/systemic inflammatory response syndrome (SIRS)
        ii. See also section below on Antifungal Therapy
7. **Prophylactic therapy**
    a. Institution of antibiotic therapy prior to surgical procedures to minimize postoperative wound infection
    b. Antibiotics given 30 to 60 minutes preoperatively associated with adequate tissue levels at the time of surgical incision
    c. Wound morbidity associated with class of procedure
        i. Clean (e.g., hernia, thoracotomy, etc.): 1% to 2%
        ii. Clean-contaminated (e.g., biliary, esophagus, gastric): 2% to 5%
        iii. Contaminated (e.g., unprepped colon, etc.): 5% to 30%
        iv. Infected (e.g., intra-abdominal abscess, etc.): >30%

B. Aminoglycosides
1. Spectrum: gram-negative aerobes and facultative anaerobes
2. Effect bacterial killing by inhibition of protein systhesis

VIII. Antibiotic Therapy

3. Single daily dose based on nomogram
4. Indications
   a. Urinary tract infection
   b. Synergistic therapy

C. Antianaerobes
1. Spectrum: anaerobe and some gram-positive pathogens
   a. Indications
      i. Intra-abdominal abscess
      ii. Oral/dental abscess
      iii. Aspiration pneumonia

D. Beta-lactams
1. **Penicillins**
   a. Inhibit bacterial cell wall synthesis
   b. Spectrum: gram-positive cocci and gram-positive bacilli
   c. Indications
      i. Clostridial myonecrosis
      ii. Streptococcal soft tissue infection
      iii. Streptococcal pneumonia

2. **Cephalosporins**
   a. **General**
      i. Mechanism: inhibition of cell wall synthesis
      ii. Bacteriocidal
   b. **First-generation**
      i. Spectrum: gram-positive pathogens
      ii. Indications
         (a) Superficial soft tissue infection
         (b) Prophylactic therapy for clean operative cases
   c. **Second-generation**
      i. Spectrum: moderate gram-positive, moderate gram-negative
      ii. Indications
         (a) Prophylactic therapy for enteric surgical procedures
         (b) Perioperative prophylaxis for suspected clean contaminated/contaminated cases
         (c) ERCP prophylaxis
         (d) Combination therapy for intra-abdominal sepsis
   d. **Third-generation**
      i. Spectrum: broad-spectrum gram-positive pathogens
      ii. Indications
         (a) Community-acquired pneumonia
         (b) *Pseudomonas* coverage; should be used in synergy with another agent
   e. **Fourth-generation**
      i. Spectrum: excellent gram-positive coverage
      ii. Indications
         (a) Resistant organisms
         (b) Nosocomial pneumonia

3. **Monobactams**
   a. **Aztreonam**
      i. Spectrum: gram-negative aerobes, including *Pseudomonas* species
      ii. Indications
         (a) Synergistic antipseudomonal therapy
         (b) Gram-negative coverage in patients with contraindications to aminoglycosides
4. **Carbapenems**
   a. **Imipenem**
      i. Spectrum: most broad coverage penicillin
      ii. Indications
         (a) Intra-abdominal sepsis
         (b) Resistant pneumonia
         (c) Synergistic antipseudomonal coverage

E. Glycopeptides
1. **Vancomycin**
   a. Spectrum: gram-positive, including *S. epidermidis*, MRSA, and *Enterococcus* species
   b. Indications
      i. Pseudomembranous enterocolitis (third-line choice)
      ii. Sternal wound infection/post-coronary artery bypass mediastinitis
      iii. MRSA
      iv. Coagulase-negative staphylococcus
      v. Ampicillin-resistant enterococcus
   c. Selective indications to prevent emergence of vancomycin-resistant *Enterococcus* species

F. Quinolones
1. Spectrum: broad gram-negative coverage, including *Pseudomonas* species
   a. Gram-positive coverage intermediate
2. Indications
   a. Nosocomial pneumonia
   b. Intra-abdominal sepsis
   c. Urinary tract infection

G. Macrolides
1. Spectrum: gram-positive organisms
2. Bacteriostatic at low concentrations/bacteriocidal at high concentrations
3. Indications
   a. Preoperative PO (oral) colon prep
   b. Synergistic combination against resistant gram-positive organisms

H. Sulfa drugs
1. Spectrum: gram-negative rods
2. Indications
   a. Urinary tract infection
   b. *Pneumocystis carinii* infection

I. Antifungal therapy[8]
1. Risk factors for disseminated fungal infection
   a. Major
      i. In hospital for 7 or more days or in intensive care unit for 3 or more days
      ii. Appropriate broad-spectrum antibiotics for 5 or more days without response
   b. Minor
      i. Immunosuppression
         (a) Trauma/burns
      ii. Multiple organ system dysfunction
      iii. Central IV line
      iv. Total parenteral nutrition
      v. Pancreatitis
      vi. Recent initiation of hemodialysis
      vii. Surgery that transects gut wall
      viii. Broad-spectrum antibiotics
   c. Empiric therapy for candidiasis in non-neutropenic patients is limited to those (1) colonized with *Candida* and (2) who meet both major and two or more minor criteria.

J. Amphotericin B
1. Indications
   a. Hematogenous fungal infection
   b. Disseminated fungal infection
2. Dose with initial 1 mg test dose. If no hypersensitivity, base daily dosing according to renal function.

K. Fluconazole
1. Indications
   a. Nonhematogenous/nondisseminated *Candida albicans* infection
   b. Limited role for treatment of invasive *Candida albicans* infection (e.g., patients with hypersensitivity to amphotericin B)
   c. Empiric therapy for inflammatory process of unknown origin in high-risk population (e.g., immunosuppression, burns, trauma, broad-spectrum antibiotics, etc.)
2. Many Candida species are resistant.

L. Caspofungin
1. Indications
   a. Similar to amphotericin B

M. Nystatin
1. Treatment of mucocutaneous candidiasis and oral thrush
2. Topical application 10 mL tid

N. Antiviral therapy
1. Acyclovir
   a. Herpes simplex virus
      i. Post-transplant
      ii. HIV
   b. Epstein-Barr virus

2. **Gancyclovir**
    a. Cytomegalovirus (CMV)
        i. Post-transplant
        ii. HIV
O. Interferon
1. Immunomodulator potentially useful against hepatitides (HCV > HBV)
P. Nucleoside analogs
1. Inhibit reverse transcription HIV virus
2. Limit retroviral replication and protein synthesis
Q. Ribavirin
1. Respiratory syncitial virus
2. Viral hepatitis

IX. REFERENCES

1. American College of Chest Physician/Society of Critical Care Medicine Consensus Conference: Definitions for sepsis and organ failure and guildellines for the use of innovative therapies in sepsis. Cril Care Med 20(6):864–874, 1992.
2. Phelan HA, Eastman AL, Fortran A, et al: Shock and hypoperfusion states. In O'Leary JP (ed): The Physiologc Basis of Surgery, 4th ed. Philadelphia, Lippincott Williams & Wilkins, 2008, pp 87–111.
3. Scott-Conner CE, Spence RK, Shander A, et al: Hemostasis, thrombosis, hematopoesis, and blood transfusion. In O'Leary JP (ed): The Physiologc Basis of Surgery, 3rd ed. Philadelphia, Lippincott Williams & Wilkins, 2002, pp 531–575.
4. De Lanzac KS, Thomas MA, Riopelle JM: Anesthesia. In O'Leary JP (ed): The Physiologc Basis of Surgery, 3rd ed. Philadelphia, Lippincott Williams & Wilkins, 2002, pp 681–704.
5. Hubmayr RD: Statement of the Fourth International Consensus Conference in Critical Care on ICU-Acquired Pneumonia. Intensive Care Medicine 28(11):1521–1536, 2002.
6. Fagon JY, Chastre J, Wolff M, et al:(2000). Invasive and noninvasive strategies for management of suspected ventilator-associated pneumonia. Ann Intern Med132:621–630, 2000.
7. Deninger RP, Levy MM, Carlet OM, et al: Surviving Sepsis Campaign: International guidelines for management of severe sepsis and septic shock. Crit Care Med 36(1): 296–327, 2008.
8. Pappas PG, Rex JH, Sobel JD, et al: Guidelines for treatment of candidiasis. Clinl Infect Dis 38:161–189, 2004.

Metabolism and Nutrition

Radha Iyengar, MD

I. POSTINJURY HYPERMETABOLIC RESPONSE

A. Balance between increased catabolism and inability to use substrate. This is classified into two phases after injury: ebb and flow.
B. Ebb: may last 24 to 72 hours and corresponds to the traumatic and initial post-traumatic period when there is usually adequate substrate (oxygen, glucose, fatty acid) to meet the diminished demand of the tissues. It is characterized by (1) changes in O_2 consumption, (2) hyperglycemia, and (3) increased vascular tone.
C. Flow: this is usually over within 2 weeks but may last up to 8 weeks or longer in more severe cases and represents the period of convalescence. It is characterized by (1) increased O_2 consumption and delivery, (2) increased body temperature, and (3) mobilization of amino acids from peripheral tissues for redistribution for gluconeogenesis, acute-phase protein production, immunologic proliferation, red blood cell production, and fibroblast proliferation.

II. ENDOCRINE RESPONSE TO STRESS AND INJURY

A. Differs from starvation (see Table 56-1)
B. Catecholamines and sympathetic nervous system: increase heart rate, contractility, vascular tone, oxygen consumption, glycogenolysis, gluconeogenesis, and lipolysis
C. Hormonal mediators
1. **Cortisol**: increases gluconeogenesis, lipolysis, and proteolysis and potentiates actions of glucagons and catecholamines
2. **Glucagon**: opposes effects of insulin; increases gluconeogenesis, lipolysis, and ketogenesis and promotes amino acid uptake by the liver
3. **Antidiuretic hormone**: acts on renal tubules to increase free water absorption; increases glycogenolysis and gluconeogenesis
4. **Insulin**: initially suppressed during first few hours of injury
5. **Growth hormone**: increases lipolysis and ketogenesis and decreases plasma insulin levels
D. Cytokines TNF, IL-6: increase resting energy expenditure, increase proteolysis, and induce liver production of acute-phase reactants

III. PROTEIN METABOLISM DURING STRESS AND INJURY

A. Protein synthesis and catabolism increase (catabolism increases more).
B. Essential amino acids, especially branched-chain acids, increase.
C. Nonessential amino acids decrease.

TABLE 56-1
METABOLIC RESPONSES TO STARVATION INJURY

Metabolic Parameter	Starvation	Hypermetabolic State (Injury)
Resting energy expenditure	Increased	Increased
Respiratory quotient	0.7 (fat is preferred fuel)	>0.8 (protein is preferred fuel)
Glucose metabolism	Hypoglycemia	Hyperglycemia
Protein metabolism	Minimal protein loss	Negative nitrogen balance
Fat metabolism	Free fatty acid primary fuel	Increased lipolysis

D. Up to 70% of amino acids are released by skeletal muscle. These are alanine and glutamine, which only make up 15% of muscle composition.
E. During stress, skeletal muscle can use branched-chain amino acids (valine, leucine, isoleucine).
F. Glutamine serves as a primary fuel for enterocytes.
G. Alanine can be recycled in liver to form glucose.
H. Synthesis of constitutive transport proteins is depressed, whereas synthesis of acute-phase proteins is increased.

IV. GLUCOSE METABOLISM DURING STRESS AND INJURY

A. Hepatic gluconeogenesis is increased despite hyperglycemia.
B. After glycogen depletion, protein serves as the substrate since fat cannot be converted to glucose.
C. Glucose infusions do not inhibit this gluconeogenesis.
D. Alanine, glutamine, lactate, and glycerol can all be used to produce glucose.

V. FAT METABOLISM IN STRESS AND INJURY

A. Enhanced lipolysis is secondary to increased levels of epinephrine, glucagons, and cortisol.
B. Plasma free fatty acid levels do no correlate with the degree of trauma.
C. All forms of intravenous fat available in the United States are omega-6 fatty acids.
D. Septic patients use fat as primary fuel as shown by the depressed RQ in these patients. As the patient recovers, the respiratory quotient increases to that of carbohydrate (1.0).

VI. NUTRITION

A. Goals
1. To provide adequate substrate for the post-injury hypercatabolic state
2. To prevent protein malnutrition that can contribute to nosocomial infections and ongoing organ dysfunction

B. Early vs delayed feeding
1. Start enteral feeds as early as possible.

2. Beware of intolerance and small bowel necrosis in patients who are incompletely resuscitated.
3. Advance feeds with caution in those patients who are heavily sedated, paralyzed, or on pressors. In this group, distal enteral feeding is encouraged at Parkland Memorial Hospital.
4. Delay enteral feeds in patients with ongoing resuscitation or those requiring initiation/escalation of pressor agents.
5. In all patient populations, total parenteral nutrition (TPN) can be instituted soon after injury (in cases where enteral feeding is not available), ideally after resuscitation is complete if the patient will not be a candidate for enteral feeding.

C. Indications for early (<48 hours) feeding
1. Major head injuries
2. Major abdominal trauma
3. Major orthopaedic trauma
4. Major chest trauma
5. Major upper gastrointestinal surgery that precludes oral intake for > 5 days
6. Burns >20% total body surface area
7. Chronically malnourished patients
   a. Albumin <2.5
   b. Recent weight loss >10%
   c. Less than 80% ideal body weight
8. Limited physiologic reserve
   a. Chronic lung, liver, or kidney disease
   b. Age >70 years

D. Route of administration
1. Parenteral vs enteral
   a. Patients with blunt and penetrating abdominal injuries sustain fewer septic complications when fed enterally as opposed to parenterally.
   b. Patients with severe head injuries have similar outcomes whether fed enterally or parenterally.
   c. In severely injured patients, TPN should be started by day 7 if enteral feeding is not successful. Patients who fail to tolerate at least 50% of their goal rate of enteral feedings by the seventh post-injury day should have TPN instituted but should be weaned when greater than 50% of enteral feedings are tolerated.
   d. This may be initiated sooner if it is clear patient will not tolerate enteral nutrition at day 7.
   e. Enteral feeding is more physiologic and less expensive than parenteral feeding.
2. Gastric vs small bowel
   a. Distal feeding (distal to ligament of Treitz) preferred over parenteral nutrition in patients not tolerating gastric or duodenal feeds
   b. Unclear as to whether stomach or small bowel feeding is preferable due to the risk of aspiration

c. Gastrointestinal injury below the site of access may slow advancement of tube feedings but is not a contraindication to direct small bowel feedings.

E. Formula selection: standard vs other

At Parkland Memorial Hospital, standard formula is used in most clinical situations. Consider the following formulas in specific patients:

1. Immune enhancing: used in patients sustaining major torso trauma who are at risk for major septic complications and multiorgan failure (injury severity score [ISS] >20, abdominal trauma index [ATI] >25)
2. Polymeric high-protein formula: for patients who have increased nitrogen requirements
3. Elemental: for pancreatitis, short gut, high-output fistula, persistent severe diarrhea, intolerance to other enteral feeds
4. Renal failure formula: for patients with progressive renal failure or for those requiring intermittent dialysis

F. Risk factors for aspiration

1. Previous episode of aspiration
2. Decreased level of consciousness (i.e., traumatic brain injury)
3. Neuromuscular disease and/or structural abnormalities of upper gastrointestinal tract
4. Endotracheal intubation
5. Persistently high gastric residuals
6. Prolonged supine positioning
7. Measurement of feeding intolerance
    a. Evaluation for vomiting, abdominal cramping or distention, tenderness, diarrhea
    b. Gastric residuals—follow trend rather than actual volume (The stomach produces 1 to 1.5 L of gastric fluid per day. Greater than 250 mL is indicative of intolerance.)

G. Parenteral nutrition

1. **Indications**
    a. Massive small bowel resection refractory to enteral feeds
    b. High-output fistula after failure of elemental diet
    c. High risk of bowel necrosis
    d. Unable to meet >50% of nutritional needs by day 7 in the intensive care unit
2. **Initiation**
    a. Can be initiated at goal rate
    b. Follow daily electrolytes
    c. Usually tapered off over two days after decision to discontinue is made
    d. Composition: carbohydrate, protein, fat, electrolytes, micronutrients
    e. Insulin, vitamins, and heparin can be added to TPN but this can make tight glycemic control difficult.
3. **Complications**
    a. Hyperglycemia
    b. Line- or access-related complications—most notably infection. This can be a significant cause of post-injury morbidity.

c. Essential fatty acid deficiency – rare if 2% to 4% of total calories are delivered as fat
   d. Zinc deficiency – rare with administration of at least 5 mg/day
   e. Fatty liver

VII. ASSESSMENT OF NUTRITIONAL REQUIREMENTS:

A. Harris-Benedict formula is used to determine basal energy. The equation estimates basic energy expenditure (BEE) in the fasted, resting, nonstressed state:

Males: BEE = 66 + (13.8 × weight) + (5 × height) − (6.8 × age)

Females: BEE = 665 + (9.6 × weight) + (1.8 × height) − (4.7 × age)

(Calculated values are increased by stress factor ranging from 1.25 to 2 and an activity factor to account for increases in metabolic rate by injury and stress.)

B. 25 to 30 non-protein kcal/kg/day or 120% to 140% of predicted BEE
C. 1.5 to 2.2 g of protein/kg/day
D. 2 to 4 g/kg/day of glucose
E. Caloric density of nutritional elements:
   1 g protein = 4 kcal
   1 g glucose = 3.4 kcal
   1 g fat = 9.1 kcal
F. Proteins, fat, and carbohydrate requirements do not appear to vary significantly according to the route of administration (enteral vs parenteral).
G. Fat or carbohydrate requirements do not appear to vary significantly according to the type of injury (e.g., burns versus physical trauma).
H. Provision of excess calories to trauma patients may induce hyperglycemia, excess CO_2 production, fluid/electrolyte abnormalities, lipogenesis, and hepatic steatosis.
I. Protein requirements in burn patients and in those with severe central nervous system injuries may be significantly greater than anticipated, up to 2.2 g/kg body weight per day.

VIII. MONITORING NUTRITIONAL SUPPORT

A. The frequency of monitoring and the efficacy of laboratory examinations to determine the adequacy of nutritional support have yet to be clearly determined.
B. Total body weight and daily intake and output should be measured regularly.
C. Ideally, prior to the initiation of nutritional support, baseline laboratory test results should be obtained: BUN, creatinine, plasma electrolytes, glucose, calcium, magnesium, inorganic phosphorus, total protein,

albumin, prealbumin, hemoglobin, white blood cell count, platelet count, triglycerides, and transaminases.
D. Nitrogen balance is the gold standard: 1 g nitrogen is produced from 6.25 g of protein.
E. Serial prealbumin measurements can be obtained weekly. When compared to other visceral proteins, serial determination of serum prealbumin is the most sensitive indicator of appropriate nutritional support. A drawback is that it can be falsely low in patient with an acute-phase response.
F. Indirect calorimetry uses expired gas analysis to determine overall resting energy expenditure. Drawbacks are that it is inaccurate in patients requiring high Fio_2 and high positive end-expiratory pressure, requires labor-intensive calculations, and may not represent total energy expenditure.

IX. HYPERGLYCEMIC PROTOCOL

A. Indications:
1. Mechanical ventilation
2. Infection
3. Steroids
4. Diabetic
B. Target range is capillary blood glucose between 80 and 110 mg/dL
C. Method of control
1. Intermittent insulin dosing
   a. May be appropriate to use initially for glycemic control, though this is in question
   b. If after 4 hours CBGs are greater than 110, switch to insulin drip.
2. Insulin infusion
   a. Titrate to keep CBGs in target range.
   b. Check CBG every hour for optimal control.

X. SUGGESTED READINGS

ASPN Board of Directors and the Clinical Guidelines Task Force: Guidelines for the Use of Parenteral and Enteral Nutrition in Adult and Pediatric Patients. JPEN 26(Suppl), 2002

Detsky AS, et al: Is this patient malnourished? JAMA 271:54–58, 1994.

Frankenfield DC, et al: Accelerated nitrogen loss after traumatic injury is not attenuated by achievement of energy balance. JPEN 21:324–320, 1997.

Jacobs DG, et al: Practice Management Guidelines for Nutritional Support of the Trauma Patient. The EAST Practice Management Guidelines Workgroup, Eastern Association for the Surgery of Trauma, 2003.

Marik PE, et al: Early enteral nutrition in acutely ill patients: A systematic review. Crit Care Med 29:2264-2270, 2001.

Organ Donation and Management of the Organ Donor

Matthias Peltz, MD

I. INTRODUCTION

- **A.** Major advances have been made in the areas of organ preservation, transplantation operative techniques, and immunosuppression that have significantly improved organ transplantation outcomes.
- **B.** The major limiting factor continues to be the shortage of donors. Nearly 90,000 individuals are currently on transplantation waiting lists. Unfortunately, the waiting list outnumbers the number of organs transplanted annually (25,461 in 2003).
- **C.** In 2003, 12,031 eligible donors were identified, 6630 consents for donation were obtained (55.1%), and 5908 patients donated one or more of their organs for a conversion rate of 49.7%. Additionally, nearly 600 non-heart-beating donors and elderly donors (age >70 years) contributed organs for transplantation.
- **D.** One-year mortality of patients waiting for life-saving organs (heart, liver, lung) ranges from 10% to 25%. Overall waiting list mortality is 7.5%.
- **E.** As severe head injury is the leading cause of death in organ donors, it is important for the trauma surgeon to recognize patients as potential donors and to refer them to the appropriate organ procurement agency.

II. LEGISLATIVE BACKGROUND

- **A.** Although many technical aspects of organ transplantation were being addressed during the 1950s and 1960s, clinically significant organ transplantation volumes were not realized until the idea of organ replacement therapy and the concept of brain death gained acceptance in medical and especially legal circles. Several pieces of legislation and policy facilitated this transition.
- **B.** The Uniform Anatomical Gift Act (1968) legalized organ donation after death and also rendered the sale of organs illegal.
- **C.** The Uniform Brain Death Act (1978) and the Uniform Determination of Death Act (1980) expanded the definition of death from cessation of cardiorespiratory function to include cessation of brain activity.
- **D.** In 1981, the President's Commission for the Study of Ethical Problems in Medicine in its report "Guidelines for the Determination of Death" established criteria for determination of brain death.

III. DONOR CRITERIA

A. The preferred candidate for organ donation is an otherwise healthy patient who has sustained irreversible brain injury due to:
1. Head trauma
2. Intracranial hemorrhage
3. Drug overdose
4. Primary brain tumor
5. Cerebral ischemia

B. Age is no longer considered an absolute exclusion criterion, and each case should be reviewed on an individual basis. Additionally, even fatally injured patients can be considered for tissue donation. At Parkland Memorial Hospital, all deaths are referred to the regional organ procurement organization to determine the patient's candidacy for donation.

C. An extensive medical and social history is essential to assess the suitability of a brain-dead patient for organ donation.

D. Absolute contraindications to donation include:
1. Malignancies other than primary brain or localized skin cancers within the past five years or with evidence of metastatic disease
2. Sepsis
3. Active tuberculosis, syphilis, human immunodeficiency virus infection, acute hepatitis B infection, or other potentially lethal, untreatable, transmittable viral infections (such as West Nile virus).
4. Prion disease
5. There should be no evidence of infection, trauma, or significant chronic disease involving the organs considered for donation.

E. Relative contraindications: risks and benefits of transplantation must be carefully evaluated prior to considering utilizing organs from afflicted potential donors.
1. Medical comorbidities such as hypertension, diabetes mellitus, coronary artery disease, or peripheral vascular disease. Careful functional evaluation, including kidney biopsy, for example, is required prior to considering organs for donation.
2. Evidence of cytomegalovirus infection, other herpes viridae infections, or bacterial/fungal infections outside the anatomic cavity of the organ considered for donation
3. Prolonged hypotension, cardiac arrest, or high-dose vasoactive pharmacotherapy
4. Chronic hepatitis B or C – can be considered for transplantation into other hepatitis B or hepatitis C infected patients
5. A recent history of IV drug use

F. Should a patient fail to meet the criteria for organ donation or die of cardiac arrest, consideration should be given for tissue donation (i.e., corneas, skin, tendons, bone, or heart valves). Satisfactory renal transplantations are being performed using organs from non-heart-beating donors, and experimental data suggest that organs from non-heart-beating donors could be used for liver, pancreas, and lung transplantation as well.

IV. ESTABLISHING BRAIN DEATH

A. Legal definition
1. A person is considered legally dead if there is irreversible cessation of spontaneous respiratory and circulatory functions.
2. If artificial means of support are utilized, a person is declared dead if there is irreversible cessation of all spontaneous brain and brainstem function. Death is then pronounced before artificial means of support are terminated.

B. Generalized criteria for brain death
1. Etiology of coma must be defined.
2. No major abnormalities in acid-base, serum electrolytes, or glucose metabolism
3. Correction of hypotension, hypothermia (>32.2°C according to the President's commission but >35°C practically), and hypoxia.
4. Absence of central nervous system depressants, neuromuscular blocking agents, and toxins
5. Absence of spontaneous movements, including posturing (Note: except for spinal cord reflexes)
6. Absent brain-stem reflexes: pupillary, corneal, gag, oculocephalic, facial motor response, and oculovestibular
7. Apnea test
8. The period of observation may range from 2 to greater than 24 hours, depending on clinical circumstances. At Parkland Memorial Hospital, typically 2 brain death examinations are performed at least 6 hours apart. The second examination is conducted by an attending neurologist, neurosurgeon, or intensivist.
9. Confirmatory tests: in the presence of confounding factors, such as certain drugs, the absence of cerebral circulation can be confirmed by cerebral angiography, radionuclide imaging, cerebral blood flow scan, or electrocerebral silence on electroencephalogram (EEG).
   a. Note: these confirmatory tests can also be used to shorten the 6-hour interval described above.
10. Pediatric patients appear more resistant to neurologic insults than adults and therefore require age-based, longer periods of observation after the intial brain death examination. Pediatric patients also require confirmatory tests prior to declaring brain death.
    a. Infants (up to 2 months) – two examinations and EEGs at least 48 hours apart
    b. 2 months to 1 year – two examinations and EEGs at least 24 hours apart
    c. Greater than 1 year – two examinations and EEGs at least 12 hours apart

V. CONSENT FOR DONATION

A. The Uniform Anatomical Gift Act allows adults to donate all or parts of their body for research, education, or transplantation. Medical facilities

in most states are legally obligated to inquire appropriate next of kin regarding organ donation. The Uniform Anatomical Gift Act also establishes a hierarchy for the next of kin from whom to obtain consent:
1. Spouse
2. Adult child
3. Either parent
4. Guardian
5. Other authorized person
- **B.** Should a discrepancy exist between the donor's and the donor's family's wishes, disagreements often can be resolved with assistance from organ procurement organization personnel and the hospital chaplain's office. In reality, the family's wishes are generally honored over the donor's – despite the prior presence of authorization for donation such as on a driver's license.
- **C.** Permission must also be granted from the medical examiner's office when appropriate.
- **D.** The family should not be approached about organ donation until brain death has been declared and they have been allowed sufficient time to accept this reality. The topic may be discussed earlier if it is brought up by the family.
- **E.** In Texas, by law the regional organ procurement organization (OPO) must be contacted when brain death is imminent or when a neurologic insult has been deemed nonsurvivable.
- **F.** Attempts by OPO personnel to obtain consent are frequently more successful than those of physicians, and they are available to assist in this matter.

VI. MANAGEMENT OF THE ORGAN DONOR

- **A.** There is a paradigm shift from preservation of life to preserving potential donor organs with declaration of brain death. Brain death results in severe physiologic disturbances that complicate management. Additionally, depending on which organs are deemed suitable for harvest, optimal support of individual organs may conflict with each other. Education of the intensive care unit service to preserve end-organ function is an important component to maximize the number of organs harvested. Consultation with the organ procurement organization is essential to support potentially transplantable organs.
- **B.** The events leading to brain death result in dramatic physiologic alterations in most organ systems. Hemodynamic instability, metabolic and electrolyte disturbances, coagulopathy, and hypoxia are common. Once consent for donation has been obtained, organ harvest should be expedited since prolonged brain death has been associated with increased donor complications and organ dysfunction after transplantation.
- **C. Cardiovascular system**: the autonomic storm precipitated by brain death results in severe cardiovascular abnormalities. Profound catecholamine

surges lead to depression of cardiac function and microvascular ischemia, resulting in myocyte necrosis, apoptosis, and proinflammatory protein expression. Goals of cardiovascular support include:

1. Maintaining mean arterial pressure greater than 60 mm Hg and systolic blood pressure greater than 90 mm Hg but less than 170 mm Hg
2. Limiting tachycardia to reduce myocardial oxygen demand
3. Maintaining adequate volume status. Diabetes insipidus in these patients is common and should be treated aggressively with desmopressin or arginine vasopressin and/or volume replacement (as free water).
4. Central venous and pulmonary artery catheter monitoring are important adjuncts to assess the patient's volume and cardiac status.
5. Pharmacologic support to treat hypo- and hypertension once the donor's volume status has been optimized
6. Arrhythmias in potential donors are common and should be managed aggressively. Of note, bradyarrhythmias are atropine resistant and should be treated with other ionotropes or chronotropes. Alterations of vasoactive drugs may be required since many of these agents are arrhythmogenic.

D. Pulmonary system

1. If lung donation is being considered, protective ventilatory strategies to minimize baro- and volutrauma should be utilized. These include limiting positive end-expiratory pressures (<7.5 cm H_2O) and peak inspiratory pressures (<30 cm H_2O) and utilizing smaller tidal volumes (6 to 8 mL/kg).
2. Pulmonary function should be supported to provide at least an arterial oxygen saturation of 90% in order to support oxidative metabolism in other organs.
3. Minimize pulmonary edema by judicious volume replacement if the patient is a potential lung donor. The central venous pressure should be maintained at 8 cm H_2O or less.
4. Continue to provide aggressive pulmonary toilet, including bronchoscopy for severe atelectasis.

E. Renal system

1. Maintain adequate renal perfusion pressure and oxygen delivery.
2. Avoid nephrotoxins. However, contrast studies sometimes are required to assess suitability for cardiac donation.

F. Hepatic system

1. Maintain hepatic perfusion although the liver may be relatively more resistant to hemodynamic changes associated with brain death than other organs.
2. Aggressively treat hypernatremia to <155 mEq/L as hepatic grafts appear quite sensitive to increased sodium levels.

G. Neuroendocrine system

1. Diabetes insipidus occurs in 75% to 80% of donors. Patients may also develop the syndrome of inappropriate antidiuretic hormone

release (SIADH) or cerebral salt wasting. Urine output, urine osmolality, urine sodium, plasma osmolality, and plasma sodium levels can distinguish between these, as noted elsewhere.
   a. Diabetes insipidus is treated with free water replacement either as 5% dextrose or by the gastrointestinal tract (if functioning), along with pharmacotherapy with desmopressin or vasopressin. Vasopressin may be a superior choice because its catecholamine-sparing pressor activity reduces myocardial oxygen demand.
   b. SIADH is managed by free water restriction.
   c. Cerebral salt wasting requires isotonic or hypertonic saline volume replacement.
2. Hyperglycemia, either as a consequence of treating diabetes insipidus and/or the high catecholamine state of the donor, is most easily managed by an insulin drip. We have found protocol-driven insulin infusion most effective.
3. Other pituitary dysfunction: thyroid-stimulating hormone and adrenocorticotropic hormone release are decreased after brain death, leading to both hypothyroidism and adrenal insufficiency. Triiodothyronine (T3) is rapidly depleted in the donor and conversion of thyroxine (T4) to T3 is impaired, resulting in metabolic disturbances and a shift to anaerobic metabolism, particularly in the myocardium. Cortisol depletion may be in part responsible for the hemodynamic instability of the organ donor.
4. Hormonal cocktails: based on the above hormonal disturbances, hormonal resuscitation packets have been recommended for managing the donor. This includes methylprednisolone (15 mg/kg bolus), T3 (4 µg bolus followed by 3 µg/hour infusion) or thyroxine, arginine vasopressin (1 U bolus then 0.5 to 4 U/hour). These protocols have resulted in increased recovery of virtually every organ evaluated.

H. Miscellaneous
1. Electrolyte abnormalities are a common occurrence after brain death. These should be treated expediently because abnormalities in potassium, hypomagnesimia, hypocalcemia, and hypophosphatemia may result in cardiac rhythm disturbances.
2. Coagulopathy in most cases is due to thromboplastin release from the lethally injured brain and not hepatic dysfunction. Factor replacement as fresh-frozen plasma, cryoprecipitate, packed red blood cells, and platelets should be administered to treat nonsurgical bleeding.
3. Hypothermia results from loss of hypothalamic thermoregulation, transfusions, and crystalloid infusion. Proactive warming of the patient and the use of warmed IV fluids is essential as hypothermia, once developed, is difficult to correct.
4. Nutritional support either by parenteral nutrition or enteric feeding should be considered if the time to organ harvest is expected to be prolonged.

VII. SUGGESTED READINGS

Klintmalm GB, Levy MF: Organ Procurement and Preservation. Austin, TX, Landes Bioscience, 1999.

Lorber MI: What's new in general surgery? Transplantation. J Am Coll Surg 198(3):424-430, 2004.

Rosendale JD, Kauffman HM, McBride MA, et al: Aggressive pharmacologic donor management results in more transplanted organs. Transplantation 75(4):482-487, 2003.

Smith M: Physiologic changes during brain stem death: Lessons for management of the organ donor. J Heart Lung Transplant 23(9S),S217-S222, 2004.

Tuttle-Newhall JE, Collins BH, Kuo PC, Schoeder R: Organ donation and treatment of the multi-organ donor. Current Prob Surg 40(5):266-310, 2003.

Index

Note: Page numbers followed by the letter f refer to figures; those followed by the letter t refer to tables.

A

Abbreviated Injury Score (AIS), 19, 21, 21f, 22f
ABCDEs, in trauma care, 31-38, 34f-37f
Abdomen
  CT scan of, 67-68
  examination of, 40-41
Abdominal abscess, 208, 221
Abdominal aorta, injury to, repair of, 268
Abdominal trauma
  in children, 413-415
  vascular, 264-272
    blunt, 264
    evaluation of, 264
    management of
      exposure and, 265-271
      in midline inframesocolic area, 267-268
      in midline supramesocolic area, 266-267
      in pelvic retroperitoneum, 269-270
      in portal area, 271
      in upper lateral retroperitoneum, 268-269
      initial, 265
    mechanisms of, 264
    morbidity/mortality of, 271-272
    penetrating, 264
Abrasions, facial, 112
Abruptio placentae, traumatic, 407
Abscess, 487
  intra-abdominal, 208
    after liver trauma, 221
  pancreatic, 198
Abuse, child, fractures associated with, 381
Accidents, motor vehicle, 2
  blunt trauma of, 24-25
Acetabular fractures
  complications of, 311
  evaluation of, 310
  pediatric, 390
  treatment of, 310-311
Acetabulum, anatomy of, 309-310

Achilles tendon, rupture of, 345
Acid burns, 185
Acid-base disturbances, 468-470
  transfusion-related, 55
Acidosis
  metabolic, 469-470
  respiratory, 469
Acromioclavicular joint, separation of, 348-349
Active core rewarming, for hypothermia, 456
Active external rewarming, for hypothermia, 455-456
Acute adrenocortical insufficiency, 459
Acute lung injury
  anesthesia management of patient with, 423f, 424
  transfusion-related, 56-57
Acute Physiology and Chronic Health Evaluation (APACHE), 19
Acute renal failure
  classification of, 470
  diagnosis of, 471
  etiology of, 470-471
  treatment of, 471-472
Acute respiratory distress syndrome, 445-447
  clinical disorders associated with, 446t
  phases of, 446
  transfusion-related, 57
  treatment of, 446-447
Acyclovir, for infection/inflammation, 493
Adrenal insufficiency, 478
  treatment of, 49
Adrenocortical insufficiency, acute, 459
Adrenocorticotropic hormone, for adrenal insufficiency, 478
Advanced trauma life support (ATLS), 16-17
Age
  chronologic vs. physiologic, 416
  physiologic changes with, 416-417
  trauma risk associated with, 2

Airway
  assessment of, 31
  compromised, in pediatric trauma patient, 410-411
  during anesthesia, 420-421
  patent, maintenance of, in pregnant trauma patient, 405
Airway maneuvers, basic, 31-34, 34f-37f
Alkali burns, 185
Alkalosis
  metabolic, 470
  respiratory, 469
Allen's test, positive, 75
Allergic reactions, transfusion-related, 54
All-hazards disaster, preparedness and mitigation of, 29-30
Alpha radiation, 27
Alveolar-arterial (A-a) gradient, 440
Aminoglycosides, for infection/inflammation, 490
Amphotericin B, for infection/inflammation, 493
AMPLE mnemonic, 38
Amputation
  of digits, 372-373
  of limbs, in children, 382
  penile, 255
Anastomotic leak, postoperative, colorectal trauma and, 241
Anatomic dead space, 439
Anesthesia
  fluid resuscitation during, 422
  for facial injury repair, 113-115
  in acute lung injury patient, 423f, 424
  in pregnant trauma patient, 424
  intraoperative techniques of, 420-422, 424
  maintenance of, 421
  massive transfusion during, 422, 422t, 424
  nerve block. *See specific nerve block.*
  preoperative preparation for, 419-420
  standard equipment for, 419
Anesthetic agents, 419-420
Angiography
  in emergency department, 68
  of splenic injury, 228
  of traumatic brain injury, 100

Animal bites. *See also* Bite(s).
  to hand, 377
  treatment of, 122
Ankle dislocation, 343
Ankle fracture, 343-344
Ankle injury
  evaluation of, 342
  management principles for, 342-343
Ankle sprain, 343
Anterior chamber, examination of, 152-153
Anterior cruciate ligament
  injury to, treatment of, 339-340
  insufficiency of, 335, 336f, 337f
  combined laxities with, 338
Anterior drawer test, for anterior cruciate ligament instability, 335, 337f
Anteroposterior compression injury, pelvic, 304, 306t
  management of, 308
Antiaerobics, for infection/inflammation, 490
Antibiotics
  for bites, 398-399
  for burns, 283
  for infection/inflammation, 489-492
  for ventilator-associated pneumonia, 451
Antifungals, for infection/inflammation, 492-493
Antihistamines, for allergic reactions, 54
Antivirals, for infection/inflammation, 493
Aorta
  abdominal, repair of, 268
  ascending, injury to, 174
  descending, injury to, 174-175
  tears of, repair of, 266
Arrhythmias, 430
Arterial blood gases, normal values of, 468
Arterial injury, signs of, in extremity trauma, 260t
Arteriography
  of extremity vascular trauma, 260-261
  of genitourinary tract trauma, 252
  of thoracic trauma, 167
Arthritis, post-traumatic, after acetabular fractures, 311
Artifact(s), imaging, 71

Aspiration
  joint, for knee ligament injuries, 334
  risk of, nutritional support and, 498
Assist-control ventilation, 442
Atriocaval shunt, for liver trauma, 219-220, 220f
Atropine, 420
  intubation attenuation with, 32
Attenuation, in ultrasonography, 71
Audit filters, in national trauma registry, 22-23
Avulsion injury
  eyelid, repair of, 118
  facial, 112-113
  scrotal, 257
Axial skeleton, radiography of, 61
Aztreonam, for infection/inflammation, 491

B

Back, examination of, 41
Bacterial contamination, of transfused blood, 55
Ballistics, 25-26
Bartonella henselae, 397
Bean-bag projectiles, 27
Beck's triad, 167
Bedrest, for fractures and dislocations, 288
Bedside procedures, in surgical intensive care unit, 434-437
Bennett's fracture, 374-375
Benzodiazepines, 420
Berkow formula, for burns, 275, 276f
Beta radiation, 27
Beta-lactams, for infection/inflammation, 490-491
Bile duct, extrahepatic, injury to, 222-223, 222t
Biliary fistula, after liver trauma, 221
Biliary tree injury scale, extrahepatic, 222t
Bite(s), 396-402
  cat, 396-397
  dog, 396
  human, 397
  monkey, 398
  rodent, 397
  snake, 400-401
    treatment of, 401-402
  to hand, 377
  treatment of, 122

Bite(s) *(Continued)*
  antibiotic, 398-399
  indications for hospital admission in, 399
  initial, 398
  rabies immunization in, 400
  tetanus immunization in, 399-400
Bladder, imaging of, 69
Blast injury, 26
Blood glucose control, for infection/inflammation, 489
Blood products
  for infection/inflammation, 489
  in transfusions, 52-53, 53t
Blood substitutes, for transfusion, 58
Blood transfusion(s). See Transfusion(s).
Blowout fracture, orbital, 131-133, 132f, 133f
Blunt trauma
  abdominal vascular, 264
  cerebrovascular, criteria for, 67t
  colorectal, 235
    evaluation and diagnosis of, 237-238
  duodenal, 199-200
  pancreatic, 195
  physics of, 24-25
  renal, 244
  scrotal and testicular, 256-257
  small bowel, 205
  splenic, 227
  survival probability vs. Injury Severity Score in, 21f
  thoracic, 165-166
Body fluids, anatomy of, 461
Boutonnière deformity, 369
Boxer's fracture, 373-374
Braces, cast, for fractures and dislocations, 289
Brain death
  generalized criteria for, 503
  legal definition of, 503
Brain injury, traumatic, 97
  evaluation of, 97-99, 98t
  imaging studies of, 99-100
  management of, 100-102
  pediatric, 412-413
Breast, examination of, 40
Breathing, in trauma care, 34-35
  of pediatric patient, 411
  of pregnant patient, 405

Bronchoscopy, fiberoptic, in surgical intensive care unit, 434-435
Systemic Inflammatory Response Syndrome (SIRS) Score, 19, 20t
Buckle fracture, 379
Buck's traction, 288
Buckshot, 27
Buffers, 468-469
Bullets, rubber, 27
Burn(s)
  chemical, 284
    esophageal, 185-187
    genitalia and perineal, 258
    ocular, 154
  complications of, 281-282
  electrical, 282-284
    genitalia and perineal, 258
  evaluation of, 273-275, 274t, 276f
  full-thickness, 273, 274f
  infection of, 281
  nutritional support for, 280
  operative management of, 279-280
  partial-thickness, 273, 274t
  pediatric, 285-286
  resuscitation therapy for, 275, 277, 278f
  thermal, 27
    genitalia and perineal, 258
  wound care of, 277-279
Burn unit referral criteria, 274t
Burst injury
  duodenal, 199
  small bowel, 205

C

Calcaneus fracture, 344
Calcium chloride, 420
Capitate fracture, 376
Carbapenems, for infection/inflammation, 491
Carbon dioxide transport, 438-439
Cardiac abnormality(ies), electrical burn–induced, 282
Cardiac arrest, pediatric patient in, 412t
Cardiac arrhythmias, 430
Cardiac function, measurement and estimation of, 428-429
Cardiac output, 428
  determinants of, 430
Cardiac support, 430-431, 432t, 433
Cardiogenic shock, 46-47, 425-426

Cardiovascular changes
  in geriatric trauma patient, 416
  in hypothermia, 454
    management of, 457
  in pregnant trauma patient, 403-404
Cardiovascular system, management of, in organ donor, 504-505
Carotid artery
  left, injury to, 176
  right, injury to, 175
Carotid-cavernous fistula, 155
Carpal fracture(s), 376
Carpometacarpal joint, injury to, 371, 372
Caspofungin, for infection/inflammation, 493
Casts, for fractures and dislocations, 289
Cat bites, 396-397. *See also* Bite(s).
Cat scratch disease, 397
Catheter(s)
  arterial, 75-76
  central venous, 79-88. *See also* Central venous catheterization.
  urinary, 89
Catheter-over-the-needle technique, of central venous catheterization, 80
Catheter-related infection, 479-480
Catheter-through-the-needle technique, of central venous catheterization, 80
Caustic ingestion
  agents in, 185
  complications of, 187
  evaluation of, 185-186
  treatment of, 186-187
Celiac artery, injury to, repair of, 266-267
Celiotomy, 229, 230f, 240
  decompressive, in surgical intensive care unit, 434
  exploratory, 265
  in pregnant trauma patient, 406
Central nervous system changes
  in geriatric trauma patient, 416-417
  in hypothermia, 454-455
Central venous catheterization, 79-88
  anatomy in, 79-80, 80f
  catheter-over-the-needle technique of, 80
  catheter-through-the-needle technique of, 80
  complications of, 86-88
  femoral vein access in, 84-85

Central venous catheterization *(Continued)*
  indications for, 79
  internal jugular vein access in
    anterior approach to, 82-83
    central approach to, 82, 84f
    posterior approach to, 83-84, 85f
  pearls and pitfalls of, 88
  pulmonary artery catheter monitoring in, 85-86
  Seldinger guide-wire technique of, 81
  subclavian vein access in
    infraclavicular approach to, 81-82, 81f
    supraclavicular approach to, 82, 83f
  ultrasound-guided, 86
Cephalosporins, for infection/inflammation, 491
Cerebral edema, 103
Cerebrovascular injury, blunt, criteria for, 67t
Cervical spine. *See also* Neck *entries.*
  assessment of, 39
  clinical clearing of, 61-63
  CT scan of, 67
  injury to, determination of level of, 106t
  radiography of, 60
  stabilization of, 31
Cesarean section, emergency, 408
Chemical burns, 284. *See also* Burn(s).
  esophageal, 185-187
  genitalia and perineal, 258
  ocular, 154
Chest. *See also* Thoracic *entries.*
  CT scan of, 67
  examination of, 40
  flail, 178
  radiography of, 60, 61t
Chest injury, in children, 413
Chest tube. *See also* Thoracostomy.
  complications of, 92
  placement of, 90-91, 91f, 166
  removal of, 91
Chest wound, open, 178
Child abuse, fractures associated with, 381
Children. *See* Pediatric *entries.*
Chlorpromazine, intravenous, for heat stroke, 459
Cholangitis, 485

Cholecystocholangiography, needle, of pancreatic injury, 196
Chronologic age, vs. physiologic age, 416
Circulation, in trauma care, 35-36
  of pediatric patient, 411-412
  of pregnant patient, 405
Clavicle fracture, 347-348
  in children, 389
Closed reduction, of mandibular fracture, 145
Closed-tube thoracostomy, 90-92, 91f
Coagulation changes, in hypothermia, 454
Coagulopathy
  correction of, 51, 51f
  in organ donor, 506
  in traumatic brain injury, 101
Cold injury, 284-285
Collateral ligament(s)
  injury to, treatment of, 339
  medial, insufficiency of, 336-337, 338f
Collisions, motor-pedestrian, blunt trauma of, 25
Colocutaneous fistula, 241
Colonic trauma. *See also* Colorectal trauma.
  destructive, 239
  nondestructive, 239
Colorectal trauma, 235-241
  blunt, 235
    evaluation and diagnosis of, 237-238
  complications of, 241
  evaluation and diagnosis of, 236-238
  management of
    nonoperative, 238
    operative, 238-240
  mechanisms of, 235-236
  penetrating, 236
    evaluation and diagnosis of, 236-237
  postoperative care for, 241
Colostomy, 239-240
Colotomy, 240
Compartment syndrome, 345, 377
  causes of, 292
  definition of, 292
  diagnosis of, 292, 293f
  pediatric, 380
  treatment of, 292-295

Compartment syndrome *(Continued)*
  forearm technique in, 294, 298f-301f
  lower leg technique in, 293, 294f-296f
  thigh technique in, 294-295
Complete blood count, in febrile patient, 476
Compression forces, in colorectal trauma, 235
Compression injury, pelvic, 304, 306t
  management of, 308
Computed tomography
  abdominal, of febrile patient, 476
  of genitourinary tract trauma, 250-251
  of pancreatic injury, 195
  of pelvic fractures, 304
  of splenic injury, 228
  of thoracic injury, 167
  of traumatic brain injury, 99-100
Condylar fracture
  humeral, 353
  in children, 386
Conjunctiva, examination of, 152
Consent, for organ donation, 503-504
Continuous arterial venous rewarming (CAVR), in surgical intensive care unit, 435-436
Contusions, 103
  facial, 111
Coral snake bites, 401. *See also* Bite(s).
Core rewarming, for hypothermia, 456
Cornea, examination of, 152
Cosyntropin stimulation test, for adrenal insufficiency, 49
Coup-contrecoup injury, 103
Cranial nerve(s). *See also specific cranial nerve.*
  examination of, in traumatic brain injury, 99
Cricothyroidotomy, 33, 35f-37f
  needle, 33-34
Crofab antivenin, 402
Crotalid(s), 401
Crotalid envenomation, grades of, 402
Cruciate ligament
  anterior. *See* Anterior cruciate ligament.
  posterior. *See* Posterior cruciate ligament.

Crush(ing) injury
  duodenal, 199
  physics of, 24
  small bowel, 205
Cryporecipitate, transfusion of, 52-53, 53t
Cullen sign, 198
Curling's ulcer, in burn patients, 281
Cytokines, in inflammatory response, 475
Cytomegalovirus (CMV) infection, transfusion-related, 55

D

Damage control surgery, 93-96
  pathophysiology involved in, 93
  stages of, 94-96
Dantrolene, for malignant hyperthermia, 457, 479
Dead space ventilation, 439
Débridement
  of pediatric open fractures, 382
  resectional, in liver trauma, 216-217
Deceleration forces, in colorectal trauma, 236
Deceleration injury(ies), renal, 244
Deep vein thrombosis, 477
  diagnosis of, 291-292
  prevention of, 291
  prophylaxis for, 107
  treatment of, 292
Degloving injury, of penile or scrotal skin, 255
Dentoalveolar fracture(s), 138
Diabetes insipidus, in organ donor, 505-506
Diagnostic peritoneal lavage
  in emergency department, 65-66
  in liver trauma, 213
  in splenic injury, 228
Diaphragmatic injury, 180-182, 181t
Diaphyseal fracture, 345
Diazepam, for sedation of burn patients, 274
Diffuse axonal injury, 103
Digital nerve(s), injury to, 370
Digital nerve blocks, 363, 365-366, 365f, 366f
Diphenhydramine, for allergic reactions, 54
Disability, in trauma care, 36
  of pediatric patient, 412, 412t

Disaster(s)
  all-hazards
    hospital space considerations for, 29-30
    inventory of available and desired supplies for, 29
  management of, 29
Disaster plans, 29
  enactment of, 30
  review of, 30
Disaster protocol, 30
Dislocation(s). *See also* Fracture(s).
  ankle, 343
  elbow, 353-354, 354f
    in children, 388
  glenohumeral, 349-350
  hip, 312-314
    in children, 391
  knee, 340-341
    in children, 393
  management of
    definitive, 288-289
    initial, 287-288
  patellar, in children, 393
  scapulothoracic, 348
  shoulder, in children, 389
  sternoclavicular, 347
  tarsometatarsal, 345
  wrist, 375-376
Displaced fracture, in children, 394
Disseminated intravascular coagulation, transfusion-related, 56
Distal interphalangeal joint
  amputation through, 372
  injury to, 370-371
Distributive shock, 48-49, 426-427
Dobutamine, for infection/inflammation, 489
Dog bites, 396. *See also* Bite(s).
Dopamine, for infection/inflammation, 488
Dorsal nasal block, for facial injury repair, 115
Drainage
  closed-tube thoracostomy, 90-92, 91f. *See also* Thoracostomy.
  of bile leaks, in liver trauma, 218
Dressing(s), for burn wounds, 279-280
Duodenum
  anatomy of, 194

Duodenum *(Continued)*
  injuries to
    blunt, 199-200
    complications of, 202-203
    diagnosis of, 199-200
    epidemiology of, 193
    grading of, 200-201
    imaging of, 200
    intraoperative evaluation of, 200-201
    mechanisms of, 199
    penetrating, 199
    treatment of, 201-202

E
Ear
  injury to, repair of, 121
  surface anatomy of, 109, 112f
Echocardiography
  in emergency department, 69
  of thoracic trauma, 168
Echogenicity, in ultrasonography, 71
Edema, cerebral, 103
Edentulous patient, mandibular fracture in, 145
Eikenella corrodens, 397
Elbow
  dislocation of, 353-354, 354f
    in children, 388
  fracture of, in children, 385
Electrical burns, 27, 282-284. *See also* Burn(s).
  to genitalia and perineum, 258
Electrocardiography, in emergency department, 69
Electrolyte(s)
  abnormal, in organ donor, 506
  daily requirement of, 461-462
Embolization, of bleeding, after hepatic trauma, 221
Embolus
  catheter-related, 76
  fat, 295-297
  pulmonary, 291-292, 477. *See also* Pulmonary thromboembolism.
Emergency cesarean section, 408
Emergency department
  diagnostic modality(ies) of, 60-70
    angiography as, 68
    computed tomography as, 67-68, 67t
    magnetic resonance imaging as, 68

Emergency department *(Continued)*
    miscellaneous, 69-70
    peritoneal lavage as, 65-66
    plain films as, 60-63, 61t, 62t
    ultrasound as, 63-65, 64f, 65f
    urologic imaging as, 68-69
  evaluation of burns in, 273-275
  thoracotomy in, 166
  treatment of fractures in, 287-288
Empyema, 483
Endocrine changes, in hypothermia, 455
  management of, 457
Endocrine response, to stress and injury, 495, 496t
Endoscopic retrograde cholangiopancreatography, of pancreatic injury, 195
Enteral nutrition. *See also* Nutrition.
  vs. parenteral nutrition, 497
Enterocolitis, pseudomembranous, 486
Ephedrine, 420
Epicondyle fracture, medial, in children, 386
Epidural hematoma, 102
Epilepsy, post-traumatic, 101
Epinephrine, 420
  for allergic reactions, 54
Escharotomy, for burns, 277, 278f
Esophageal injury, 162-163, 183-187
  caustic ingestion in, 185-187
  evaluation of, 183-184
  incidence of, 183
  management of, 184
  outcome of, 184
Esophagography, 183
  barium, of thoracic trauma, 167-168
  in emergency department, 69
Esophagoscopy, 183
Etomidate, 419
  sedation/paralysis with, 32
Euvolemic hypernatremia, 463-464
Excision, of burns, 279
Exposure, in trauma care, 36, 38
Extensor tendon(s)
  injury to, 368-369
  zones of, 367, 369f
External fixation
  of fractures, 289
  of pelvic fractures, 307

External rewarming, for hypothermia
  active, 455-456
  passive, 455
Extracellular fluid, 461
Extrahepatic bile duct, injury to, 222-223, 222t
Extraocular movements, examination of, 148-150
Extremity(ies). *See also specific part.*
  CT scan of, 68
  examination of, 41
  lower, fractures and dislocations of, 312-346
    pediatric, 390-395
  radiography of, 61
  upper, fractures and dislocations of, 347-359
    pediatric, 382-390
  vascular trauma of, 259-263
    epidemiology of, 259
    evaluation of, 259-261, 260f
    management of, 261-263
    mechanisms of, 259
    pathophysiology of, 259
    postoperative care for, 263
Eye(s). *See also specific part.*
  anatomy of, 148, 149f
  multiple injuries to, examination of, 148-154
Eyebrow injury, repair of, 116-117
Eyelid(s)
  anatomy of, 117, 118f, 119f
  avulsion injury to, repair of, 118
  examination of, 150-151, 151f
  laceration of, repair of, 117

F
Face
  CT scan of, 67
  sensory anatomy within, 109, 114f
  soft tissue injuries to, 109-122. *See also* Soft tissue trauma, facial.
  surface anatomy of, 109, 110f
Facial avulsion injury, 112-113
Facial fracture(s). *See also at specific anatomic site.*
  mandibular, 142-146
  maxillary and midface, 137-142
  upper, 123-136
Facial nerve, branches of, 109, 113f
Factor VII, activated, transfusion of, 53

Falls, 3
  blunt trauma of, 25
Fascial compartments, of leg, 294f
Fasciotomy, 263
Fat embolism syndrome, 295-297
Fat metabolism, during stress and injury, 496
Fatalities
  firearm-related, 3
  non-CNS traumatic, comparison of, 6t
Febrile reactions
  evaluation of, 475-476
  transfusion-related, 54
Femoral artery, catheterization of, 75
Femoral fracture(s)
  subtrochanteric, 317-318
  supracondylar, 321-325
    classification of, 322-323, 322f-324f
    complications of, 325
    evaluation of, 322
    treatment of, 323-325
Femoral neck fracture
  classification of, 315, 315f
  complications of, 316-317
  treatment of, 315-316
Femoral nerve trauma, in hip dislocation, 312
Femoral shaft fracture
  complications of, 319-320
  in children, 391-392
  occurrence of, 318
  special situations associated with, 320-321
  treatment of, 319
Femoral vein
  access to, in central venous catheterization, 84-85
  anatomy of, 80
Fentanyl, intubation attenuation with, 32
Fetal injury, 408
Fiberoptic bronchoscopy, in surgical intensive care unit, 434-435
Finger tip amputation, 372
Firearm-related fatalities, 3
Fistula
  biliary, after liver trauma, 221
  carotid-cavernous, 155
  colocutaneous, 241
  duodenal, 203
  pancreatic, 198
  small bowel, 208

Flail chest, 178
Flaps, in facial soft tissue injury repair, 116
Flexor tendon(s), 366-367, 367f
  injury to, 367-368
  zones of, 367, 368f
Flexor tenosynovitis, 378
Fluconazole, for infection/inflammation, 493
Fluid(s)
  daily requirement of, 461
  loss of, replacement of, 463
Fluid resuscitation
  during anesthesia, 422
  for burn patients, 283
  for pediatric burn patients, 285-286
  for shock, 43
Fluid volume disorders, 462
Flumazenil, for facial injury repair, 113
Focused Assessment for Sonographic Examination of Trauma Patient (FAST), 63
  for blunt abdominal wounds, 64, 65f
  for penetrating torso wounds, 63, 64f
Foot fracture, 344-345
Foot injury(ies)
  evaluation of, 342
  management principles for, 342-343
Forced inspiratory oxygen (FiO_2), 443
Forearm fracture, 356, 357f
Foreign body(ies), rectal, 240
Formula, selection of, in nutritional support, 498
Fracture(s). *See also at anatomic site for details; specific type of fracture.*
  acetabular, 309-311
  concomitant, management of, 262-263
  facial
    mandibular, 142-146
    maxillary and midface, 137-142
    upper, 123-136
  lower extremity, 312-346
  management of, 41
    definitive, 288-289
    initial, 287-288
  pediatric, 379-395. *See also Pediatric fracture(s).*
  pelvic, 303-309
  penile, 254
  rib, 177

Fracture(s) (Continued)
skull, 102
sternal, 177-178
ultrasonography of, 74
upper extremity, 347-359
Frequency, in ultrasonography, 71
Fresh frozen plasma, transfusion of, 51, 52, 53t
Frontal sinus, anatomy of, 123
Frontal sinus fracture, 123-124, 126
cranialization of, 126f
treatment algorithm for, 125f
Frostbite, 284-285
Frykman classification, of distal radial fractures, 358t

G

Galeazzi fracture, 356
in children, 385
Gallbladder injury, 221-222
Gamma radiation, 27
Gancyclovir, for infection/inflammation, 493
Garden classification, of femoral neck fractures, 315, 315f
Gastric artery(ies), 226
Gastric feeding, vs. small bowel feeding, 497-498
Gastric trauma, 188-192
diagnosis of, 189-190
epidemiology of, 188
grading of, 190
management of, 190-191
mechanisms of, 188-189
pearls and pitfalls of, 192
postoperative care of, 191
Gastrointestinal changes
in hypothermia, 455
in pregnant trauma patient, 404
Gastrointestinal ulceration, in burn patients, 281
Gender, trauma risk associated with, 2
Genitalia, chemical, electrical, and thermal injury to, 258
Genitourinary changes, in pregnant trauma patient, 404
Genitourinary trauma
diagnostic studies of, 250-253
imaging of, indications for, 250
Geriatric trauma, 25
demographics of, 416

Geriatric trauma (Continued)
physiologic changes associated with, 416-417
treatment of, 417
Gilles approach, to zygomaticomaxillary complex fracture, 135
Glasgow Coma Scale, 97-99, 98t
Glasgow Come Score, 18, 18t
adapted for children, 412t
Glenohumeral joint, dislocation of, 349-350
Globe, ruptured, 155
Glucose metabolism, during stress and injury, 496
Glycopeptides, for infection/inflammation, 491-492
Gout, 478
Grafts, in facial soft tissue injury repair, 116
Great auricular block, for facial injury repair, 115
Great vessels, injury to, 174
radiographic abnormalities associated with, 61t
Greenstick fracture, 379, 384, 394
Grey-Turner sign, 198
Gunshot wounds, 103. See also Penetrating trauma.
thoracoabdominal, 165

H

Hamate fracture, 376
Hand
anatomy of, 366-367
extensor tendon zones of, 367, 369f
extensor tendons of, injury to, 368-369
flexor tendon zones of, 367, 368f
flexor tendons of, 366-367, 367f
injury to, 367-368
fracture of, 373-375
in children, 382-383
infections of, 377-378
Hand injury(ies)
anesthetic techniques for, 363, 364f-366f, 365-366
involving blood vessels, 370
involving extensor and flexor tendons, 367-369
involving ligaments, 370-372
involving nerves, 370
mechanisms of, 360

Hand injury(ies) *(Continued)*
  physical examination of, 360-361, 361f, 362f, 363
Harris-Benedict formula, for nutrition, 499
Head
  CT scan of, 67
  penetrating injuries to, 103-104
Heat stroke, 458-459
  complications of, 459-460
Hematoma
  epidural, 102
  subdural, 102-103
Hematopoietic changes, in pregnant trauma patient, 404
Hemobilia, after liver trauma, 221
Hemodialysis, for acute renal failure, 472
Hemolytic reactions, transfusion-related, 54
Hemopneumothorax, 178-179
Hemorrhage
  in pelvic fractures, 309
  recurrent, after liver trauma, 221
  retrobulbar, 155
Hemorrhagic pancreatitis, 198-199
Hemorrhagic (hypovolemic) shock, 44-46, 45t, 425, 426t
Hemothorax, traumatic, ultrasonography of, 74
Heparin, unfractionated, for pulmonary thromboembolism, 449
Hepatic. *See also* Liver *entries*.
Hepatic artery
  injury to, repair of, 271
  ligation of, 217
Hepatic system, management of, in organ donor, 505
Hepatic vein, injury to, liver trauma and, 218-219
Hepatitis B, transfusion-related, 55
Hepatitis C, transfusion-related, 55
Hepatotomy, with vascular ligation, 216, 217f
Herniation, uncal, 155
Herpetic whitlow, 377-378
High pressure injection injury, to hand, 378
Hindfoot fractures, 344
Hip dislocation, 312-314
  in children, 391
Hip fracture, 314, 317
  in children, 390-391

Homicide, 1, 4
Hospital admission, indications for, bites and, 399
Hospital disaster committee, 29
Host defense, 475
Human bites, 397. *See also* Bite(s).
  to hand, 377
Human immunodeficiency virus (HIV) infection, transfusion-related, 55
Humeral fracture(s)
  diaphyseal, 352
  distal, 352-353
    in children, 385-386
  proximal, 350, 351f, 352
    in children, 389
Humeral shaft fracture, in children, 388
Hydrocortisone
  for acute adrenocortical insufficiency, 459
  for adrenal insufficiency, 49
  for allergic reactions, 54
Hypercalcemia, 466
Hypercapnia, 441
Hyperflexion injury, in children, 414-415
Hyperglycemia, in organ donor, 506
Hyperglycemic protocol, 500
Hyperkalemia, 464-465
  transfusion-related, 55
Hypermagnesemia, 467
Hypermetabolic response, postinjury, 495
Hypernatremia, 463-464
Hyperphosphatemia, 468
Hyperthermia
  complications of, 459-460
  etiology of, 477
  in intensive care unit, 457-460
  malignant, 457-458, 479
    complications of, 460
Hypertonic hyponatremia, 464
Hyperventilation, in traumatic brain injury, 101
Hypervolemic hypernatremia, 464
Hypocalcemia, 466-467
  transfusion-related, 55
Hypokalemia, 465-466
Hypomagnesemia, 467
Hyponatremia, 464
Hypophosphatemia, 468
Hypothermia
  cardiovascular changes in, 454

Hypothermia *(Continued)*
  central nervous system changes in, 454-455
  coagulation changes in, 454
  diagnosis of, 455
  endocrine changes in, 455
  etiology of, 453
  gastrointestinal changes in, 455
  in intensive care unit, 453-457
  in organ donor, 506
  oxygen consumption in, 453-454
  pathophysiology of, 453-455
  renal changes in, 455
  respiratory changes in, 454
  transfusion-related, 56
  treatment of, 455-457
Hypotonic hyponatremia, 464
Hypovolemia, 462
Hypovolemic hypernatremia, 463
Hypovolemic (hemorrhagic) shock, 44-46, 45t, 425, 426t
Hypoxemia, 440-441

I

Iatrogenic injury, thoracic, 166
Ileum, anatomy of, 204
Ileus, in burn patients, 281
Iliac artery, injury to, repair of, 270
Iliac vein, injury to, repair of, 270
Iliosacral screw fixation, of pelvic fractures, 307
Immunosuppression, transfusion-related, 54
Infection(s). *See also specific infection.*
  antibiotics in, 489-492
  catheter-related, 76
  definition of, 474
  etiology of, 479-488
  in surgical intensive care unit, 474-493
  of burn wounds, 281
  of hand, 377-378
  transfusion-related, 55
  treatment of, 488-489
    antibiotics in, 489-492
    antifungals in, 492-493
    antivirals in, 493
Inferior vena cava, injury to
  liver trauma and, 218-219
  repair of, 268

Inflammation
  definition of, 474
  etiology of, 479-488
  response to, 475
  treatment of, 488-489
Infraorbital nerve block, for facial injury repair, 114-115
Infratrochlear nerve block, for facial injury repair, 115
Inhalational anesthetic agents, 420
Injury. *See* Trauma *entries; at anatomic site; specific type of injury.*
Injury Severity Score (ISS), 19, 21t
  vs. survival probability, 21f, 22f
Innominate artery, injury to, 175
Innominate vein, injury to, 175
Intensive care unit
  cardiovascular support and management in, 425-433
  surgical
    bedside procedures in, 434-437
    infection in, 474-493
    thermoregulatory disorders in, 453-460
Intercostal nerve block, 173-174, 173f
Interferon, for infection/inflammation, 493
Intermittent mandatory ventilation (IMV), 442
Internal fixation, of fractures, 289
Internal jugular vein
  access to
    anterior approach to, 82-83
    central approach to, 82, 84f
    posterior approach to, 83-84, 85f
  anatomy of, 79-80
Intertrochanteric hip fracture, 317
Intra-abdominal abscess, 208
  after liver trauma, 221
Intra-abdominal infections, 484-485
Intracellular fluid, 461
Intracranial pressure, monitoring of, 101-102
Intrapulmonary shunt, 439-440
Intravascular volume, restoration of, 50
Intubation
  indications for, in pediatric trauma patient, 411
  rapid sequence, 31-32
Inverse-ratio ventilation, 442
Iris, examination of, 153
Isotonic hyponatremia, 464

J

Jejunum, anatomy of, 204
Joint(s). *See also named joint.*
  aspiration of, for knee ligament injuries, 334
Jones fracture, 345

K

Kanavel's cardinal signs, of tenosynovitis, 378
Ketamine, 419
Kidney(s). *See also Renal entries.*
  anatomy of, 243
  imaging of, 68
Knee dislocation, 340-341
  in children, 393
Knee ligament injury(ies), 334-340
  classification of, 334-335
  evaluation of, 334
  in children, 393
  mechanisms of, 335t
  stability testing of, 335-339
    combined laxities in, 338-339
    isolated laxities in, 335-337, 336f-338f
  treatment of, 339-340

L

Lacerations
  facial, 112-113
  perineal, 257
  scrotal, 257
  tendon, 345
  testicular, 257
Lachman test, for anterior cruciate ligament instability, 335, 336f
Lacrimal apparatus, repair of, 118
Laryngeal injury, 161-162
Lateral compression injury, pelvic, 304, 306t
  management of, 308
Lateral condylar fracture, in children, 386
Lawn mower injury(ies), 346
Le Fort I fracture, 138, 140f
Le Fort II fracture, 138, 140f
Le Fort III fracture, 139, 140f
Left upper quadrant, ultrasonography of, 72, 73f
Leg, fascial compartments of, 294f
Legislation, trauma, 5, 7
Lens, examination of, 153-154
Lidocaine, intubation attenuation with, 32
Life support, advanced trauma, 16-17
Ligament(s). *See named ligament.*
Ligament injury(ies)
  in dislocations, 340-341
  of hand, 370-373
  of knee, 334-340. *See also* Knee ligament injury(ies).
Lightning injuries, 283-284
Limb amputation, in children, 382
Lip(s), laceration of, repair of, 119-120
Lisfranc injury, 345
Liver. *See also* Hepatic; Hepatitis; Hepato- *entries.*
  anatomy of, 210, 211f
Liver injury scale, 212t
Liver suturing, deep, 216
Liver transplantation, after hepatic trauma, 220
Liver trauma, 210-221
  classification of, 210, 212t
  complex injury in, operative management of, 215-216
  complications of, 221
  diagnosis and assessment of, 212-213
  management of
    initial, 210-212
    nonoperative, 214
    operative, 214-221, 217f, 219f
  pearls and pitfalls of, 223
  simple injury in, operative management of, 215
Local anesthesia, for facial injury repair, 114-115
Lorazepam, 420
Lower extremity(ies). *See also specific part.*
  fractures and dislocations of, 312-346
  pediatric, 390-395
Lunate fracture, 376
Lung(s). *See also* Pulmonary; Respiratory *entries.*
  protective strategy for, in mechanical ventilation, 443-444
Lymphatics, of neck, injury to, 164

M

Macrolides, for infection/inflammation, 492
Mafenide acetate, for burn wounds, 279

Magnetic resonance imaging
    in emergency department, 68
    of knee ligament injuries, 334
Maintenance anesthetic agents, 420
Malignant hyperthermia, 457-458, 479
    complications of, 460
Mallet finger, 282
Mandible
    anatomy of, 143, 143f
    innervation of, 143-144
Mandibular block, for facial injury
        repair, 115
Mandibular fracture(s), 142-146
    in edentulous patient, 145
    management of, 144-145
    pediatric, 145
    postoperative care for, 145-146
    surgical complications of, 146
Mannitol, in prevention of secondary
        brain injury, 101
Massive transfusion protocol, 57-58, 58t
Maternal death, impending, 408
Mattox maneuver, 266
Maxillary fracture
    classification of, 137-139, 140f
    clinical presentation of, 139, 141
    complications of, 142
    management of, 141-142
Maxillofacial assessment, in trauma
        care, 39
Mean arterial pressure, 430
Mechanical ventilation
    lung mechanics in, 441-442
    modes of, 442-443
    protective lung strategy in, 443-444
    ventilator settings in, 443
    weaning from, guidelines for, 444-445,
        444t
Medial collateral ligament, insufficiency of
    with valgus or medial laxity, 336, 338f
    with varus or lateral laxity, 336-337
Medial condylar fracture, in children, 386
Medial epicondyle fracture, in children,
        386
Median nerve block, 363, 364f
Mediastinitis, 483
Mediastinum, widened, multiple injuries
        to, 177
Meleney's ulcer, 488
Meningitis, 486-487
Mental nerve block, for facial injury
        repair, 115

Mesenteric artery, superior
    anatomy of, 204
    repair of injury to, 267
Mesenteric vein, superior
    anatomy of, 204
    repair of injury to, 267
Metabolic acidosis, 469-470
Metabolic alkalosis, 470
Metabolism, during stress and injury,
        495-496
Metacarpal head fracture, 373
Metacarpal neck fracture, 373-374
Metacarpal shaft fracture, 374
Metaphyseal fractures, 371-372
    in children, 388
Metatarsal fractures, 344-345
Methylprednisolone, intravenous, for
        spinal cord injury, 107
Midazolam, 420
    sedation/paralysis with, 32
Midface, anatomy of, 137, 138f,
        139f
Midface fractures
    classification of, 137-139, 140f
    clinical presentation of, 139, 141
    complications of, 142
    management of, 141-142
Midfoot fractures, 344
Military conflicts, development of
        organized trauma care from, 5
Miniplate fixation, of midface fractures,
        142
Missiles, penetrating, characteristics of
        damage from, 26
Mixed venous oxygen saturation,
        428-429
Monkey bites, 398. *See also* Bite(s).
Monobactams, for
        infection/inflammation, 491
Monteggia fracture
    in children, 385
    types of, 356, 357f
Morbidity and mortality, of abdominal
        vascular trauma, 271-272
Morphine, for sedation of burn patients,
        274
Motor examination, of spinal cord injury,
        105-106
Motor vehicle accidents, 2
    blunt trauma of, 24-25
Motor-pedestrian collisions, blunt
        trauma of, 25

Multiple organ dysfunction syndrome (MODS), definition of, 474-475
Musculoskeletal trauma
  complication(s) of, 290-302
    compartment syndrome as, 292-295, 293f-296f, 298f-301f
    fat embolism syndrome as, 295-297
    rhabdomyolysis as, 297, 301-302
    thromboembolic disease as, 290-292
  in children, 415
  to neck, 163-164

N

Nailbed injury, 372
Naloxone, for facial injury repair, 114
Nasal fracture, 126-128, 128f
Nasogastric tubes, types of, 90
Naso-orbito-ethmoid complex, fractures of, 128-131
  classification of, 130
Nasotracheal intubation, 32-33
National trauma registry, 22-23
Neck. *See also* Cervical spine.
  anatomic zones of, 158-159, 158f
  CT scan of, 67, 67t
  sensory anatomy within, 109, 114f
Neck trauma, 157-164
  assessment of, 157-158
  esophageal, 162-163
  laryngeal, 161-162
  lymphatic, 164
  musculoskeletal, 163-164
  pearls and pitfalls of, 164
  pharyngeal, 161
  tracheal, 162
  vascular, 159-161
Needle cholecystocholangiography, of pancreatic injury, 196
Needle cricothyroidotomy, 33-34
Neer classification, of proximal humeral fracture, 350, 351f
Nerve block(s). *See specific nerve block.*
Nerve injury
  in hand, 370
  in knee dislocation, 340
Neuroendocrine system, management of, in organ donor, 505-506
Neurogenic shock, 48, 427
Neuroleptic malignant syndrome, 458
  complications of, 460
Neurologic assessment, in trauma care, 41

Neurologic trauma, 97-108
  electrical burns with, 283
  extremity vascular trauma with, management of, 263
  imaging studies of, 99-100
  initial evaluation of, 97-99, 98t
  management of, 100-102
    ICP monitoring in, 101-102
    prevention of secondary injury in, 100-101
    surgical, 104-105
  specific injuries in, 102-104
  spinal cord injuries in, 105-108, 106t
Neuromuscular blocking agents, 419-420
Neutron radiation, 28
Night stick fracture, 356
Nondisplaced fracture, in children, 394
Nonlethal weapons, 27
Norepinephrine, for infection/inflammation, 489
Nose. *See also* Nasal; Naso- *entries.*
  anatomy of, 126-127
  injury to, repair of, 119
  surface anatomy of, 109, 111f
Nuclear radiation, 27-28
Nucleoside analogs, for infection/inflammation, 493
Nursemaid's elbow, 388
Nutrition, 496-499
  aspiration risk associated with, 498
  early vs. delayed, 496-497
  goals of, 496
  hyperglycemic protocol in, 500
  indications for, 497
  monitoring of, 499-500
  parenteral, 498-499
  requirements for, assessment of, 499
  route of administration of, 497-498
Nutritional support
  for burn patient, 280
  for organ donor, 506
  formula selection for, 498
Nystatin, for infection/inflammation, 493

O

Obstructive shock, 47-48
Olecranon fracture, 355
  in children, 388
Open fracture(s)
  ankle, 344
  pediatric, 381-382
  pelvic, 309

Open plate fixation, of pelvic fractures, 307
Open reduction, of mandibular fracture, 145
Ophthalmic injury(ies), 148-156
  examination of, 148-154
  imaging of, 154
  pearls and pitfalls of, 156
  vision-threatening, recognition of, 154-155
Optic neuropathy, traumatic, 154-155
Oral mucosa lacerations, repair of, 121-122
Orbit, anatomy of, 131
Orbital fracture, 131-134
  blowout, 131-133, 132f, 133f
Orbital rim, examination of, 150
Organ donation
  consent for, 503-504
  contraindications to, 502
  donor criteria in, 502-503
  establishing brain death in, 503
  legislative background to, 501
Organ donor(s)
  criteria for, 502-503
  management of, 504-506
  shortage of, 501
Orotracheal intubation, 32
Ossification, heterotopic, after acetabular fractures, 311
Ottawa ankle rules, for sprains, 343
Overwhelming postsplenectomy infection (OPSI), 233
Oxygen consumption, 429
  in hypothermia, 453-454
    management of, 456-457
Oxygen content (CaO_2), 438
Oxygen delivery (DO_2), 429, 438
Oxygen extraction ratio (O_2ER), 438
Oxygen uptake (VO_2), 438
Oxygen-carrying capacity, restoration of, 50

P

Packed red blood cells, transfusion of, 52, 53t
Palsy, sciatic nerve, after acetabular fractures, 311
Pancreas, anatomy of, 193
Pancreatic trauma, 194-199
  blunt, 195

Pancreatic trauma (Continued)
  classification of, 196-197
  complications of, 198-199
  epidemiology of, 193
  imaging of, 195
  mechanisms of, 194
  operative evaluation of, 195-196
  penetrating, 194
  treatment of, 197-198
Pancreatitis, 198, 485
  hemorrhagic, 198-199
Pancuronium, 420
Parenteral nutrition, 498-499. See also Nutrition.
  vs. enteral nutrition, 497
Parkland formula, for burn resuscitation, 275, 277
Parotid duct
  anatomy of, 120-121
  injury to, repair of, 121
Passive external rewarming, for hypothermia, 455
Pasteurella multocida, 396, 397
  antibiotics for, 399
Patellar dislocation, in children, 393
Patellar fracture, 325-326
  in children, 393
Patient safety improvement, trauma performance and, 11-15. See also Trauma performance.
Pediatric burns, 285-286
Pediatric fracture(s), 379-395
  etiology of, 379
  in child abuse, 381
  management of, principles in, 380
  of acetabulum, 390
  of lower extremity, 390-395
  of mandibe, 145
  of pelvis, 390
  of upper extremity, 382-390
  open, 381-382
  pathophysiology of, 379
  patterns of, 379-380
Pediatric trauma, 25, 410-415
  anatomic differences in, 410
  occult, 410
  physiologic differences in, 410
  primary survey of, 410-412, 411t, 412t
  specific injuries in, 412-415
Pediatric Trauma Score (PTS), 21

Pelvic binder, 304, 307
Pelvic fractures, 303-309
  classification of, 304, 306t
    Young-Burgess, 62t, 304, 305f, 306t
  evaluation of, 303-304
  pediatric, 390
  trauma team management of, 307-308
  treatment of, 304, 307
    of anteroposterior compression types, 308
    of lateral compression types, 308
    of vertical shear types, 308
    special situations in, 309
Pelvis
  anatomy of, 303
  CT scan of, 68
  radiography of, 60-61
  ultrasonography of, 72, 73f
Penetrating trauma
  abdominal vascular, 264
  colorectal, 236
    evaluation and diagnosis of, 236-237
  duodenal, 199
  pancreatic, 194
  penile, 255-256
  physics of, 25-26
  rectal, 236
  scrotal and testicular, 257
  small bowel, 204-205
  splenic, 227
  survival probability vs. Injury Severity Score in, 22f
  thoracic, 166
  to head, 103-104
Penicillin, for infection/inflammation, 490
Penile trauma, 254-256
  penetrating, 255-256
Percutaneous screw fixation, of pelvic fractures, 307
Pericardiocentesis, 171-172
Pericarditis, 483-484
Pericardium, ultrasonography of, 72
Perihepatic packing, 218
Perineum
  examination of, 41
  injury to, 257
    chemical, electrical, and thermal, 258
    lacerations of, 257

Peripheral nerve(s), injury to, 370
Peripheral perfusion, measurement and estimation of, 428-429
Peritoneal dialysis, for acute renal failure, 472
Peritoneal lavage, diagnostic, in emergency department, 65-66
Permanent cavity, from penetrating missiles, 26
Phalanx
  distal, fracture of, 374
    in children, 383
  middle
    amputation through, 372
    fracture of, 374
  proximal, fracture of, in children, 383
Pharyngeal injuries, 161
Phenylephrine, 420
  for infection/inflammation, 489
Physeal fracture(s), pediatric, 380
Physical examination
  of extremity vascular trauma, 259-260, 260t
  of febrile patient, 475-476
  of knee ligament injuries, 334
  of pelvic fractures, 303
Physical therapy, for burn patients, 280
Physiologic age, vs. chronological age, 416
Physiologic dead space, 439
Piezoelectric effect, in ultrasonography, 71
Pilon fracture, of ankle, 343
Pisiform fracture, 376
Pit viper bites, 401, 402. *See also* Bite(s).
Pit viper venom, 401
Pituitary dysfunction, in organ donor, 506
Placental abruption, traumatic, 407
Plate fixation
  of midface fractures, 142
  of pelvic fractures, 307
Platelet(s), transfusion of, 51, 52, 53t
Pneumonia, 481-482
  in burn patients, 281
  ventilator-associated, 450-452, 482-483
    definition of, 450
    diagnosis of, 450, 451t
    prevention of, 452
    treatment of, 450-451
Pneumothorax, ultrasonography of, 74
Porta hepatis injury, 223
Portal vein, injury to, repair of, 271

Positive end-expiratory pressure (PEEP), 443
Posterior cruciate ligament
  injury to, treatment of, 340
  insufficiency of, 335-336
    posterolateral complex with, 338-339
Postinjury hypermetabolic response, 495
Postsplenectomy infection, overwhelming, 233
Pregnant patient
  anatomic and physiologic changes in, 403-404
  trauma in, 403-408
    anesthesia management in, 424
    etiology of, 403
    evaluation of
      primary survey in, 404-405
      secondary survey in, 405-406
    obstetric emergencies in, 407-408
    operative management of, 406
Preoxygenation, 32
Pressure-controlled ventilation, 442
Pressure-support ventilation, 442-443
Pringle maneuver, 211f, 216
Proctoscopy, rigid, in emergency department, 70
Prolapse, umbilical cord, 408
Protein metabolism, during stress and injury, 495-496
Proximal interphalangeal joint
  amputation proximal to, 372-373
  amputation through, 372
  injury to, 371
Prune test, of hand, 363
Pseudocysts, pancreatic, 199
Pseudomembranous enterocolitis, 486
Pulmonary artery, injury to, 176
Pulmonary artery catheter monitoring, in central venous catheterization, 85-86
Pulmonary artery wedge pressure (PAWP), 428
Pulmonary changes, in pregnant trauma patient, 404
Pulmonary disorders, miscellaneous, 445-452. *See also specific disorder.*
Pulmonary embolus, 477
  diagnosis of, 292
  treatment of, 292-293
Pulmonary function, in spinal cord injury, 107-108
Pulmonary infection score, clinical, 451t, 482t
Pulmonary system, management of, in organ donor, 505
Pulmonary thromboembolism, 447-450
  diagnosis of, 448-449
  pathophysiology of, 447
  prevention of, 449-450
  risk factors for, 447-448
  treatment of, 449
Pulmonary vein, injury to, 176
Pulse-echo principle, in ultrasonography, 71
Pupil(s), examination of, 150
Pyelography, retrograde, of genitourinary tract trauma, 252

Q

Quinolones, for infection/inflammation, 492

R

Rabies immunization, 400
Radial artery, catheterization of, 75-76
Radial fracture(s), distal, 356, 358f-359f, 358t
  in children, 383-384
Radial head fracture, 355
  in children, 386
Radial head subluxation, in children, 388
Radial neck fracture, in children, 387
Radial shaft fracture, in children, 384-385
Radiation, nuclear, 27-28
Radiography
  chest, of febrile patient, 476
  in emergency department, 60-63, 61t, 62t
  of hand injuries, 363
  of knee ligament injuries, 334
  of pelvic fractures, 303-304
  of spinal cord injury, 106-107
  of splenic injury, 227
Range of motion, of hand and wrist, 360, 361f, 362f
Rapid sequence intubation, 31-32
Recombinant human activated protein C, for infection/inflammation, 489

Rectal trauma, 235. *See also* Colorectal trauma.
 management of, 240
 penetrating, 236
Rectum
 examination of, 41
 foreign bodies in, 240
Reduction, of mandibular fracture, 145
Reflexes, in spinal cord injury, 106
Regionalized care, rationale for, 5, 6t, 7
Renal artery, injury to, repair of, 269
Renal changes
 in geriatric trauma patient, 416
 in hypothermia, 455
Renal failure, acute, 470-472
Renal system, management of, in organ donor, 505
Renal trauma, 243-249
 blunt, 244
 classification of, 244t
 deceleration, 244
 epidemiology of, 243
 evaluation of, 244-245
 in children, 414
 management of, 245-248
  nonoperative, 247
  operative, 247-248
  specific scenarios in, 246-247
 mechanisms of, 243-244
 penetrating, 243-244
 postoperative care for, 248-249
Renal vein, injury to, repair of, 269
Replantation, of digits, 373
Respiratory acidosis, 469
Respiratory alkalosis, 469
Respiratory changes, in hypothermia, 454
Respiratory failure, acute, 440-441
 definition of, 440
Respiratory physiology, 438-441
 acute failure in, 440-441
 carbon dioxide transport in, 438-439
 tissue oxygenation in, 438
 ventilation-perfusion balance in, 439-440
Respiratory rate, 443
Resuscitation. *See also* Fluid resuscitation.
 of burn patients, 275, 277, 278f
 volume, for infection/inflammation, 488

Resuscitation agents, 420
Resuscitative thoracotomy, 172
Retrobulbar hemorrhage, 155
Retrograde pyelography, of genitourinary tract trauma, 252
Retrograde urethrography, of genitourinary tract trauma, 252-253
Revised Trauma Score (RTS), 18-19, 19t
 vs. survival probability, 20f
Rewarming, of hypothermia patient, methods of, 454-455
Rhabdomyolysis, 297, 301-302
 definition of, 297
 diagnosis of, 297, 301
 treatment of, 301-302
Rib fracture, 177
Ribavirin, for infection/inflammation, 493
Right upper quadrant, ultrasonography of, 72, 73f
Right ventricular end-diastolic volume (RVEDV), 428
Rigid sigmoidoscopy, in emergency department, 70
Rocuronium, 420
Rodent bites, 397. *See also* Bite(s).
Rubber bullets, 27
Rupture
 Achilles, 345
 testicular, 256-257
 uterine, 407

S

Salter-Harris fractures, 380
Saphenous vein cutdown, 76-79, 77f-79f
Scalp
 injury to, repair of, 116
 layers of, 116, 117f
Scaphoid fracture, 376
 in children, 389-390
Scapular fracture, 349
Scapulothoracic dislocation, 348
Schatzker classification, of tibial plateau fractures, 327, 327f-328f
Sciatic nerve palsy, after acetabular fractures, 311
Sciatic nerve trauma, in hip dislocation, 312
Sclera, examination of, 152
Scrotal trauma
 blunt, 256-257
 penetrating, 257

Sedation, for facial injury repair, 113-114
Sedatives, 419
Seizure(s), post-traumatic, 101
Seizure prophylaxis, 101
Seldinger guide-wire technique, of
    central venous catheterization, 81
Sensory examination, of spinal cord
    injury, 106
Sepsis
  colorectal trauma and, 241
  definition of, 474
Septic shock, 48, 426-427
  definition of, 474
Shear(ing) injury
  duodenal, 199
  physics of, 24
  small bowel, 205
Shock, 43-49
  assessment of, 43
  cardiogenic, 46-47, 425-426
  definition of, 43
  distributive, 48-49, 426-427
  etiology of, 425-427
  hypovolemic (hemorrhagic), 44-46,
      45t, 425, 426t
  neurogenic, 427
  obstructive, 47-48
  septic, 426-427
    definition of, 474
  spinal, 49, 107
  treatment of, 43-44
    vasoactive agents in, 432t
Shock states
  characteristics of, 44t
  differential diagnosis of, 427t
Shoulder dislocation, in children, 389
Shunt
  atriocaval, 219-220, 220f
  intrapulmonary, 439-440
Sigmoidoscopy, rigid, in emergency
    department, 70
Silver sulfadazine, for burn wounds, 279
Sinusitis, 486
Skeletal traction, for pelvic fractures, 307
Skeleton, axial, radiography of, 61
Skin flaps, in facial soft tissue injury
    repair, 116
Skin grafts, in facial soft tissue injury
    repair, 116
Skull
  fracture of, 102
  frontal view of, 138f

Small bowel, anatomy of, 204
Small bowel feeding, vs. gastric feeding,
    497-498
Small bowel trauma, 204-208
  complications of, 208
  diagnosis of, 205-206
  epidemiology of, 204
  management of, 206-207
  mechanisms of, 204-205
  pearls and pitfalls of, 208
  postoperative care for, 207-208
Snake bites, 400-401. *See also* Bite(s).
  treatment of, 401-402
Soft tissue trauma
  facial, 109-122
    physical examination of, 109-111,
        114f
    repair of
      anesthesia for, 113-115
      structural, 116-122, 117f-120f
      wound closure techniques in,
          115-116
    types of, 111-113
  wounds in, 480-481
Spinal cord trauma
  cervical, determination of level of, 106t
  examination of, 105-106
  general principles of, 105
  incomplete, 106
  management of, 107
  pulmonary function in, 107-108
  radiographic studies of, 106-107
  shock in, 107
  surgical intervention for, 108
Spinal shock, 49, 107
Spine
  cervical. *See* Cervical spine.
  injury to, in children, 413
Spleen
  accessory, 227
  anatomy of, 225-227, 226f
Splenectomy, 229
  overwhelming infection after, 233
Splenic artery, 226, 226f
Splenic injury grading system, 229t
Splenic trauma, 225-233
  blunt, 227
  diagnosis of, 227-228
  epidemiology of, 227
  history of, 225
  injury grading system of, 228-229,
      229t

Splenic trauma *(Continued)*
  penetrating, 227
  postoperative complications of, 232-233
  treatment option(s) for, 229, 230f-232f, 230t, 231-232
    celiotomy as, 229, 230f
    nonoperative, 231-232
    splenectomy as, 229
      overwhelming infection after, 233
    splenorrhaphy as, 229, 231f, 232f
Splenic vein, 226f, 227
Splenorrhaphy, 229, 231f, 232f
Splint(s), for fractures and dislocations, 288
Sprain(s)
  ankle, 343
  wrist, 375
Stab wounds. *See also* Penetrating trauma.
  hepatic, 212-213
  thoracoabdominal, 165
Stability testing, of knee ligament injuries, 335-339
  combined laxities in, 338-339
  isolated laxities in, 335-337, 336f-338f
Sternal fracture, 177-178
  ultrasonography of, 74
Sternoclavicular joint, dislocation, 347
Sternotomy
  exposure considerations in, 168
  indications for, 168
Stomach. *See also* Gastric *entries.*
  anatomy of, 188
Strangulation, penile, 255
Stress
  endocrine response to, 495, 496t
  fat metabolism during, 496
  glucose metabolism during, 496
Subclavian artery
  left, injury to, 176
  right, injury to, 175
Subclavian vein
  access to
    infraclavicular approach to, 81-82, 81f
    supraclavicular approach to, 82, 83f
  anatomy of, 79, 80f
Subdural hematoma, 102-103
Subluxation, of radial head, in children, 388

Subtrochanteric femoral fracture, 317-318
Subxiphoid exploration, 172-173
Succinylcholine, 419
  sedation/paralysis with, 32
Suicide, 1, 4
Sulfa drugs, for infection/inflammation, 492
Superior mesenteric artery
  anatomy of, 204
  injury to, repair of, 267
Superior mesenteric vein
  anatomy of, 204
  injury to, repair of, 267
Supracondylar femoral fracture, 321-325
  classification of, 322-323, 322f-324f
  complications of, 325
  evaluation of, 322
  in children, 392-393
  treatment of, 323-325
Supracondylar humeral fracture, 352-353
  in children, 385-386
Supraglottic intubation, 33, 34f
Supraorbital nerve block, for facial injury repair, 115
Supratrochlear nerve block, for facial injury repair, 115
Surgical control, of infection/inflammation, 489
Symphyseal plate fixation, of pelvic fractures, 307
Systemic inflammatory response syndrome (SIRS), definition of, 474
Systemic Inflammatory Response Syndrome (SIRS) Score, 19, 20t
Systemic vascular resistance (SVR), 429

T
Talus fracture, 344
Tamponade, internal, for liver trauma, 218, 219f
Tarsometatarsal dislocations, 345
TASERs, 27
Temperature, in febrile patient, 475
Temperature homeostasis, in intensive care unit, 453
Temporary cavity, from penetrating missiles, 26
Tendon(s). *See also named tendon.*
  laceration of, 345
Tenosynovitis, flexor, 378
Tensile injury, physics of, 24

Testicular trauma
  blunt, 256-257
  penetrating, 257
Tetanus, 487-488
Tetanus immunization, 399-400
Thermal burns, 27. *See also* Burn(s).
  to genitalia and perineum, 258
Thermoregulatory disorders, in intensive care unit, 453-460
Thoracic. *See also* Chest *entries*.
Thoracic duct, injury to, 179
Thoracic trauma, 165-179
  anatomy in, 165
  diagnosis of, 166-167
  diagnostic studies in, 167-168
  exposure considerations in, 168
  flail chest in, 178
  hemopneumothorax in, 178-179
  incidence of, 165
  management of
    initial, 166
    intraoperative, 169
    invasive procedures in, 169-174, 171f, 173f
    postoperative, 169
  mechanisms of, 165-166
  multiple injuries in, 177
  open chest wound in, 178
  rib fracture in, 177
  specific injuries in, 174-176
  sternal fracture in, 177-178
  thoracic duct injuries in, 179
  thoracotomy or sternotomy in, indications for, 168
Thoracoabdominal gunshot wounds, 165
Thoracoabdominal stab wounds, 165
Thoracostomy
  closed-tube, 90-92, 91f
  tube insertion in, 169-170
    principles of, 169-170
  tube management in, 170, 171f
  tube removal in, 170-171
Thoracotomy
  exposure considerations in, 168
  in emergency department, 166
  indications for, 168
  resuscitative, 172
Thromboembolic disease
  pulmonary, 447-450
  risk factors for, 290
  treatment of, 291-292

Thrombosis
  catheter-related, 76
  deep vein, 291-292, 477
    prophylaxis for, 107
Thumb
  amputation of, 373
  fractures of, 374-375
  joints of, injury to, 371-372
Thyroid storm, 478
Tibial epiphyseal fracture, in children, 393-394
Tibial metaphyseal fracture, in children, 394
Tibial physeal fracture, distal, in children, 394-395
Tibial plateau fracture, 326-330
  complications of, 330
  evaluation of, 326-327
  Schatzker classification of, 327, 327f-328f
  treatment of, 328-330
Tibial shaft fracture
  complications of, 332
  in children, 394
  treatment of, 330-332
Tibial spine fracture, in children, 393
Tibial tubercle fracture, in children, 394
Tidal volume, 443
Tissue damage, chemical burn–related, 284
Tissue oxygenation, 438
Tissue pressure, Whitesides' method of measuring, 293f
Tongue lacerations, repair of, 122
Toxic shock syndrome, 487
Tracheal injury, 162
Traction
  for fractures and dislocations, 288
  skeletal, for pelvic fractures, 307
Transatrial shunt, for liver trauma, 219-220, 220f
Transcondylar fracture, humeral, 353
Transfusion(s), 50-58
  blood products in, 52-53, 53t
  blood substitutes for, 58
  complication(s) of, 53-57
    acute lung injury as, 56-57
    acute respiratory distress syndrome as, 57
    disseminated intravascular coagulation as, 56

Transfusion(s) *(Continued)*
   iatrogenic, 53-54
   immunologic, 54
   infectious, 55
   metabolic, 55-56
  for shock, 43-44
  indications for, 50-52
  massive
   during anesthesia, 422, 424
   protocol for, 422t
  pearls and pitfalls of, 58
  protocol for, 57-58, 58t
Transfusion reactions, 477
Transfusion triggers, 50, 51-52
Trapezium fracture, 376
Trapezoid fracture, 376
Trauma. *See also at anatomic site; specific type of injury.*
  anesthesia in, 419-424. *See also Anesthesia.*
  endocrine response to, 495, 496t
  epidemiology of, 1-4
  fat metabolism during, 496
  geriatric, 25, 416-417
  glucose metabolism during, 496
  impact of, 3
  incidence of, 1
  mechanisms of, 24-28
   blunt injury physics in, 24-25
   general aspects of, 24
   miscellaneous, 26-28
   penetrating injury physics in, 25-26
  neurologic, 97-108. *See also Neurologic trauma.*
  patterns of, 2-3
  pediatric, 410-415. *See also Pediatric trauma.*
  prevention of, 3-4
  protein metabolism during, 495-496
  ultrasonography in, 71-74. *See also Ultrasonography.*
  unintentional, 1
Trauma care
  airway in, 31-34, 34f-37f
  breathing in, 34-35
  circulation in, 35-36
  disability in, 36
  exposure in, 36, 38
Trauma centers, essential and desirable characteristics of, 7t-10t
Trauma patient, assessment of
  primary survey in, 31-38, 34f-37f
  secondary survey in, 38-42
Trauma performance
  and patient safety improvement, 11-15
  diversion review of, 15
  improvement report of, 13-14
  monitoring of, 15
  protocol for, 11-13
  purpose of, 11
  record keeping of, 14
  registry review of, 14
Trauma Performance Improvement (TPI) Protocol, 11-13
Trauma personnel, definitions of, 11
Trauma scoring systems, 18-23
  common, 18-19, 18t, 19t, 20f-22f, 20t, 21, 21t
  national registry of, 22-23
  overview of, 18
  quality improvement of, 22
Trauma systems, 5-10
  historical development of, 5
  regionalized care in, rationale for, 5, 6t, 7
  structure of, 7, 7t-10t
Trauma team management, of pelvic fractures, 307-308
Trauma transfers, 13
Traumatic deaths, non-CNS, comparison of, 6t
Triage, in geriatric trauma, 417
Trigeminal nerve, distribution of, 109, 114f
Triquetrum fracture, 376

U

Ulcer
  Curling's, in burn patients, 281
  Meleney's, 488
Ulnar fracture, distal, in children, 383-384
Ulnar nerve block, 363, 364f
Ulnar shaft fracture, in children, 384-385
Ultrasonography
  advantages and disadvantages of, 71
  basic definition of, 71
  bedside, of febrile patient, 476
  cardiac, 166
  essential principles of, 71

Ultrasonography (Continued)
focused assessment of, for trauma, 72-73, 73f
in emergency department, 63-65, 64f, 65f
of extremity vascular trauma, 260
of genitourinary tract trauma, 251-252
of pancreatic injury, 195
of splenic injury, 227-228
Umbilical cord prolapse, 408
Uncal herniation, 155
Uniform Anatomical Gift Act (1968), 501
Uniform Brain Death Act (1978), 501
Unstable fracture, in children, 394
Upper extremity(ies). *See also* specific part.
fractures and dislocations of, 347-359
pediatric, 382-390
Ureter(s), imaging of, 68
Urethra, imaging of, 69
Urethrography, retrograde, of genitourinary tract trauma, 252-253
Urinalysis, in febrile patient, 476
Urinary catheter, 89
Urinary tract infections, 484
Urine output, in burn patients, 283
Urologic imaging, in emergency department, 68-69
Urologic injury, in pelvic fractures, 309
Urologic trauma series, 251
Uterine rupture, 407

V

Vaccine (vaccination)
rabies, 400
tetanus, 399-400
Vancomycin, for infection/inflammation, 491-492
Vascular access, for shock, 43
Vascular assessment, in trauma care, 41-42
Vascular trauma
abdominal, 264-272. *See also* Abdominal trauma, vascular.
extremity, 259-263. *See also* Extremity(ies), vascular trauma of.
in knee dislocation, 340
of hand, 370
of neck, 159-160
operative management of, 160-161
pediatric, 380

Vasopressors, 420
for infection/inflammation, 488-489
Vecuronium, 420
sedation/paralysis with, 32
Vena cava
inferior, injury to, 218-219, 268
thoracic, injury to, 176
Venography, of genitourinary tract trauma, 252
Venous oxygen saturation (Svo_2), mixed, 428-429
Venous thrombosis, deep, 291-292, 477
prophylaxis for, 107
Ventilation, mechanical, 441-445. *See also* Mechanical ventilation.
Ventilation-perfusion balance, 439
Ventilator settings, 443
Ventilator-associated pneumonia, 450-452, 482-483
definition of, 450
diagnosis of, 450, 451t
prevention of, 452
treatment of, 450-451
Vertical shear injury, pelvic, 304, 306t
management of, 308
Violence, incidence of, 1
Vision-threatening emergencies, recognition of, 154-155
Visual acuity, examination of, 148
Visual fields, examination of, 148
Vital signs
assessment of, 38-39
in febrile patient, 475
Volume deficits, 462
Volume overload, 462
Volume resuscitation, for infection/inflammation, 488
Volume status, monitoring of, 462

W

Warfarin, for pulmonary thromboembolism, 449
Water, daily requirement of, 461
Weaning, for mechanical ventilation, guidelines for, 444-445, 444t
Weapons, nonlethal, 27
Wharton's duct, injury to, repair of, 122
Whitesides' method, of measuring tissue pressure, 293f
Whole blood, transfusion of, 52, 53t

Withdrawal of care, in geriatric trauma patient, 417
Wound(s)
  bite. See Bite(s).
  burn. See also Burn(s).
    care of, 277-279
    complications of, 281-282
    infection of, 281
  gunshot, 103
    thoracoabdominal, 165
  local exploration of, 69
  open chest, 178
  soft tissue, 480-481. See also Soft tissue trauma.
  stab
    hepatic, 212-213
    thoracoabdominal, 165

Wrist dislocation, 375-376
Wrist fracture, 376
Wrist nerve blocks, 363, 364f
Wrist sprain, 375

Y

Young-Burgess classification, of pelvic fractures, 62t, 304, 305f, 306t

Z

Zygoma, articulations of, 134, 135f
Zygomaticofacial block, for facial injury repair, 115
Zygomaticomaxillary complex, fracture of, 134-136